Handbook of
Gastroenterology
Second Edition

EDITOR

Tadataka Yamada, M.D.

Adjunct Professor
Department of Internal Medicine
Division of Gastroenterology
University of Michigan Health System
Ann Arbor, Michigan

SPECIAL EDITORS

William L. Hasler, M.D.
Associate Professor
Department of Internal Medicine
Division of Gastroenterology
University of Michigan Health System
Ann Arbor, Michigan

John M. Inadomi, M.D.
Associate Professor
Department of Internal Medicine
Division of Gastroenterology
University of Michigan Health System
Chief, Endoscopy
Veterans Affairs Ann Arbor Healthcare System
Ann Arbor, Michigan

ASSISTANT SPECIAL EDITORS

Michelle A. Anderson, M.D.
Assistant Professor
Department of Internal Medicine
Division of Gastroenterology
University of Michigan Health System
Ann Arbor, Michigan

Robert S. Brown, Jr., M.D., M.P.H.
Associate Professor of Medicine and Surgery
Department of Medicine
Columbia University College of Physicians
    & Surgeons
Chief, Division of Hepatobiliary and
    Abdominal Transplant Surgery
Center for Liver Disease
    and Transplantation
New York-Presbyterian Hospital
New York, New York

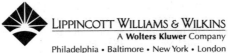

LIPPINCOTT WILLIAMS & WILKINS
A **Wolters Kluwer** Company
Philadelphia • Baltimore • New York • London
Buenos Aires • Hong Kong • Sydney • Tokyo

Executive Editor: Charles W. Mitchell
Managing Editor: Lisa R. Kairis
Project Manager: Nicole Walz
Senior Manufacturing Manager: Ben Rivera
Marketing Manager: Angela Panetta
Design Coordinator: Holly Reid McLaughlin
Cover Designer: Andrew Gatto
Production Service: TechBooks, Inc.
Printer: RR Donnelley, Crawfordsville

© 2005 by LIPPINCOTT WILLIAMS & WILKINS
530 Walnut Street
Philadelphia, PA 19106 USA
LWW.com

Printed in the United States of America

Library of Congress Cataloging-in-Publication Data

Handbook of gastroenterology / editor, Tadataka Yamada ; special editors, William L. Hasler, John M. Inadomi ; assistant special editors, Michelle A. Anderson, Robert S. Brown, Jr.–2nd ed.
    p. ; cm.
    Includes index.
    ISBN 0-7817-5460-7
1. Gastroenterology–Handbooks, manuals, etc.   2. Gastrointestinal–system–Diseases–Handbooks, manuals, etc. I. Yamada, Tadataka.
    [DNLM: 1. Gastrointestinal Diseases–Handbooks. WI 39 H2354 2005]
RC801.H28   2005
616.3′3–dc22

                                                                 2005006419

Care has been taken to confirm the accuracy of the information presented and to describe generally accepted practices. However, the authors, editors, and publisher are not responsible for errors or omissions or for any consequences from application of the information in this book and make no warranty, expressed or implied, with respect to the currency, completeness, or accuracy of the contents of the publication. Application of this information in a particular situation remains the professional responsibility of the practitioner.

The authors, editors, and publisher have exerted every effort to ensure that drug selection and dosage set forth in this text are in accordance with current recommendations and practice at the time of publication. However, in view of ongoing research, changes in government regulations, and the constant flow of information relating to drug therapy and drug reactions, the reader is urged to check the package insert for each drug for any change in indications and dosage and for added warnings and precautions. This is particularly important when the recommended agent is a new or infrequently employed drug.

Some drugs and medical devices presented in this publication have Food and Drug Administration (FDA) clearance for limited use in restricted research settings. It is the responsibility of the health care provider to ascertain the FDA status of each drug or device planned for use in their clinical practice.

10 9 8 7 6 5 4 3 2

Contents

Preface   xi

CHAPTER 1
Psychosocial Factors in the Care of Patients with Gastrointestinal
Disorders   1

CHAPTER 2
Approach to the Patient with Dysphagia or Odynophagia   4

CHAPTER 3
Approach to the Patient with Chest Pain   9

CHAPTER 4
Approach to the Patient with Gross Gastrointestinal Bleeding   14

CHAPTER 5
Approach to the Patient with Occult Gastrointestinal Hemorrhage   26

CHAPTER 6
Approach to the Patient with Unexplained Weight Loss   32

CHAPTER 7
Approach to the Patient with Nausea and Vomiting   37

CHAPTER 8
Approach to the Patient with Abdominal Pain   45

CHAPTER 9
Approach to the Patient with Acute Abdomen   54

CHAPTER 10
Approach to the Patient with Gas and Bloating   61

CHAPTER 11
Approach to the Patient with Ileus or Obstruction   68

CHAPTER 12
Approach to the Patient with Diarrhea   76

CHAPTER 13
Approach to the Patient with Constipation   87

CHAPTER 14
Approach to the Patient with an Abdominal Mass   94

CHAPTER 15
Approach to the Patient with Ileostomy or Ileal Pouch   100

CHAPTER 16
Approach to the Patient with Jaundice   105

CHAPTER 17
Approach to the Patient with Abnormal Liver Chemistry Values   113

CHAPTER 18
Approach to the Patient with Ascites   124

CHAPTER 19
Approach to Gastrointestinal Problems in the Elderly   133

CHAPTER 20
Approach to Gastrointestinal and Liver Diseases in the Female Patient   140

CHAPTER 21
Approach to the Patient Requiring Nutritional Support   151

CHAPTER 22
Approach to the Patient with Alcohol or Drug Dependency   162

CHAPTER 23
Advice to Travelers   168

CHAPTER 24
Nosocomial Infections and Risks to Health Care Providers   174

CHAPTER 25
Structural Anomalies and Miscellaneous Disorders
of the Esophagus   182

CHAPTER 26
Motor Disorders of the Esophagus   193

CHAPTER 27
Reflux Esophagitis and Esophageal Infections   203

CHAPTER 28
Esophageal Tumors   216

CHAPTER 29
Structural Disorders and Miscellaneous Disorders of the Stomach   223

CHAPTER 30
Disorders of Gastric Emptying   231

CHAPTER 31
Acid Peptic Disorders and Zollinger-Ellison Syndrome   240

CHAPTER 32
Surgery for Peptic Ulcer Disease and Postgastrectomy Syndromes   253

CHAPTER 33
Functional Dyspepsia   259

CHAPTER 34
Gastritis, Duodenitis, and Associated Ulcerative Lesions   262

CHAPTER 35
Tumors of the Stomach   271

CHAPTER 36
Structural Anomalies and Miscellaneous Diseases
of the Small Intestine 279

CHAPTER 37
Dysmotility and Bacterial Overgrowth of the Small Intestine 288

CHAPTER 38
Infections of the Small Intestine with Bacterial and Viral Pathogens 298

CHAPTER 39
Celiac Disease 308

CHAPTER 40
Disorders of Epithelial Transport in the Small Intestine 313

CHAPTER 41
Short Bowel Syndrome 320

CHAPTER 42
Tumors and Other Neoplastic Diseases of the Small Intestine 325

CHAPTER 43
Structural Anomalies and Diverticular Disease of the Colon 331

CHAPTER 44
Irritable Bowel Syndrome and Motor Disorders of the Colon 340

CHAPTER 45
Bacterial Infections of the Colon 349

CHAPTER 46
Inflammatory Bowel Disease 357

CHAPTER 47
Miscellaneous Inflammatory and Structural Disorders of the Colon 373

CHAPTER 48
Colonic Polyps and Polyposis Syndromes 384

CHAPTER 49
Malignant Tumors of the Colon 399

CHAPTER 50
Anorectal Diseases 409

CHAPTER 51
Structural Anomalies and Hereditary Diseases of the Pancreas 419

CHAPTER 52
Acute Pancreatitis 427

CHAPTER 53
Chronic Pancreatitis 435

CHAPTER 54
Pancreatic Adenocarcinoma 441

CHAPTER 55
Endocrine Neoplasms of the Pancreas 447

CHAPTER 56
Structural Anomalies, Tumors, and Diseases of the Biliary Tract 454

CHAPTER 57
Biliary Tract Stones and Postcholecystectomy Syndrome 462

CHAPTER 58
Abdominal Cavity: Structural Anomalies, Hernias, Intra-Abdominal
Abscesses, and Fistulae 470

CHAPTER 59
Diseases of the Mesentery, Peritoneum, and Retroperitoneum 480

CHAPTER 60
Cholestatic Syndromes 490

CHAPTER 61
Drug-Induced Hepatic Injury 496

CHAPTER 62
Viral Hepatitis 502

CHAPTER 63
Nonviral Hepatitis 512

CHAPTER 64
Autoimmune Liver Disease 517

CHAPTER 65
Alcoholic Liver Diseases 522

CHAPTER 66
Cirrhosis, Portal Hypertension, and End-Stage Liver Disease 529

CHAPTER 67
Primary Hepatic Neoplasms 539

CHAPTER 68
Gastrointestinal Complications of the Acquired Immunodeficiency
Syndrome 547

CHAPTER 69
Parasitic Diseases: Protozoa and Helminths 555

CHAPTER 70
Gastrointestinal Manifestations of Systemic Diseases 567

CHAPTER 71
Gastrointestinal Manifestations of Immunologic Disorders 580

CHAPTER 72
Skin Lesions Associated with Gastrointestinal
and Liver Diseases 589

CHAPTER 73
Vascular Lesions: Ectasias, Tumors, and Malformations 598

CHAPTER 74
Mesenteric Vascular Insufficiency 605

CHAPTER 75
Radiation Injury   611

CHAPTER 76
Endoscopy   615

CHAPTER 77
Imaging Procedures   628

Subject Index   639

Preface

The practice of gastroenterology has evolved dramatically during the past three decades. The science of the alimentary canal has advanced rapidly, and new diagnostic and therapeutic techniques have been added to our clinical methods, almost daily. Recognizing the need to advance current teaching materials for gastroenterology incorporating this new knowledge, we undertook editing of the *Handbook of Gastroenterology*. The success of the past four editions of the *Textbook of Gastroenterology* attested to the demand for information on the modern practice of gastroenterology. Because of the encyclopedic scope of the *Textbook* and the increasing demand for new knowledge in gastroenterology among trainees and medical students at the earliest level, we developed this *Handbook*. Our aim is to present the quality and depth of the *Textbook* in a more concise and portable form. The *Handbook* focuses on the practical clinical aspects of the *Textbook*, making it particularly useful to the medical student, house officer, and advanced trainee. Of course, we hope that the clarity and completeness of the newly updated *Handbook* will also make it a useful resource for all physicians who treat patients with gastrointestinal and liver disorders.

The associate editors and I are greatly indebted to William Hasler, John Inadomi, Michelle Anderson, and Robert Brown, who served as special editors of the *Handbook*. We hope that their careful editing and attention to detail, as well as their obvious mastery of the practice of gastroenterology, have made the *Handbook* a useful guide to this discipline.

Tadataka Yamada, M.D.

Handbook of
Gastroenterology
Second Edition

CHAPTER 1

Psychosocial Factors in the Care of Patients with Gastrointestinal Disorders

Human illness results from a complex interplay of clinical, biologic, psychological, and sociologic variables. The clinician's understanding of these diverse yet interacting variables is critical for adequate diagnosis and treatment of gastrointestinal disease. Diagnostic findings of endoscopy, manometry, or radiography may not explain the degree or even the presence of selected gut symptoms. Failure to link physical and psychological components of a clinical disease presentation may reduce the likelihood of successful treatment of the condition and its manifestations.

PSYCHOPHYSIOLOGICAL FACTORS

Previously healthy persons may experience abdominal discomfort and altered bowel patterns during periods of emotional distress. Furthermore, stressful stimulation alters intestinal vascularity, secretion, motor activity, and pain perception and can modify a person's actions, evoking striking autonomic responses and emotional changes (e.g., increased anxiety). In a reciprocal manner, primary alterations in bowel function can affect emotional centers in the brain, such as the locus ceruleus. Various stressors modify humoral and cellular immunity, including delayed responsiveness to mitogens and antigens, reduced lymphocyte-mediated cytotoxicity, and suppression of delayed hypersensitivity, potentially increasing a person's susceptibility to inflammatory or infectious disease. Conversely, successful behavioral treatment has been shown to increase natural killer cytotoxic activity, leading to lower mortality from certain malignancies.

These effects are mediated by bidirectional interconnecting pathways that link the cognitive and emotional centers in the brain with the neuroendocrine axis, the enteric nervous system, and the immune system by means of specific brain-gut neurotransmitters. Descending pathways from the brainstem to the dorsal horn of the spinal cord modulate the information that projects to the brain, while ascending arousal systems from the brainstem to the cortex regulate the perception of visceral sensation. Functional bowel disorders, including irritable bowel syndrome (IBS), may result from dysregulation of these brain-gut neuroenteric systems. Patients with IBS exhibit exaggerated responsiveness to lumenal distention and other stimuli. Furthermore, life stressors predict the development of IBS after infectious gastroenteritis. Brain regions involved in the emotional aspects of visceral pain show altered function in patients with IBS, providing a physiological correlate to these observations. Psychoimmune factors also may modify clinical features of inflammatory bowel disease. Although not initiated by psychosocial stressors, dysregulation of immune function can prolong or exacerbate inflammatory and infectious conditions, producing an inability to clear or suppress the agent or stimulus that activated the immune response.

THE ILLNESS EXPERIENCE

After an illness is established, cultural norms, family beliefs, personality, prior history of abuse or stress, and previous illness experiences affect a patient's reaction to the new illness and impact symptom severity, psychological distress, quality of life, and the use of health care. Because attention to psychosocial features may improve the response to treatment, clinicians should address the contribution of these factors in managing the underlying condition. To establish an effective therapeutic relationship with the patient, the caregiver should consider guidelines that include the following recommendations: listen and provide empathy, identify the patient's expectations and concerns, provide education and reassurance, establish limits and reinforce health-promoting behavior, and guarantee continuity of care.

INTERVIEWING THE PATIENT WITH GASTROINTESTINAL OR HEPATIC DISEASE

The medical interview is the process by which the clinician obtains initial data to diagnose, directly manage, and determine the prognosis of a gastrointestinal illness. The physician should strive to understand the illness from the patient's perspective and then generate a medical knowledge base organized into disease-related and behavioral categories. Questions should be posed in an open-ended format, especially for patients with unexplained or chronic symptoms. Psychosocial and biomedical data are acquired concurrently because the patient often cannot separate an emotional response to illness from the strict biologic factors that produce clinical disease. Moreover, addressing the patient's emotional state and underlying concerns facilitates a positive therapeutic relationship with the caregiver.

Once the medical and psychosocial data are obtained, their contribution to biologic illness must be determined. Patients with long-standing, unexplained symptoms may not be given a specific diagnosis, and thus psychosocial factors are likely to be major contributors to disease expression. Prominent extraintestinal complaints concurrent with a history of gastrointestinal symptoms and numerous prior health care visits predict a lesser response to specific medical or surgical therapy. Unresolved loss or previous physical or sexual abuse can affect the timing of presentation and the severity of clinical symptoms. Many patients with chronic illness have unrealistic expectations of cure. Some persons with persistent, unresolved symptoms acquire abnormal illness behaviors that prolong and embellish the symptom constellation (e.g., disability disproportionate to detectable disease, placement of responsibility on the physician, a sense of entitlement to be cared for by others, avoidance of health-promoting activities, and behavior that sustains the sick role).

For any illness, the clinician must decide if and when behavioral intervention is required. For patients with chronic disease, this issue is best addressed in the context of the effect on daily life. It is important to consider the possibility of concurrent psychiatric diagnoses (including depression, anxiety, somatization, or factitious disorders), which may be subtle in presentation. Participation of other factors, including cultural or ethnic beliefs, family involvement, and community support systems, must be considered. If there are no alarming findings of organic disease (e.g., weight loss, bleeding, abnormal laboratory tests), the clinical course may be followed over time before one embarks on an aggressive diagnostic evaluation. When psychosocial factors dominate the clinical presentation, referral to a mental health specialist should be considered.

TREATMENT

Pharmacotherapy

Antidepressants, including tricyclics, selective serotonin reuptake inhibitors (SSRIs), and newer agents (e.g., venlafaxine, mirtazapine), may offer several benefits, including (1) treatment of underlying psychiatric comorbidity; (2) alteration of gut physiology, including visceral sensation, motility, and secretion; (3) reduction of visceral pain perception; and (4) improvement of vegetative symptoms (i.e., sleep disturbances, anorexia, weight loss, and decreased activity level). Tricyclic agents (e.g., amitriptyline, doxepin) control pain and may promote sleep if taken at bedtime. Desipramine and nortriptyline have fewer sedating and anticholinergic side effects but still relieve chronic pain. The SSRIs fluoxetine and sertraline have fewer side effects than tricyclic agents, but their efficacy in treating gastrointestinal pain syndromes is less well established. Antidepressants usually are continued for 6 to 12 months before dose tapering is considered. Poor clinical responses can result from inadequate dosing and noncompliance.

Other psychopharmacological agents have been used for gastrointestinal disorders. Benzodiazepines have anxiolytic properties, but using them for chronic gastrointestinal conditions is discouraged because they can cause drug dependence and may worsen underlying depression. The serotonin agonist buspirone elicits relaxation of the gut smooth muscle and may reduce symptoms in some patients with functional bowel disorders; however, further investigation is needed to define its clinical role. Major tranquilizers or neuroleptics (e.g., phenothiazines or butyrophenones) usually are useful only when disordered thought is present. Because of their abuse potential, opiate agents have little or no role in treating chronic abdominal pain.

Psychological Treatments

Psychological treatments by psychologists, social workers, nurses, or physicians can reduce anxiety and pain levels, teach patients to promote their own health, and give them control over their treatment programs. Relaxation techniques, including biofeedback, meditation, and autogenic training, can alleviate stressors that contribute to biologic illness. Biofeedback involves patient monitoring of physiological activity, which may then be modified using visual or auditory cues. This technique has proved especially useful for bowel disturbances such as fecal incontinence or refractory constipation. Hypnotherapy involves eye fixation or hand levitation to increase the patient's openness to relaxation. Cognitive-behavioral treatment identifies maladaptive perceptions and behaviors and "reframes" them to increase symptom control. Dynamic psychotherapy to prevent disease recurrence addresses difficulties in interpersonal relationships that underlie symptoms. Psychotherapy should be considered if the patient has a treatable psychiatric disorder or an illness that impairs daily functioning, or if the patient is motivated to address psychological functioning. Behavior modification may be effective for patients with long-standing, maladaptive illness behavior. Successful programs include withdrawal from narcotics addiction and bowel retraining for severe constipation.

CHAPTER 2

Approach to the Patient with Dysphagia or Odynophagia

DIFFERENTIAL DIAGNOSIS

Dysphagia is the sensation of food hindered in its passage from the mouth to the stomach. Dysphagia is differentiated from odynophagia (pain on swallowing) and from globus sensation (perception of a lump, tightness, or fullness in the throat that is temporarily relieved by swallowing). The act of swallowing has four phases—the oral preparation phase, the oral transfer phase, the pharyngeal phase, and the esophageal phase. An interplay of cranial nerves and motor and sensory pathways mediates all of them. An abnormality of any of the phases can produce dysphagia. Dysphagia is usually divided into two categories: (1) illnesses involving the oral preparation, oral transfer, or pharyngeal phases of swallowing; and (2) conditions involving dysfunction of the esophageal phase (Table 2-1).

Oropharyngeal Dysphagia

Defects in Oral Preparation
The oral preparation phase consists of coordinated actions of the lips, jaw, buccal and facial muscles, tongue, and soft palate to break down food and mix it with saliva to obtain a particle size and consistency appropriate for swallowing. Neurological diseases that impair orofacial coordination, oral tumors that physically impede food breakdown, poor dentition, and poor saliva output can affect oral preparation of ingested food.

Defects in Oral Transfer
The oral transfer phase is initiated by the movement of the tongue upward and backward against the palate, which results in propulsion of the food bolus into the pharynx in a rapid symmetric action lasting less than 1 second. Disorders of the oral phase include neurological or neoplastic conditions that produce dysfunctional tongue movements, incomplete bolus clearance from the mouth, delayed oral transit, and a sensation that swallowing requires increased effort.

Pharyngeal Disorders
The pharyngeal phase coordinates pharynx and tongue movements to prevent reflux of the food bolus into the nose or penetration into the larynx and to deliver the ingested bolus through an open cricopharyngeus (upper esophageal sphincter [UES]) into the esophagus in a rapid response that lasts less than 1 second. This process requires respiratory cessation, velopharyngeal and laryngeal closure, pharyngeal peristalsis, and elevation and anterior movement of the larynx. Delays in the pharyngeal phase predispose to filling of an inactive pharynx against a closed

TABLE 2-1
Causes of Dysphagia

Oropharyngeal Dysphagia
  Neuromuscular diseases
    Cerebrovascular accident
    Parkinson disease
    Amyotrophic lateral sclerosis
    Brainstem tumors
    Bulbar poliomyelitis
    Myasthenia gravis
    Muscular dystrophies
    Polymyositis
    Metabolic myopathy
    Amyloidosis
    Systemic lupus erythematosus
  Local mechanical lesions
    Inflammation (pharyngitis, abscess, tuberculosis, radiation, syphilis)
    Neoplasm
    Congenital webs
    Extrinsic compression (thyromegaly, cervical spine hyperostosis, adenopathy)
    Radiation or caustic damage
  Upper esophageal sphincter disorders
    Primary cricopharyngeal dysfunction
    Cricopharyngeal bar
    Zenker diverticulum

Esophageal Dysphagia
  Motor disorders
    Achalasia
    Scleroderma
    Diffuse esophageal spasm
    Other spastic motor disorders
    Other rheumatic conditions
    Chagas disease
  Intrinsic mechanical lesions
    Benign stricture (peptic, lye, radiation)
    Schatzki ring
    Carcinoma
    Esophageal webs
    Esophageal diverticula
    Benign tumors
    Foreign bodies
  Extrinsic mechanical lesions
    Vascular compression
    Mediastinal abnormalities
    Cervical osteoarthritis

UES that produces dysphagia, tracheal aspiration, nasal regurgitation, or bolus retention in the vallecula or piriform sinuses. Defects in the pharyngeal phase include neurological or structural diseases of the pharynx and rare disorders of the UES. Increased UES pressure is measured in some patients with globus sensation or with gastroesophageal reflux. Patients with primary cricopharyngeal dysfunction may present with impaired UES relaxation with poor transfer of swallowed material from the pharynx to the upper esophagus. However, more common causes of incomplete UES relaxation include central nervous system lymphoma and oculopharyngeal dystrophy. Cricopharyngeal bars are prominent muscle structures that prevent complete UES opening. Zenker diverticulum is an outpouching of one or more layers of the esophagus above the UES that produces pharyngeal dysphagia, coughing, regurgitation, and aspiration. Findings of radiographic and manometric tests suggest that Zenker diverticula result from UES inelasticity.

Esophageal Dysphagia

The esophageal phase of swallowing involves coordinated peristalsis of the esophageal body with simultaneous relaxation of the lower esophageal sphincter (LES) that requires 7 to 15 seconds. This pattern, known as *primary peristalsis*, milks the food bolus into the stomach with minimal resistance. Secondary peristalsis refers to propulsive esophageal body contractions generated by retained food in the esophagus, and tertiary contractions signify uncoordinated, nonpropulsive motor activity that is observed in neuromuscular esophageal disease.

Obstructive Esophageal Lesions

Most often, esophageal dysphagia is caused by structural lesions that physically impede bolus transit. Patients with esophageal strictures secondary to acid peptic damage may present with progressive dysphagia after a long history of heartburn. These strictures usually are located in the distal esophagus. More proximal strictures develop above the transition point to columnar mucosa in patients with Barrett esophagus. A Schatzki ring, a thin, circumferential mucosal structure at the gastroesophageal junction, causes episodic and nonprogressive dysphagia that often occurs during rushed ingestion of poorly chewed meat. Patients with squamous cell carcinoma also report progressive dysphagia, similar to peptic disease, but affected patients often are older and have had long-standing exposure to tobacco or alcohol and no prior pyrosis. Esophageal adenocarcinoma develops in areas of Barrett metaplasia resulting from prolonged gastroesophageal reflux. Other mechanical lesions (e.g., abnormal great vessel anatomy, mediastinal lymphadenopathy, and cervical vertebral spurs) can rarely cause dysphagia.

Motor Disorders of the Esophagus

Primary and secondary disorders of esophageal motor activity represent the other main etiology of esophageal dysphagia. Primary achalasia is an idiopathic disorder characterized by esophageal body aperistalsis and failure of LES relaxation on swallowing with or without associated LES hypertension. Conditions that mimic primary achalasia include secondary achalasia, a disorder with identical radiographic and manometric characteristics caused by malignancy at the gastroesophageal junction or by paraneoplastic effects of a distant tumor, and Chagas disease, which results from infection with *Trypanosoma cruzi*. Other spastic esophageal dysmotilities, such as diffuse esophageal spasm, have also been associated with dysphagia.

Systemic diseases (e.g., scleroderma and other rheumatic diseases) also cause dysphagia because of reduced rather than spastic esophageal motor function.

Odynophagia

Oropharyngeal odynophagia most commonly results from malignancy, foreign body ingestion, or mucosal ulceration. Esophageal odynophagia usually is a consequence of caustic ingestion, infection (e.g., *Candida albicans,* herpes simplex virus, cytomegalovirus), radiation damage, pill esophagitis, or ulcer disease induced by acid reflux.

WORKUP

History

A history establishes whether dysphagia or odynophagia is oropharyngeal or esophageal in location and structural or neuromuscular in origin. If dysphagia occurs within 1 second of swallowing or is associated with drooling, choking, coughing, aspiration, nasal regurgitation, or tossing movements of the head, an oropharyngeal process is likely. Conversely, an esophageal cause is probable if dysphagia occurs more than 1 second after swallowing, if there is retrosternal pain or if there is regurgitation of unchanged food. Dysphagia perceived in the retrosternal or subxiphoid area is nearly diagnostic of an esophageal source. Dysphagia perceived in the cervical area may result from either oropharyngeal or esophageal disease. Structural esophageal disorders generally produce solid food dysphagia with progression to liquid dysphagia only if lumenal narrowing becomes severe. Patients with neuromuscular disorders of the esophagus usually report both liquid and solid dysphagia from the onset of symptoms. Both structural and neuromuscular oropharyngeal disorders produce early liquid dysphagia. In patients with odynophagia, risk factors for opportunistic infection should be assessed and a careful medication history is warranted if pill esophagitis is a consideration.

Physical Examination

The head and neck must be examined for sensory and motor function of the cranial nerves, masses, adenopathy, or spinal deformity. The patient is observed swallowing water to visualize the coordinated symmetric action of the neck and facial musculature. The clinician should examine for evidence of systemic disease, including sclerodactyly, telangiectasias, and calcinosis in scleroderma; neuropathies or muscle weakness from generalized neuromuscular disease; and hepatomegaly or adenopathy due to esophageal malignancy. The presence of oral thrush suggests candidal infection as a cause of odynophagia.

Additional Testing

If dysphagia is believed to be oropharyngeal, barium swallow radiography or endoscopy of the pharynx and esophagus may show occlusive lumenal lesions. Transnasal or peroral endoscopy also may reveal vocal cord paralysis, indicating neural dysfunction (Fig. 2-1). Videofluoroscopy of mastication and swallowing of three different preparations (thin liquid, thick liquid, barium cookie) are helpful in examining the coordination of the swallowing process in patients with suspected

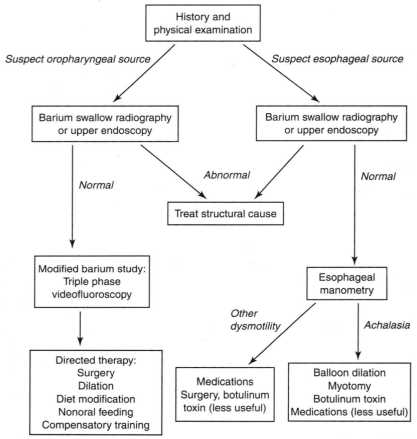

FIGURE 2-1. Workup of a patient with dysphagia.

neuromuscular disease. In some instances, specialized manometry can reveal abnormal UES relaxations. Ultrasound can examine tongue and laryngeal movement during swallowing.

For dysphagia of presumed esophageal origin, barium swallow radiography or endoscopy may reveal occlusive lesions such as carcinomas, strictures, rings, or webs. Barium swallow testing also can show the characteristic bird's beak deformity of achalasia. The addition of a solid bolus (e.g., a marshmallow or barium pill) can increase the detection of subtle abnormalities during contrast radiography. Upper endoscopy affords the additional capability to perform a biopsy of any suspicious areas. If structural testing is nondiagnostic, manometry of the esophageal body and LES may detect the characteristic findings of achalasia, systemic diseases such as scleroderma, and other primary and secondary esophageal motor disorders.

Endoscopy is the procedure of choice for both oropharyngeal and esophageal odynophagia. Plain radiography of the neck may detect pharyngeal foreign bodies.

PRINCIPLES OF MANAGEMENT

Selected causes of oropharyngeal dysphagia, including Parkinson disease, hypothyroidism, polymyositis, and myasthenia gravis, may have specific therapies. Surgical myotomy may benefit patients with Zenker diverticulum or cricopharyngeal achalasia. A few limited studies suggest that myotomy also may be useful in treating selected cases of neuromuscular disease. For untreatable neuromuscular conditions, consultation with a speech pathologist may afford development of a rehabilitation program to improve swallowing. Techniques include altering food consistency, motor retraining, controlled breathing, coughing, and head positioning. When adequate nutrition cannot be maintained, alternate enteral feedings through a gastrostomy may be indicated.

Management of esophageal dysphagia depends on its cause. Benign strictures, webs, and rings are dilated by bougienage. Early malignancies may be surgically resected, whereas dilation, cautery, laser, stenting, or radiation therapy may be used for unresectable lesions. Achalasia can be treated with botulinum toxin injection into the LES, endoscopic dilation, or surgical myotomy. Other primary esophageal dysmotilities may respond to nitrates, calcium channel antagonists, and, in rare instances, botulinum toxin or surgical myotomy.

Therapy for odynophagia secondary to opportunistic infection relies on anti-infective treatments, whereas pill esophagitis and caustic ingestion may be managed with medications to reduce acid reflux and to coat the irritated esophagus.

COMPLICATIONS

The most serious complication of oropharyngeal dysphagia is tracheal aspiration, with development of cough, asthma, or pneumonia. Esophageal dysphagia results in a failure to thrive because of reduced oral intake.

CHAPTER 3

Approach to the Patient with Chest Pain

DIFFERENTIAL DIAGNOSIS

Chest pain most often is attributed to cardiac etiologies. However, 20% to 30% of patients who undergo cardiac catheterization for chest pain exhibit patent coronary arteries. These patients with noncardiac chest pain experience symptoms as a consequence of diseases of the cardiopulmonary system, musculoskeletal structures, gastrointestinal tract, and central nervous system (Table 3-1). Less common causes

---

TABLE 3-1
Causes of Chest Pain

Cardiopulmonary Disease
  Coronary artery disease
  Coronary artery spasm
  Microvascular angina
  Mitral valve prolapse
  Aortic valve disease
  Pericarditis
  Dissecting thoracic aortic aneurysm
  Mediastinitis
  Pneumonia
  Pulmonary embolus

Musculoskeletal Causes
  Costochondritis
  Fibromyalgia
  Arthritis
  Nerve entrapment or compression

Esophageal Disease
  Gastroesophageal reflux
  Achalasia
  Diffuse esophageal spasm
  Other spastic motor disorders
  Infectious or pill-induced esophagitis
  Food impaction

Neuropsychiatric Causes
  Panic disorder
  Anxiety disorder
  Depression
  Somatization

Miscellaneous
  Varicella-zoster virus reactivation

---

include biliary tract disease, pleural and mediastinal inflammation, dissecting aortic aneurysm, and varicella-zoster virus infection of the chest wall.

Cardiac Disease

Cardiac etiologies must be considered in a patient with unexplained chest pain, even in the absence of coronary atherosclerosis. Coronary artery spasm in response to ergonovine is reported in some individuals with chest pain. Exertional chest pain may be a consequence of abnormalities of the smaller endocardial vasculature without evidence of fixed lesions or spasm of the epicardial vessels, a condition termed *microvascular angina* or *syndrome X*. Diagnosis of this disorder requires measuring cardiac lactate production and coronary sinus blood flow during fasting and after rapid atrial pacing followed by intravenous ergonovine challenge. Microvascular angina should be considered in patients with ischemic ST segment changes on electrocardiography or if left ventricular ejection fractions decrease in response to exercise on echocardiography or radionuclide ventriculography. The relationship of chest pain to mitral valve prolapse is controversial. Furthermore, esophageal motor abnormalities may coexist with both microvascular angina and mitral valve prolapse that make the cause of chest pain uncertain in affected individuals.

Musculoskeletal Causes

Musculoskeletal conditions account for 10% to 30% of cases of noncardiac chest pain. Chest pain from musculoskeletal sources (e.g., costochondritis [Tietze syndrome], fibromyalgia, inflammatory arthritis, osteoarthritis, thoracic spinal disease) is characterized by localized chest wall tenderness and definable trigger points and may be reported at rest, with movement, or during sleep.

Neuropsychiatric Causes

Panic disorder presents with at least three attacks in as many weeks of intense fear or discomfort accompanied by at least four of the following symptoms: chest pain, restlessness, choking, palpitations, sweating, dizziness, nausea or abdominal distress, paresthesia, flushing, trembling, and a sense of impending doom. Of all cases of noncardiac chest pain, 34% to 59% result from panic disorder. In addition to increased anxiety, these patients also exhibit increased incidence of depression and somatization.

Esophageal Disease

Esophageal disorders, the most common causes of noncardiac chest pain, account for 20% to 60% of cases. Although heartburn is more prevalent, chest pain is a common atypical symptom of gastroesophageal reflux disease. In some cases, acid reflux may be induced by exercise. A small percentage of these patients exhibits altered esophageal motor patterns on acid perfusion. In most patients, however, there is a poor correlation between chest pain and acid reflux episodes. Primary spastic esophageal motor disorders are found in less than 50% of patients with noncardiac chest pain. One such condition, diffuse esophageal spasm, accounts for 5% of cases and is characterized by the presence of high-amplitude, nonperistaltic esophageal contractions on manometry. Esophageal hypersensitivity to balloon distention may correlate better with symptoms in patients with noncardiac chest pain than motor disturbances, which suggests that a primary disturbance of esophageal afferent neural function is pathogenic. Miscellaneous gastroesophageal sources of chest pain include infectious or pill-induced esophagitis, food impaction, and proximal gastric ulcers.

WORKUP

History

Chest pain from esophageal causes commonly is described as squeezing or burning, is substernal in location, and may last from minutes to hours. Noncardiac chest pain from esophageal sources may radiate in a pattern indistinguishable from angina and may not be related to swallowing. Symptoms can be exacerbated by ingesting cold or hot liquids or by stress and can awaken the patient from sleep. In contrast to cardiac chest pain, exertion only rarely triggers esophageal chest pain. Relief may be provided by antacid ingestion or nitroglycerin administration. Pain that lasts for hours, that is related to meals, that does not radiate laterally, and that is relieved by acid suppressants suggests an esophageal origin.

Physical Examination

Physical examination occasionally helps to delineate the cause of chest pain. Reproduction of symptoms by chest wall palpation suggests a musculoskeletal source. Auscultation of pleural friction rubs or decreased breath sounds infers pleuropulmonary disease. Cutaneous eruptions in a dermatomal pattern indicate probable varicella-zoster virus reactivation. A characteristic midsystolic click and murmur may suggest mitral valve prolapse. Abdominal tenderness raises concern for peptic or biliary tract disease.

Additional Testing

Initial diagnostic tests involve exclusion of cardiac disease. Most patients should undergo electrocardiography, exercise stress testing, echocardiography, or coronary arteriography, depending on their age and risk factors, because the presence of coronary artery disease cannot be established reliably from the history (Fig. 3-1). An ergonovine test may be used to elicit coronary spasm in some patients. Once cardiac disease is excluded, noncardiac sources for chest pain may be evaluated. Musculoskeletal causes usually are detected on physical examination, whereas psychogenic causes may require referral to a mental health specialist for assessment.

Barium swallow radiography or upper endoscopy is used to exclude esophageal mucosal sources of chest pain. Radiographic techniques may observe subtle strictures or dysmotilities, whereas endoscopy is superior for detecting esophagitis and affords the capability to perform a biopsy of suspicious mucosa. When structural studies are normal, gastroesophageal reflux disease should be excluded because of its prevalence as a cause of chest pain. The best test for correlating symptoms with acid reflux is ambulatory pH monitoring of the esophagus using a probe positioned 5 cm above the lower esophageal sphincter. With this procedure, episodes may relate temporally to periods in which esophageal pH decreases. An esophageal pH less than 4 for longer than 5% of total exposure time infers a diagnosis of gastroesophageal reflux disease with a sensitivity of 85% and a specificity of 95%. If ambulatory pH testing is unavailable, an acid perfusion test can be performed. With this technique, known as the Bernstein test, alternating infusions of 0.1 normal hydrochloric acid and normal saline should reproduce and then relieve the patient's chest pain. An empirical trial of high-dose proton pump inhibitor therapy represents an alternative to this test and can be expected to relieve symptoms in 80% of patients with noncardiac chest pain and underlying acid reflux.

Esophageal manometry may define an underlying esophageal dysmotility syndrome. By itself, manometry detects potentially pathogenic motor abnormalities in only a minority of patients with noncardiac chest pain. The diagnostic accuracy of manometry may be enhanced by pharmacological challenge with the α-adrenergic stimulant erogonovine, the cholinergic agonist bethanechol, or the cholinesterase inhibitor edrophonium. However, these agents provoke significant side effects—especially in those individuals with underlying cardiac disease. Furthermore, their

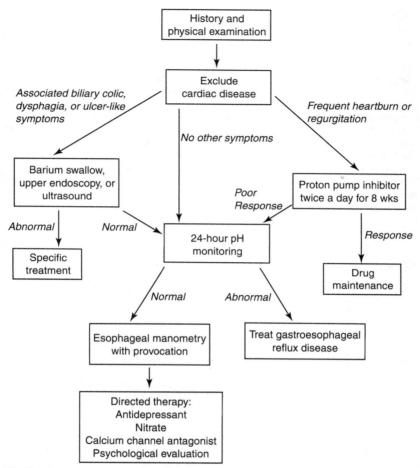

FIGURE 3-1. Workup of a patient with chest pain.

clinical utility is unproved. Thus, provocative testing is falling out of favor at many institutions. In some patients, balloon distention of the esophagus reproduces the presenting complaint, which suggests a visceral afferent disturbance as a cause of symptoms. Some centers use this test in their diagnostic evaluations.

PRINCIPLES OF MANAGEMENT

Treatment of esophageal chest pain may be unsatisfactory because of diagnostic uncertainties, the intermittent nature of symptoms, the side effect profiles of available pharmaceutical agents, and the awareness that many of these conditions improve spontaneously without treatment. After a careful diagnostic examination, many patients respond to physician reassurance that no dangerous condition exists. For underlying gastroesophageal reflux disease, long-term treatment with a potent acid-suppressing medication such as a proton pump inhibitor (e.g., omeprazole) may be needed. Patients who respond poorly to medical therapy can be considered for antireflux surgery. For painful esophageal dysmotility, nitrates and calcium channel blockers may be considered, although response rates for these agents are low. Many of these patients respond instead to antidepressant agents (e.g., amitriptyline, imipramine, desipramine, trazodone) at doses lower than those used to treat endogenous depression. One study has shown improvement in chest pain with the selective serotonin reuptake inhibitor sertraline. Uncontrolled studies suggest that injecting botulinum toxin into the esophageal body may decrease symptoms caused by diffuse esophageal spasm. In rare cases of refractory esophageal motor dysfunction, esophageal dilation or surgical myotomy may relieve symptoms. For panic disorders, anxiolytics (e.g., benzodiazepines or buspirone) may be effective. However, these agents have abuse potential, may induce tolerance, and may exacerbate underlying depression. Cognitive and behavioral therapy may produce significant improvements in chest pain, functional disability, and psychological distress in selected patient populations with psychogenic etiologies of chest pain.

Complications

Chest pain of esophageal origin rarely has long-term sequelae. The major risk in evaluating a patient with unexplained chest pain is the premature exclusion of coronary ischemia, which may have life-threatening consequences.

CHAPTER 4

Approach to the Patient with Gross Gastrointestinal Bleeding

Gastrointestinal (GI) bleeding is a common problem. Its severity ranges from life-threatening hemorrhage to insidious occult blood loss. In approaching the patient with GI bleeding, it is important to assess the severity as well as the site of blood loss. Hematemesis (vomiting of bright-red blood or coffee ground–colored matter) indicates an upper GI source proximal to the ligament of Treitz. Melena (black, malodorous, tarry stools that indicate intestinal degradation of blood) usually results from acute upper GI bleeding, although bleeding from the small intestine and the right colon also produces melena. Hematochezia (bright-red rectal bleeding) usually indicates a colonic source, although brisk bleeding from an upper GI site may also produce hematochezia or maroon-colored stools. During the past decade, hospitalization rates for GI bleeding have decreased significantly. Most patients with upper GI bleeding undergo endoscopy within 24 hours of admission. Mortality from upper GI sources is 3.5% to 7%, whereas mortality from lower GI bleeding is 3.6%.

ACUTE UPPER GASTROINTESTINAL BLEEDING

Differential Diagnosis

The most common causes of upper GI hemorrhage are peptic ulcer disease, gastropathy (or gastric erosions), and sequelae of portal hypertension (i.e., esophageal and gastric varices, portal gastropathy). Other disorders comprise a small minority of cases (Table 4-1).

TABLE 4-1
Causes of Gross Gastrointestinal Hemorrhage

Upper Gastrointestinal Sources
　　Peptic ulcer disease (duodenal, gastric, stomal)
　　Gastritis (NSAID-, stress-, chemotherapy-induced)
　　Varices (esophageal, gastric, duodenal)
　　Portal gastropathy
　　Mallory-Weiss tear
　　Esophagitis and esophageal ulcers (acid reflux, infection, pill-induced,
　　　　sclerotherapy, radiation-induced)
　　Neoplasms
　　Vascular ectasias and angiodysplasias
　　Gastric antral vascular ectasia
　　Aortoenteric fistula
　　Hematobilia
　　Hemosuccus pancreaticus
　　Dieulafoy erosion

Lower Gastrointestinal Sources
　　Diverticulosis
　　Angiodysplasia
　　Hemorrhoids
　　Anal fissures
　　Neoplasms
　　Inflammatory bowel disease
　　Ischemic colitis
　　Infectious colitis
　　Radiation-induced colitis
　　Meckel diverticulum
　　Intussusception
　　Aortoenteric fistula
　　Solitary rectal ulcers
　　NSAID-induced cecal ulcers

Peptic Ulcer Disease

Duodenal, gastric, and stomal ulcers cause 50% of upper GI bleeding. Bleeding occurs if an ulcer erodes into the lateral wall of a vessel, which may loop into the floor of the ulcer crater, forming an aneurysmal dilation. Most cases of peptic ulcer disease result from gastric infection with *Helicobacter pylori* or from chronic use of aspirin or nonsteroidal antiinflammatory drugs (NSAIDs). Stigmata of recent bleeding from ulcer sources on endoscopy that are predictors of poor outcome include active arterial spurting, oozing of blood, a visible vessel (an elevated red, blue, or gray mound that resists washing), and adherent clot. Other prognostic indicators include amount of blood lost, patient age, concomitant disease, onset of bleeding while hospitalized, giant ulcers larger than 2 cm, and need for emergency surgery.

Gastropathy

Gastropathy may be produced by several mechanisms. Endoscopically, gastropathy may be visualized as mucosal hemorrhages, erythema, or erosions. An erosion, in contrast to an ulcer, represents a break in the mucosa of less than 5 mm that does not traverse the muscularis mucosae. In addition to causing ulcers, NSAIDs produce erosions most often in the antrum that usually resolve after removing the offending agent. Ethanol is a gastric mucosal irritant when administered in high concentrations. However, it is uncertain if chronic ethanol intake causes damage in amounts usually ingested during binge drinking or if bleeding is a consequence of portal hypertensive gastropathy secondary to unsuspected liver disease. Stress gastritis develops in patients in the intensive care unit who have underlying respiratory failure, hypotension, sepsis, renal failure, burns, peritonitis, jaundice, or neurological trauma. Although most patients in the intensive care unit have gastric mucosal abnormalities on endoscopy, only 2% to 10% develop gross hemorrhage. The hallmark of stress gastritis is the presence of multiple bleeding sites, which limit the therapeutic options. A rare cause of gastropathy is chemotherapy delivered hrough the hepatic artery, which may induce mucosal necrosis of the stomach and duodenum.

Hemorrhage Secondary to Portal Hypertension

Patients with portal hypertension are predisposed to hemorrhage from esophageal and gastric varices and portal hypertensive gastropathy. However, up to 50% of upper GI bleeds in patients with cirrhosis do not result from these causes. One fourth to one third of patients with cirrhosis experience variceal hemorrhage on at least one occasion. Thirty percent of patients die of their initial esophageal variceal hemorrhage, and two-thirds die within 1 year. A portal pressure of 12 mm Hg or higher must be present for varices to develop. Absolute pressures above this level correlate poorly with the propensity for bleeding. Variceal size is the best predictor of esophageal variceal hemorrhage because wall tension is determined by the diameter of a hollow vessel. Other predictors of esophageal variceal bleeding include the red color sign, which is the result of microtelangiectasia; red wale marks, which appear as whip marks; hemocystic spots, which appear as blood blisters; and diffuse redness. The white nipple sign, a platelet-fibrin plug, is diagnostic of previous hemorrhage but does not predict rebleeding.

Gastric varices are present in 20% of patients with portal hypertension and develop in another 8% after esophageal variceal obliteration. Most gastric varices involving the fundus and cardia span the gastroesophageal junction and merge with esophageal columns. Isolated gastric varices suggest splenic vein thrombosis, which may be a consequence of pancreatic disease and is treated by splenectomy. Ectopic varices elsewhere in the stomach and duodenum rarely bleed. Portal hypertensive gastropathy appears endoscopically as a mosaic, snakeskin-like mucosa as a result of engorged mucosal vessels that may bleed briskly or produce insidious iron deficiency anemia.

Miscellaneous Causes of Upper Gastrointestinal Bleeding

Mallory-Weiss tears are linear breaks in the mucosa of the gastroesophageal junction that are induced by retching, often in patients who have consumed alcohol. Most Mallory-Weiss tears resolve spontaneously with conservative management. Esophagitis and esophageal ulcers result from acid reflux, radiation therapy, infections with *Candida albicans* and herpes simplex virus, pill-induced damage, or iatrogenic sources (e.g., sclerotherapy). Hemorrhage from erosive duodenitis is similar to duodenal ulcer bleeding but usually is less severe because the lesions are shallower. Neoplasms most commonly bleed slowly but occasionally exhibit massive hemorrhage. Vascular ectasia and angiodysplasia occur less commonly in the stomach and duodenum than in the colon and cause recurrent acute GI hemorrhage that may require frequent blood transfusions. Angiodysplasias often occur as a consequence of advanced age, but also are associated with chronic renal failure, aortic valve disease, and prior radiation therapy. Hereditary hemorrhagic telangiectasia, or Osler-Weber-Rendu syndrome, is an autosomal dominant disorder with telangiectasia of the tongue, lips, conjunctiva, skin, and mucosa of the gut, bladder, and nasopharynx. Gastric arteriovenous ectasia (GAVE), or watermelon stomach, has the appearance of columns of vessels along the tops of the antral longitudinal rugae. Biopsies show dilated mucosal capillaries with focal thrombosis and fibromuscular hyperplasia of lamina propria vessels. Aortoenteric fistulae may produce fatal hemorrhage from the third portion of the duodenum in patients who have undergone prior synthetic aortic graft surgery. This patient may present with a minor "herald" hemorrhage before fatal exsanguination occurs. Hematobilia and hemosuccus pancreaticus present with hemorrhage from the ampulla of Vater and are complications of liver trauma or biopsy, malignancy, hepatic artery aneurysm, hepatic abscess, gallstones, and pancreatic pseudocyst. Bleeding in a Dieulafoy lesion results from pressure erosion of the overlying epithelium by an ectopic artery in the proximal stomach without surrounding ulceration or inflammation. Some patients present with upper GI bleeding from epistaxis, hemoptysis, oral lesions, or factitious blood ingestion.

Workup

History

In a patient with hemodynamically significant upper GI bleeding, volume replacement with intravenous fluids and blood products is of paramount importance. While resuscitation is under way, a directed history usually can be obtained. Prior peptic disease or dyspeptic symptoms suggest ulcer bleeding. Recent ingestion of aspirin, NSAIDs, alcohol, or caustic substances should be ascertained. Chronic ethanol consumption or known liver disease raises the possibility of varices or portal gastropathy. Prior aortic surgery, coagulopathies, neoplasm, or recent nosebleeds may suggest specific diagnoses.

Physical Examination

Various physical findings point to the cause of upper GI bleeding. Cutaneous stigmata of cirrhosis or malignancy may be present. Multiple cutaneous telangiectases suggest hereditary hemorrhagic telangiectasia. Lymphadenopathy, hepatosplenomegaly, and abdominal masses raise the possibility of malignancy. Hepatosplenomegaly, ascites, or dilated abdominal wall vessels suggest portal hypertension. Demonstration of maroon or melenic stools on rectal examination in the patient with upper GI bleeding indicates significant hemorrhage.

Additional Testing

Laboratory studies.   A hematocrit, platelet count, and coagulation studies should be part of the initial laboratory evaluation. The first hematocrit may not reflect the degree of blood loss because acute hemorrhage produces loss of both erythrocytes and volume, and thus the ratio of the two parameters is not altered. As intravascular volume is replenished with endogenous and exogenous fluids, the hematocrit decreases gradually to a stable level after 24 to 48 hours. A low hematocrit with microcytosis suggests chronic blood loss, which can be confirmed with iron studies or ferritin measurement. Thrombocytopenia may be a consequence of bone marrow disease, autoimmune disorders, or portal hypertension with splenomegaly. Prothrombin time prolongation results from liver disease, warfarin, or malnutrition. With massive upper GI bleeding, azotemia reflects intestinal absorption of nitrogenous breakdown products of blood, although azotemia with creatinine elevation suggests renal insufficiency. Abnormal liver chemistry levels raise concern about possible cirrhosis with portal hypertension.

Upper endoscopy.   Urgent upper endoscopy is indicated for hemorrhage that does not stop spontaneously or in patients with suspected cirrhosis or aortoenteric fistulae. If bleeding stops, endoscopy may be postponed up to 24 hours without compromising care. Upper endoscopy is contraindicated when perforation is suspected and is relatively contraindicated in patients with compromised cardiopulmonary status or depressed consciousness. In such cases, endotracheal intubation with mechanical ventilation may enhance the safety of the technique. Upper GI barium radiography is not performed in the acute setting in a potentially unstable patient because it offers no therapeutic capability and may obscure endoscopic or angiographic visualization of the bleeding site.

Scintigraphy and angiography.   When hemorrhage is so brisk that it obscures endoscopic visualization, scintigraphic and angiographic studies may be indicated. Scintigraphic ^{99m}Tc-sulfur colloid– or ^{99m}Tc-pertechnetate–labeled erythrocyte scans can localize bleeding to an area of the abdomen if the rate of blood loss exceeds 0.5 mL/min. They are used to determine if angiography is feasible and to direct the angiographic search and minimize any dye load. Angiography can localize the bleeding site if the rate of blood loss is greater than 0.5 mL/min and can offer therapeutic capability. Angiography also identifies the bleeding site in hemobilia or hemosuccus pancreaticus and can detect vascular ectasia in patients with intermittent hemorrhage who have normal findings on upper endoscopy.

Other radiographic studies.   If an aortoenteric fistula is suspected, a vigorous diagnostic approach, including abdominal computed tomographic or magnetic resonance imaging studies, should be pursued after endoscopy has excluded other bleeding sources.

Principles of Management

Resuscitation

The first step in managing a patient with upper GI bleeding is to assess the urgency of the clinical condition (Fig. 4-1). Hematemesis, melena, or hematochezia suggest major hemorrhage, whereas pallor, hypotension, and tachycardia indicate

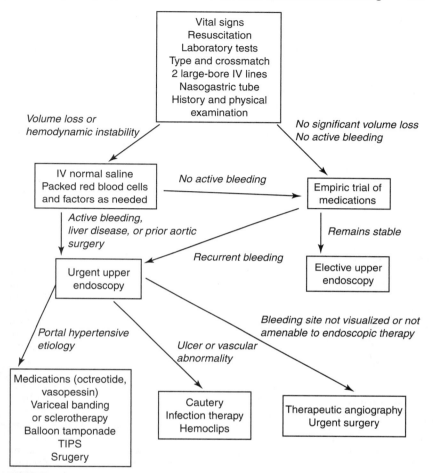

FIGURE 4-1. Workup of a patient with acute upper gastrointestinal bleeding (*IV*, intravenous; *TIPS*, transjugular intrahepatic portosystemic shunt).

substantial blood volume loss (>40% of total volume) and mandate immediate volume replacement. Postural hypotension of greater than 10 mm Hg indicates a lesser blood loss (20% blood volume reduction), but acute volume replacement usually is still required. A patient with GI bleeding and postural or supine hypotension must be admitted to an intensive care unit. Two large-bore intravenous catheters should be inserted. In cases of shock, a central venous line may afford more aggressive volume replacement. Fragile patients with cardiopulmonary disease may require capillary wedge pressure measurement. A nasogastric tube is placed. A bright-red aspirate that does not clear with lavage of room temperaure water is an indication for urgent endoscopy because it is associated with a 30% mortality, whereas coffee ground–colored material that clears permits further assessment in a hemodynamically stable patient. A clear aspirate is found in some patients with duodenal bleeding. Thus, the clinician cannot be complacent if unstable hemodynamic parameters indicate ongoing blood loss. In addition to diagnostic laboratory testing, blood samples are sent for blood typing and cross matching. Intravascular volume should be replenished with normal saline while awaiting the availability of blood products.

Transfusion of Blood Products
The need for blood transfusion is influenced by patient age, coexistent cardiovascular disease, and persistent hemorrhage. Generally, the hematocrit should be maintained above 30% in elderly patients and above 20% in younger patients. Packed erythrocytes are preferred for blood transfusion to avoid fluid load. If coagulation studies are abnormal, as in cirrhosis, fresh frozen plasma or platelets also may be needed. Patients without coagulopathy may need fresh frozen plasma and platelet transfusion if multiple transfusions have been given, because transfused blood is deficient in some clotting factors. Warmed blood should be transfused in patients with massive blood loss (>3 L) to prevent hypothermia. Some individuals with massive bleeding also require supplemental calcium to counter the calcium-binding effects of preserved blood.

Medications
Empiric medical treatment is often given before the evaluation is complete. For presumed peptic disease, intravenous proton pump inhibitor therapy may be given. Studies demonstrate that high doses of omeprazole reduce rates of rebleeding from ulcers. Proton pump inhibitors also play prominent roles in prophylaxis against development of erosions in patients on NSAIDs. Patients with *H pylori* infection should be given combined therapy including antibiotics to eradicate the organism, even those who may have mucosal injury secondary to NSAIDs. Prophylaxis against stress gastropathy should be provided for patients at risk in intensive care units and may include histamine H_2 receptor antagonists, proton pump inhibitors, and sucralfate. For presumed varices or portal gastropathy, intravenous octreotide is begun when bleeding is diagnosed. Vasopressin can also be given with or without nitroglycerin; however, this therapy has higher complication rates. Metoclopramide has been used to increase lower esophageal sphincter pressure to reduce variceal blood flow. Chronic use of β-adrenergic blockers with or without nitroglycerin may reduce rates of rebleeding from varices. Intravenous or oral estrogens may be of some benefit in bleeding from angiodysplasia. However, in the acutely bleeding patient, these agents have limited effect and do not substitute for more aggressive means of controlling hemorrhage.

Therapeutic Endoscopy
Urgent upper endoscopy is performed for upper GI bleeding in the setting of presumed liver disease, a suspected aortoenteric fistula, or bleeding that does not abate spontaneously. Before endoscopy, the stomach should be lavaged through a large-bore orogastric tube with room temperature saline or water to enhance mucosal visualization. Bleeding esophageal varices may be managed by endoscopic placement of rubber bands to constrict the bleeding site or by direct injection of a sclerosant solution such as sodium morrhuate. These therapies have initial success rates of 85% to 95% for controlling active hemorrhage. Band ligation may exhibit lower complication rates compared to sclerotherapy. Multiple courses of banding or sclerotherapy can be recommended to reduce rates of rebleeding. The role of endoscopy in managing gastric varices is less well established, although sclerotherapy, thrombin injection, cyanoacrylate injection, and snare ligation have been reported to be effective in small studies. For nonvariceal hemorrhage, local injection, placement

of hemoclips, or cautery may provide effective initial hemostasis and reduce the risk of rebleeding. Additional meta-analyses also suggest reductions in mortality with endoscopic therapy. Solutions that stop bleeding from nonvariceal disease when injected include sclerosants (ethanolamine), vasoconstrictors (epinephrine), and normal saline. Thermal methods of cautery include bipolar electrocautery, heater probe application, argon plasma coagulation, and Nd:YAG laser therapy. Endoscopic visualization of a nonbleeding visible vessel or an adherent clot increases the risk of rebleeding in the patient with ulcer hemorrhage. Thus for major hemorrhage secondary to ulcer disease, endoscopic therapy should be performed for active bleeding sites as well as visible vessels and adherent clots, which, when washed off, reveal visible vessels or active bleeding. Other sources amenable to cautery include refractory Mallory-Weiss tears, neoplasms, angiodysplasia, or Dieulafoy lesions. Patients with stress gastritis, gastropathy resulting from analgesics, and portal gastropathy usually present with multiple bleeding sites that cannot be controlled endoscopically. Fortunately, bleeding stops spontaneously in many of these individuals.

Mechanical Compression
When endoscopic therapy of variceal hemorrhage fails, balloon tamponade with a Sengstaken-Blakemore or Linton-Nachlas tube achieves initial hemostasis in 70% to 90% of cases. However, rebleeding rates are high after removing the device. Most patients benefit from prophylactic endotracheal intubation before balloon tamponade. Initial inflation of the gastric balloon controls hemorrhage in some patients, but many require controlled inflation of both the gastric and esophageal balloons for optimal hemostasis.

Therapeutic Angiography
Angiography is effective for many cases when endoscopic therapy fails or is not indicated. In peptic ulcer hemorrhage refractory to endoscopic control, angiographic embolization with microcoils, absorbable gelatin sponge (Gelfoam), or autologous clot may be attempted. This treatment is best for patients who are not surgical candidates. Intra-arterial vasopressin or embolization is useful for some patients with stress gastritis bleeding, as well as in those with bleeding from esophageal sources, refractory Mallory-Weiss tears, neoplasms, hematobilia, and hemosuccus pancreaticus. Angiographic placement of a portocaval shunt (transjugular intrahepatic portosystemic shunt, or TIPS) can effectively control bleeding secondary to gastric varices, portal hypertensive gastropathy, and refractory esophageal varices. With TIPS, an expandable metal stent is placed between the hepatic and portal veins to reduce portal pressure. Other angiographic methods to control variceal hemorrhage are available but are not commonly used because of their technical difficulty and complication rates.

Surgery
When endoscopy or angiography fail, emergency surgery may be required. Early operative intervention is indicated for persistent or recurrent bleeding from ulcers, Mallory-Weiss tears, Dieulafoy syndrome, or for "herald" bleeding from aortoenteric fistulae. Antrectomy may be required for GAVE. Hemorrhage from portal gastropathy, or gastric varices may need urgent portocaval shunting or esophageal devascularization in patients in whom TIPS is unsuccessful or not available, although the mortality rate for these procedures exceeds 50%. However, many patients experience worsening liver function or hepatic encephalopathy after portocaval shunts. Recurrent variceal hemorrhage is considered an indication for hepatic transplantation in patients with advanced liver disease. Splenectomy can control hemorrhage from isolated gastric varices secondary to splenic vein thrombosis.

Complications

The most serious complication of upper GI bleeding is exsanguination and death. Mortality from acute upper GI hemorrhage increases from 8% to 10% to 30% to 40% in patients with persistent or recurrent bleeding. Thus, a major focus of research has been on means to prevent initial or recurrent hemorrhage. For bleeding from ulcers, treatments directed to causes such as *H pylori* are indicated. Prostaglandin analogs (e.g., misoprostol) and proton pump inhibitors have demonstrated efficacy in preventing NSAID-induced gastropathy and ulcers. Stress gastritis prophylaxis includes proton pump inhibitors, H_2 receptor antagonists, high-dose antacids, or sucralfate. Sucralfate therapy may be associated with lower rates of nosocomial pneumonias in mechanically ventilated patients. Chronic estrogen-progesterone therapy may reduce transfusion requirements in patients with angiodysplasia.

Because of the high mortality of hemorrhage secondary to portal hypertension, prevention of rebleeding is crucial. Obliteration of varices with multiple courses of endoscopic variceal band ligation or sclerotherapy reduces rebleeding rates, although the effects on mortality are less certain. Meta-analyses suggest that propranolol therapy to reduce portal pressures reduces the probability of initial and recurrent hemorrhage from esophageal varices. Propranolol has also shown efficacy in preventing rebleeding from portal gastropathy.

ACUTE LOWER GASTROINTESTINAL BLEEDING

Differential Diagnosis

Bleeding colonic diverticula, angiodysplasia, and ischemic colitis are the major causes of acute lower GI bleeding (see Table 4-1). Chronic or recurrent lower GI hemorrhage is most often due to hemorrhoids and colonic neoplasia. Unlike upper GI bleeding, most lower GI bleeding is slow and intermittent and does not require hospitalization.

Diverticulosis

Diverticular bleeding usually is painless and occurs in 3% of patients with diverticulosis. Red or maroon stools usually are passed, although melena may occur. Despite the preponderance of diverticula in the sigmoid colon, many bleeding diverticula are right-sided. Most cases spontaneously resolve and do not recur. Therefore no specific therapy is indicated for the majority of patients.

Angiodysplasia

Angiodysplasia is responsible for 10% to 40% of acute lower GI bleeding episodes. Angiodysplasia is also a common cause of chronic blood loss. Colonic angiodysplasias usually are multiple in number, small (<5 mm in diameter), and localized to the right colon and cecum. As with gastroduodenal vascular ectasia, colonic lesions are associated with advanced age, renal insufficiency, prior irradiation, and aortic valve disease, although the latter association has been questioned.

Ischemic Colitis

Most cases of ischemic colitis present in the setting of reduced visceral blood flow and do not involve any underlying fixed narrowing of the mesenteric vasculature. Nevertheless, most patients with ischemic colitis are elderly with significant concurrent disease. Other causes include sepsis, hemorrhage from other causes, and dehydration.

Perianal Disease

Hemorrhoids and anal fissures usually result in small volumes of bright-red blood on toilet paper or on but not mixed in stool. In contrast, hemorrhage from rectal varices in patients with portal hypertension may be life-threatening. Because polyps and carcinoma may present similarly to hemorrhoids or fissures, these causes need to be excluded in appropriate patient populations.

Colonic Neoplasia

Benign and malignant colonic neoplasms are common in elderly patients and usually are associated with small degrees of intermittent bleeding or occult blood loss. In contrast, small intestinal neoplasms are rare disorders that have increased incidence in inflammatory conditions (e.g., Crohn's disease or celiac sprue).

Miscellaneous Causes of Lower Gastrointestinal Bleeding

Colitis secondary to inflammatory bowel disease, infection (*Campylobacter jejuni*, *Salmonella* spp., *Shigella* spp., *Escherichia coli*), and radiation therapy (acute or chronic) rarely lead to bleeding that is more than small to moderate in volume. Meckel diverticulum, a congenital ileal diverticulum resulting from incomplete obliteration of the vitelline duct, may bleed profusely because acid-producing gastric-type mucosa within the lesion causes peptic ulceration. Patients usually present in childhood with painless red or melenic bleeding, which has been described as having a "currant jelly" appearance. Intussusception presents with maroon stools and crampy pain and usually occurs at the site of a polyp or malignancy in adults. Portal hypertension may predispose to development of ileocolonic and anorectal varices, which may cause voluminous, brisk, blood loss. Portal colonopathy appears as multiple colonic vascular ectasias. Other rare causes of lower GI bleeding include aortoenteric fistulae, solitary rectal ulcers (caused by constipation-induced rectal prolapse), and cecal ulcers (most often caused by NSAIDs).

Workup

History and Physical Examination

A thorough history and physical examination may point to the correct diagnosis. A history of hemorrhoids or inflammatory bowel disease is important to note. Abdominal pain or diarrhea suggests colitis or neoplasm. Malignancy also may be indicated by weight loss, anorexia, lymphadenopathy, or palpable masses.

Additional Testing

Endoscopy. When lower GI bleeding is slow or has stopped, colonoscopy is the diagnostic procedure of choice because it is highly accurate in detecting potential bleeding sites and affords therapeutic capability. Colonoscopy can document the presence of diverticula; however, it frequently does not identify the actual bleeding site. With brisk bleeding, colonoscopy attempted after a rapid purge may provide diagnostic accuracy similar to or greater than angiography. In contrast, barium enema radiography may miss up to 20% of endoscopically identifiable lesions, especially angiodysplastic lesions, and can prevent therapies directed by colonoscopy or angiography. Thus, the technique is rarely useful in patients with unexplained lower GI bleeding. In patients with presumed GI bleeding distal to the ligament of Treitz who have undergone a colonoscopy with negative results, peroral enteroscopy or capsule endoscopy may detect small intestinal angiodysplastic lesions or other subtle lesions. Therapy may be provided by enteroscopy, although the capsule technique is purely a diagnostic modality. Enteroscopy may be performed intraoperatively at the time of laparotomy in rare cases in which an elusive bleeding source produces recurrent hemodynamically significant hemorrhage.

Scintigraphy and angiography. For cases with rapid hemorrhage where colonoscopy is nondiagnostic or cannot be performed, angiography can provide important information. With bleeding rates greater than 0.5 mL/min, lumenal blood extravasation from diverticula, angiodysplasia, neoplasia, Meckel diverticula, or aortoenteric fistulae may be observed. In rare cases, angiodysplasia or neoplasms in the small intestine and colon may be detected from the angiographic blush pattern in the absence of active bleeding. Prior to angiography, a scintigraphic bleeding scan may be needed to confirm ongoing bleeding and to direct the angiographer to the anatomic region where bleeding is occurring. When a bleeding site cannot be defined, some have advocated an aggressive angiographic approach with administration of heparin or streptokinase to increase the bleeding rate with the hope of enhancing the detection rate of the test. Helical computed tomography angiography also can detect angiodysplasia. Meckel diverticula can be diagnosed with Meckel scanning, which uses a radiolabeled technetium compound that accumulates in acid-producing mucosa in the diverticulum.

Other radiographic studies. Barium enema radiography may be useful for both diagnosing and treating intussusception. Dedicated small intestinal barium radiography may demonstrate a Meckel diverticulum. Detection of selected unusual bleeding sites in the small intestine may require enteroclysis, a barium study of the small intestine that involves perfusing barium, water, and methylcellulose through a tube fluoroscopically advanced to the ligament of Treitz to create a double-contrast image. If enteroscopy, colonoscopy, and barium radiography do not identify the source in such a case but iron supplementation compensates for the blood loss, no further intervention is required.

Principles of Management

Resuscitation
Resuscitation in acute lower GI bleeding follows protocols similar to those for upper GI hemorrhage, with prompt correction of volume deficits and stabilization of hemodynamic variables (Fig. 4-2). Because extremely brisk upper GI hemorrhage also may present with red rectal bleeding, a nasogastric tube may need to be placed and upper endoscopy performed in any patient with a potential upper GI source. Laboratory studies provide the same information as with upper GI sources, although azotemia resulting from intralumenal blood degradation usually does not occur. Urgent therapeutic measures are needed when more than three units of packed erythrocytes are transfused.

Medications
Certain lower GI sources are amenable to specific medication therapy. Hemorrhoids, anal fissures, and solitary rectal ulcers benefit from bulk-forming agents, sitz baths, and avoidance of straining. Steroid-containing ointments and suppositories are often used, but their efficacy is questioned. Estrogen-progesterone

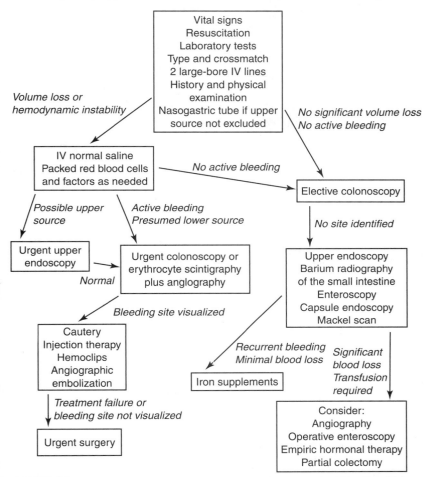

FIGURE 4-2. Workup of a patient with acute lower gastrointestinal bleeding (IV, intravenous).

combinations reduce bleeding in some patients with angiodysplasia. Inflammatory bowel disease usually responds to specific antiinflammatory drug therapy. Intrarectal formalin may reduce bleeding secondary to radiation proctitis. Similar responses to hyperbaric oxygen have been anecdotally noted.

Therapeutic Endoscopy

Colonoscopic bipolar cautery, monopolar cautery, heater probe application, argon plasma coagulation, and Nd:YAG laser have all been used successfully to treat angiodysplasia and the vascular changes that occur with chronic radiation proctocolitis. Colonoscopy also may be used to ablate or resect bleeding polyps or to reduce hemorrhage associated with colonic malignancy. Sigmoidoscopy can treat bleeding internal hemorrhoids with banding or thermal techniques.

Therapeutic Angiography

When colonoscopy fails or cannot be performed, angiography may offer important therapeutic capability. Selective arterial embolization with polyvinyl alcohol particles or microcoils is replacing intra-arterial vasopressin to control lower GI bleeding. Angiographic embolization in the colon is considered a last resort because of a 13% to 18% risk of bowel infarction.

Surgery

For certain diagnoses (e.g., Meckel diverticulum or some malignancies), surgery is the appropriate primary therapy after stabilizing a patient. Emergency surgery carries high morbidity and mortality that increase as the clinical condition deteriorates. For cases of recurrent significant bleeding without a defined source of hemorrhage, right hemicolectomy or subtotal colectomy may be indicated in some patients with good overall prognoses.

Complications

As with upper GI sources, massive lower GI bleeding can have profound sequelae. Chronic or recurrent lower GI bleeding is associated with significant morbidity and subjects the patient to the risks of frequent transfusions. It can also use significant health care resources. Persistent bleeding usually results from small intestinal sources that remain relatively inaccessible to endoscopic therapy despite advances in diagnostic capability.

CHAPTER 5

Approach to the Patient with Occult Gastrointestinal Hemorrhage

DIFFERENTIAL DIAGNOSIS

Occult gastrointestinal (GI) hemorrhage is bleeding that is not apparent on visual stool inspection. Its prevalence is as high as 1 in 20 adults. Up to 150 mL of blood may be lost in the proximal gut without reliably producing melena. Most occult GI bleeding is chronic and, if significant, can produce marked iron deficiency anemia. An extensive list of disorders, including inflammatory disorders, infectious causes, vascular diseases, neoplasms, and other conditions, may produce occult bleeding with or without iron deficiency anemia (Table 5-1).

| **TABLE 5-1** |
| Causes of Occult Gastrointestinal Blood Loss |

Tumors and Neoplasms
   Primary adenocarcinoma
   Metastases
   Large polyps
   Lymphoma
   Leiomyoma
   Leiomyosarcoma
   Lipoma

Infectious Causes
   Hookworm
   Strongyloidiasis
   Ascariasis
   Tuberculous enterocolitis
   Amebiasis

Miscellaneous Causes
   Medications (NSAIDs)
   Long-distance running
   Gastrostomy tubes and other appliances

Vascular Causes
   Angiodysplasia and vascular ectasia
   Portal hypertensive gastropathy
   Hemangiomas
   Blue rubber bleb nevus syndrome
   Gastric antral vascular ectasia

Inflammatory Disorders
   Acid peptic disease
   Hiatal hernia (Cameron erosions)
   Inflammatory bowel disease
   Celiac sprue
   Whipple disease
   Eosinophilic gastroenteritis
   Meckel diverticulum
   Solitary rectal ulcer
   Cecal ulcer

Inflammatory Causes

Acid peptic diseases, including erosions or ulcers of the esophagus, stomach, and duodenum, are the most common causes of occult GI bleeding and are associated with iron deficiency in 30% to 70% of cases. Longitudinal erosions within the large hiatal hernia sac, known as Cameron erosions, may cause up to 10% of the cases of iron deficiency anemia. Other inflammatory causes of occult bleeding include inflammatory bowel disease, celiac sprue, Meckel diverticulum, eosinophilic gastroenteritis, radiation enteritis, colorectal ulcers, and Whipple disease.

Infectious Causes

In the United States, infectious causes of occult GI bleeding are uncommon, but organisms such as hookworms, *Mycobacterium tuberculosis*, amebas, and *Ascaris* species cause chronic blood loss in several hundred million people worldwide.

Vascular Causes

Vascular malformations cause up to 6% of all cases of iron deficiency anemia. Some of these are acquired lesions, such as sporadic telangiectasia, postradiation telangiectasia, scleroderma, and gastric antral vascular ectasia (GAVE, also known as watermelon stomach, a vascular ectasia that appears as jagged stripes and is due to longitudinal vessels on the tops of antral rugae). Alternatively, inherited conditions of vascular ectasia (e.g., hereditary hemorrhagic telangiectasia [Osler-Weber-Rendu disease], Turner syndrome, and Klippel-Trénaunay syndrome) can bleed in occult fashion. In patients with portal hypertension, portal hypertensive gastropathy commonly causes occult blood loss and iron deficiency.

Tumors and Neoplasms

GI tumors are the second most prevalent cause of occult bleeding in the United States after acid peptic disease. Colorectal carcinoma and adenomatous polyps are the most common neoplasms, followed by gastric, esophageal, and ampullary malignancies. Other tumors, such as lymphomas, metastases, leiomyomas and leiomyosarcomas, and juvenile polyps, also produce occult blood loss.

Other Causes of Occult Gastrointestinal Bleeding

Medications are important causes of occult bleeding. Ulcerations and erosions of the stomach, small intestine, and colon can result from NSAIDs. Other drugs that cause occult bleeding include potassium preparations, certain antibiotics, and antimetabolites. Anticoagulants (e.g., warfarin) cause an increased incidence of occult bleeding, although anticoagulants more commonly increase the rate of blood loss from preexisting lesions. Esophageal webs, as in the Plummer-Vinson or Paterson-Kelly syndrome, are associated with iron deficiency. Iron deficiency anemia also develops in long-distance runners, possibly secondary to mechanical jarring or to subclinical mesenteric ischemia. Non-GI causes such as hemoptysis, oral bleeding, epistaxis, and factitious blood ingestion can mimic occult GI blood loss.

WORKUP

History

Patients with chronic occult blood loss most often are asymptomatic or report fatigue secondary to anemia. Palpitations, postural lightheadedness, and exertional dyspnea suggest more significant anemia. Some patients exhibit pica, or compulsive ingestion of ice or soil, with iron deficiency. Dyspepsia, abdominal pain, heartburn, or regurgitation suggests possible peptic causes, whereas weight loss and anorexia raise concern for malignancy. Recurrent episodes of occult blood loss in elderly patients without other symptoms are consistent with angiodysplasia or other vascular ectasias.

Physical Examination

Profound iron deficiency may present with pallor, tachycardia, postural or supine hypotension, and a hyperdynamic heart caused by high cardiac output. Other rare findings include papilledema, hearing loss, cranial nerve palsies, retinal hemorrhages, as well as koilonychia (brittle, furrowed, and spooned nails), glossitis, and cheilosis. Lymphadenopathy, masses, hepatosplenomegaly, or jaundice suggest possible malignancy, whereas epigastric tenderness is found with peptic disease. Splenomegaly, jaundice, or spider angiomata raise the possibility of blood loss secondary to portal hypertensive gastropathy. Numerous cutaneous telangiectasias are suggestive of possible hereditary hemorrhagic telangiectasia.

Additional Testing
Fecal Blood Testing

Guaiac preparations, such as Hemoccult cards, are the most widely used fecal blood tests because of their simplicity and portability. The leuco dye guaiac is a colorless compound that turns blue on exposure to blood. However, peroxidase-containing foods such as radishes, turnips, cantaloupe, bean sprouts, cauliflower, broccoli, and grapes also cause the color change, as can medications (sucralfate, cimetidine), halogens, and toilet bowl sanitizers. Iron, however, causes a green, not blue, color change. Conversely, ascorbic acid, antacids, heat, and acid pH inhibit guaiac reactivity and obscure the diagnosis of fecal blood loss. In general, fecal blood loss must exceed 10 mL/d (normal <2 mL/d) for Hemoccult cards to produce positive findings 50% of the time. Guaiac testing should be performed on a diet low in red meats and devoid of NSAIDs to prevent false-positive results. Wetting the card before addition of the peroxide catalyst may increase the sensitivity of Hemoccult testing but raises false-positive rates to levels considered unacceptable by some.

Other available fecal blood tests have not achieved widespread use. Immuno-chemical tests are very sensitive to fresh blood. However, these techniques are less useful for upper GI sources because gut metabolism of globin compromises its immunologic detection. Fluorometric assays of heme and heme-derived porphyrin, such as HemoQuant, are sensitive to both upper and lower GI bleeding sources, but the requirement to send stool samples to reference laboratories is a disincentive for test performance for most clinicians. Fecal recovery of intravenously injected ^{51}Cr-labeled erythrocytes is the standard for quantifying enteric blood loss, but it is impractical in most clinical settings.

Tests for Iron Deficiency

Hypochromic, microcytic anemia, determined by visual or automated peripheral smear analysis, provides evidence of occult GI bleeding, although it may not develop until significant blood loss has occurred. Anisocytosis, or variability of cell size reflected by the red cell distribution width, also often increases with iron deficiency. In addition to these measured variables of complete blood count analysis, values of serum iron and transferrin may be obtained. With iron deficiency, the iron level is low with a compensatory increase in transferrin concentration, resulting in a reduced percentage of transferrin saturation. Low values for serum iron and transferrin saturation also may be seen in anemia of chronic disease. Serum ferritin levels correlate better with tissue iron stores and may decrease before anemia develops, although inflammatory conditions can falsely elevate ferritin levels because this marker is an acute phase reactant. In questionable cases, determination of bone marrow iron stores remains the gold standard for diagnosing iron deficiency anemia.

Endoscopy and Radiography

For the patient with asymptomatic guaiac-positive stools with no anemia and normal ferritin, colonoscopy is the appropriate diagnostic procedure because most studies show little risk of upper GI malignancies in this setting. In large, population-based screening studies, 2% to 10% of patients with guaiac-positive stools have colorectal cancer, although a much higher percentage have nonmalignant polyps. Sigmoidoscopy plus barium enema radiography is inferior to colonoscopy because it has significantly lower sensitivity in detecting colonic neoplasia.

With iron deficiency anemia and occult GI bleeding, the approach shown in Figure 5-1 is recommended. With this protocol, a GI lesion will be found in 66% to 97% of men and postmenopausal women. An initial colonoscopy is performed. If no lesion is detected, upper endoscopy is performed immediately. In cases of unexplained iron deficiency anemia but no positive fecal blood testing, small intestinal biopsies may be performed to exclude celiac disease. If both endoscopic investigations fail to reveal a bleeding source, barium radiography of the small intestine is performed. In patients with specific GI symptoms, the sequence of diagnostic testing should be directed to the anatomic site from which symptoms appear to arise. If no lesion is found using this protocol, further evaluation is indicated only if oral iron fails to correct the patient's anemia. Enteroclysis, a double-contrast radiography technique for the small intestine involving fluoroscopic infusion of barium, methylcellulose, and water, provides greater mucosal detail than standard single-contrast procedures, but it is technically demanding. Push enteroscopy can visualize the proximal small intestine usually to the level of the midjejunum and offers steerability and a central channel for therapeutic options. Capsule endoscopy is a new technique that affords the ability to visualize the entire length of the small intestine, although no therapy is possible with this test. In rare instances, angiography may demonstrate mucosal blush patterns in patients with occult angiodysplasia. Abdominal computed tomographic scanning may define intra-abdominal disease undetected by lumenal investigations. Advances in helical computed tomography have enhanced the capability of this imaging technique to detect small intestinal angiodysplasia.

PRINCIPLES OF MANAGEMENT

Treatment of occult GI bleeding is dictated by the diagnostic evaluation. Peptic disease is managed according to its cause and usually involves short-term or long-term courses of acid-suppressive medications with possible addition of therapies to eradicate *Helicobacter pylori* infection, if present. Many premalignant colon polyps and some pedunculated malignant polyps can be removed colonoscopically. Angiodysplasia may be cauterized endoscopically or treated medically with estrogen-progesterone preparations if the lesions are the source of significant anemia. Portal hypertensive gastropathy may respond to measures designed to reduce portal

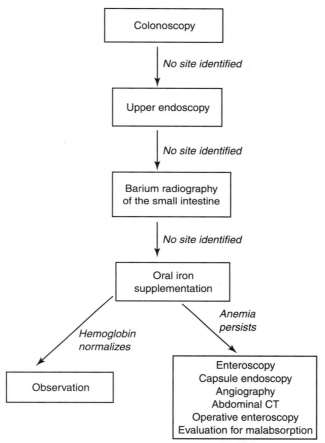

FIGURE 5-1. Workup of a patient with occult gastrointestinal bleeding (CT, computed tomography).

hypertension. If medications are the cause of occult blood loss, withdrawing them may correct the problem.

Some conditions of chronic blood loss require long-term iron supplementation. Oral ferrous sulfate at a dose of 325 mg three times daily is preferred in most patients because it is inexpensive, effective, and well tolerated. Other oral preparations include ferrous fumarate, ferrous gluconate, and preparations with added ascorbic acid to enhance absorption. Repletion of iron stores may take 3 to 6 months, although reticulocytosis peaks within 10 days and the hemoglobin level normalizes within 2 months. Parenteral iron, in complexed form, is indicated for patients who cannot absorb or do not tolerate oral iron. Usually 7 to 10 intramuscular injections of 250 mg elemental iron are required for moderate anemia. In some instances, iron may be administered intravenously. Parenteral preparations may result in rare anaphylaxis, and 10% of patients develop serum sickness–like reactions.

COMPLICATIONS

Chronic occult GI blood loss usually is well tolerated in young individuals; however, older patients or those with underlying cardiorespiratory disease may deteriorate because of the reduced oxygen-carrying capacity of their blood.

CHAPTER 6

Approach to the Patient with Unexplained Weight Loss

DIFFERENTIAL DIAGNOSIS

Unexplained weight loss may result from combinations of biologic and behavioral factors. Hunger is a consequence of physiological processes, whereas appetite is more heavily influenced by environmental and psychological input, including the aroma and appearance of food and a person's mood. Weight loss may result from decreased caloric intake, increased metabolism, or urinary or fecal loss of calories. In general, a person's weight fluctuates by as much as 1.5% per day. A sustained weight loss greater than 5% warrants concern and possible investigation. In addition to anorexia, other symptom complexes contribute to weight loss, including nausea, vomiting, early satiety, postprandial abdominal pain, and altered consciousness. A variety of general medical, gastrointestinal (GI), and behavioral illnesses produce unexplained weight loss (Table 6-1). About half of all cases of unexplained weight loss are attributable to organic disease, whereas psychiatric conditions, especially in the elderly, comprise the majority of the remaining cases. Parkinson disease and Alzheimer disease are common neurological etiologies of weight loss.

General Medical Disorders

Because of its gravity, malignancy should be considered early in evaluating weight loss, although neoplasm is not prevalent in patients without specific signs or symptoms. Endocrinopathies such as thyrotoxicosis, diabetes, and Addison disease produce weight loss by varying mechanisms. Chronic infections (e.g., tuberculosis, fungal diseases, subacute bacterial endocarditis, and AIDS) can cause weight loss. In elderly patients, weight loss results from physiological changes, reduced taste or smell, neuropsychiatric syndromes, effects of medication, poor dentition, and lack of available food. Chronic obstructive lung disease and congestive heart failure produce weight loss by increasing caloric demands, by causing anorexia, or by increasing the work of eating.

TABLE 6-1
Causes of Weight Loss

General Medical Disorders
Endocrinopathies (thyrotoxicosis, diabetes mellitus, Addison disease)
Chronic infections (tuberculosis, fungal infections, endocarditis, AIDS)
Malignancy (carcinoma, lymphoma, leukemia)
Medications
Inadequate intake (immobility, impaired consciousness, dementia)

Behavioral Disorders
Depression
Schizophrenia
Anorexia nervosa
Bulimia nervosa
Adult rumination syndrome

Gastrointestinal Disease
Gastrointestinal obstruction (stricture, adhesions, neoplasm)
Motility disorders (achalasia, gastroparesis, intestinal pseudoobstruction)
Pancreaticobiliary disease (biliary colic, chronic pancreatitis, pancreatic carcinoma)
Chronic hepatitis
Malabsorption in the small intestine
Bacterial overgrowth
Chronic mesenteric ischemia

Gastrointestinal Disorders

Abdominal diseases cause weight loss in several ways. Lumenal obstruction usually is associated with exacerbation of symptoms on meal ingestion, either immediately (esophageal stricture or cancer, achalasia), 1 to 3 hours postprandially (gastric or proximal intestinal blockage), or several hours later (distal ileitis, colon cancer). Motor disorders such as gastroparesis have similar effects. Likewise, pain from pancreaticobiliary sources may worsen after food ingestion, thus reducing intake. Malabsorption may result from disease of the small intestine or pancreas. Weight loss occurs in ulcer disease because of meal-evoked pain. Constipation may cause anorexia.

Behavioral Disorders

looseness-1Depression is the most common behavioral disorder that decreases food intake and also is characterized by mood changes, sleep disruption, anhedonia, and low self-esteem. Alcoholism produces weight loss by mechanisms independent of its common association with depression. Weight loss may also occur with thought disorders (e.g., schizophrenia) as a consequence of distorted perception about food or eating.

Eating Disorders

Eating disorders such as anorexia nervosa and bulimia nervosa, both of which may affect up to 5% to 10% of young women, are distinguished by the patient's desire to maintain thinness and an altered body image. Adult rumination syndrome also produces weight loss and is often unrecognized.

Anorexia Nervosa

Anorexia nervosa is characterized by distortion of body image, inability to interpret hunger and satiety with a preoccupation with eating, and a sense of ineffectiveness. Patients are not truly anorectic but struggle against hunger to achieve an unrealistic degree of weight loss through dietary restriction and exercise, as well as self-induced vomiting or laxative abuse. The condition affects predominantly young women of all ethnic groups and socioeconomic levels. There is significant concordance of anorexia nervosa in identical twins and a 6% prevalence in siblings of affected patients, suggesting genetic components as well. Other psychosocial factors, including low self-esteem, obsessive-compulsive and avoidant personality traits, and perfectionistic tendencies, participate in disease pathogenesis.

Bulimia Nervosa

Bulimia nervosa is characterized by repetitive binges of overeating followed by acts to avert weight gain (e.g., self-induced emesis, laxative or diuretic abuse, excessive exercise) and occurs almost exclusively in women younger than 30 years, with a prevalence of 1% to 10%. Partial syndromes with occasional binge eating then purging behavior may be present in up to 19% of college age women. There is a strong association of bulimia with affective disorders, low self-esteem, and family histories of mood disturbances, alcoholism, and drug addiction. Binge episodes typically last for 1 to 2 hours, during which up to 4,000 calories are ingested.

Adult Rumination Syndrome

Rumination syndrome, or merycism, is an eating disorder in which the patient repetitively regurgitates food from the stomach, rechews it, and then reswallows it. Adult patients generally report weight loss, regurgitation, and vomiting and are concerned about medical rather than psychiatric causes. The episodes are initiated by belching or swallowing and creating a common esophageal and gastric channel by reducing lower esophageal sphincter pressure. Diaphragmatic and rectus abdominis muscle contraction produces regurgitation, expelling gastric contents into the mouth, where they are rechewed and ingested. The differential diagnosis includes esophageal strictures, gastroesophageal reflux disease, GI dysmotility syndromes, and lumenal obstruction. Characteristic manometric patterns may be seen in some patients with rumination syndrome.

WORKUP

History

The first step in evaluation is documenting weight loss because this symptom is not corroborated by objective records in 50% of patients who report weight loss. Once documented, the history can provide important clues to the etiology of weight loss. Medications (e.g., procainamide, theophylline, thyroxin, and nitrofurantoin) may be factors in older patients. Fever or chills may suggest infectious causes, whereas selected risk factors raise the possibility of AIDS. Nausea or pain is reported with GI obstruction, whereas masses or jaundice suggests underlying malignancy. Bulky, foul-smelling, greasy stools indicate probable malabsorption. Other systemic diseases are suggested by specific symptom profiles.

The history should also include a search for psychiatric causes, including alcoholism and depression. Psychomotor retardation or lack of interest in daily activities is characteristic of depression. A denial of significant weight loss is common in anorexia nervosa, whereas secretive purging is classic in bulimia. Anorexia nervosa may also be associated with symptoms of altered gut function (e.g., early satiety, bloating, vomiting, constipation) and endocrine activity (e.g., amenorrhea, loss of libido, symptoms of hypothyroidism).

Physical Examination

Physical findings of weight loss relate to its cause and the degree of malnutrition. Attention should be given to overall appearance as well as mood and affect. Cutaneous examination may suggest endocrine disease or AIDS (Kaposi sarcoma). Jaundice reflects hepatic disease. Malignancy is suggested by lymphadenopathy, occult fecal blood, or masses, whereas obstruction produces abdominal distention and high-pitched bowel sounds. Demonstrably impaired mental function may be an underlying factor in older patients. Gross GI bleeding may be seen as a result of emesis-induced esophageal damage.

Manifestations of severe malnutrition include hypothermia, bradycardia, arrhythmias, hypotension, hypothermia, and dehydration, especially in patients with anorexia nervosa. Brittle hair or nails, decreased fat stores, acrocyanosis, downy hair, yellow cutaneous discoloration (from hypercarotenemia), and loss of secondary sexual characteristics may be seen, especially in young patients with anorexia nervosa. Self-induced vomiting or regurgitation produces halitosis, pharyngitis, gingival or dental erosions from reflux of gastric acid, and also may lead to parotid swelling and abrasion or scarring of the knuckles from inserting the fingers into the mouth.

Additional Testing

Laboratory, radiologic, and endoscopic evaluations are guided by the history and physical examination, including associated symptoms, patient age, symptom duration, prior medical conditions, degree of malnutrition, and emotional factors (Fig. 6-1). Laboratory studies should include a complete blood count; sedimentation rate, electrolytes, blood urea nitrogen, creatinine, total protein, and albumin; urinalysis; and liver chemistries. Radiography of the chest and abdomen can detect malignancy or obstruction. Specific blood testing can screen for thyroid disease, and human immunodeficiency virus assays or placement of a purified protein derivative can test for infectious causes (e.g., AIDS and tuberculosis). In the absence of specific findings, routine screening for malignancy is indicated, including Papanicolaou smear in women, colonoscopy in persons older than 50 years, mammography in women older than 40 years, and prostate specific antigen in men older than 50 years.

Other tests for organic disease may be indicated in some patients. If malabsorption is suspected, screening tests such as qualitative fecal fat, serum carotene, and prothrombin time are obtained. Specific tests for small intestinal or pancreatic causes of malabsorption are ordered if results of screening tests are positive or if suspicion of malabsorption is high. If structural disease is suspected, abdominal computed tomography or ultrasonography may detect underlying malignancies, whereas barium radiography and endoscopy may define sites of obstruction. In patients with suspected anorexia nervosa, structural evaluation of the GI tract is considered because Crohn's disease is in the differential diagnosis. Upper endoscopy or barium radiography should be performed with suspected rumination because esophageal disease can mimic this disorder.

When biologic disease has been excluded, referral to a mental health specialist should be contemplated to exclude psychiatric causes of weight loss. Establishing a specific diagnosis using strict criteria (e.g., *Diagnostic and Statistical Manual [of Mental Disorders]-IV*) benefits the patient by directing psychosocial treatment of the underlying condition.

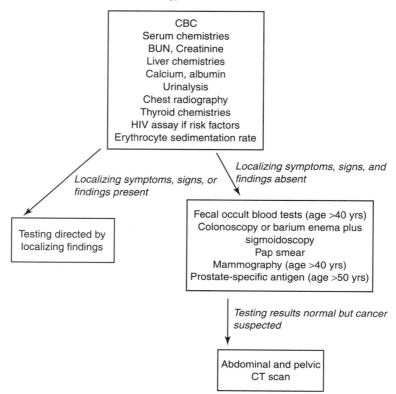

FIGURE 6-1. Workup of a patient with unexplained weight loss (CBC, complete blood count; BUN, blood urea nitrogen; HIV, human immunodeficiency virus; CT, computed tomography).

PRINCIPLES OF MANAGEMENT

Specific therapies are available for many organic diseases that cause weight loss. If test results are negative, a period of observation is indicated because more than 65% of these individuals do well on follow-up. For individuals with minor degrees of weight loss, offering favorite foods or snacks may be adequate. With severe malnutrition (<70%–75% of ideal body weight), hospitalization is necessary. Enteral refeeding may be attempted. If enteral feedings are poorly tolerated or refused, central or peripheral parenteral nutrition may be required. In severe malnutrition, rapid refeeding should be avoided because of potential gastroduodenal dilation and refeeding pancreatitis or diarrhea. For anorexia nervosa, feedings are reestablished at 200 to 250 calories above the intake at time of presentation and are increased by 250 to 300 calories every 5 days to ensure a weekly weight gain of 1.5 kg as an inpatient and 0.75 to 1.0 kg as an outpatient. The goal for refeeding is to achieve 90% to 100% of ideal body weight.

Medical and psychological management of behavioral disease should be initiated immediately along with any refeeding program. Potassium supplements may be needed for patients with anorexia or bulimia nervosa. Antidepressant medications may produce striking weight gain in depressed patients. Prokinetic medications and laxatives may reduce GI symptoms in anorexia nervosa, thus aiding the overall treatment plan. Antidepressants may reduce binge episodes and impulsive behavior in some patients with bulimia but play little role in anorexia nervosa. Psychological therapy for eating disorders addresses distorted beliefs about weight and eating, body image, fear of weight gain, self-criticism, and poor self-regulation. Therapies that have been efficacious for carefully selected patients with eating disorders include individual psychotherapy, interpersonal therapy, family therapy, and cognitive-behavioral therapy. For patients with adult rumination syndrome, behavior modification and biofeedback appear to be the most effective approaches.

COMPLICATIONS

Profound weight loss has significant complications regardless of its cause. Cardiac complications include arrhythmias and sudden death, caused by either the primary disorder or by metabolic consequences secondary to purging. Electrocardiographic changes include bradycardia, decreased QRS amplitude, QT prolongation, ST segment changes, and U waves secondary to hypokalemia. Liver chemistry abnormalities result from hepatic steatosis. Fecal impaction can result from many of the causes of weight loss as well as from decreased oral intake and dehydration. Clinical features of hypothyroidism may develop, although free thyroxin levels usually are normal. Bulimia patients may develop pseudo-Bartter syndrome with fluid retention and peripheral edema after abruptly discontinuing diet pills and laxatives.

The prognosis of a patient with unexplained weight loss depends on the cause. Many organic conditions, especially malignancies, are fatal. For patients with anorexia nervosa, the recovery rate ranges from 32% to 71% at 20 years although up to 5% die from complications of malnutrition. Nearly 75% of adolescents with anorexia nervosa continue to suffer from psychiatric diseases. Recovery rates for bulimia are 50% to 60%, although the condition is fatal in 1% to 5%.

CHAPTER 7

Approach to the Patient with Nausea and Vomiting

DIFFERENTIAL DIAGNOSIS

Nausea is the subjective sensation of an impending urge to vomit, and vomiting (emesis) is the forceful ejection of gastric contents from the mouth. Before vomiting occurs, there is a characteristic preejection phase that lasts minutes to hours and consists of licking and salivation associated with tachycardia and tachypnea. Retching may precede vomiting but involves no discharge of upper gut contents. Other symptoms may be misinterpreted by the patient as nausea or vomiting. Regurgitation is the effortless return of gastric or esophageal contents in the absence of nausea or involuntary spasmodic muscular contractions. Rumination is characterized by regurgitation of food into the mouth, where it is rechewed and reswallowed. Anorexia refers to loss of appetite. Early satiety is the sensation of gastric fullness before a meal is completed. Nausea may be part of a general complaint of indigestion that includes abdominal discomfort, heartburn, anorexia, and bloating. The differential diagnosis of nausea and vomiting includes medications, gastrointestinal and intraperitoneal disease, neurological disorders, metabolic conditions, and infections (Table 7-1).

Medications

Drug reactions are among the most common causes of nausea and vomiting, especially within days after initiating therapy. Chemotherapeutic agents such as cisplatin and cyclophosphamide are potent emetic stimuli that act on central and peripheral neural pathways. Emesis from chemotherapy may be acute, delayed, or anticipatory. Analgesics such as aspirin or NSAIDs induce nausea by direct gastrointestinal mucosal irritation. Other classes of medications that produce nausea include cardiovascular drugs (e.g., digoxin, antiarrhythmics, antihypertensives), diuretics, hormonal agents (e.g., oral antidiabetics, contraceptives), antibiotics (e.g., erythromycin), and gastrointestinal medications (e.g., sulfasalazine).

Disorders of the Gastrointestinal Tract and Peritoneum

Gut and peritoneal disorders represent prevalent causes of nausea and vomiting. Gastric outlet obstruction often produces intermittent symptoms, whereas small intestinal obstruction is usually acute and associated with abdominal pain. Disorders of gut motor activity (e.g., gastroparesis and chronic intestinal pseudoobstruction) evoke nausea because of an inability to clear retained food and secretions. Gastroparesis occurs with systemic diseases (e.g., diabetes, scleroderma, lupus, amyloidosis, pancreatic adenocarcinoma, ischemia) or it may be idiopathic, occurring after a viral prodrome in some cases. Nausea is reported by half of patients with functional dyspepsia as well as some patients with gastroesophageal reflux, in individuals with both normal and delayed gastric emptying. Chronic intestinal pseudoobstruction may be hereditary, result from systemic disease, or occur as a paraneoplastic response to malignancy (most commonly, small cell lung carcinoma). Superior mesenteric artery syndrome, developing after severe weight loss, recent surgery, or prolonged bed rest, occurs when the duodenum is compressed and obstructed by the superior mesenteric artery as it originates from the aorta. Other rare mechanical causes of nausea and vomiting include gastric volvulus and antral webs. Inflammatory conditions (e.g., pancreatitis, appendicitis, and cholecystitis) irritate the peritoneal surface, whereas biliary colic produces nausea by activating the afferent neural pathways. Fulminant hepatitis causes nausea, presumably because of accumulation of emetic toxins and increases in intracranial pressure.

Central Nervous System Causes

Conditions with increased intracranial pressure, such as tumors, infarction, hemorrhage, infections, or congenital abnormalities, produce emesis with and without

---

TABLE 7-1
Causes of Nausea and Vomiting

Medications
  NSAIDs
  Cardiovascular drugs (e.g., digoxin, antiarrhythmics, antihypertensives)
  Diuretics
  Hormonal agents (e.g., oral antidiabetics, contraceptives)
  Antibiotics (e.g., erythromycin)
  Gastrointestinal drugs (e.g., sulfasalazine)

Central Nervous System Disorders
  Tumors
  Cerebrovascular accident
  Intracranial hemorrhage
  Infections
  Congenital abnormalities
  Psychiatric disease (e.g., anxiety, depression, anorexia nervosa, bulimia nervosa, psychogenic vomiting)
  Motion sickness
  Labyrinthine causes (e.g., tumors, labyrinthitis, Ménière disease)

Miscellaneous Causes
  Posterior myocardial infarction
  Congestive heart failure
  Excess ethanol ingestion
  Jamaican vomiting sickness
  Prolonged starvation
  Cyclic vomiting syndrome

Gastrointestinal and Peritoneal Disorders
  Gastric outlet obstruction
  Obstruction of the small intestine
  Superior mesenteric artery syndrome
  Gastroparesis
  Chronic intestinal pseudoobstruction
  Pancreatitis
  Appendicitis
  Cholecystitis
  Acute hepatitis
  Pancreatic carcinoma

Endocrinologic and Metabolic Conditions
  Nausea of pregnancy
  Uremia
  Diabetic ketoacidosis
  Thyroid disease
  Addison disease

Infectious Disease
  Viral gastroenteritis (e.g., Hawaii agent, rotavirus, reovirus, adenovirus, Snow Mountain agent, Norwalk agent)
  Bacterial causes (e.g., *Staphylococcus* spp., *Salmonella* spp., *Bacillus cereus, Clostridium perfringens*)
  Opportunistic infection (e.g., cytomegalovirus, herpes simplex virus)
  Otitis media

---

nausea. Emotional responses to unpleasant smells or tastes induce vomiting, as can anticipation of cancer chemotherapy. Psychiatric causes of nausea include anxiety, depression, anorexia nervosa, and bulimia nervosa. Young women with psychiatric illness or social difficulty may present with psychogenic vomiting. Labyrinthine etiologies of nausea include labyrinthitis, tumors, and Ménière disease. Motion sickness is induced by repetitive movements that result in activating vestibular nuclei.

Endocrinologic and Metabolic Conditions

First-trimester pregnancy is the most common endocrinologic cause of nausea. This condition, occurring in 50% to 70% of pregnancies, usually is transitory and is not associated with poor fetal or maternal outcome. However, 1% to 5% of cases progress to hyperemesis gravidarum, which may produce dangerous fluid losses and electrolyte disturbances. Other endocrinologic and metabolic conditions associated with vomiting include uremia, diabetic ketoacidosis, thyroid and parathyroid disease, and Addison disease.

Infectious Causes

Infectious illness produces nausea and vomiting, usually of acute onset. Viral gastroenteritis may be caused by rotaviruses, and the Hawaii, Snow Mountain, and Norwalk agents. Bacterial infection with *Staphylococcus* or *Salmonella* organisms, *Bacillus cereus*, and *Clostridium perfringens* also produces nausea and vomiting, in many cases via toxins that act on the brainstem. Nausea in immunosuppressed patients may result from gastrointestinal cytomegalovirus or herpes simplex infections. Infections not involving the gastrointestinal tract, such as hepatitis, otitis media, and meningitis, may also elicit nausea.

Miscellaneous Causes of Nausea and Vomiting

Other common causes of symptoms include abdominal radiation therapy and postoperative nausea and vomiting. Nausea may be a manifestation of posterior wall myocardial infarction as well as of congestive heart failure. Acute graft-versus-host disease is the dominant cause of nausea and vomiting in bone marrow transplant recipients. Excess ethanol intake evokes nausea by acting on the central nervous system. Cyclic vomiting syndrome is a condition of unknown etiology characterized by episodes of emesis with intervening asymptomatic periods. Excess vitamin intake and prolonged starvation also cause nausea. Jamaican vomiting sickness results from ingesting unripe ackee fruit.

WORKUP

History

Acute vomiting (for 1 to 2 days) most often results from infection, a medication or toxin, or accumulation of endogenous toxins, as in uremia or diabetic ketoacidosis. Chronic vomiting (longer than 1 week) usually results from a long-standing medical or psychiatric condition. Vomiting soon after eating suggests gastric outlet obstruction or inflammatory conditions (e.g., cholecystitis and pancreatitis), whereas delayed vomiting is characteristic of gastroparesis or more distal obstruction.

Psychogenic vomiting may occur soon after eating, but most patients control their emesis until the gastric contents can be expelled into a toilet or other receptacle. Early morning nausea characterizes endocrine conditions, such as pregnancy. Meals may relieve nausea associated with peptic ulcer or esophagitis.

The character of the vomitus can provide diagnostic clues. Vomiting of undigested food is seen with Zenker diverticulum and achalasia. Partial digestion is observed with gastric obstruction and gastroparesis. Bilious vomiting excludes proximal obstruction, whereas vomiting of blood suggests mucosal damage. Voluminous acidic emesis is observed with gastrinomas, whereas feculent emesis occurs in distal obstructions, bacterial overgrowth, and gastrocolic fistulae.

Associated symptoms should be investigated. Pain is reported with ulcer disease, obstruction, or inflammatory disorders. Diarrhea, fever, or myalgias suggest possible infection. Weight loss occurs in many patients with chronic nausea. However, patients with psychogenic vomiting usually maintain stable weight. Headaches, visual changes, altered mentation, and neck stiffness raise the possibility of central nervous system etiologies, whereas tinnitus or vertigo indicate labyrinthine causes. Light-headedness, palpitations, and dry mucous membranes suggest severe dehydration.

Physical Examination

A physical examination assists in diagnosing and managing nausea and vomiting. Fever suggests inflammation or infection. Tachycardia, orthostatic hypotension, loss of skin turgor, and dry mucous membranes indicate dehydration. Oral examination may reveal loss of dental enamel, a common finding in bulimia. Sclerodactyly and jaundice are characteristic skin findings in scleroderma and hepatobiliary disease, respectively. Adenopathy and masses suggest malignancy; hepatomegaly is also found in malignancy and in benign hepatic disease. An absence of bowel sounds signifies ileus, whereas high-pitched hyperactive bowel sounds with a distended abdomen are consistent with intestinal obstruction. A succussion splash on side-to-side movement is found in gastric obstruction and gastroparesis. Abdominal tenderness is noted with inflammation, infection, and lumenal distention, whereas gross or occult fecal blood prompts evaluation for ulcer, inflammation, or malignancy. On neurological examination, focal signs, papilledema, and impaired mentation suggest central nervous system disease. Asterixis is present in metabolic conditions such as uremia and hepatic failure. Gut motility disorders may be associated with peripheral and autonomic neuropathy.

Additional Testing

A thorough history and physical examination will provide sufficient information to diagnose and treat most patients with nausea and vomiting. If there is a clear temporal association of the onset of vomiting with myalgias, cramps, and diarrhea or with initiation of a new medication, no further workup is needed. However, some patients require blood studies, structural evaluation, or assessment of gut function for appropriate treatment.

Laboratory Studies

Several blood tests assist in evaluating the patient with nausea and vomiting (Fig. 7-1). With long-standing symptoms or dehydration, serum electrolytes may show hypokalemia or an elevated blood urea nitrogen relative to creatinine. Metabolic alkalosis may result from loss of hydrogen ions in the acidic vomitus and contraction of the extracellular space from dehydration. A complete blood

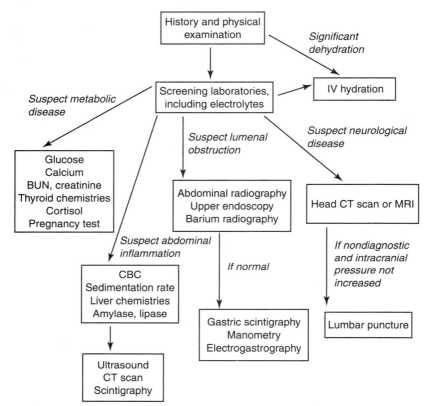

FIGURE 7-1. Workup of a patient with nausea and vomiting (BUN, blood urea nitrogen; CT, computed tomography; MRI, magnetic resonance imaging; CBC, complete blood count).

count rules out anemia from inflammation or blood loss, leukocytosis from inflammation, or leucopenia from viral infection. Blood loss may be further suggested by a low serum iron level and iron saturation of transferrin and by a low ferritin level. Hypoalbuminemia results from chronic disease and gut protein loss. Amylase, lipase, and liver chemistry determinations are obtained for suspected pancreaticobiliary or hepatic disease. Metabolic causes can be assessed through pregnancy and thyroid tests, blood urea nitrogen, creatinine, glucose, calcium, and plasma cortisol. Specific serologic markers can screen for presumed collagen vascular diseases, and antineuronal antibodies are positive with malignancy-associated motility disorders. Meningitis may be confirmed by lumbar puncture.

Structural Studies

Structural investigation may be needed to exclude organic illness as a cause of vomiting. Flat and upright abdominal radiographs are obtained as a screening examination. Small intestinal air-fluid levels with absent colonic air suggest obstruction, whereas diffuse distention is consistent with ileus. Contrast radiography of the small intestine may confirm partial obstruction. If symptoms are intermittent, enteroclysis may provide more detailed assessment of the small bowel. Upper endoscopy can assess possible gastric outlet obstruction and affords the ability to perform biopsy of suspicious lesions. Retained food in the absence of obstruction is seen in gastroparesis. For suspected pancreaticobiliary disease, ultrasound, computed tomography, endoscopic ultrasound, hepatobiliary scintigraphy, or magnetic resonance cholangiopancreatography may be useful. Computed tomographic and magnetic resonance imaging (MRI) of the head may be indicated for suspected central nervous system sources. Angiography or MRI can detect mesenteric ischemia.

Functional Studies

When lumenal obstruction is excluded, gastroparesis and intestinal pseudoobstruction are considered causes of symptoms. Gastroparesis is diagnosed by demonstrating delayed emptying of an ingested meal. Scintigraphic measures of emptying of solid (^{99m}Tc-sulfur colloid in eggs) or liquid (^{111}In-DTPA in water) radionuclides are most commonly used, although office-based breath tests using ^{13}C-labeled foods show promise. When scintigraphy incompletely characterizes the cause of nausea and vomiting, other functional tests may be offered in specialized gastrointestinal physiology laboratories. Manometry of the stomach and duodenum can evaluate motor patterns under fasting and fed conditions. These patterns are reasonably specific for neuropathic and myopathic causes of gastroparesis and pseudoobstruction. Intestinal manometry complements findings from barium radiography of the small intestine, which can reveal slow transit and lumenal dilation in cases of severe dysmotility. Electrogastrography measures electrical pacemaker activity of the stomach through electrodes affixed to the abdomen. Some clinical conditions produce pacemaker rhythms that are too rapid (tachygastria) or slow (bradygastria) that are postulated to underlie development of nausea and vomiting. In rare cases of severe unexplained dysmotility, a surgical full-thickness intestinal biopsy is required to show degeneration of nerve or muscle layers.

PRINCIPLES OF MANAGEMENT

The first decision in treating the patient with vomiting is to determine if intravenous resuscitation is needed. Poor skin turgor or orthostatic pulse or blood pressure changes indicate that more than 10% of body fluids have been lost, mandating intravenous infusion of saline. Potassium supplements may be started for hypokalemia when urine output is adequate. If prospects for oral replenishments are uncertain, hospitalization should be considered. The threshold for hospitalization is lower for diabetic patients, those with concurrent diarrhea or other chronic debilitating disease, and very young or old patients. Nasogastric suction may provide benefit in patients with obstruction or ileus. If the patient can be discharged, a liquid diet low in fat and indigestible residue is recommended because such a diet empties from the stomach more briskly. Medications that inhibit gastric motor function should be discontinued if possible. Diabetics should strive for optimal glycemic control because elevated blood glucose impairs gut motor function.

When feasible, medical treatment for nausea should be directed at the underlying illness. However, many patients benefit from medications that suppress emesis and correct aberrant gastrointestinal function. Antiemetic drugs acting on central nervous system muscarinic cholinergic, histamine, or dopamine receptors reduce symptoms in many cases. Antihistamines (e.g., meclizine, dimenhydrinate) are useful for labyrinthine disorders such as motion sickness or inner ear disease as well as uremic or postoperative vomiting. Sedation and dryness of the mouth may limit their use in some cases. Anticholinergic medications (e.g., scopolamine) also are effective in motion sickness when given orally or transdermally; however, these agents produce numerous side effects, including dry mouth, headache, urinary retention, and constipation. Antidopaminergics (e.g., phenothiazines, butyrophenones) are the most commonly prescribed antiemetics. These drugs act directly on the brainstem regions that mediate emesis in response to a diverse range of peripheral stimuli and are thus useful for many causes of nausea and vomiting including gastroenteritis, toxins, medications, abdominal radiation, and surgery. Antidopaminergics produce many side effects in the central nervous system, including sedation, agitation, mood changes, dystonias, parkinsonian symptoms, irreversible tardive dyskinesia, and hyperprolactinemic symptoms (galactorrhea, sexual dysfunction, amenorrhea). Other drug classes that have been suggested as generalized antiemetics include serotonin ($5\text{-}HT_3$) receptor antagonists (e.g., ondansetron, granisetron) and tricyclic antidepressants (e.g., nortriptyline, amitriptyline).

Gut motility disorders may respond to drugs known as prokinetic agents, which stimulate gastric emptying and intestinal transit. The most widely prescribed prokinetic medication is metoclopramide, which acts via serotonin ($5\text{-}HT_4$) receptor facilitation of gastric cholinergic function as well as by antidopaminergic effects in the stomach and brainstem. This drug enhances gastric emptying and reduces symptoms in gastroparesis but is poorly tolerated by 20% of patients because of significant antidopaminergic side effects, including extrapyramidal reactions, dystonias, and galactorrhea. Domperidone is a peripheral dopamine antagonist with prokinetic properties that does not cross the blood-brain barrier and thus has fewer side effects. This drug is prescribed throughout much of the world but is not approved for prescription in the United States by the Food and Drug Administration. The macrolide antibiotic erythromycin stimulates gastric emptying by action on receptors for the hormone motilin, which is the endogenous mediator of fasting gastrointestinal motility. However, erythromycin often is poorly tolerated because it can exacerbate nausea or induce abdominal pain. The $5\text{-}HT_4$ receptor agonist-tegaserod stimulates gastric emptying in patients with gastroparesis and is under investigation in this condition. Pyloric injection of botulinum toxin reduces pylorospasm and improves symptoms in some patients with gastroparesis. The somatostatin analog octreotide is useful in some cases of intestinal pseudoobstruction as a result of selective effects to stimulate contractile activity of the small intestine.

Extensive investigation has focused on drugs to prevent vomiting after cancer chemotherapy. $5\text{-}HT_3$ antagonists, such as ondansetron and granisetron, provide significant benefit with the most emetogenic treatments. Other drugs useful in this setting include high-dose metoclopramide, corticosteroids, and cannabinoids (e.g., tetrahydrocannabinol, nabilone). Benzodiazepines (e.g., lorazepam) are especially effective for anticipatory nausea and vomiting. Recently introduced neurokinin (NK_1) receptor antagonists (e.g., aprepitant) are useful for both acute as well as delayed emesis caused by chemotherapy.

Nonmedication therapies can be considered for some conditions of chronic nausea and vomiting. Acupuncture and acupressure have been used to treat nausea of pregnancy, motion sickness, and postoperative nausea. Ginger and pyridoxine have been proposed for nausea of pregnancy. Jejunostomy feedings may improve overall health in patients with advanced gastroparesis, whereas intravenous hyperalimentation may be needed for severe forms of intestinal dysmotility. Gastric neurostimulation delivered by an implantable device may reduce nausea and vomiting in patients with gastroparesis who are unresponsive to medications. Surgical resections only rarely benefit patients with nausea and vomiting secondary to dysmotility.

COMPLICATIONS

Chronic nausea and vomiting can produce dehydration, weight loss, and electrolyte abnormalities (e.g., hypokalemia and metabolic alkalosis), which may have significant morbidity in some patients. Increased intrathoracic pressure during vomiting produces purpura on the face and neck, whereas retch-induced Mallory-Weiss tears across the esophagogastric junction may present as upper gastrointestinal hemorrhage. The Boerhaave syndrome is a more severe complication that results when vomiting ruptures the esophagus, leading to mediastinitis or peritonitis. In patients with impaired mentation, emesis may cause pulmonary aspiration, producing chemical pneumonitis.

CHAPTER 8

Approach to the Patient with Abdominal Pain

Abdominal pain is caused by conditions that range from trivial to life-threatening illness. Pain originates from activation of nociceptive nerve fibers with endings in the serosal, muscular, and mucosal layers by mechanical (stretch or spasm) or chemical (inflammation or ischemia) stimuli. Two types of nerve fibers carry pain impulses: rapidly conducting A-delta fibers that yield a well-localized sensation and slowly conducting C fibers that yield a dull, poorly localized pain. Most fibers supplying the abdominal viscera are of the C type, which are few in number; thus, visceral pain is dull, gnawing, or burning and poorly localized. Visceral pain elicited by spasm, distention, ischemia, or necrosis may be accompanied by autonomic disruption, including nausea, diarrhea, pallor, and diaphoresis. The parietal peritoneum has both A-delta and C fibers; thus, pain with parietal peritoneal inflammation is better localized and more distinctly described than visceral pain. Autonomic disturbances with parietal pain are less common. In solid organs such as the liver or kidney, nociceptive nerve endings are restricted to the capsule; thus, pain is elicited only if the capsule is invaded or stretched by a large lesion. Pain fibers from both the visceral organs and peipheral somatic sites terminate in the same regions of the dorsal horn of the spinal cord, explaining the phenomenon of referred pain. Cerebral cortical function is important for modulating pain perception. Patients with impaired mentation may not exhibit typical pain responses. Severe pain may not be perceived on a battlefield, after hypnotism, or after a placebo. Conversely, anxiety may increase the level of discomfort.

DIFFERENTIAL DIAGNOSIS

The differential diagnosis of abdominal pain includes pathological processes within and outside the abdomen (Table 8-1). Generally, pain from diseases of the hollow organs (e.g., gut, urinary tract, pancreaticobiliary tree) results from obstruction, ulceration, inflammation, perforation, or ischemia. Pain from disorders of solid organs (e.g., liver, kidneys, spleen) is caused by distention from infection, obstruction to drainage, or vascular congestion. In women, the adnexa and uterus are potential

TABLE 8-1
Causes of Abdominal Pain

Intra-abdominal
 Parietal inflammation
  Perforated viscus
  Spontaneous bacterial peritonitis
  Appendicitis
  Diverticulitis
  Pancreatitis
  Cholecystitis/cholangitis
  Pelvic inflammatory disease
  Familial Mediterranean fever
 Visceral mucosal disorders
  Peptic ulcer disease
  Inflammatory bowel disease
  Infectious colitis
  Esophagitis
 Visceral obstruction
  Intestinal obstruction (adhesions, hernia, volvulus, intussusception, malignancy)
  Biliary obstruction (stone, tumor, stricture)
  Renal colic (stone, tumor)
 Capsular distention
  Hepatitis
  Budd-Chiari syndrome
  Pyelonephritis
  Tubo-ovarian abscess
  Ovarian cyst
  Endometritis
  Ectopic pregnancy
 Vascular disorders
  Intestinal ischemia
  Abdominal aortic aneurysm
  Splenic infarction
  Tumor necrosis
 Visceral motor and functional disorders
  Irritable bowel syndrome
  Functional dyspepsia
  Esophageal dysmotility
  Viral gastroenteritis
Extra-abdominal
 Neurological
  Radiculopathy
  Varicella-zoster virus reactivation
 Musculoskeletal
  Trauma
  Fibromyalgia

(continued)

| **TABLE 8-1** |
| *(Continued)* |

Cardiothoracic
  Pneumonia
  Myocardial infarction
  Pneumothorax
  Empyema
  Pulmonary infarction
Toxic/metabolic
  Uremia
  Diabetic ketoacidosis
  Porphyria
  Lead poisoning
  Reptile venom, insect bite
  Addison disease

sources of pain. Lung or cardiac abnormalities may secondarily cause referred pain in the upper abdomen. Metabolic conditions (e.g., lead poisoning, diabetic ketoacidosis) cause diffuse or localized abdominal pain. Acute intermittent porphyria, a disorder of heme biosynthesis that results in accumulation of toxic intermediates, causes colicky abdominal pain, ileus, and psychiatric disturbances. Familial Mediterranean fever produces painful inflammation of joints, skin, and serosal surfaces in the abdomen and the chest. Degenerative disk disease, tabes dorsalis, and varicella-zoster virus reactivation elicit superficial abdominal wall pain.

The acuity of the clinical presentation restricts the possible differential diagnoses. With acute abdominal pain, the clinician should quickly establish an accurate diagnosis and implement specific measures to reduce pain and treat the underlying cause if possible. Recurrent pain that lasts hours to days with intervening asymptomatic periods represents a diagnostic challenge in some cases. Many such patients are ultimately diagnosed as having a functional abdominal pain syndrome which is defined as at least 6 months of nearly continuous pain with poor relationship to physiological events such as eating or defecation, some loss of daily function, no evidence of malingering, and insufficient criteria to satisfy other functional or organic diagnoses. Patients with functional abdominal pain syndrome often exhibit evidence of psychosocial dysfunction, including anxiety, depression, somatization, or hypochondriasis. Functional abdominal pain often occurs in individuals with prior childhood abdominal pain or with a history of physical or sexual abuse. Aberrant illness behaviors may be prominent in these patients. Chronic, continuous abdominal pain often has an obvious cause such as disseminated malignancy, chronic pancreatitis, or less serious illnesses with concurrent depression.

WORKUP

History

The location, character, intensity, and timing of pain as well as factors that enhance or minimize the pain are obtained from the history. Symptoms pertinent to past or present illnesses also are evaluated.

Pain Localization

Pain from esophagitis, esophageal dysmotility, or esophageal neoplasm usually is substernal and may radiate to the back, jaw, and left shoulder and arm. The usual pain of peptic ulcer disease is epigastric. Radiation of ulcer pain to the back suggests a posterior penetrating duodenal ulcer. Small intestinal disease most commonly produces periumbilical pain, although ileal lesions may elicit hypogastric symptoms. Colonic pain may be perceived in any region of the abdomen or back. Liver capsular distention produces right upper quadrant pain. Gallbladder and bile duct pain is experienced in the epigastrium and right upper quadrant. Pancreatic pain typically is felt in the epigastrium with radiation to the back. Left upper quadrant pain suggests pancreatic disease but may also result from greater curvature gastric ulcers, splenic lesions, perinephric disease, and colonic splenic flexure lesions. Renal pain from acute pyelonephritis or obstruction of the ureteropelvic junction usually is sensed in the costovertebral angle or flank, although upper abdominal pain is not unusual. Ureteral pain may be referred to the testicle or thigh. Uterine lesions produce midline lower abdominal pain, whereas adnexal pain localizes to the ipsilateral lower quadrant. Pelvic pain may radiate to the back. Migration of pain with disease evolution suggests underlying inflammation. Cholecystitis may begin in the epigastrium and migrate to the right upper quadrant, whereas appendicitis may start in the midline and then move to the McBurney point in the right lower abdomen.

Pain Quality

Esophagitis produces burning or warm pain, whereas peptic ulcer pain is dull or gnawing. Pain from small intestinal obstruction or inflammation is colicky or crampy and may be associated with abdominal distention and audible bowel sounds. Pain from appendicitis may be colicky, but usually is a constant dull ache. Despite use of the terms biliary colic and renal colic, obstruction of these organs more often produces a steady rather than colicky pain. Acute cholecystitis leads to squeezing pain, whereas acute pancreatitis results in penetrating or boring pain. Nephrolithiasis evokes a sharp or cutting pain.

Pain Intensity

Extremely severe abdominal pain is produced by peptic ulcer perforation, acute pancreatitis, or passage of a renal stone, whereas severe acute pain is evoked by small intestinal obstruction, cholecystitis, and appendicitis. Causes of more moderate acute pain include peptic ulcer disease, gastroenteritis, and esophagitis. Intensity of chronic abdominal pain is more difficult to assess because psychological factors can modify pain perception. Then, indirect questions about interference with sleep or daily function may provide useful information about pain severity.

Pain Chronology

Peptic ulcer pain may be intermittent and often occurs in the morning or before meals. Posterior penetration should be considered when peptic ulcer pain becomes constant.

Acute cholecystitis commonly develops during sleep and may be preceded by months of intermittent biliary colic. Nocturnal pain rarely occurs in patients with irritable bowel syndrome or functional abdominal pain. Appendicitis typically presents as progressive pain for 10 to 15 hours without remission. Pain reaching peak intensity within minutes is more characteristic of ulcer perforation, abdominal aortic aneurysm rupture, passage of renal stones, or ruptured ectopic pregnancy. In acute pancreatitis, intestinal obstruction, cholecystitis, or mesenteric arterial occlusion, peak pain intensity is reached in 10 to 60 minutes. A gradual onset of pain for hours is reported in appendicitis, some cases of cholecystitis, diverticulitis, and mesenteric venous occlusion. The pain of irritable bowel syndrome is chronic and may be most intense after meals. In women, pain at monthly intervals suggests endometriosis or ovulation-related symptoms. Pain after starting medication raises the possibility of acute intermittent porphyria (barbiturates) or pancreatitis (steroids, tetracycline, thiazides).

Alleviating and Aggravating Factors

Antacids or acid-suppressing medications may relieve the pain of esophagitis or peptic ulcer disease. Ingesting food can relieve discomfort from a duodenal ulcer but may aggravate pain because of gastric body ulcers. The pain of pancreatic disease almost always is intensified by meal ingestion, as is discomfort from intestinal obstruction or mesenteric ischemia. Duodenal obstruction provokes pain within minutes of eating, whereas ileal lesions cause pain 1 to 2 hours after a meal. Pain from mesenteric ischemia is intensified after meals due to the inability of the impaired blood supply to satisfy the metabolic demands of the gut. Lactase deficiency may produce discomfort that is specific to consumption of dairy products. Heartburn may be aggravated by reclining or straining. Pancreatic pain is worse in the supine position and is relieved by leaning forward. In contrast, back pain in irritable bowel syndrome may be relieved by hyperextension of the spine. Psoas muscle irritation, as with a psoas abscess in Crohn's disease, often causes the patient to lie supine with the right leg flexed at the hip and knee. The pain of nerve root compressions and other musculoskeletal conditions may worsen with some movements. Abdominal pain in irritable bowel syndrome may be ameliorated by massaging the abdominal wall or by passing feces or flatus. Alternatively, irritable bowel pain is aggravated by eating or stress. Passage of diarrheal stools may reduce cramping in colitis.

Associated Symptoms

Abdominal pain usually precedes nausea in conditions that ultimately require surgery, whereas nausea may occur first in disorders not requiring surgery. Diarrhea typically indicates a nonsurgical condition such as gastroenteritis, although appendicitis is an exception to this rule. In elderly patients with acute left-sided pain and bloody stools, ischemic colitis should be considered. Chronic abdominal pain with rectal bleeding suggests colonic neoplasm or inflammatory bowel disease. Abdominal pain with the recent onset of constipation is consistent with colonic obstruction, whereas longstanding constipation is a feature of irritable bowel syndrome. Anorexia and weight loss raise concern for malignancy, whereas high fevers ($>39.5°C$) early in the course of a painful condition suggest cholangitis, urinary tract infection, infectious enteritis, or pneumonia. Late fevers suggest a localized infection such as diverticulitis, appendicitis, or cholecystitis. Jaundice suggests disease of the liver, biliary tree, or pancreas. Many but not all women report abnormal or absent menses with ectopic pregnancy.

Risk Factors

Heavy alcohol intake for prolonged periods can lead to acute pancreatitis, whereas analgesic intake predisposes to ulcer disease. Cocaine abuse may cause mesenteric ischemia. A patient with gallstones may present with distal intestinal obstruction secondary to gallstone ileus. Cardiovascular disease predisposes to mesenteric ischemia, whereas prior abdominal surgery increases the likelihood of intestinal obstruction.

Patients with cirrhosis and ascites develop spontaneous bacterial peritonitis. During pregnancy, abdominal pain results from appendicitis, pyelonephritis, cholelithiasis, pancreatitis, and adnexal disease. The presence of a gravid uterus may modify the symptom presentation or findings of physical examination. Immunocompromised individuals are susceptible to common causes of abdominal pain as well as neutropenic enterocolitis, opportunistic infections such as cytomegalovirus, and graft-versus-host disease in patients who have undergone bone marrow transplantation. The typical signs of peritonitis may be absent in these patients.

Physical Examination

A comprehensive extra-abdominal physical examination is required to provide insight into the cause of abdominal pain. A writhing, diaphoretic, pale patient usually is more ill than one who is resting comfortably, although some individuals with peritonitis may lie motionless to avoid abdominal irritation. Fever or tachycardia may point to an acute infectious or inflammatory process. Hypotension raises concern for an abdominal catastrophe such as a ruptured aneurysm. Scleral icterus or jaundice suggests cholestasis or biliary obstruction. Adenopathy, masses, and hepatomegaly suggest malignancy. A chest examination may reveal pneumonia as the cause of pain, whereas an irregular heart rhythm might suggest new-onset atrial fibrillation as a source of mesenteric arterial embolism. Radiculopathy as a cause of pain is suspected with asymmetric strength or sensation on neurological examination. Peripheral or autonomic neuropathies are found in some patients with gastrointestinal dysmotility. The presence of occult fecal blood on rectal examination raises the possibility of malignancy, ischemia, ulcer disease, and inflammation. Right-sided tenderness on rectal examination may also be found with appendicitis. Perianal fistulae, fissures, and abscesses suggest Crohn's disease. In women, a pelvic examination is used to evaluate possible adnexal or uterine causes of abdominal pain.

Abdominal, rectal, genital, and pelvic examinations are mandatory in a patient with acute abdominal pain. Intestinal obstruction is considered if scars are observed on inspection and if auscultation reveals high-pitched bowel sounds. In contrast, a silent distended abdomen suggests ileus secondary to intra-abdominal inflammation or peritonitis. A right upper quadrant friction rub or bruit suggests a possible hepatic tumor, whereas bruits elsewhere may indicate mesenteric insufficiency. Abdominal palpation should begin in an area distant from the reported site of pain to prevent conscious guarding. Involuntary guarding suggests peritonitis. Rebound tenderness suggests peritoneal inflammation but also may be elicited in noninflammatory conditions such as irritable bowel syndrome and thus has been considered an unreliable sign. It is often useful to shake the patient's bed gently from side to side, which may be a more subtle means of detecting peritonitis. Severe pain with little tenderness or guarding is consistent with intestinal infarction or early acute pancreatitis. The Carnett test can distinguish intra-abdominal discomfort from abdominal wall pain. Increased tenderness upon raising the head and tensing the abdomen suggests a superficial abdominal wall source. Discrepancies between tenderness elicited with pressure from the stethoscope and that from the examining hand suggest possible functional abdominal pain. Fecal occult blood raises concern for malignancy, ischemia, ulcer disease, or inflammatory conditions, whereas perianal fistulas, abscess, or inflammation suggests possible Crohn's disease. Rectal examination also may detect an intra-abdominal inflammatory process such as an appendiceal abscess that is not palpable over the anterior abdominal wall. Inguinal hernias as a cause of intestinal obstruction may be detected on genital examination, whereas pelvic examination of women is essential for diagnosing adnexal masses and pelvic inflammatory disease.

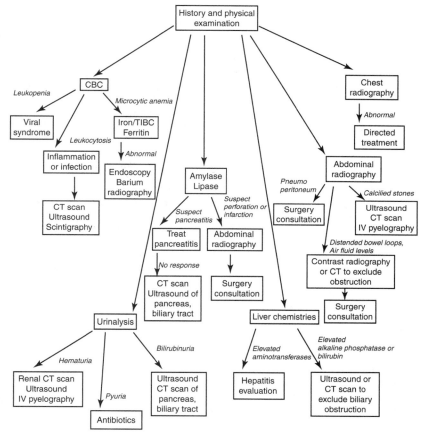

FIGURE 8-1. Workup of a patient with abdominal pain (CBC, complete blood count; TIBC, total iron-binding capacity; CT, computed tomography; IV, intravenous).

Additional Testing

Determining the cause of abdominal pain commonly requires laboratory testing (Fig. 8-1). However, diagnostic testing in the patient with chronic functional pain should be directed by alarm findings on exam and screening blood tests to avoid reinforcing the patient's conviction that there is something organically wrong. A complete blood count may show leukocytosis, indicating an inflammatory condition, or leukopenia, suggesting a viral syndrome. Microcytic anemia raises the possibility of gut blood loss. The sedimentation rate may be elevated in inflammatory conditions. Electrolytes, blood urea nitrogen, and creatinine are measured to assess fluid status and renal function. Elevated serum amylase or lipase or both usually are observed early in acute pancreatitis. Perforated ulcers, diabetic ketoacidosis, or mesenteric infarction also may cause hyperamylasemia. Elevated levels of bilirubin or alkaline phosphatase suggests disease of the pancreas or biliary tract, whereas aminotransferase elevations indicate hepatocellular disease. Serum pregnancy testing is performed in women of reproductive potential who present with unexplained abdominal pain. Specific laboratory tests can assist in diagnosing acute porphyria or heavy metal intoxication. Urinalysis may show erythrocytes or crystals, suggesting calculi; leukocytes or bacteria, suggesting infection; or bilirubin, suggesting pancreaticobiliary disease. Patients with ascites and abdominal pain should undergo paracentesis to exclude spontaneous bacterial peritonitis. Culdocentesis can aid in assessing intra-abdominal hemorrhage.

Supine and upright (or decubitus) abdominal plain radiography is essential in all patients with acute abdominal pain and can detect pneumoperitoneum from lumenal perforation, calcified gallstones or renal stones, air-fluid levels with intestinal obstruction, generalized or localized distention with ileus, pneumobilia with biliary disease, and a ground-glass appearance with ascites. Barium radiographs may complement the findings of plain films when mechanical obstruction is suspected. Chest radiographs can eliminate pulmonary sources of acute abdominal pain.

Other imaging studies complement findings of the examination, laboratory testing, and plain films. Ultrasound is useful for suspected cholelithiasis, biliary dilation, ovarian cysts, abscess formation, and ectopic pregnancy, whereas computed tomography (CT) is more sensitive for pancreatic disease, retroperitoneal collections, intra-abdominal abscess, some vascular processes, trauma-induced hematomas, and changes in the mesentery or intestinal wall resulting from ischemia or inflammation (as with diverticulitis). Scintigraphy with ^{99m}Tc-iminodiacetic acid derivatives detects cystic duct obstruction from cholecystitis. Angiography or mesenteric resonance angiography may be indicated for suspected vascular occlusion. Ultrasound is sensitive for diagnosing the impending rupture of an abdominal aortic aneurysm, but further study with aortography may delay definitive therapy and should be performed in the operating room, if indicated, because of the risk of exsanguination. Upper endoscopy is performed for chronic epigastric pain that suggests uncomplicated peptic ulcer, but is contraindicated with suspected perforation. Sigmoidoscopy or colonoscopy is helpful with lower abdominal pain secondary to suspected ischemia, infection, volvulus, drug-induced colitis, or inflammatory bowel disease. Endoscopic retrograde cholangiopancreatography (ERCP) may be required for suspected cholangitis, whereas ERCP and endoscopic ultrasound (EUS) are sensitive for detecting choledocholithiasis. ERCP, EUS, and magnetic resonance cholangiopancreatography may provide complementary information in diagnosing chronic pancreatitis. Laparoscopy may be performed on an emergency basis in extremely ill patients or electively for chronic abdominal pain where the diagnosis is elusive after extensive diagnostic testing.

PRINCIPLES OF MANAGEMENT

Under ideal conditions, therapy is directed at eliminating the cause of abdominal pain. If this is not possible, efforts are aimed at decreasing pain perception and removing factors that exacerbate pain. Patients with pain from fever, vomiting, orthostatic hypotension, tachycardia, rebound, leukocytosis, new hyperbilirubinemia, or impaired mentation may need hospitalization. The threshold for hospital admission is lowered for the very young or old and for immunocompromised individuals. Specific therapy exists for many conditions such as acid suppressants for gastroesophageal reflux or surgery for appendicitis or cholecystitis, but the diagnosis must be accurate. Some conditions that cause chronic pain may not be curable. NSAIDs are often prescribed for chronic pain. However, because many chronic conditions have little tissue damage or inflammation, it is not surprising that NSAIDs are often ineffective. Opioid agents are useful for managing pain that is secondary to unresectable malignancy, but prescribing them for chronic nonmalignant states is controversial. Regardless of the indication, narcotics are best administered within an integrated treatment program. The use of opioids at regular intervals, rather than on an as-needed basis, is often more effective for treating severe pain. Pain cocktails that incorporate opioids, acetaminophen, and antiemetics allow flexible dosing that prevents mental clouding, respiratory depression, nausea, and constipation. Tricyclic antidepressants have analgesic effects that are independent of their mood-elevating effects. Agents with serotonergic and noradrenergic activity (e.g., amitriptyline, doxepin) exhibit the greatest effects, often at doses lower than required to treat depression. Conversely, although anxiolytics may reduce anxiety, they have little long-term efficacy in managing chronic abdominal pain and may actually worsen symptoms because of depleted brain serotonin levels.

Nonmedical treatments also are useful in treating chronic pain. Patients with pain secondary to unresectable neoplasm may benefit from referral to a mutlidisciplinary pain clinic. Celiac plexus blockade is effective therapy for selected patients with pancreatic adenocarcinoma but is less likely to control pain from chronic pancreatitis. Local neural blockade of trigger points may provide benefit in some cases of abdominal wall pain. Rhizotomy and cordotomy involve severing the neural pathways that sense pain and are indicated only for conditions in which life expectancy does not exceed 6 months because of significant complications, including bowel and bladder dysfunction, dysesthesias, and exacerbation of the pain. Transcutaneous electrical nerve stimulation and dorsal column stimulation reduce pain in some chronic conditions, presumably because pain inhibitory nerve fibers are stimulated and endogenous opioid production is activated. Acupuncture may work by similar mechanisms. Unfortunately, these techniques have not shown significant efficacy in treating chronic pain that is secondary to intra-abdominal causes.

Like most chronic illnesses, irritable bowel syndrome and functional abdominal pain have no cure. Thus, efforts should be directed to enhancing the quality of the patient's life. The physician must establish a good working relationship with the patient and acknowledge the reality of the pain and the suffering that it causes. Scheduling of frequent brief visits and directed appropriate diagnostic evaluation are important. The emphasis then shifts from diagnosis to treatment with a realization by the patient that a cure is not possible and an understanding that a major part of the treatment process will be to minimize the impact of the pain on daily life. Psychological or psychiatric consultation is appropriate when the clinician suspects a concurrent, major affective or personality disorder. Tricyclic agents represent the main form of medication therapy. Meta-analyses of tricyclic agents used to treat functional causes of abdominal pain showed significant therapeutic benefits compared with a placebo. Most other drug classes provide little or no benefit in this condition. Opioid agents should be avoided in these patients because of drug dependency. Relaxation training, biofeedback, and hypnosis have shown benefit in small trials. Behavioral therapy reduces chronic pain behavior by rewarding the patient's expression of well behavior. Cognitive therapies promote healthy behavior by increasing the patient's awareness of situations that increase pain, with the goal of increasing the patient's control over these situations. Subsets of patients may benefit from formal psychotherapy.

COMPLICATIONS

The potential for complications depends on the cause of the pain. Failure to diagnose peritonitis, a ruptured ectopic pregnancy, or an aortic aneurysm can have fatal consequences. Other inflammatory conditions (e.g., pancreatitis, inflammatory bowel disease, or pelvic inflammatory disease) may require prolonged courses of treatment, producing debilitating symptoms and loss of productivity at home and work. Renal stones may lead to infection and renal insufficiency. The prognosis is excellent for many patients with chronic noninflammatory abdominal pain, including those with irritable bowel syndrome, endometriosis, and nerve root compression syndromes.

CHAPTER 9

Approach to the Patient with Acute Abdomen

DIFFERENTIAL DIAGNOSIS

The term *acute abdomen* denotes a disorder of sudden onset with a duration less than 24 hours that is manifested as abdominal pain and associated gastrointestinal symptoms. Surgical management is often but not always needed and must be completed without inordinate delay when indicated. The differential diagnosis of the acute abdomen is nearly as extensive as that for abdominal pain itself and includes intra-abdominal and extra-abdominal disease processes (Table 9-1).

Acute Appendicitis

Acute appendicitis, the most common cause of acute abdomen in the United States, results from obstruction of the appendiceal lumen by a fecalith, calculus, or hyperplastic submucosal lymphatic tissue. The disorder initially presents with periumbilical pain, low-grade fever, and anorexia with or without vomiting. Over several hours, the pain migrates into the right lower quadrant where tenderness classically is elicited at the McBurney point. However, the site of maximal tenderness depends on the location of the appendix. If the appendix is in the pelvis, tenderness is greatest on rectal examination. A retrocecal appendix produces flank tenderness, whereas a medial appendix causes psoas muscle inflammation resulting in pain on hip flexion (psoas sign). Two percent to 3% of patients with appendicitis present with an abdominal mass, signifying phlegmon or abscess development secondary to perforation. This complication is suspected if the pain has lasted longer than 24 hours, the patient's temperature is higher than 38°C, and if the leukocyte count is greater than 15,000 cells per μL.

Perforated Duodenal Ulcer

A patient with a perforated ulcer commonly presents with the sudden onset of severe upper abdominal pain followed by progression to more diffuse pain that is exacerbated by respiration or movement because of peritoneal inflammation. Because gastric secretions are nearly sterile, the risk of peritoneal infection relates

---

TABLE 9-1
Causes of Acute Abdomen That May Require Surgical Intervention

---

Gastrointestinal
Appendicitis
Perforated peptic ulcer
Intestinal obstruction
Intestinal ischemia
Diverticulitis
Inflammatory bowel disease
Meckel diverticulitis

Pancreaticobiliary Tract, Liver, Spleen
Acute pancreatitis
Calculous cholecystitis
Acalculous cholecystitis
Acute cholangitis
Hepatic abscess
Ruptured hepatic tumor
Splenic rupture

Urinary Tract
Renal/ureteral stone

Gynecologic
Ectopic pregnancy
Tubo-ovarian abscess
Ovarian torsion
Uterine rupture
Ruptured ovarian cyst or follicle

Retroperitoneum
Abdominal aortic aneurysm

Supradiaphragmatic
Pneumothorax
Pulmonary embolus
Acute pericarditis
Empyema

---

to the time that elapses before definitive treatment is provided. Less than half of cases exhibit positive peritoneal fluid cultures within 12 hours of perforation. Two-thirds of patients report prior dyspepsia or a history of ulcer disease. Bowel sounds are usually absent, and the liver span may not be detectable by percussion because of air interposed between the liver and the abdominal wall.

Obstruction of the Small Intestine

In the United States, 70% to 80% of the cases of small intestinal obstruction result from postoperative adhesions. Other causes include primary and metastatic carcinoma, external and internal hernias, Crohn's disease, prior radiation therapy, intussusception, endometriosis, volvulus, and congenital abnormalities. The condition presents with periods of crampy midabdominal pain interspersed with nearly asymptomatic intervals, which may progress to unrelenting pain. Vomiting may transiently relieve the pain. Complete obstruction produces constipation or obstipation. In cases of bowel strangulation, signs of peritonitis, an abdominal mass, tachycardia, and fever may be noted. With prolonged obstruction, bacterial overgrowth develops and leads to feculent emesis.

Colonic Diverticulitis

Although colonic diverticula are common, diverticulitis is rare with a lifetime risk of 5%. Acute diverticulitis occurs when the ostia of one or more diverticula, usually in the sigmoid colon, become obstructed with feces and develop local inflammation, which may progress to peritonitis or local pericolic abscess formation. In complicated cases, peridiverticular abscesses can erode into the adjacent bladder to produce recurrent urinary tract infections and pneumaturia. Most cases present with lower abdominal pain, fever, and obstipation with minimal nausea. Distention is variable, and examination may reveal a palpable, tender mass in the lower abdomen. Leukocytosis is so common that the diagnosis should be questioned in its absence.

Acute Cholecystitis

Gallstone impaction in the cystic duct elicits biliary colic, characterized by epigastric or right upper quadrant pain. Continued cystic duct obstruction initiates an inflammatory response in the gallbladder wall, which distinguishes acute cholecystitis from biliary colic. Although 95% of cases of acute cholecystitis relate to gallstones, some individuals with severe systemic disease develop acalculous cholecystitis. Acute cholecystitis commonly presents with right upper quadrant pain 1 to 2 hours after eating and is often accompanied by nausea and vomiting. The pain reaches maximum intensity rapidly and may persist for a prolonged period, often with shoulder radiation. Patients may report a prior history of biliary colic or intolerance to fatty food. Tenderness and guarding in the right upper quadrant are elicited on physical examination, and there may be sufficient inflammation of the parietal peritoneum to produce sudden arrest of inflammation (Murphy sign). Low-grade fever is common and jaundice occurs in 10% of cases.

Acute Pancreatitis

The causes of acute pancreatitis are extensive, although most cases in the United States relate to long-standing alcohol intake or gallstones. The condition presents with epigastric and left upper quadrant pain radiating to the back. In severe cases, hypovolemia, hypotension, or respiratory distress may ensue. Tenderness out of proportion to abdominal wall rigidity may be present on examination. If a peripancreatic phlegmon dissects down either paracolic gutter, the presentation may be confused with that of acute appendicitis or diverticulitis.

Mesenteric Ischemia

The four major ischemic syndromes are mesenteric embolism, acute mesenteric thrombosis, low-flow mesenteric ischemia, and iatrogenic mesenteric ischemia. Each may produce life-threatening disease. Mesenteric embolism, which accounts for 50% of cases of mesenteric ischemia, often derives from cardiac sources such as mural thrombi from recent myocardial infarction or atrial fibrillation. Commonly, the embolus lodges at branch points of the superior mesenteric artery (SMA) distal to its origin. Affected patients present with sudden, severe epigastric and midabdominal pain with forceful vomiting and defecation. Classically, the early examination is unremarkable. Distention, guarding, and an absence of bowel sounds imply intestinal infarction. Laboratory findings may show progressive hemoconcentration, leukocytosis, and acidosis. Mesenteric thrombosis occurs with critical atherosclerotic narrowing of the SMA, usually at its origin from the aorta. Many patients report prior postprandial abdominal pain and weight loss consistent with chronic intestinal angina. Nonocclusive ischemia with intestinal vasoconstriction occurs in low-flow states such as shock, reduced cardiac output, and dehydration and usually responds to measures that restore intravascular volume and hemodynamic stability. Iatrogenic mesenteric ischemia may occur after angiographic dislodgment of an atheroma or induction of vascular dissection.

Abdominal Aortic Aneurysm

Expansion, rupture, dissection, distal embolism, or thrombosis of an abdominal aortic aneurysm may present with the sudden onset of symptoms. Severe pain in the back, flank, or abdomen occurs with aneurysmal expansion or small tears. Aneurysmal rupture may produce sudden exsanguination and rapid hypovolemic shock. The most important physical finding is a palpable, pulsatile abdominal mass.

Ectopic Pregnancy

An intra-abdominal catastrophe occurs when a tubal pregnancy ruptures into the peritoneum. Sudden lower abdominal pain is followed by generalized peritonitis and hypovolemic shock from intra-abdominal hemorrhage. Pelvic examination may reveal a blue-colored cervix or blood at the cervical os. The uterus may be enlarged and a hematoma may be palpated in the cul-de-sac.

Other Causes of Acute Abdomen

Other conditions may elicit an acute abdomen. The Charcot triad of right upper quadrant pain, jaundice, and fever characterizes acute cholangitis secondary to choledocholithiasis or bile duct obstruction, although the triad is present in only 60% of cases. Esophageal rupture from instrumentation or forceful vomiting (Boerhaave syndrome) produces pneumomediastinum or pneumoperitoneum and peritonitis with development of subcutaneous emphysema, pleural effusions, friction rubs, and pneumothorax on examination. Neutropenic colitis presents with diffuse pain, fever, and diarrhea in individuals with very low absolute neutrophil counts secondary to hematologic disease or cancer chemotherapy. On pathological examination, the condition is characterized by mucosal ulceration and invasive infection with enteric organisms.

WORKUP

History

A systematic approach to interviewing the patient with acute abdomen is critical in obtaining an accurate diagnosis. The potential for rapid progression and development of complications places time constraints on diagnosis and treatment. The nature and timing of pain should be characterized. Pain from ulcer perforation or abdominal aortic aneurysm rupture is sudden and incapacitating. In contrast, the pain of appendicitis may increase over several hours. Biliary colic may resolve after a few hours, whereas pancreatitis pain is unrelenting. Ulceration of the duodenum, an embryological foregut structure, is experienced as epigastric discomfort, whereas early appendicitis produces periumbilical pain that corresponds to the embryological midgut origin of the appendix. With progressive inflammation, the adjacent parietal peritoneum becomes irritated and the site of maximal pain may migrate. In appendicitis, the pain shifts from the periumbilical region to the right lower quadrant. Pain referral patterns can suggest specific diagnoses. Gallbladder disease may elicit right shoulder pain, whereas renal colic may radiate to the groin or testicle.

Symptoms other than pain provide useful diagnostic clues. The diagnosis of appendicitis should be questioned in the absence of anorexia. In contrast, anorexia is uncommon in urologic or gynecologic conditions that produce acute abdomen. Whereas vomiting may relieve pain from intestinal obstruction, vomiting provides little benefit in inflammatory conditions such as pancreatitis or cholecystitis. Constipation is produced by obstruction and by inflammatory disorders that produce ileus, although some partial obstructions permit limited passage of intestinal contents. Watery diarrhea suggests gastroenteritis, whereas bloody diarrhea results from infectious colitis, inflammatory bowel disease, and mesenteric ischemia. Jaundice occurs with hepatic and pancreaticobiliary disease or with sepsis. Urinary frequency, dysuria, hematuria, and suprapubic or flank pain suggest urologic disease.

Confounding factors can complicate the diagnosis in selected patient populations. Levels of diagnostic inaccuracy are high in young women. Thus, careful sexual and menstrual histories must be taken, and possible ectopic pregnancy, ovarian cyst, salpingitis, or tubo-ovarian abscess must be considered. In pregnancy, diagnosis of acute abdomen may be difficult because of uterine displacement of intraperitoneal structures. Likewise, the diagnosis of acute abdomen may be challenging in patients at the extremes of age. Because infants lack the ability to communicate and their abdominal walls are poorly developed, peritonitis may go undetected. Elderly patients have reduced febrile and inflammatory responses that can mislead the clinician about the severity of the underlying condition. Immunosuppressed or diabetic patients may report reduced clinical responses to acute intraperitoneal inflammation. Reliable symptoms and signs may not develop in patients with impaired mentation or spinal cord injury. In such individuals, fever, leukocytosis, and hypotension may be the only presenting findings of an acute abdomen. A record of prior surgical procedures is needed to confirm or exclude certain causes. Prior laparotomy increases the risk of obstruction secondary to adhesions. Previous cholecystectomy and appendectomy eliminate the possibilities of cholecystitis and appendicitis, respectively. Abdominal pain in the immediate postoperative period raises concern for ileus, abscess, acalculous cholecystitis, and anastomotic dehiscence. Family histories of sickle cell anemia or familial Mediterranean fever should be elicited. Certain medications can produce acute abdomen; for example, oral contraceptives can lead to hepatic adenoma rupture.

Physical Examination

A patient with acute abdomen appears anxious with a pale, diaphoretic face, dilated pupils, and shallow respirations. Parietal peritoneal inflammation causes the patient to lie quietly. In contrast, the patient with renal colic or mesenteric ischemia may appear restless. Fever, tachypnea, tachycardia, or hypotension may be present. The abdomen is carefully inspected for surgical scars. Distention results from mechanical obstruction, ileus, or ascites. Bluish discoloration of the flanks or the periumbilical region is evidence of retroperitoneal or intra-abdominal hemorrhage. An absence of bowel sounds after 2 minutes of auscultation suggests ileus, whereas a high-pitched, hyperactive bowel raises suspicion of intestinal obstruction. Bruits suggest the possibility of vascular insufficiency. The abdomen is percussed beginning in the quadrant farthest from the site of the pain. Gentle palpation is performed last to assess for mass lesions or fullness in addition to point tenderness, rigidity, and involuntary guarding. Point tenderness, as found in parietal inflammatory processes, is elicited by one-finger palpation. Although often elicited in the patient with acute abdomen, rebound tenderness is a nonspecific finding in inflammatory and functional abdominal disorders. Rectal examination can detect point tenderness as well as assess for occult fecal blood. Pelvic examination in women evaluates for adnexal and uterine enlargement or tenderness that suggests ectopic pregnancy, salpingitis, or tubo-ovarian abscess. Bluish cervical discoloration typifies ectopic pregnancy whereas cervical displacement or discharge is seen with inflammatory conditions.

Additional Testing

Initial Studies

Laboratory testing of the patient with acute abdomen is performed in all cases (Fig. 9-1). A complete blood count detects anemia, leukocytosis, or leukopenia, whereas levels of serum electrolytes, blood urea nitrogen, and creatinine reflect the metabolic consequences of associated vomiting or diarrhea. Urinalysis is useful in diabetic ketoacidosis, urinary infection, or nephrolithiasis. Amylase and lipase are elevated in acute pancreatitis, whereas liver chemistry levels increase with hepatobiliary disease. Pregnancy testing is performed in women of child-bearing potential with acute abdomen. Microscopic examination and culture of cervical discharges can assist in diagnosing gynecologic causes of acute abdomen. Abdominal radiographs are obtained, including supine, upright, and right or left lateral decubitus

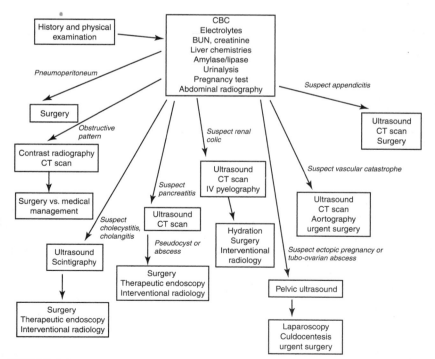

FIGURE 9-1. Workup of a patient with acute abdomen (CBC, complete blood count; BUN, blood urea nitrogen; CT, computed tomography; IV, intravenous).

views. Free subdiaphragmatic air is seen on upright or decubitus views in 75% of patients with ulcer perforation. Pneumoperitoneum may be more pronounced with colonic perforation. Gas in the biliary tree suggests a fistulous tract from the gut or, alternatively, a gas-forming biliary infection. Gas in the intestinal wall or portal vein raises concern for intestinal infarction. Ileus manifests as diffusely dilated loops of the small intestine and colon, whereas obstruction is characterized by proximal distention and air-fluid levels with little or no air distal to the blockage. Abdominal radiography may also demonstrate localized ileus in patients with pancreatitis or abdominal aortic aneurysmal calcification.

Imaging Studies

In some cases, the initial data gleaned from the history, examination, and screening diagnostic tests will provide the information needed to proceed to immediate surgery. In many other instances, sufficient time will be afforded to complete the diagnostic evaluation with selected imaging techniques. Although appendicitis is usually a clinical diagnosis, ultrasound may be useful for atypical presentations, and computed tomographic (CT) scanning can distinguish periappendiceal phlegmon from abscess. Likewise, the diagnosis of acute diverticulitis is primarily clinical, although CT scanning may show colonic thickening, mesenteric edema, abscesses, or phlegmon formation when the diagnosis is uncertain or if complications are suspected. Barium radiography and colonoscopy are generally contraindicated in suspected acute diverticulitis. With incomplete mechanical obstruction, barium radiography, CT scanning, or endoscopy may be indicated to characterize the site and cause of blockage. Ultrasound is the preferred modality for suspected gallstones, gallbladder wall inflammation, biliary dilation, or liver lesions. In some cases of acute cholecystitis, a sonographic Murphy sign is elicited by compression of the right upper quadrant by the ultrasound transducer. Biliary scintigraphy may indicate cystic duct obstruction in acute cholecystitis. Endoscopic retrograde cholangiopancreatography (ERCP), magnetic resonance cholangiopancreatography (MRCP), or percutaneous transhepatic cholangiography may facilitate diagnosis of bile duct obstruction. Endoscopic ultrasound can screen for bile duct stones not detected by other modalities. Mesenteric angiography is diagnostic of mesenteric embolism or thrombosis. When abdominal aortic aneurysm leakage is suspected, ultrasound or aortography may provide diagnostic information. However, these procedures should be performed in the operating room because of the risk of exsanguination. CT scanning excludes abscess, hemorrhage, and pseudocyst in complicated pancreatitis, whereas ERCP can exclude biliary calculi. Renal ultrasound, intravenous pyelography or CT scanning can reveal ureteral stones, whereas pelvic ultrasound provides images of the adnexa in women with suspected tubo-ovarian abscess or ectopic pregnancy. Culdocentesis can aid in assessing intraperitoneal hemorrhage. In some cases, no combination of laboratory or imaging studies can confidently provide a diagnosis for the cause of acute abdomen. In such a setting, the importance of laparoscopy or laparotomy in establishing a diagnosis should not be overlooked.

PRINCIPLES OF MANAGEMENT

To manage a patient with acute abdomen, the nature of the pathological process must be determined. Once a diagnosis is made, it is important to decide if immediate surgery is required. Usually there is sufficient time to obtain laboratory and imaging studies, although a ruptured aortic aneurysm may mandate immediate transfer to the operating room for emergency vascular grafting. Similarly, a young woman with peritonitis, a positive pregnancy test, and hypotension requires immediate laparotomy to control bleeding from a ruptured ectopic pregnancy. Urgent surgery is needed to treat lumenal perforation, appendicitis, and intestinal obstruction, but diagnostic evaluation usually can be completed before operative intervention.

Operative intervention can be deferred in other settings. For cholecystitis or cholangitis, definitive surgery generally is not performed until after stabilization with intravenous antibiotics and fluids. However, some unstable patients may need operations more urgently. Some appendiceal masses or abscesses are initially treated nonsurgically with percutaneous drainage and intravenous antibiotics, and appendectomy is reserved until a later date. Before surgical management of intestinal obstruction, abdominal decompression with nasogastric suction is instituted. In contrast to appendicitis, many cases of mild diverticulitis are managed nonoperatively with intravenous antibiotics, bowel rest, and intravenous fluids. Mesenteric ischemia from embolism and thrombosis may be controlled operatively and with angiographic angioplasty techniques. Nonocclusive mesenteric ischemia commonly resolves with hemodynamic stabilization. Acute pancreatitis usually responds to intravenous hydration, parenteral narcotics, and restriction of oral intake. Surgery for neutropenic colitis is indicated if perforation is suspected, but recovery correlates more closely with normalization of the neutrophil count.

COMPLICATIONS

Complications of acute abdomen relate to the underlying disease process. In extreme circumstances, for example, aortic aneurysm rupture or an ectopic pregnancy, rapid exsanguination and death are possible. In visceral perforation, the probable outcome is generalized peritonitis followed by systemic infection and death if surgery is not performed. With inflammatory conditions (e.g., appendicitis, diverticulitis, and cholecystitis), the major risk is the spread of infection resulting in intra-abdominal or hepatic abscess, followed by sepsis. Local complications of acute pancreatitis include pseudocyst formation or pancreatic ascites, whereas generalized consequences include hypocalcemia, acidosis, and respiratory insufficiency. Intestinal obstruction may result in pulmonary aspiration from intractable vomiting. Renal calculi may be complicated by pyelonephritis or renal failure.

CHAPTER 10

Approach to the Patient with Gas and Bloating

The intestine of a normal person typically contains 200 mL of gas, and flatus evacuation averages 600 mL per day. The principal gases in flatus are nitrogen (90% of expelled gas), oxygen, carbon dioxide, hydrogen, and methane. Nitrogen and oxygen content in flatus reflects the contribution from swallowed air, whereas the other gases result from bacterial fermentative processes in the colon. Expelled

---

TABLE 10-1
Causes of Gas and Bloating

Eructation
Involuntary postprandial belching
Magenblase syndrome
Aerophagia (e.g., as from gum chewing, smoking, oral irritation)
Gastroesophageal reflux
Biliary colic

Bacterial Overgrowth
Intestinal or colonic obstruction
Diverticula of the small intestine
Hypochlorhydria
Chronic intestinal pseudoobstruction
Cologastric fistula
Coprophagia

Functional Bowel Disorders
Irritable bowel syndrome
Nonulcer dyspepsia
Idiopathic constipation
Functional diarrhea

Carbohydrate Malabsorption
Lactase deficiency
Fructose, sorbitol, and starch intolerance
Bean and legume ingestion

Gas-bloat Syndrome
Postfundoplication

Miscellaneous Causes
Hypothyroidism
Medications (e.g., anticholinergics, opiates, calcium channel antagonists, antidepressants)

---

hydrogen is generated by bacterial breakdown of dietary carbohydrates and endogenous glycoproteins. Methane is a highly volatile metabolite produced by anaerobic methanogenic bacteria (e.g., *Methanobrevibacter smithii*). Carbon dioxide in expelled flatus derives from bacterial fermentation of dietary carbohydrates, fats, and proteins. Flatus odor correlates with sulfur-containing compounds in the expelled gas. Various clinical syndromes are associated with complaints of gas and bloating (Table 10-1).

Lumenal gas produces several clinical syndromes. Eructation, or belching, is the retrograde expulsion of esophageal and gastric gas from the mouth. Involuntary belching after eating is a normal phenomenon caused by the release of swallowed air during decompression of the distended stomach. It is exacerbated by foods that reduce lower esophageal sphincter tone. The Magenblase syndrome is defined as epigastric fullness and bloating relieved by belching. Most upper gastrointestinal air accumulates because of aerophagia, which is worsened by stimuli that evoke hypersalivation, including gum chewing, smoking, and oral irritation. Flatulence is the volitional or involuntary release of gas from the anus. On average, healthy young men pass flatus 14 times per day; some individuals report up to 25 daily gas expulsions. Bloating is the perception of retained excess gas within the gut lumen. Women more often report bloating than men. Although some conditions lead to increased gas production, many individuals with bloating exhibit normal gut gas volumes.

DIFFERENTIAL DIAGNOSIS

Carbohydrate Maldigestion

Malabsorption of small amounts of carbohydrates, demonstrated by increased breath hydrogen excretion, may produce eructation, bloating, abdominal pain, and flatulence. Lactase deficiency is the most common form of carbohydrate intolerance, affecting approximately 20% of the population in the United States. Certain ethnic groups such as African Americans and Asians exhibit far greater rates of lactose intolerance. Fructose is naturally found in honey and fruits and is used as a sweetener in many commercial soft drinks. Sorbitol is also present in fruits and is used as a sweetener in dietetic candies and chewing gum. Malabsorption of as little as 37.5 g of fructose and 5 g of sorbitol may produce significant gaseous symptoms. Other poorly absorbed carbohydrates include xylitol and isomalt. To date, there is no convincing evidence to suggest that gaseous symptoms in irritable bowel syndrome result from abnormal metabolism of these ingested simple carbohydrates. The autosomal recessive hereditary syndrome sucrase-isomaltase deficiency typically presents in infancy with malabsorption of sucrose. Of the complex carbohydrates, only rice and gluten-free wheat are completely absorbed in healthy individuals, whereas up to 20% of the carbohydrates from whole wheat, oat, potato, and corn flour are maldigested and can contribute to gas generation. Nondigestible oligosaccharides (e.g., stachyose, raffinose, and verbascose) abundant in beans and legumes are avidly fermented by colonic bacteria to produce voluminous quantities of intestinal gas. Fiber intake correlates with flatus production in some individuals, although other studies suggest that fiber only increases the sensation of bloating without increasing gas production.

Small Intestinal Bacterial Overgrowth

The stomach and small intestine are relatively sterile compared with the colon. Small intestinal bacterial overgrowth may complicate mechanical obstruction of the gut from postoperative adhesions, Crohn's disease, radiation enteritis, ulcer disease, or malignancy. Other organic abnormalities that predispose to bacterial overgrowth include small intestinal diverticula and gastric achlorhydria most often secondary to surgical vagotomy. Motor disorders of the gut are associated with overgrowth because of an impaired ability to clear organisms from the gut. Forty-three percent of cases of diabetic diarrhea are attributable to bacterial overgrowth. The purported association of small intestinal bacterial overgrowth with irritable bowel syndrome is unproven. Disorders that increase bacterial delivery to the upper gut (e.g., cologastric fistulae and coprophagia) can overwhelm normal defenses against infection.

Dysmotility Syndromes

Conditions that alter gut motor function produce prominent gas and bloating. Bloating is reported by patients with gastroparesis and by those with fat intolerance and rapid gastric emptying. A consequence of fundoplication for gastroesophageal reflux disease is an inability to belch or vomit secondary to an unyielding wrap of gastric tissue around the distal esophagus. In the initial months after fundoplication, up to 70% of patients experience bloating, upper abdominal cramping, and flatulence, a constellation of symptoms known as *gas-bloat syndrome*. Surgical revision is rarely necessary because symptoms usually improve with time. Intestinal pseudoobstruction leads to gaseous symptoms because of delayed small bowel transit of gas and development of bacterial overgrowth. Bloating also is reported by patients with chronic constipation.

Functional Bowel Disorders

Complaints of excess gas are prevalent in patients with functional bowel disorders such as irritable bowel syndrome and functional dyspepsia. Older studies that used argon washout techniques reported normal intra-abdominal gas volumes in patients with functional disease; however, more recent investigations of transit of jejunally perfused gas mixtures report retarded gas expulsion by these individuals. Others have suggested that an additional factor of visceral hypersensitivity contributes to a sensation of retained gas in addition to abnormal gut motor function. Historical diagnoses of hepatic and splenic flexure syndromes in patients with purported gas trapping in these sites probably represent subsets of functional bowel disorders.

Miscellaneous Causes

Aerophagia during gum chewing, smoking, or oral irritation produces significant gas symptoms, especially eructation. Patients who have undergone laryngectomy experience eructation from swallowing air for esophageal speech. Patients with intestinal obstructions may infrequently present only with symptoms of gas and bloating. Small bowel malabsorptive conditions including celiac sprue may produce gaseous manifestations that may predominate or be part of a larger constellation of symptoms. Individuals with peptic ulcer, gastroesophageal reflux, or biliary colic may belch to relieve their other symptoms. Gaseous complaints may be reported as consequences of endocrinopathies such as hypothyroidism. Many medications (e.g., anticholinergics, opiates, calcium channel antagonists, and antidepressants) produce gas by retarding gut transit.

WORKUP

History

Patients with complaints of excess gas also commonly report associated symptoms including pain, bloating, halitosis, anorexia, early satiety, nausea, belching, loud borborygmi, constipation, and flatulence, which suggest a diagnosis of a functional bowel disorder. Thus, the clinician must be alert for warning symptoms or signs that indicate an underlying organic condition. Relief of symptoms with defecation or passage of flatus is consistent with a functional disorder, as is the absence of symptoms that awaken the patient from deep sleep. Conversely, the presence of associated vomiting, fever, weight loss, nocturnal diarrhea, steatorrhea, and rectal bleeding indicate probable organic disease. Medical conditions that predispose to bacterial overgrowth and use of medications that delay gut transit should be determined from the history. Selected carbohydrate malabsorptive conditions are hereditary, whereas others (e.g., lactase deficiency) are more prevalent in some ethnic groups. Anxiety disorders and other psychiatric conditions predispose to aerophagia and functional bowel disorders.

A precise dietary history may correlate specific foods with symptoms. Ingestion of legumes, fruits, unrefined starches, and lactose-containing foodstuffs should be addressed, as should consumption of diet foods and candies and soft drinks containing fructose. Gum chewing, smoking, and chewing tobacco predispose to aerophagia.

Physical Examination

Physical findings are usually normal in patients with complaints of excess gas. On assessment of general appearance, the patient with functional disease may exhibit anxiety, hyperventilation, and air swallowing. Other findings suggest organic disease, including sclerodactyly with scleroderma, peripheral or autonomic neuropathy with dysmotility syndromes, and cachexia, jaundice, and palpable masses with malignant intestinal obstruction. Visible scars on abdominal inspection may be evidence of prior fundoplication with subsequent induction of gas-bloat syndrome or other laparotomy with development of obstructing intra-abdominal adhesions. Abdominal auscultation can assess for absent bowel sounds with ileus or myopathic dysmotility, high-pitched bowel sounds with intestinal obstruction, or a succussion splash with gastric obstruction or gastroparesis. Abdominal percussion and palpation may reveal tympany and distention in mechanical obstruction or intestinal dysmotility. Ascites should be excluded on abdominal examination because patients occasionally misinterpret the fluid accumulation as excess gas. Occult fecal blood on rectal examination indicates mucosal damage, as occurs with ulceration, inflammation, and neoplasm.

Additional Testing

Laboratory Studies

Screening laboratory tests are useful in excluding organic disease (Fig. 10-1). Normal values for a complete blood count, electrolytes, glucose, albumin, total protein, and sedimentation rate exclude most inflammatory and neoplastic conditions. In selected patients, calcium and phosphate levels, renal function, liver chemistry values, and thyroid function tests may be needed. Patients with diarrhea should undergo stool examination for ova and parasites to rule out giardiasis. Endomysial or tissue transglutaminase antibodies can screen for celiac disease.

Structural Studies

Supine and upright plain abdominal radiographs may reveal generalized lumenal distention with ileus, diffuse haziness in ascites, and air-fluid levels in mechanical obstruction. Barium radiography and endoscopy are considered for patients with suspected obstruction, pseudoobstruction, or an intralumenal inflammatory or neoplastic process. Small bowel biopsies are performed to confirm a diagnosis of celiac disease. Other tests such as ultrasound and computed tomography can be used to assess the patient for other intra-abdominal disorders that might predispose the patient to complaints of excess gas.

Functional Studies

Gastric emptying scintigraphy or manometry of the esophagus, stomach, and small intestine can be performed when an underlying motility disorder is considered.

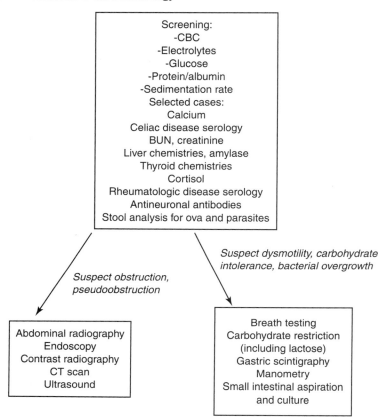

FIGURE 10-1. Workup of a patient with gas and bloating (CBC, complete blood count; BUN, blood urea nitrogen; CT, computed tomography).

Hydrogen breath testing to detect monosaccharide or disaccharide malabsorption confirms associations between symptoms and specific foods. Conceptually, this technique relies on the ability of lumenal bacteria to produce hydrogen gas when metabolizing ingested substrates and the concurrent inability of human tissue to use similar metabolic pathways. Expired breath samples are obtained before and after ingesting an aqueous solution of the sugar that is presumed to be malabsorbed. In some cases, breath hydrogen measurements can be extended for up to 10 hours if testing is performed to exclude malabsorption of complex carbohydrates (e.g., starch). An increase in breath hydrogen of greater than 20 parts per million within 120 minutes of lactose ingestion distinguishes biopsy-proven, lactase-deficient persons from lactase-sufficient persons with a sensitivity of 90%. Elevations in fasting breath hydrogen before substrate ingestion and early rises within 30 minutes of sugar ingestion raise the possibility of small intestinal bacterial overgrowth. Glucose, the most commonly used sugar for breath hydrogen testing in suspected bacterial overgrowth, provides a diagnostic sensitivity of 70% to 90%. Other centers have relied on ^{14}C- or ^{13}C-labeled substrates; however, special facilities are needed to measure breath

$^{14}CO_2$ or $^{13}CO_2$. Patients can be tested for fructose or sorbitol malabsorption using hydrogen breath testing; however, the normal values of these tests are not well established.

PRINCIPLES OF MANAGEMENT

Any underlying disorder responsible for symptoms of excess gas should be specifically managed whenever possible. Mechanical obstruction is usually managed surgically. Surgeries to vent the gut may help selected individuals with gas-bloat syndrome or intestinal pseudoobstruction. Lactase deficiency is controlled by excluding lactose from the diet or by supplementing the diet with exogenous lactase. Acid-suppressive medications may reduce eructation associated with gastroesophageal reflux disease. Single or intermittent courses of oral antibiotics may control small intestinal bacterial overgrowth.

For complaints of excess gas for which no organic disorder is defined after appropriate diagnostic testing, attempts are made to decrease intestinal gas and to regulate bowel function. Aerophagia may be controlled by cessation of gum chewing and smoking and improving oral hygiene. The chronic belcher may be aided by self-observation in a mirror to demonstrate aerophagia. Dietary restriction of legumes, beans, fruits, soft drinks, dietetic candies and gums, and complex carbohydrates may benefit some individuals. Patients with constipation may experience reductions in gaseous symptoms when fiber products and gas forming sugar laxatives such as lactulose, sorbitol, or prune juice are replaced by osmotic laxatives or prokinetic agents such as tegaserod.

Medications may provide benefits for some individuals with gas and bloating. Simethicone alters the elasticity of mucus-covered intralumenal gas bubbles and promotes their coalescence. Activated charcoal sometimes reduces breath hydrogen and symptoms caused by ingesting indigestible carbohydrates. Bacterial α-galactosidase (Beano) has been marketed to reduce symptoms after ingesting legumes high in indigestible oligosaccharides, presumably by hydrolyzing these sugars in the lumen of the small intestine before they are fermented by colonic bacteria. Probiotic compounds purportedly repopulate the gut with nonpathogenic organisms that do not generate gas. In healthy individuals, pancreatic enzyme preparations, bismuth subsalicylate, and nonabsorbable antibiotics reportedly reduce gas production or odor. However, none of these agents have been subjected to rigorous investigation to verify their utility in patient populations who complain of excess gas. The prokinetic drug tegaserod reduces bloating in patients with irritable bowel syndrome and constipation.

COMPLICATIONS

Few complications occur in patients with gas and bloating caused by functional disease. However, complications from organic disease usually are manifestations of the underlying disease rather than of the gas itself. There have been rare case reports of explosions resulting from ignition by tobacco smoking of feculent gas expelled during eructation in patients with gastrointestinal obstruction and proximal bacterial overgrowth. Similarly, colonic explosions with perforation have been reported in patients undergoing colonoscopy with intracolonic cautery. In general, these vanishingly rare complications result from inadequate bowel cleansing or the use of mannitol or sorbitol purging solutions, both of which generate hydrogen gas.

CHAPTER 11

Approach to the Patient with Ileus or Obstruction

DIFFERENTIAL DIAGNOSIS

Acute ileus is a potentially reversible state of inhibited motor activity in the gastrointestinal tract. Toxic megacolon is a special form of ileus in which severe transmural inflammation produces colonic atony, systemic toxemia, and a high risk of spontaneous perforation. Chronic pseudoobstruction is a functional abnormality of longer duration that simulates mechanical obstruction but has no anatomic cause and may exhibit clinical manifestations similar to ileus. Obstruction implies complete or partial blockage of the gut at one or more levels. Acute ileus, chronic pseudoobstruction, and mechanical obstruction have numerous causes (Table 11-1).

Acute Ileus and Chronic Pseudoobstruction

Acute Ileus

Several conditions have been associated with the development of acute ileus. Ileus also is the normal physiological response to laparotomy. The neural mechanisms underlying development of ileus are poorly understood. Gastric and small intestinal motility recover in the first postoperative day, whereas colonic contractions return in 3 to 5 days. Postoperative ileus beyond that time is considered pathological and warrants a search for surgical complications. Other intra-abdominal causes of acute ileus include abdominal trauma and inflammatory gut disorders (e.g., ulcer perforation, bile or chemical peritonitis, toxic megacolon, pancreatitis, cholecystitis, appendicitis, diverticulitis, and inflammatory bowel disease). Noninflammatory conditions (radiation damage and mesenteric ischemia) and retroperitoneal disorders (e.g., renal calculi, pyelonephritis, renal transplantation, and retroperitoneal hemorrhage) can also produce acute ileus. Extra-abdominal causes of ileus include reflex inhibition of gut motility by craniotomy, fractures, myocardial infarction, heart surgery, pneumonia, pulmonary embolus, and burns. Medications (e.g., anticholinergics, opiates, calcium channel antagonists, chemotherapeutic agents, and antidepressants) may inhibit motor activity, as may metabolic abnormalities, including electrolyte disturbances, sepsis, uremia, diabetic ketoacidosis, sickle cell anemia, respiratory insufficiency, porphyria, and heavy metal intoxication.

Chronic Intestinal Pseudoobstruction

Chronic intestinal pseudoobstruction is a consequence of a variety of conditions. Chronic idiopathic pseudoobstruction often presents after a viral prodrome, suggesting an infectious etiology. Hereditary conditions such as familial visceral

TABLE 11-1
Causes of Ileus and Obstruction

Acute Ileus
Postoperative ileus
Abdominal trauma
Ulcer perforation
Bile or chemical peritonitis
Toxic megacolon
Pancreatitis
Cholecystitis
Appendicitis
Diverticulitis
Inflammatory bowel disease
Radiation therapy
Mesenteric ischemia
Retroperitoneal disorders (e.g., renal calculi, pyelonephritis, renal transplant, hemorrhage)
Extra-abdominal sources (e.g., craniotomy, fractures, myocardial infarction, cardiac surgery, pneumonia, pulmonary embolus, burns)
Metabolic disorders (e.g., electrolyte abnormalities, uremia, sepsis, diabetic ketoacidosis, sickle cell anemia, respiratory insufficiency, porphyria, heavy metal toxicity)
Medications (e.g., anticholinergics, opiates, calcium channel antagonists, chemotherapy, antidepressants)

Chronic Intestinal Pseudoobstruction
Hereditary diseases (e.g., familial visceral neuropathy, familial visceral myopathy)
Diabetes mellitus
Rheumatologic disorders (e.g., scleroderma, systemic lupus erythematosus, amyloidosis)
Endocrinopathies (e.g., hypothyroidism, hyperparathyroid disease or hypoparathyroid disease, Addison disease)
Neuromuscular diseases (e.g., muscular dystrophy, myotonic dystrophy)
Chagas disease
Infectious pseudoobstruction
Pheochromocytoma
Paraneoplastic pseudoobstruction

Mechanical Obstruction
Adhesions
Congenital bands (e.g., Ladd bands)
Hernias (e.g., external, internal, diaphragmatic, pelvic)
Volvulus (e.g., colon, small intestine, stomach)
Obstructive lumenal tumors
Inflammatory bowel disease
Diverticulitis
Mesenteric ischemia
Radiation injury
Intussusception
Congenital conditions (e.g., hypertrophic pyloric stenosis, Hirschsprung disease, intestinal atresia/agenesis)
Fecal impaction
Gallstone ileus
Retained barium
Gastric bezoars

myopathies and neuropathies produce pseudoobstruction at early ages. In addition to gastroparesis, long-standing, poorly controlled diabetes mellitus may disrupt motor function in the small intestine. Rheumatologic disorders (e.g., scleroderma, systemic lupus erythematosus, and amyloidosis) and some endocrinopathies (e.g., hypothyroidism, hyperparathyroidism or hypoparathyroidism, and Addison disease) can lead to chronic pseudoobstruction. Neuromuscular diseases (e.g., myotonic dystrophy or muscular dystrophy) chronically disrupt motor activity. In selected geographic locations, Chagas disease represents an infectious cause of pseudoobstruction that occurs after exposure to *Trypanosoma cruzi*. Viral pseudoobstruction in immunosuppressed patients has been reported as a consequence of infection with cytomegalovirus and other agents. Pheochromocytoma produces chronic intestinal hypomotility, probably because of the motor inhibitory effects of circulating catecholamines. Chronic intestinal pseudoobstruction can be a paraneoplastic manifestation of small cell lung carcinoma and, less commonly, other malignancies. Paraneoplastic pseudoobstruction results from malignant invasion of the celiac axis or, alternatively, from plasma cell infiltration of the myenteric plexus, leading to the loss of enteric neural function.

Mechanical Obstruction

The causes of mechanical intestinal obstruction may be divided into extrinsic lesions, intrinsic lesions, and intralumenal objects.

Extrinsic Lesions

Extrinsic adhesions are the most common cause of small intestinal obstruction in adults, but they rarely occlude the colon. Adhesions become clinically apparent at times ranging from a few days to 20 years postoperatively. They also may occur in nonoperative conditions after intra-abdominal infection or abdominal irradiation. Congenital bands behave similarly and may occur in association with malrotation (Ladd bands). Hernias represent another extrinsic cause of obstruction that may be external (protruding through the abdominal wall), internal, diaphragmatic (usually paraesophageal), or pelvic. Internal and pelvic hernias usually are identified at the time of surgery. Volvulus is an abnormal torsion of the bowel that produces a closed and obstructed loop of bowel, associated with an impairment of blood flow. Colonic volvulus involves the cecum in 10% to 20% and the sigmoid colon in 70% to 80% of cases and manifests as sudden abdominal pain followed by distention. Gastric volvulus occurs with diaphragmatic defects, congenital malformations, and large paraesophageal hernias.

Intrinsic Lesions

Intrinsic lesions are less common causes of mechanical obstruction. Benign and malignant tumors can obstruct the lumen or provide a leading point for intussusception. Primary small intestinal malignancies are rare and include lymphoma, adenocarcinoma, and carcinoids, whereas adenocarcinoma represents the most common obstructing colonic neoplasm. Metastatic tumors usually tether and fix the bowel rather than obstruct the lumen. Inflammatory processes and ischemia cause obstructing strictures, whereas blunt trauma may produce an intramural hematoma. In addition to neoplasm, a Meckel diverticulum may initiate intussusception. In children, there usually is no underlying mucosal or submucosal lesion that predisposes to intussusception.

Intralumenal Objects

Intralumenal objects represent the least common causes of mechanical obstruction. Fecal impaction may produce colonic obstruction in patients who are dehydrated or immobile, who have underlying constipation, or who take medications that slow colonic transit. Rarely, large gallstones erode through the gallbladder into the gut lumen, where they migrate to obstruct the intestine, usually at the level of the distal ileum. Barium from radiographic procedures may obstruct the colon in patients with underlying colonic motility disorders. Gastric bezoars and ingested foreign bodies may occlude the gut lumen in select cases.

WORKUP

History

Patients with ileus, pseudoobstruction, and obstruction may present with similar symptoms (e.g., pain, nausea, vomiting, abdominal distention, and obstipation). Acute ileus and gastric or duodenal obstruction cause little associated abdominal pain, whereas distal intestinal and colonic obstructions elicit greater discomfort. Upper and midabdominal pain are characteristic of obstruction proximal to the transverse colon, whereas left colonic blockage produces lower abdominal discomfort. The pain of mechanical obstruction is dull, ill-defined, or squeezing. True colic or intermittent waves of pain may be prominent.

Distention may be pronounced with ileus and with distal obstruction, whereas gastric obstruction produces little distention. Audible bowel sounds may be present with intestinal obstruction but are reduced or absent with acute ileus. Copious vomiting of clear liquid characterizes gastric obstruction, whereas marked bilious emesis occurs with duodenal blockage. Distal obstruction and ileus produce only mild nausea and vomiting. The pain of proximal, not distal, obstruction is often relieved by vomiting. If mechanical obstruction is incomplete or if ileus is mild, pain and distention may be intermittent and aggravated by fiber-rich, poorly digestible foods. Complete obstruction usually produces obstipation and the inability to expel flatus. Conversely, watery diarrhea is noted with partial obstruction and fecal impaction. Children with intussusception may pass bloody mucus that resembles red currant jelly.

Clues about the cause of ileus or obstruction can be determined from the history. Careful family, medication, endocrine, immunologic, and metabolic histories should be obtained from a patient with ileus, and the clinician should be alert to thyroid and parathyroid disorders, diabetes, scleroderma, heavy metal intoxication, and porphyria. Prior surgery raises the possibility of adhesions, and reports of abdominal wall bulging suggest hernias as a possible cause of obstruction. Histories of malignancy, radiation, inflammatory bowel disease, ulcer disease, gallstones, diverticular disease, pancreatitis, motility disorders, and foreign body ingestion suggest specific causes. Exacerbation of pain with menses is consistent with endometriosis.

Before making management decisions, it is important to determine if complications such as peritonitis, perforation, sepsis, or strangulation have occurred. Constant localized pain, fever, rigors, and sudden clinical deterioration suggest bowel ischemia and infarction, although strangulation with necrosis may be present before these symptoms develop. Therefore, a high degree of suspicion must be maintained and the clinician must be ready to intervene if the status of the patient changes.

Physical Examination

Careful examination of the patient is necessary to determine the appropriate diagnostic and therapeutic plans. A patient with obstruction usually appears to be in great distress, whereas a patient with ileus may be more comfortable despite the obvious distention. Cutaneous findings with selected causes of obstruction include pyoderma gangrenosum and erythema nodosum with inflammatory bowel disease, Cullen sign or Grey-Turner sign with pancreatitis, vesicles and bullae with some forms of porphyria, acanthosis nigricans with gastrointestinal malignancy, butterfly dermatitis with systemic lupus erythematosus, and sclerodactyly and telangiectasias with scleroderma.

An abdominal examination provides crucial diagnostic information about a patient with ileus or obstruction. Inspection may reveal scars and visible distention. Gentle palpation may detect subtle hernias that are not obvious on inspection. Hepatosplenomegaly, lymphadenopathy, and masses raise concern for malignancy, although tender masses may be present in inflammatory diseases (e.g., Crohn's disease). Tympany accompanies both ileus and obstruction, whereas shifting dullness and a fluid wave characterize ascites. Auscultation usually reveals hypoactive or absent bowel sounds with ileus, whereas obstruction produces louder, high-pitched, hyperactive bowel sounds that may have a musical or tinkling quality. Shaking of the abdomen while listening through a stethoscope may reveal a succussion splash, which is rarely found with gastric obstruction and gastroparesis. Rectal examination may detect occult fecal blood with inflammatory, neoplastic, infectious, or ischemic disease. Digital rectal and pelvic examinations may also detect subtle masses not found on abdominal palpation or may reveal obturator or sciatic hernias. Repeated abdominal examinations are essential for surveillance of complications. If fever, hypotension, or signs of sepsis or peritonitis develop or if bowel sounds disappear, the viscus may be ischemic and operative intervention may be urgently indicated.

Additional Testing
Laboratory Studies
Blood tests aid in establishing the cause of mechanical obstruction only in rare cases related to inflammation, infection, or neoplasm. In contrast, laboratory studies are essential in discovering the cause of ileus (Fig. 11-1). Abnormal electrolyte (including calcium, phosphate, and magnesium), blood urea nitrogen, or creatinine values support a clinical impression of dehydration. Progressive dehydration also promotes development of hemoconcentration, as indicated by increases in hemoglobin and albumin levels. Leukocytosis may be present with inflammation or infection. Measurement of arterial blood gases may be necessary to evaluate the acid-base balance. With an ischemic or infarcted bowel, elevations in amylase, alkaline phosphatase, creatine phosphokinase, aspartate and alanine aminotransferase, and lactate dehydrogenase may be evident, although these enzymes also increase with hepatic and pancreaticobiliary disease.

Plain Radiographic Studies
Plain radiographs should be the initial structural studies performed on patients with suspected ileus or obstruction. Chest radiography can detect pneumonia, evaluate cardiorespiratory status, and detect free subdiaphragmatic air, whereas supine and upright abdominal plain films show intra-abdominal gas distribution. Left lateral decubitus abdominal radiographs may be obtained on patients who cannot assume an upright position. In general, the jejunum lies in the left upper and central abdomen, the ileum in the right central and lower abdomen, and the colon in the flanks and right iliac fossa. In early or partial obstruction, lumenal distention occurs, but air may still be evident distal to the blockage. With complete occlusion of the small intestine, the lumen is widely distended and the valvulae conniventes are observed to span the lumenal air column. Upright or decubitus views commonly demonstrate air-fluid levels in a stepladder configuration. With complete small intestinal obstruction, the colon empties and collapses within 12 to 24 hours and no colonic air is radiographically visible. With colonic obstruction, the colon

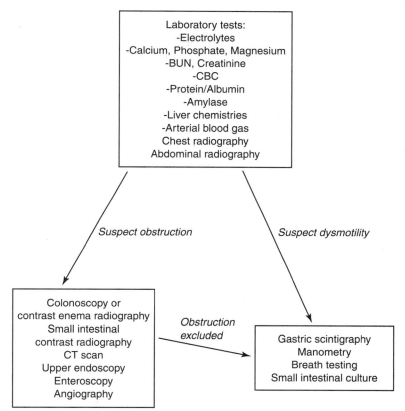

FIGURE 11-1. Workup of a patient with ileus or obstruction (BUN, blood urea nitrogen; CBC, complete blood count; CT, computed tomography).

proximal to the blockage dilates and the characteristic incomplete and scalloped indentations of the haustra are visible. With advanced strangulation, the bowel wall becomes edematous, exhibiting a thumbprint pattern on radiographs, and air in the intestinal wall, portal vein, and peritoneal cavity may be observed.

In ileus, lumenal dilation may be generalized or it may only manifest adjacent to an inflammatory site, producing a sentinel loop, as in appendicitis or pancreatitis. With concurrent peritonitis, the bowel wall may thicken. Colonic gas usually is more prominent in ileus than with small intestinal obstruction. Pure colonic dilation, most pronounced in the cecum, is the defining feature of acute colonic pseudoobstruction. Stepladder air-fluid levels may be observed with either ileus or obstruction, but they are more well defined and longer with obstruction. A string-of-beads pattern of the air-fluid interfaces is most suggestive of high-grade obstruction of the small intestine. A diffusely hazy pattern with central localization of bowel loops is characteristic of ascites.

Additional Structural Studies
Contrast radiography should be performed to localize the anatomic site of partial obstruction or if the ileus and obstruction cannot be differentiated. Barium is the

superior contrast agent, but a water-soluble agent should be used if perforation is suspected because barium elicits an intense peritoneal inflammatory reaction. If there is doubt about the site of obstruction, contrast enema radiography or lower endoscopy should be performed before upper gastrointestinal barium radiography to exclude a colonic cause. Upper endoscopy is useful with suspected esophageal, gastric, or duodenal lesions and offers the additional capability of therapeutic dilation of any stricture. Push enteroscopy provides similar diagnostic and therapeutic capabilities to the proximal jejunum. Computed tomography scanning techniques are increasingly used to define the site of obstruction and to exclude selected underlying disease processes (i.e., inflammation vs. neoplasm). Conversely, ultrasound is generally not useful because of the obscuring effects of intralumenal gas. Angiography or magnetic resonance angiography may be useful for patients with suspected mesenteric ischemia and infarction.

Functional Studies

Functional testing of gut motility may be considered for patients with prolonged ileus or suspected chronic intestinal pseudoobstruction. Gastric emptying scintigraphy may document gastroparesis, whereas esophageal or gastroduodenal manometry may show the characteristic hypomotility pattern of visceral myopathy or the random, intense bursts of contractions in visceral neuropathy. Some centers have proposed using gastroduodenal manometry for suspected obstruction of the small intestine if radiographic studies are normal. In these instances, manometry shows clusters of contractions separated by periods of quiescence, called the *minute rhythm.*

PRINCIPLES OF MANAGEMENT

Fluid Replacement

Correction of fluid, electrolyte, and acid-base imbalances is guided by the physical findings coupled with laboratory determination of hematocrit, electrolyte, blood urea nitrogen, creatinine, and blood gas levels. With severe hypovolemia, fluid resuscitation should be performed with concurrent monitoring of urine output, central venous pressure, and blood pressure. In patients with superimposed cardiorespiratory or renal disease, a Swan-Ganz catheter may be needed. In mild to moderate hypovolemia, one half of the fluid deficit should be replaced using crystalloid solutions (e.g., lactated Ringer solution, normal saline) within 24 hours, and one half in the second 24 hours. Maintenance fluid requirements average 1500 to 2500 mL per day in an afebrile person with normal renal function. Additional fluids are given with fever or with fluid losses, as for nasogastric suction. With gastric outlet obstruction, potassium chloride is often needed after establishing normal urine output because renal potassium losses are high in this condition. Sodium bicarbonate is given for profound metabolic acidosis (e.g., pH <7.1). The bicarbonate deficit can be calculated as follows: $24 \text{ mEq/L} - [HCO_3^-] \times 0.6$ body weight. One half of the deficit should be given to raise plasma bicarbonate to 16 mEq/L in the first 12 to 24 hours. Overaggressive correction of acidosis can produce intracellular volume depletion, neurological dysfunction, and decreased blood oxygen delivery.

Bowel Decompression

Abdominal distention increases gastrointestinal secretion and causes nausea and vomiting, thereby increasing the risk of aspiration. Nasogastric suction is appropriate in ileus and obstruction. The use of longer tubes (e.g., Cantor, Miller-Abbott) is controversial. The patient should be given nothing by mouth, and intravenous fluids with or without parenteral nutrients should be administered to maintain adequate hydration and nutrition. For patients with acute colonic pseudoobstruction, some clinicians advocate therapeutic colonoscopic decompression, although few objective data support this practice. Placing a rectal tube or administering tap water enemas may reduce colonic distention in some patients. In patients without significant cardiovascular disease, the acetylcholinesterase inhibitor neostigmine may promote gas expulsion when administered in a controlled setting with cardiac monitoring. Drugs that inhibit motor activity should be withheld.

Surgical Management

As a rule, complete obstruction is an indication for urgent surgery as soon as resuscitation is completed and nasogastric decompression is achieved, because strangulation cannot be excluded using clinical criteria in this setting. Antibiotics are given preoperatively to reduce the likelihood of wound infections resulting from enterotomy of an unprepared bowel. With strangulation, any necrotic bowel should be resected. Intraoperative Doppler ultrasound and fluorescein dye injection can be used to assess the viability of the adjacent intestine. In questionable cases, a second-look laparotomy may be needed. With partial obstruction, immediate surgery and antibiotics are of no proven benefit. However, if fever, peritoneal signs, leukocytosis, or hyperamylasemia develop, laparotomy is indicated. With multiple prior operations, immediate surgery usually is not indicated because bowel fixation from intraperitoneal scarring makes strangulation unlikely. Colonic obstruction nearly always requires surgery; nasogastric suction may have little effect in this setting. If the bowel cannot be cleansed, many surgeons perform a two-stage operation with initial resection of the obstructed segment and placement of a diverting colostomy followed by reanastomosis at a later date to reduce wound infection.

Nonsurgical Management

Nonsurgical therapy is useful in some settings. Sigmoid volvulus is treated by gentle endoscopic detorsion with aspiration of retained gas or by gentle hydrostatic pressure provided by rectally introduced contrast agents. Endoscopic dilation of adhesions or radiation-induced strictures may be possible. Inoperable colorectal cancer may be palliatively treated by Nd:YAG laser recanalization of the colonic lumen or by placing expandable intralumenal stents. The use of prokinetic agents in ileus (e.g., metoclopramide and erythromycin) has been advocated by some, although studies documenting their efficacy are inconclusive. Prokinetic drugs such as metoclopramide, erythromycin, and octreotide may have greater value for patients with chronic intestinal pseudoobstruction. Unfortunately, in advanced cases, no medical therapy provides impressive relief and total parenteral nutrition may be required.

COMPLICATIONS

The most serious complication of obstruction or ileus is bowel infarction, with resulting peritonitis and possible death. Other complications include aspiration pneumonia, electrolyte abnormalities, and malnutrition. All may have serious consequences for unstable patients who have other concurrent disease. Many of the diseases that produce ileus and obstruction have serious sequelae, in addition to those that result from involvement of the bowel.

CHAPTER 12

Approach to the Patient with Diarrhea

Diarrhea is one of the most common complaints evaluated by physicians. Patients may describe diarrhea as bowel movements that are increased in frequency, larger in size, loose in consistency, or associated with urgency or incontinence. The range of normal bowel patterns is broad, but 99% of the population in Western societies defecates between three times a week and three times a day. The normal daily stool weight is 100 to 200 g, although individuals on high fiber diets may pass 500 g per day. In the United States, a daily stool weight of more than 200 g is considered abnormal.

DIFFERENTIAL DIAGNOSIS

High-output diarrhea of more than 200 g daily arises from two pathophysiological mechanisms: increased anion secretion and decreased absorption of electrolytes. Increased anion secretion may result from enterotoxins, endogenous hormones or neuropeptides, inflammatory mediators, bile salts, laxatives, and medications. Decreased water and electrolyte absorption develop from enterotoxins, decreased mucosal absorptive surface area, acceleration of transit with inadequate time for absorption, impaired mucosal barrier function, and ingestion of poorly absorbed osmotically active solutes. Conditions that produce high-output diarrhea are divided into osmotic, secretory, and mucosal injury categories (Table 12-1). Some diseases produce diarrhea by more than one mechanism. For example, intestinal pseudoobstruction is a primary motor disorder that leads secondarily to bacterial overgrowth and malabsorption. Furthermore, small intestinal bacteria deconjugate bile acids, which in turn stimulate colonic water and electrolyte secretion. Patients with normal stool output of less than 200 g daily may also complain of diarrhea. Normal-output diarrhea most often results from anorectal disease, hormonally induced hyperdefecation, or functional bowel disorders in which gut sensorimotor defects alter perception and transit of lumenal contents (Table 12-1).

Osmotic Diarrhea

Under normal conditions, most ingested food is absorbed before it reaches the colon. In many diarrheal disorders, undigested nutrients are not absorbed and act as osmotic agents to draw free water into the intestinal lumen. The most common cause of osmotic diarrhea is lactase deficiency. In this condition, lactose in dairy products remains unhydrolyzed because of reduced brush border disaccharidase activity and acts as an osmotically active agent. In the colon, lactose is further metabolized by lumenal bacteria to short-chain fatty acids that further increase

TABLE 12-1
Causes of Diarrhea

Osmotic Diarrhea
  Nonabsorbed solutes
    Saline and phosphate laxatives
    Sorbitol, fructose, lactulose
  Disaccharidase deficiency
    Lactase deficiency
    Isomaltase-sucrase deficiency
    Trehalase deficiency
  Small intestinal mucosal disease
    Celiac sprue
    Tropical sprue
    Viral gastroenteritis
    Whipple disease
    Amyloidosis
    Intestinal ischemia
    Lymphoma
    Giardiasis
    Intestinal radiation
    Mastocytosis
    Eosinophilic gastroenteritis
    Abetalipoproteinemia
    Lymphangiectasia
  Pancreatic insufficiency
    Chronic pancreatitis
    Pancreatic carcinoma
    Cystic fibrosis
  Reduced intestinal surface area
    Small intestinal resection
    Enteric fistulae
    Jejunoileal bypass
  Bile salt malabsorption
    Bacterial overgrowth
    Ileal resection
    Crohn's disease
  Other medications
    Olestra and orlistat

Secretory Diarrhea
  Laxatives
    Bisacodyl
    Ricinoleic acid
    Dioctyl sodium sulfosuccinate
    Senna and aloe
    Oxyphenisatin
  Medications
    Diuretics
    Thyroid supplements
    Theophylline
    Colchicine
    Quinidine
    Selective serotonin reuptake inhibitors

(continued)

TABLE 12-1
(*Continued*)

Bacterial toxins
  Vibrio cholerae
  Toxigenic *Escherichia coli*
  Clostridium perfringens
Hormonally induced
  Vasoactive intestinal polypeptide
  Serotonin
  Calcitonin
  Glucagon
  Gastrin
  Substance P
  Prostaglandins
Defective neural control
  Diabetic diarrhea
Bile acid diarrhea
  Ileal resection
  Crohn's disease
  Bacterial overgrowth
  Postcholecystectomy
Mucosal inflammation
  Collagenous colitis
  Lymphocytic colitis
Defective transport
  Congenital chloridorrhea
Villous adenoma

Mucosal Injury Diarrhea
Inflammatory bowel disease
  Crohn's disease
  Ulcerative colitis
Acute infections
  Viruses (rotavirus, Norwalk agent)
  Parasites (*Giardia, Cryptosporidium, Cyclospora*)
  E coli
  Shigella
  Salmonella
  Campylobacter
  Yersinia enterocolitica
  Entamoeba histolytica (amebiasis)
Chronic infections
  E histolytica (amebiasis)
  Clostridium difficile
  Nematode infestation
Ischemia
  Atherosclerosis
  Vasculitis

Normal-volume Diarrhea
Functional bowel disorders
  Irritable bowel syndrome
Endocrinopathies
  Hyperthyroidism

TABLE 12-1
(*Continued*)

Proctitis
  Ulcerative proctitis
  Infectious proctitis
Fecal incontinence
  Surgical and obstetrical trauma
  Hemorrhoids
  Anal fissures
  Perianal fistulae
  Anal neuropathy (diabetes)

the number of osmotically active particles. Ethnic groups with high risk for lactase deficiency include Asians and Native Americans (90% prevalence), African Americans, Jews, Hispanics, and southern Europeans (60% to 70%). Conversely, individuals of northern European descent exhibit prevalence rates of 10% to 15%. Causes of osmotic diarrhea in persons with normal gut absorptive function include nonabsorbable laxatives, magnesium-containing antacids, medications (orlistat, olestra, colchicine, neomycin), and candies or soft drinks that contain the poorly absorbed sugars fructose and sorbitol. Sorbitol also is responsible for diarrhea after ingestion of elixir forms of certain medications (e.g., potassium chloride and theophylline). Congenital defects of carbohydrate absorption include sucrase-isomaltase deficiency, trehalase deficiency, and glucose-galactose malabsorption.

Some small intestinal diseases produce osmotic diarrhea from maldigestion or malabsorption. Celiac sprue develops from hypersensitivity to dietary gluten. Patients with this disease may be asymptomatic, may exhibit iron deficiency anemia, or may develop diarrhea and malabsorptive symptoms because of profound villous flattening in the small intestine. Tropical sprue is an infectious disease of unknown origin that is observed on the Indian subcontinent, Asia, the West Indies, northern South America, central and southern Africa, and Central America. It produces diarrhea and malabsorption in persons who have resided in these regions for as little as 1 to 3 months. Villous atrophy may be present; treatment involves a combination of tetracycline and folic acid. Crohn's disease involving the small intestine may lead to malabsorption and diarrhea. Whipple disease, caused by infection with *Tropheryma Whippelii*, is diagnosed by demonstration of characteristic periodic acid–Schiff (PAS)-positive macrophages on examination of small intestinal mucosal biopsies. Associated neurological symptoms (e.g., hypersomnolence and oculofacial-skeletal myorhythmias), arthralgias, fever, hypotension, and lymphadenopathy commonly are present. Children with the congenital defect of chylomicron formation, abetalipoproteinemia, present with steatorrhea, red blood cell acanthocytosis, ataxia, and retinitis pigmentosa. Congenital or acquired (secondary to trauma, lymphoma, or carcinoma) intestinal lymphangiectasia causes protein-losing enteropathy with steatorrhea as a result of obstructed lymphatic channels. In this condition, amino acid and carbohydrate absorption are normal because lymphatic pathways do not participate in their uptake. Bacterial overgrowth produces steatorrhea from bile salt deconjugation, brush border injury, and mucosal inflammation. Intestinal infection with *Giardia, Cryptosporidium, Isospora*, or *Mycobacterium avium* complex produces brush border and intramucosal damage. Systemic mastocytosis and eosinophilic gastroenteritis grossly distort the intestinal mucosa and promote nutrient malabsorption. Short bowel syndrome and fistulae reduce the villous surface area available for nutrient uptake. Other conditions (e.g., postvagotomy diarrhea and thyrotoxicosis) accelerate intestinal transit, leaving inadequate time for nutrient assimilation. Adrenal insufficiency causes generalized disturbances in mucosal absorption.

Pancreaticobiliary diseases also are common causes of osmotic diarrhea with maldigestion and malabsorption. Chronic pancreatitis, malignancy, cystic fibrosis, and somatostatinomas lead to steatorrhea as a result of the impaired delivery of pancreatic enzymes to the intestine. Cirrhosis and bile duct obstruction can rarely produce maldigestion because of the impaired delivery of bile salt to the small intestine, which then leads to poor micelle formation with ingested fats.

Secretory Diarrhea

Under physiological conditions, only 1.5 of the 9 L of fluid that pass the ligament of Treitz daily reach the proximal colon. The colon absorbs all but 100 to 200 mL of this fluid before defecation. Diarrhea results when this net absorption is converted to net secretion. The most common causes of acute secretory diarrhea are enterotoxins released by infectious organisms (*Vibrio cholerae*, enterotoxigenic *Escherichia coli*, *Staphylococcus aureus*, *Bacillus cereus*, and *Clostridium perfringens*). Viruses (e.g., rotavirus, Norwalk agent) are also likely to act through toxins. Prolonged diarrhea also may be caused by organisms yet to be identified (e.g., Brainerd diarrhea associated with consumption of raw milk). In some AIDS patients, secretory diarrhea results from defined organisms (*Cryptosporidium, Mycobacterium avium* complex), but other cases are idiopathic. Laxatives (ricinoleic acid, bisacodyl, senna, cascara, aloe, rhubarb, frangula, danthron, and dioctyl sodium sulfosuccinate) represent the other common cause of secretory diarrhea.

Rare cases of secretory diarrhea result from overproduction of circulating agents that stimulate secretion. Carcinoid syndrome classically presents with watery diarrhea, flushing, skin changes, bronchospasm, and cardiac murmurs, which are consequences of secreting serotonin, histamine, catecholamines, kinins, and prostaglandins by the tumor masses. One third of patients with carcinoid syndrome present only with diarrhea. Diarrhea is the major symptom in 10% of patients with gastrinoma and exhibits both secretory and osmotic characteristics. Overproduction of vasoactive intestinal polypeptide (VIP) by VIPoma tumors produces the syndrome of watery diarrhea, hypokalemia, and achlorhydria (WDHA), in which patients often pass more than 3 L of stool daily. Pain and flushing may also be reported in WDHA syndrome. Medullary carcinoma of the thyroid, which may be sporadic or part of the multiple endocrine neoplasia (MEN type IIA) syndrome, causes secretory diarrhea because of the release of calcitonin, although these tumors also produce prostaglandins, VIP, kinins, and serotonin. Glucagonoma patients report mild diarrhea as well as characteristic rashes (migratory necrolytic erythema), glossitis, cheilitis, neuropsychiatric manifestations, and thromboembolism. Systemic mastocytosis produces a mixed secretory and osmotic diarrhea associated with flushing, tachycardia, hypotension, headache, cognitive dysfunction, nausea, ulcer disease, syncope, and urticaria. Histamine and prostaglandins have been proposed as mediators of this condition. Villous adenomas larger than 3 cm in diameter produce secretory diarrhea, possibly secondary to prostaglandin production.

Other disorders also cause secretory diarrhea. The mucosal inflammatory conditions, collagenous and lymphocytic colitis, induce active colonic secretion of water and electrolytes. Bile salt diarrhea results from stimulation of colonic secretion. Diabetic diarrhea presents in patients with long-standing diabetes and characteristically is profuse, watery, nocturnal, and associated with severe urgency. Multiple factors contribute to the pathogenesis of diabetic diarrhea; however, the response of this condition to the somatostatin analog octreotide suggests a prominent secretory component. Furthermore, improvement in diabetic diarrhea on the α-adrenoceptor agonist, clonidine, suggests a pathogenic imbalance between absorptive adrenergic and secretory cholinergic mucosal function. Chronic alcoholics may develop severe watery diarrhea, which may be partly secretory. Ten percent to 25% of long-distance runners develop diarrhea, which is postulated to result from release of gastrin, motilin, VIP, or prostaglandins. Congenital causes of secretory diarrhea include congenital chloridorrhea, congenital sodium diarrhea, and microvillous inclusion disease. A small subset of patients exhibits chronic idiopathic secretory diarrhea or pseudopancreatic cholera syndrome, which is a diagnosis of exclusion, is often self-limited, and disappears spontaneously in 6 to 24 months.

Mucosal Injury Diarrhea

Conditions that injure the small intestinal or colonic mucosa lead to passive secretion of fluids from damaged epithelia and alterations in electrolyte and water absorption. Epithelial destruction may be a consequence of infection with *Shigella* and *Salmonella* spp., enteroinvasive or enterohemorrhagic *E coli*, *Campylobacter jejuni*, *Clostridium difficile*, or *Entamoeba histolytica*). Affected patients may present with watery or bloody diarrhea with or without systemic symptoms of fever, chills, or abdominal pain. Small intestinal infections that produce mucosal injury diarrhea include yersiniosis, tuberculosis, and histoplasmosis. Proctitis from infection with gonorrhea, herpes, syphilis, *Chlamydia*, or amebiasis may be a consequence of anal intercourse. Chronic mucosal injury diarrhea may result from inflammatory bowel diseases such as Crohn's disease and ulcerative colitis, ischemic colitis, and radiation enterocolitis. Other diseases that manifest as inflammatory diarrhea include eosinophilic gastroenteritis, milk and soy protein allergy, Behçet syndrome, Cronkhite-Canada syndrome, graft-versus-host disease, and Churg-Strauss syndrome.

Normal-Output Diarrhea

It is not uncommon for patients with chronic diarrhea to present with stools of normal daily volume. Many of these individuals pass frequent, small, well-formed stools that are associated with urgency and a sense of incomplete evacuation. The most common cause of chronic diarrhea in the United States is irritable bowel syndrome. Some patients with irritable bowel syndrome complain of intermittent diarrhea alternating with constipation. Endocrinopathies such as hyperthyroidism alter colonic motor activity leading to passage of multiple low-volume stools. Proctitis also is a common cause of low-volume, frequent stools. A short distal segment of inflammation sufficient to cause tenesmus and urgency may not be extensive enough to lead to active secretion or loss of absorption. Fecal impaction in institutionalized or hospitalized patients may cause diarrhea from flow of fluid around the obstructing bolus. Incontinence of stool secondary to anal disease, instrumentation, surgery, or neuropathy may be misinterpreted as diarrhea by some patients.

WORKUP

History

A thorough history provides important clues about the cause of diarrhea. Diarrhea can be acute (<3 weeks in duration) or chronic (>3 weeks). Acute diarrhea usually is due to an infectious agent, although drugs or osmotically active compounds may be the culprit. The patient should be questioned about recent travel; sexual practices; ingestion of well water or poorly cooked food and shellfish; and exposure to high-risk persons in day-care centers, hospitals, mental institutions, and nursing homes. The characteristics of the diarrhea provide clues to the causative organism. Watery diarrhea with nausea but little pain is most consistent with toxin-producing bacteria, whereas invasive bacteria may produce more pain and bloody diarrhea. Viruses induce watery diarrhea in association with pain, fever, and mild to moderate vomiting. Homosexual men, prostitutes, and intravenous drug abusers are prone to diarrhea acquired through fecal-oral transfer. Antibiotic-associated colitis must be suspected if there is a history of recent antibiotic use. Recently initiated medication regimens or inadvertent use of over-the-counter preparations with laxative effects (e.g., antacids containing magnesium) should be determined. Common drugs that produce diarrhea include antiarrhythmics, antihypertensives, diuretics, central nervous system drugs, antiarthritics, cholesterol-lowering medications, and theophylline.

The differential diagnosis of chronic diarrhea is more extensive, and the history must be detailed. Frequent passage of voluminous stools that do not abate with food avoidance is consistent with a secretory process, whereas passage of low-volume, loose stools at a normal frequency may be secondary to a motor disturbance. Foul-smelling, bulky, greasy stools suggest fat malabsorption. Soft stools that float or disperse in the toilet water and resolve with fasting are reported by some patients with carbohydrate malabsorption, especially if they occur after ingesting specific foodstuffs such as dairy products or fruits. However, mild degrees of malabsorption, as with bile duct obstruction or mild chronic pancreatitis, may be asymptomatic and suspected only if complications supervene (e.g., anemia, bleeding, osteopenia, tetany, and amenorrhea). Fever, bleeding, pain, and weight loss raise concern for a mucosal injury etiology. Severe pain also may be present with pancreatic disease. Fecal incontinence raises the question of a neuropathic disorder.

Determination of risk factors is important in diagnosing the cause of diarrhea. Diabetes and scleroderma are associated with intestinal dysmotility and bacterial overgrowth. Heat intolerance, palpitations, and weight loss suggest possible hyperthyroidism, whereas flushing and wheezing are reported by some patients with carcinoid syndrome. Histories of radiation therapy or atherosclerotic disease may pertain to the cause of symptoms. Chronic diarrhea may be a consequence of selected abdominal surgeries including vagotomy and cholecystectomy. Long-standing ethanol abuse impairs small intestinal function and promotes development of pancreatic exocrine insufficiency. A family history of diarrheal illness warrants evaluation for inflammatory bowel disease, celiac sprue, hereditary pancreatitis, or multiple endocrine neoplasia.

Physical Examination

The physical examination can aid in diagnosing diarrhea and determines the severity of illness. Orthostatic pulse or blood pressure changes, decreased skin turgor, and dry mucous membranes indicate the need for intravenous hydration and possible hospital admission, especially in individuals at high risk for severe dehydration (e.g., the very young or very old, patients with mental impairment, those with high fever or those who are unable to tolerate oral intake, and persons with precarious cardiorespiratory or renal disease who cannot tolerate small changes in intravascular volume). Emaciation, edema, peripheral neuropathy, cheilosis, and glossitis result from severe malabsorption. Relevant skin findings include dermatitis herpetiformis with celiac sprue, pyoderma gangrenosum with inflammatory bowel disease, and sclerodactyly with scleroderma. Arthritis may complicate inflammatory bowel disease or Whipple disease. Resting tachycardia suggests hyperthyroidism, whereas pulmonic stenosis and tricuspid regurgitation are found in carcinoid syndrome.

Peripheral or autonomic neuropathy suggests diabetes or intestinal pseudoobstruction. Neuropsychiatric findings are characteristic of Whipple disease. An abdominal mass suggests the presence of malignancy, Crohn's disease, or diverticulitis. Localized abdominal tenderness implicates an inflammatory condition. Rectal examination may reveal perianal disease with Crohn's disease, reduced sphincter tone that could lead to incontinence, and occult or gross fecal blood suggestive of mucosal injury.

Additional Testing

Acute Diarrhea

The management of acute diarrhea depends on its duration and severity. With severe dehydration or hemorrhage, serum electrolytes and a complete blood count should be obtained. Noninfectious causes (e.g., a medication) should be identified and corrected without further investigation. For acute infectious diarrhea without bleeding, severe dehydration, or host factors that impair the ability to clear the infection, the patient should be treated symptomatically with antidiarrheal agents and rehydration if necessary. With complicated or prolonged infection unresponsive to supportive care, liquid stools should be sent for culture, especially if there has been recent travel or there is a suspicion of food-borne illness. Routine stool cultures are readily available for detecting *Salmonella*, *Shigella*, or *Campylobacte.* Special culture techniques are needed to diagnose *Yersinia* and *Plesiomonas* and enterohemorrhagic *E coli.* If parasitic disease is suspected, stool samples may be examined for ova and parasites to find *Giardia*, *Cryptosporidium*, *E. histolytica*, or *Strongyloides.* Not infrequently, parasites are difficult to detect in the stool, and aspiration of duodenal juice or biopsy of the small intestine by endoscopy or fluoroscopy is required. Stool antigen tests also are available for *Giardia.* In individuals with recent antibiotic use, stools should be sent for *C difficile* culture and toxin determination. Twenty percent to 40% of cases of acute infectious diarrheas remain undiagnosed despite laboratory evaluation.

Screening Evaluation of Chronic Diarrhea

Most patients with chronic diarrhea require additional tests to complement the history and physical examination findings (Fig. 12-1). Stools can be examined for leukocytes to provide evidence of mucosal injury. Qualitative stool examination for fat droplets (Sudan stain) serves as a crude screen for malabsorption. Fresh, loose stool samples should be directly examined for parasites, or in rare instances, sent for culture. *Clostridium difficile* can be a cause of chronic as well as acute diarrhea; thus, stool should be tested if there is a history of recent antibiotic use. Serum electrolyte values and a complete blood count are routinely obtained. An elevated erythrocyte sedimentation rate or C-reactive protein raises concern for inflammatory disease. Serum albumin and globulin may be reduced by malabsorption, malnutrition, or protein-losing enteropathy. Protein and hemoglobin levels tend to be lower with small intestinal versus pancreatic etiologies of malabsorption. Endomysial or tissue transglutaminase antibodies are positive in many cases of celiac sprue. Other blood tests that may be abnormal with maldigestion or malabsorption include carotene, iron, folate, vitamin B_{12}, cholesterol, alkaline phosphatase, and prothrombin time. Thyroid hormone testing is indicated in some individuals. Lower endoscopy is advocated to exclude proctitis, pseudomembranes, or melanosis coli secondary to anthracene laxative abuse. If the endoscopic appearance of the colon is normal, random biopsies are performed to test for collagenous and lymphocytic colitis. In patients with normal screening studies, no alarm symptoms to suggest severe organic disease, and relatively low-volume diarrhea, irritable bowel syndrome can be confidently diagnosed.

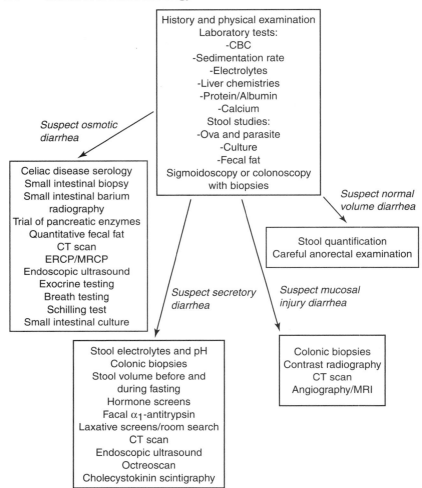

FIGURE 12-1. Workup of a patient with diarrhea (CBC, complete blood count; ERCP/MRCP, endoscopic retrograde cholangiopancreatography/magnetic resonance cholangiopancreatography; CT, computed tomography).

Directed Evaluation of Chronic Diarrhea

If initial testing is unrevealing, subsequent evaluation is directed by the history and examination findings. To evaluate for malabsorption, a 72-hour stool specimen is obtained for fecal fat testing, although the values often will be normal in mild cases of disease of the small intestine or pancreatic insufficiency. If a small intestinal etiology of malabsorption is suspected, duodenal or jejunal biopsies can provide definitive diagnoses of mucosal inflammatory or infiltrative etiologies. An endoscopic appearance of scalloping or a mosaic pattern of the duodenal mucosa suggests possible celiac disease, although other small bowel conditions can give similar appearances. Barium radiography of the small intestine occasionally is useful to evaluate for mucosal diseases, jejunal diverticula with bacterial overgrowth, or fistulae. Suspected Crohn's disease, ulcerative colitis, or infectious processes may warrant further evaluation by colonoscopy or barium radiography. Small bowel aspiration may facilitate the diagnosis of giardiasis or bacterial overgrowth. Breath testing also is used to detect bacterial overgrowth as well as lactase deficiency. Arteriography or mesenteric resonance imaging may be necessary to confirm the diagnosis of mesenteric ischemia. In selected instances, ^{14}C-triolein breath tests can provide evidence of fat malabsorption, whereas D-xylose testing can screen for small intestinal mucosal disease. Schilling tests help distinguish small bowel disease, bacterial overgrowth, and pancreatic disease as causes of malabsorption. Pancreatic etiologies, including chronic pancreatitis and pancreatic neoplasms, can be evaluated by abdominal radiography, endoscopic retrograde pancreatography, endoscopic ultrasound, or exocrine pancreatic function tests in selected referral centers.

Even after careful, directed investigation, a small subset of patients exhibits diarrhea of an elusive nature. Many of these individuals have irritable bowel syndrome, or they abuse laxatives or diuretics. Nevertheless, rarer causes of diarrhea need to be considered. Quantification of stool volume may provide useful diagnostic information. A normal stool volume strongly suggests irritable bowel syndrome. Diarrhea of more than 1 L daily that is unresponsive to fasting suggests a secretory process, whereas osmotic and mucosal injury diarrheas typically exhibit lesser volumes that decrease upon fasting. Secretory diarrhea that abates with nasogastric suction suggests a gastric source such as a gastrinoma. Stool electrolyte and pH values sometimes are obtained as well. Osmotic diarrhea from malabsorption typically is acidic, whereas secretory processes produce stools of neutral pH. A stool osmolarity of 100 mOsm greater than twice the sum of stool sodium and potassium suggests an osmotic cause, whereas lower values are seen with secretory diarrhea. When a secretory process is suggested by these investigations, serum gastrin, VIP, serotonin, calcitonin, histamine, and prostaglandins and urine 5-hydroxyindoleacetic acid can screen for endocrine neoplasia. Further evaluation with abdominal computed tomography, endoscopic ultrasound, and somatostatin receptor scintigraphy is performed to localize the tumor(s) and direct therapy. Octapeptide (^{111}In-OTPA) cholecystokinin analog scanning has been used for medullary thyroid carcinoma. Rare patients will benefit from ^{111}In-labeled leukocyte tests for inflammatory disease or ^{51}Cr-albumin or α_1-antitrypsin tests that demonstrate protein-losing enteropathy. If the entire workup is negative, surreptitious laxative abuse is a serious consideration. A stool osmolarity value less than that of the plasma indicates addition of free water to a fecal specimen. Stool or urine samples can be analyzed for sulfate, magnesium, phosphate, bisacodyl, castor oil, or anthracene derivatives. The role of inpatient room searches by the clinician for hidden laxatives is controversial.

PRINCIPLES OF MANAGEMENT

Therapy for diarrhea depends on its severity and its cause. Fluid resuscitation is crucial in cases of severe diarrhea, especially in infants and elderly patients because they are least able to maintain hydration independently. Oral rehydration solutions maximize intestinal absorption and should be started early in the course of illness. Intravenous crystalloid solutions are indicated for hypotensive patients or those who cannot drink. Serum electrolytes should be closely monitored. Zinc and magnesium losses may be significant with chronic diarrhea, thus specific replacement therapy may be needed.

Whenever possible, the therapy of diarrhea is directed to the underlying cause. Lactose restriction is indicated for lactase deficiency, whereas a gluten-free diet is the appropriate treatment for celiac disease. Inflammatory bowel diseases are treated with specific antiinflammatory medications, whereas pancreatic enzyme replacement is indicated for chronic pancreatitis. Antibiotic therapy of acute infectious diarrhea depends on the causative organism. Antibiotics are indicated for shigellosis, cholera, some cases of traveler's diarrhea, antibiotic-associated colitis, parasites, and sexually transmitted infections. Treatment with an antibiotic is usually recommended for noncholera vibrios; prolonged *Yersinia* infection; early *Campylobacter, Aeromonas,* and *Plesiomonas* infections; and day-care outbreaks of enteropathogenic *E coli.* Antibiotic treatment of O157:H7 enterohemorrhagic *E coli* infection is not recommended because it may predispose to development of hemolytic uremic syndrome. Antibiotics also are indicated for chronic diarrhea secondary to bacterial overgrowth, tropical sprue, and Whipple disease. Viral diarrhea and cryptosporidiosis usually are not treated specifically. For secretory diarrhea secondary to endocrine neoplasia, AIDS, or diabetes, the somatostatin analog octreotide has antisecretory and motor-retarding properties that provide effective antidiarrheal action. Octreotide may also prevent other manifestations of hormone oversecretion such as flushing and tachycardia with carcinoid syndrome. Parenteral calcitonin has shown utility in controlling diarrhea from VIPoma and carcinoid tumors. The α-adrenoceptor agonist clonidine treats diabetic diarrhea and diarrhea associated with opiate withdrawal. Indomethacin is occasionally effective for diarrhea secondary to endocrine tumors and food allergy. Lithium carbonate, bromocriptine, nicotinic acid, phenothiazines, calcium channel antagonists, and serotonin receptor antagonists such as methysergide and cyproheptadine are used in rare cases.

For diseases that do not have a specific treatment, therapy relies on medications that stimulate absorption, inhibit secretion, or retard transit to afford time for improved fluid absorption. The antidiarrheal effects of bismuth subsalicylate in traveler's diarrhea may stem from both antimicrobial and antisecretory properties. Over-the-counter kaolin-pectin preparations are promoted in commercial advertisements, but they exhibit only modest efficacy. The opiate derivatives loperamide, diphenoxylate, codeine, and paregoric are the most common nonspecific treatments for diarrhea and act to retard gut transit by evoking a segmenting motor pattern to promote increased fluid absorption. Diphenoxylate has fewer central nervous system effects than codeine; however, it is sold in combination with atropine so that anticholinergic side effects prevent its abuse. Loperamide does not cross the blood-brain barrier and has minimal central nervous system side effects. Cholestyramine binds bile acids and some toxins and may be useful in some cases. Diarrhea secondary to irritable bowel syndrome may be controlled with antispasmodic drugs such as hyoscyamine, a tricyclic antidepressant, or a serotonin receptor antagonist such as alosetron in cases refractory to opiate agents.

COMPLICATIONS

Most cases of diarrhea in the United States result only in loss of productive work and personal time. However, in other regions of the world and in high-risk patients in the United States (e.g., persons with AIDS), diarrhea is a major cause of morbidity and mortality, especially in children. Diarrhea causes up to 8 million deaths of children yearly because of severe volume depletion or electrolyte disturbances. This group requires aggressive fluid and electrolyte replacement, intravenously with crystalloid formulations, or orally with glucose-electrolyte combinations (e.g., the World Health Organization solution) or commercial formulas (e.g., Pedialyte and Infalyte).

CHAPTER 13

Approach to the Patient with Constipation

DIFFERENTIAL DIAGNOSIS

Constipation, the most prevalent digestive complaint in the United States, is defined as a symptomatic decrease in stool frequency to fewer than three bowel movements per week. Some patients with normal stool frequency report constipation if they pass dry stools, strain during defecation, or experience a sense of incomplete fecal evacuation. The causes of constipation are numerous, including secondary causes and idiopathic disorders, and relate either to impairment of colonic transit or to structural or functional obstruction to fecal evacuation (Table 13-1).

Mechanical Colonic Obstruction

Colonic obstruction may result from mechanical narrowing of the distal colon or anus or from functional outlet obstruction. The most important mechanical cause is colon carcinoma, which typically presents in individuals over age 50 or in selected high-risk groups. Although colon cancer often presents with gross or occult fecal bleeding, a subtle decrease in stool frequency or caliber for weeks to months may be the only initial complaint. Benign colonic strictures resulting from diverticulitis, ischemia, or inflammatory bowel disease produce similar symptoms. Anal strictures, foreign bodies, or spasm from painful fissures or hemorrhoids also may interrupt stool expulsion.

Neuropathic and Myopathic Disorders

Diseases of the extrinsic or the enteric innervation of the colon and anus may produce constipation. Constipation with transection of the sacral nerves or cauda equina, lumbosacral spinal injury, meningomyelocele, or low spinal anesthesia result from colonic hypomotility and dilation, decreased rectal tone and sensation, and impaired defecation. Colonic reflexes are preserved with high spinal lesions; thus, digital stimulation can trigger defecation. However, patients with spinal injury have reduced meal-induced colonic motor activity and impaired rectal sensation and compliance that can contribute to constipation. Constipation is prevalent with multiple sclerosis, cerebrovascular accidents, Parkinson disease, and dysautonomias, including Shy-Drager syndrome.

Hirschsprung disease is the best characterized enteric nervous system disease that presents with constipation. Most commonly, affected infants present with obstipation and proximal colonic dilation at birth. With Hirschsprung, the internal anal sphincter does not relax normally with rectal stimulation because of an absence

TABLE 13-1
Causes of Constipation

Colonic Obstruction
Colorectal neoplasms
Benign strictures (e.g., diverticulitis, ischemia)
Inflammatory bowel disease
Endometriosis
Anal strictures or neoplasms
Rectal foreign bodies
Anal fissures and hemorrhoids

Neuropathic and Myopathic Disorders
Peripheral and autonomic neuropathy
Hirschsprung disease
Chagas disease
Neurofibromatosis
Ganglioneuromatosis
Hypoganglionosis
Intestinal pseudoobstruction
Multiple sclerosis
Spinal cord lesions
Parkinson disease
Shy-Drager syndrome
Transection of sacral nerves or cauda equina
Lumbosacral spinal injury
Meningomyelocele
Low spinal anesthesia
Scleroderma
Amyloidosis
Polymyositis/dermatomyositis
Myotonic dystrophy

Metabolic and Endocrine Disorders
Diabetes mellitus
Pregnancy
Hypercalcemia
Hypothyroidism
Hypokalemia
Porphyria
Glucagonoma
Panhypopituitarism
Pheochromocytoma

Medications
Opiates
Anticholinergics
Tricyclic antidepressants
Antipsychotics
Antiparkinsonian agents
Antihypertensives
Ganglionic blockers
Vinca alkaloids
Anticonvulsants

(continued)

TABLE 13-1
(Continued)

Calcium channel antagonists
Iron supplements
Aluminum antacids
Calcium supplements
Barium sulfate
Heavy metals (i.e., lead, arsenic, mercury)

Idiopathic Constipation
Colonic inertia
Megarectum/megacolon
Rectosphincteric dyssynergia
Rectocele/rectal prolapse
Irritable bowel syndrome

---

of enteric ganglion cells which functionally blocks fecal expulsion. Some individuals with very short segment involvement present with constipation in adulthood or, in rare instances, incontinence. Other enteric nervous system diseases include zonal colonic aganglionosis (in which patchy areas of the colon are devoid of neurons either congenitally or secondary to ischemia), chronic intestinal pseudoobstruction (myopathic and neuropathic), and Chagas disease (resulting from infection with *Trypanosoma cruzi*). Neurofibromatosis, long-standing laxative abuse, and diabetes mellitus may lead to enteric neuronal damage. Idiopathic megacolon is divided into primary and secondary disorders. Primary megacolon is thought to be associated with neuropathic dysfunction. Secondary megacolon and megarectum develop later in life, usually in response to chronic fecal retention. This disorder may be confused with Hirschsprung disease on anorectal manometry, if large enough volumes of rectal distention are not used to elicit anal relaxation on reflex testing.

Rheumatologic disorders evoke a generalized slowing of colonic transit. Dermatomyositis and myotonic dystrophy produce myopathic dysfunction. Amyloidosis and scleroderma may produce either myopathic or neuropathic disease. Constipation in systemic lupus erythematosus has multiple mechanisms, including local ischemia secondary to vasculitis.

Metabolic and Endocrine Disorders

The most common endocrine causes of constipation are diabetes, pregnancy, and hypothyroidism. Although symptoms usually are mild, life-threatening megacolon may develop in myxedema. Other endocrine causes of constipation include hypercalcemia, hypokalemia, porphyria, panhypopituitarism, pheochromocytoma, and glucagonoma.

Medications

Many medications produce mild or severe constipation that may limit their use. Drug classes that slow colonic transit include antispasmodics, tricyclic antidepressants, antipsychotics, anti-parkinsonian agents, opiates, certain antihypertensives, ganglionic blockers, vinca alkaloids, anticonvulsants, and calcium channel antagonists. Cation-containing agents include iron, aluminum antacids, calcium, barium, and heavy metals (i.e., arsenic, lead, mercury).

Idiopathic and Functional Causes

In most patients with constipation, no organic abnormality can be identified that causes their symptoms. The majority of young to middle-aged adults with chronic constipation are women. The most common cause of constipation in association with abdominal pain in this age group is irritable bowel syndrome, which is defined by specific symptom criteria. Thirty percent of patients who complain of infrequent defecation have normal colonic transit on quantitative testing. Many of these individuals exhibit evidence of psychosocial stress and have irritable bowel syndrome as a cause of symptoms. Many individuals with delayed colonic transit exhibit a generalized disorder of propulsion in the colon and are given a diagnosis of slow transit constipation or colonic inertia. Some patients with colonic inertia also exhibit dysmotility of the esophagus, small intestine, or bladder that suggests the presence of a systemic disorder of smooth muscle function. Other persons with delayed colonic transit exhibit a functional impediment to defecation at the level of the anorectum. Causes of outlet obstruction include rectal prolapse, rectal intussusception, rectocele, megarectum, and rectosphincteric dyssynergia. Normal defecation involves the coordinated relaxation of the puborectalis muscle and anal sphincter. With rectosphincteric dyssynergia, ineffective defecation is associated with impaired relaxation or paradoxical contraction of the puborectalis muscle or anal sphincter.

Childhood constipation often manifests as fecal impaction with rectosigmoid dilation. The cause of childhood constipation is uncertain; impaired rectal sensation and altered anal tone are not reliably demonstrable. Many children exhibit evidence of rectosphincteric dyssynergia upon attempted defecation, which may be a learned behavior in response to prior painful defecation problems.

Constipation in the elderly also has several potential etiologies, including mechanical factors, hormonal disturbances, impaired motor function, and effects of medication. Straining with defecation is more commonly reported than infrequent stool passage in the elderly, possibly explaining the high rates of laxative use in this age group. In elderly institutionalized patients, fecal impaction is a common problem because of mental confusion, immobility, or inadequate toilet arrangements.

WORKUP

History

In evaluating constipation, a directed history may uncover evidence of organic or functional disease as well as medication use. Lifelong constipation usually suggests a congenital disorder of coloanal motor function. In adults, a recent change in bowel habits warrants exclusion of organic obstructive disease, whereas a several year history is more consistent with functional disease. Bleeding or anal pain suggests a structural cause of symptoms. Other symptoms (e.g., straining, abdominal pain, bloating, a sense of incomplete evacuation) or associated extracolonic manifestations (e.g., heartburn, nausea, dyspepsia, early satiety, and genitourinary symptoms) are more common with functional disorders such as irritable bowel syndrome. Reports of skin or hair changes, temperature intolerance, or weight gain suggest possible hypothyroidism, whereas weight loss raises concern for malignancy. Underlying systemic illness (e.g., diabetes or a rheumatologic condition) should be determined. A careful history of medication use, including laxative use, is essential. In children, inquiry should be made regarding nightmares, enuresis, school performance, and family tension.

Physical Examination

The examination includes a search for gastrointestinal and nongastrointestinal diseases that can cause constipation. Abdominal masses, hepatomegaly, or lymphadenopathy suggest possible obstructing malignancy. Demonstration of a peripheral or autonomic neuropathy may suggest a neuropathic motility disorder. The anorectal examination can detect tumors, strictures, fissures, hemorrhoids, and rectal prolapse. Occult or gross fecal blood warrants a search for neoplasm or inflammatory disease, although local anorectal disease commonly produces blood loss. Anorectal neuromuscular function is tested by assessing basal anal tone; adequacy of maximal anal squeeze;, and perianal cutaneous sensation, including the anal wink. Long-standing constipation with straining and prolapse may produce anal or perineal nerve damage that leads to reduced anal pressure and fecal incontinence. Examination during attempted defecation maneuvers can suggest rectal prolapse and evidence of rectosphincteric dyssynergia. Pelvic examination in women may demonstrate a rectocele with straining.

Additional Testing

Laboratory Studies

If the history or examination suggests systemic or local anorectal disease, further evaluation may be needed (Fig. 13-1). Detecting microcytic anemia from a complete blood count raises concern for colonic neoplasm or inflammatory disease. Other screening tests include measuring serum calcium to exclude hyperparathyroidism and thyroid stimulating hormone levels to exclude hypothyroidism. Specific serologic tests can detect rheumatologic disease, Chagas disease, or paraneoplastic pseudoobstruction, whereas other assays are used for catecholamines, porphyrins, and glucagon.

Structural Studies

Endoscopic or radiographic evaluation is performed on any individual with suspected mechanical obstruction as a cause of constipation. In young patients, flexible sigmoidoscopy excludes distal occlusive lesions and can detect melanosis coli, a brown-black mucosal discoloration from chronic anthraquinone laxative use. For patients older than 40 to 45 years or if alarm findings such as bleeding are present, it is important to evaluate the entire colon by colonoscopy because of the increased risk of colorectal neoplasm. Barium enema radiography can show proximal colonic dilation as well as persistent contraction of the denervated segment in Hirschsprung disease. Deep rectal biopsy specimens obtained at least 3 cm above the anal verge are obtained to exclude Hirschsprung disease, when indicated.

Functional Studies

After structural diseases have been excluded, empiric trials of medical therapy are offered. For a patient whose condition is refractory to standard treatment, additional evaluation may be indicated to assess the functional integrity of the colon and anorectum. The transit of stool through different colonic regions can be quantified by obtaining serial abdominal radiographs after ingesting plastic radiopaque markers. Marker studies can distinguish between slow transit constipation (also known as colonic inertia), in which transit is delayed in all colonic regions, and functional outlet obstruction, where marker passage is selectively retarded at the level of the anorectum. Colonic transit is tested concurrently with a bowel diary to quantify defecation frequency. In some cases, marker elimination is normal, even though the patient denies stool output. Such individuals often exhibit psychological

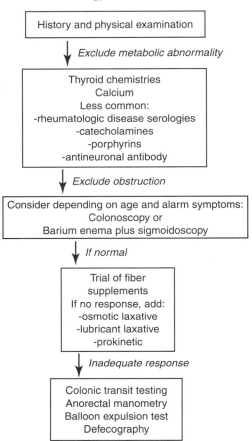

FIGURE 13-1. Workup of a patient with constipation.

disturbances that contribute to their symptoms. Some referral centers perform colonic transit scintigraphy. However, this technique offers few advantages over radiopaque marker studies and is not widely used.

Anorectal manometry assesses anorectal function in patients with straining and suspected functional outlet obstruction. Rectal sensation is quantified during progressive rectal balloon inflation. Some patients with irritable bowel syndrome tolerate balloon distention poorly, whereas individuals with megarectum accommodate large balloon volumes without sensing a need to defecate. Measurement of anal tone during rectal balloon inflation detects a volume-dependent relaxation, a phenomenon known as the *rectoanal inhibitory reflex*. Loss of this reflex suggests possible Hirschsprung disease, The diagnosis must be confirmed by deep rectal biopsy because falsely absent rectoanal inhibitory reflexes are present with megarectum if inadequate rectal volumes are delivered. Attempted defecation maneuvers, including expulsion of a rectal balloon, can help to assess for abnormalities of anal relaxation. Rectosphincteric dyssynergia is suggested by manometric demonstration of increased anal tone with attempted defecation. Manometry is complemented by electromyography of the anal sphincter in some centers.

Defecography involves cinefluoroscopic recording of the attempted defecation of barium paste which is infused into the rectum. Structural abnormalities, including rectoceles and rectal prolapse or intussusception, can be diagnosed by this technique. Defecography also quantifies the anorectal angle at rest and with defecation. Rectosphincteric dyssynergia is characterized by a paradoxical decrease in this angle during defecation, which precludes evacuation of the rectal contrast material.

PRINCIPLES OF MANAGEMENT

Dietary and Behavioral Approaches

Once structural and metabolic causes of constipation are excluded and offending medications are withdrawn, dietary and lifestyle changes can be offered. Many persons respond to increasing fiber intake to 20 to 30 g per day. Wheat bran is most effective in increasing stool weight and accelerating colonic transit, followed by fruits and vegetables, oats, corn, cellulose, soya, and pectin. In patients with irritable bowel syndrome, fiber should be gradually increased to minimize bloating. Establishing routine defecation after meals is recommended to take advantage of the gastrocolonic reflex, the increase in colonic motility that occurs in the initial postprandial hour. Daily exercise, such as walking or running, is encouraged.

Pharmacological Therapy

Bulk-forming agents such as psyllium, methylcellulose, and polycarbophil may be given to patients who do not respond to dietary measures. These agents increase stool volume, improve fecal hydration, and increase colonic bacterial mass, leading to acceleration of colonic transit and reduced straining. If bulking agents are ineffective or produce unacceptable gas and bloating, hypertonic cationic and anionic (magnesium hydroxide), lubricant (mineral oil), or hyperosmotic sugar (sorbitol, lactulose) laxatives or stool softeners (docusate salts) may be useful. Cationic laxatives increase intralumenal water content by their osmotic effects. The use of magnesium products should be avoided in renal failure. Many such agents also can be given in the enema form to effect prompt defecation. Mineral oil penetrates and softens the stool but may reduce absorption of vitamins A, D, and K. Sorbitol and lactulose are nonabsorbable sugars that are degraded by colonic bacteria to increase stool osmolarity. Docusate salts are anionic surfactants that reduce fecal surface tension, allowing better mixing of aqueous and fatty substances thereby softening the stool. Stimulant laxatives include castor oil, anthraquinones (e.g., cascara, senna, casanthranol, and danthron), and phenylmethanes (e.g., phenolphthalein and bisacodyl). Anthraquinones may produce melanosis coli, whereas danthron has reported hepatotoxic effects. Phenolphthalein has been associated with nongastrointestinal neoplasms in rodents and has been removed from the U.S. market. The use of some stimulant laxatives purportedly produces long-term damage of colonic enteric nerves.

Other medications are useful in selected patients. Isotonic electrolyte solutions containing polyethylene glycol may promote a gentle laxative effect without uncomfortable side effects in patients who develop cramping with hypertonic laxatives. The prokinetic drug tegaserod increases stool frequency, improves stool consistency, and reduces bloating and straining in patients with chronic constipation as well as those with constipation-predominant irritable bowel syndrome. For patients with more refractory constipation, the prostaglandin analog misoprostol and the antigout drug colchicine exhibit impressive stimulatory effects on colonic function.

However, these agents may produce significant cramping in some individuals. Furthermore, misoprostol should be used with care in women of reproductive potential because of its abortifacient properties.

Nonpharmacological Treatment

Nonmedication treatments are more appropriate for some causes of constipation. Biofeedback techniques using manometry or electromyography are indicated for selected conditions of anorectal dysfunction that do not respond to laxative therapy. With these methods, rectal sensation can be enhanced and paradoxical anal contractions with defecation can be corrected with learned behaviors. Surgery is indicated for Hirschsprung disease. Anal myotomy may be beneficial with short segment involvement, whereas resection, bypass, or endorectal pull-through procedures are performed for more typical presentations of the disease. Subtotal colectomy with ileorectal anastomosis may be beneficial in carefully selected patients with severe colonic inertia that is unresponsive to medications. Surgical resection or reduction of large rectoceles is considered in patients when digital pressure on the pelvis or posterior vaginal wall results in improved fecal evacuation. Rectal prolapse may be surgically repaired with suspension or rectopexy, although these operations often have no effect on the underlying defecation problem. Surgery for rectosphincteric dyssynergia is contraindicated because of a high risk of postoperative incontinence.

COMPLICATIONS

Chronic constipation may lead to rectal prolapse, hemorrhoidal bleeding, or development of an anal fissure. Fecal impaction may produce colonic obstruction or stercoral ulcers, which can bleed or perforate. Large fecalomas may cause extrinsic ureteral compression, resulting in recurrent urinary infections. Fecal incontinence results from anal sphincter damage or perineal nerve dysfunction from straining or prolapse.

CHAPTER 14

Approach to the Patient with an Abdominal Mass

Mass lesions in the abdomen may arise from localized infection or from inflammation, trauma, vascular disease, or neoplasm. These can be difficult to distinguish from the history and physical examination alone, given that the clinical presentation often is nonspecific. Careful radiologic or endoscopic characterization of the lesion is important because the etiology determines the clinical management and prognosis.

DIFFERENTIAL DIAGNOSIS

The differential diagnosis of abdominal masses is broad (Table 14-1). The likelihood of finding unresectable neoplasm also is highly variable, depending on the anatomic site of its origin. Many intra-abdominal masses present with pain, whereas others present with bleeding, systemic symptoms such as weight loss or fever, or obstruction. Others are detected while still asymptomatic as part of a routine health care surveillance program.

Liver Masses

Both solid and cystic masses may develop in the liver. Causes of single solid hepatic masses include hemangiomas, adenomas, focal nodular hyperplasia, focal fatty infiltration, leiomyomas, teratomas, hepatocellular carcinoma, lymphomas, sarcomas, and solitary metastases from distant cancer. The presence of multiple solid lesions should prompt a search for extrahepatic malignancy, most commonly from the breast, colon, or lung. Cystic masses include benign cysts, bacterial liver abscesses (which may be multiple), amoebic abscess, and *echinococcal cysts*.

Pancreaticobiliary Masses

Most solid masses in the pancreas are malignant. Pancreatic adenocarcinoma usually arises from pancreatic ductal epithelium. Other solid pancreatic masses include lymphoma, solid and papillary epithelial neoplasms, and neuroendocrine tumors (insulinomas, gastrinomas, glucagonomas, somatostatinomas, VIPomas). Pancreatic masses with cystic components include pancreatic pseudocysts complicating pancreatitis, mucinous or serous cystadenoma, cystadenocarcinoma, and intraductal papillary mucinous tumors.

Masses of the biliary tree also may be cystic or solid. Cystic lesions include choledochal cysts and Caroli disease, which is characterized by segmental dilation of the intrahepatic bile ducts. Cholangiocarcinoma is the most common malignant tumor of the bile ducts. Other biliary tumors include gallbladder carcinoma, bile duct adenomas, cystadenomas, and granular cell tumors.

Gastrointestinal Masses

Masses involving the lumenal gastrointestinal tract are prevalent. Adenocarcinoma accounts for 95% of gastric cancers. Lymphoma is the second most common cell type. Small intestinal masses more commonly are benign and include adenomas, hamartoma, fibromas, and angiomas. Adenocarcinoma, leiomyosarcoma, and lymphoma are malignancies that arise from the small intestine. The most common colorectal masses are benign polyps including nonadenomatous (hyperplastic, hamartoma) and adenomatous growths. Polyps may be sporadic, occur in those with risk factors such as a positive family history or long-standing colitis, or arise as part of a hereditary polyposis syndrome. Adenocarcinomas constitute the majority of colorectal cancers, although lymphoma and Kaposi sarcoma also occur. Benign colonic masses may be due to perforation of an inflamed appendix, selected infections (e.g. amebiasis), or inflammation from Crohn's disease. The appearance of colorectal cancer can be mimicked by colitis cystica profunda, a benign disease characterized by submucosal mucus-filled cysts. Carcinoids arise most commonly in the appendix, followed by the ileum, rectum, and stomach. Gastrinomas may originate in the pancreas or in the proximal bowel wall. Tumors originating from

TABLE 14-1
Causes of Abdominal Masses

Hepatic Masses
Hemangioma
Adenoma
Focal nodular hyperplasia
Focal fatty infiltration
Hepatocellular carcinoma
Lymphoma
Sarcoma
Leimyoma
Teratoma
Metastatic tumor
Abscess
Benign cysts
Echinococcal cyst

Pancreaticobiliary Masses
Pancreatic adenocarcinoma
Lymphoma
Neuroendocrine tumors
Pseudocysts
Abscess
Mucinous and serous cystadenoma
Cystadenocarcinoma
Intraductal papillary mucinous tumors
Bile duct adenoma
Choledochocele
Cholangiocarcinoma
Gallbladder carcinoma
Granular cell tumor

Gastrointestinal Masses
Adenocarcinoma
Adenoma
Lymphoma
Hyperplastic polyps
Hamartoma
Leiomyoma
Leiomyosarcoma
Leioblastoma
Kaposi sarcoma
Carcinoid
Colitis cystica profunda
Lipoma
Liposarcoma
Angioma
Neuroma
Schwannoma
Inflammatory mass (Crohn's disease, appendicitis)
Abscess

(continued)

TABLE 14-1
(Continued)

Miscellaneous Masses

Renal cell carcinoma
Renal cyst
Transitional cell carcinoma of the renal pelvis
Renal lymphoma
Mesenteric cyst
Cystic teratoma
Mesothelioma
Hematoma
Abdominal aortic aneurysm
Ovarian carcinoma
Ovarian cyst
Uterine fibroma
Uterine carcinoma
Tuboovarian abscess
Ectopic pregnancy

smooth muscle (leiomyoma, leiomyosarcoma) or fat (lipoma, liposarcoma) may be seen throughout the digestive tract. Less common cell types include neurofibromas, schwannomas, and leioblastomas.

Miscellaneous Masses

Miscellaneous lesions may present as abdominal masses. Renal masses may be infectious, neoplastic, or congenital. The most common malignancy is renal cell carcinoma. Other neoplasms include transitional cell carcinoma of the renal pelvis with parenchymal invasion, lymphoma, and renal oncocytoma. Renal cysts most commonly are benign but may harbor carcinoma especially in patients with von Hippel-Lindau or tuberous sclerosis. Cystic masses in the mesentery include mesenteric cysts, cystic teratomas, and cystic mesotheliomas. A hematoma is considered in any patient with a history of blunt abdominal trauma. Abdominal aortic aneurysms may be detected as pulsatile abdominal masses. Gynecologic masses involving the ovaries or uterus may be palpable on abdominal examination.

WORKUP

History

The history provides important clues to the etiology of an abdominal mass. Pain related to meals or defecation suggests a lumenal origin, whereas gross or occult fecal bleeding or alterations in bowel function suggest either a primary source within or invasion of a lumenal site. Nausea and vomiting with abdominal distention raise concern for an obstructive process within the proximal gut. Dysuria or hematuria may indicate involvement of the urinary tract either by primary disease or by local irritation, as with Crohn's disease. Jaundice suggests benign or malignant obstruction at the level of the pancreas or bile ducts. Impingement of a large mass on surrounding vasculature may present with lower extremity edema or intestinal ischemia. Ascites may indicate peritoneal metastases from an intra-abdominal malignancy or a worsening of liver function in a cirrhotic patient with hepatocellular carcinoma. High fever points toward an intra-abdominal abscess, whereas unexpected loss of more than 5% of body weight raises suspicion of malignancy. Medications may predispose to selected liver masses (e.g., hepatic adenoma with oral contraceptive use). Paraneoplastic syndromes may suggest specific malignancies: pseudoachalasia may relate to hepatocellular carcinoma, dermatomyositis may develop with lumenal cancer, seborrheic keratoses (Leser-Trélat sign) or acanthosis nigricans are seen with gastric cancer, and deep venous thromboses (Trousseau syndrome) are found with intra-abdominal adenocarcinoma. A family history of neoplasia or inflammatory bowel disease may suggest these as etiologies.

Physical Examination

A general physical examination as well as directed assessment of the mass complements the history. Scleral icterus or jaundice suggests liver infiltration versus biliary obstruction from a bile duct or pancreatic tumor. Temperature higher than 38°C is consistent with an infectious or inflammatory process such as an intra-abdominal abscess. Lower fevers may accompany some neoplasms. If the mass is tender as with Crohn's disease, this suggests that the mass is inflammatory. Lymphadenopathy raises concern for metastatic malignancy. Palpable supraclavicular (Virchow) or periumbilical (Sister Mary Joseph) nodes are found with gastric cancer. Rectal examination detects approximately half of all rectal neoplasms. Occult fecal blood is highly predictive of malignancy in a patient with a known abdominal mass.

Additional Testing

Laboratory Studies

Laboratory tests are important in evaluating selected abdominal masses. A complete blood count can test for anemia due to blood loss or chronic disease or for leukocytosis with inflammation or localized infection such as an abscess. Liver chemistry levels are abnormal with some hepatobiliary neoplasms. Determination of chronic liver chemistry abnormalities with the new onset of a liver mass suggests possible hepatocellular carcinoma arising in preexisting cirrhosis. Amylase and lipase values may be elevated in some pancreatic cancers. Endocrine neoplasms may secrete hormones that can be detected by specific blood tests or measurement of urinary metabolites. Serum tumor markers may provide adjunctive information in the diagnostic workup. CA 19-9 and CA 242 are reasonably sensitive for detecting pancreatic adenocarcinoma but are not specific. Carcinoembryonic antigen is elevated with colon cancer as well as with benign liver and pancreatic diseases. Alpha fetoprotein is secreted by larger hepatocellular carcinomas. Ovarian tumors are suggested by elevations of CA 125. If ascites is present, cytological examination may reveal malignant cells. Serologies for infections such as echinococcosis may be obtained for suspicious cystic liver masses. A high level of triglycerides in the ascitic fluid indicates chylous ascites possibly due to lymphoma. Hematuria is worrisome for urologic malignancy versus bladder or uerteral involvement by intra-abdominal tumors. Aspiration of pus with Gram stain and culture can provide both a diagnosis and treatment of selected intra-abdominal abscesses.

Structural Studies

Endoscopy of the gastrointestinal tract is useful in evaluating suspected lumenal masses because of the ability to visualize suspicious lesions directly and because of the capability of obtaining biopsies. Routine upper endoscopy evaluates to the descending duodenum. Enteroscopy can be used to evaluate more distal small intestinal masses. Push enteroscopy can reach lesions in the upper jejunum. When there is no evidence of obstruction, capsule endoscopy may detect unsuspected small bowel tumors in patients with unexplained blood loss. Sigmoidoscopy examines the colon distal to the splenic flexure in optimally prepared patients, whereas colonoscopy visualizes the entire organ as well as the distal ileum. Endoscopic retrograde cholangiopancreatography defines filling defects within the pancreas or biliary tree and can obtain diagnostic brushings in approximately 50% of pancreaticobiliary neoplasms. Endoscopic ultrasound provides additional detail in characterizing tumors of the gut lumen and pancreaticobiliary tree and can determine if local disease extension precludes surgical resection.

Radiologic and radionuclide imaging techniques are useful for evaluating suspected masses in the solid organs of the abdomen, pelvis, and retroperitoneum and in regions of the gut lumen that are poorly investigated by endoscopic techniques. Ultrasound is an effective screening examination for imaging the biliary tree and liver. Computed tomography provides a more detailed and comprehensive evaluation of suspected neoplasia in many organs. Specialized dedicated protocols have been developed to focus on selected regions such as the pancreas. Both techniques are of value in diagnosing intra-abdominal abscess as well. Both modalities can be used to direct needle aspiration or biopsy of suspected lesions. Magnetic resonance imaging is especially useful in the study of selected liver masses and can help delineate the presence of hemangiomas, focal nodular hyperplasia, adenomas, and other abnormalities. Magnetic resonance cholangiopancreatography can assess for abnormalities within the bile and pancreatic ducts. Selected nuclear medicine tests are indicated in evaluating certain abdominal masses. Octreoscanning has assumed a crucial role in investigating suspected endocrine neoplasia. ^{111}In-labelled leukocyte scans may define the extent and locations of intra-abdominal abscesses. ^{18}F-fluorodeoxyglucose positron emission tomography is emerging as a promising modality for characterizing selected intra-abdominal malignancies.

Histopathological Evaluation

In many instances, tissue must be obtained to distinguish accurately between a malignant and a noncancerous etiology of a radiographically or endoscopically detected mass. For solitary liver lesions, a directed biopsy can be obtained under laparoscopic guidance. If radiographic testing suggests hepatic adenoma, surgical resection is advised rather than biopsy due to the risk of hemorrhage. When multiple liver lesions suggest metastases, computed tomography or ultrasound can be used to direct percutaneous biopsy. Percutaneous biopsy is not recommended for suspected renal cell cancer because of the risk of seeding the needle tract with malignant cells. For suspected resectable pancreatic cancer, tissue is best obtained using endoscopic retrograde cholangiopancreatography or endoscopic ultrasound. Mucosal masses in the stomach, colon, and rectum often are easily accessible to endoscopy for biopsy. Tissue from submucosal biopsies may be obtained by endoscopic ultrasound.

PRINCIPLES OF MANAGEMENT

Management of an intra-abdominal mass depends on the nature of the mass and whether it is malignant, has disseminated, and is no longer surgically resectable. In general, solitary neoplasms are best cured by operative removal. Additional benefit may be obtained with adjuvant chemotherapy with or without concomitant radiotherapy in some settings, as with certain colorectal carcinomas. Intra-abdominal carcinomas with local or distant spread that preclude resection may be subjected to systemic chemotherapy with variable, often disappointing results. Other multifocal neoplasms such as lymphomas may be more responsive to cytotoxic chemotherapy. Some endocrine tumors may respond to hormonal suppression using chronic therapy with the somatostatin analog octreotide. Abdominal abscesses should be drained percutaneously or surgically and therapy should be directed at the underlying cause (e.g., active Crohn's disease). Pancreatic pseudocysts can be drained percutaneously, endoscopically, or surgically. Finally, endoscopy can be used to remove large polyps (including some with superficial carcinoma) using a snare and retrieval technique.

COMPLICATIONS

The complications associated with an abdominal mass depend on its location and histological characteristics. Lumenal obstruction results from gut mucosal tumors, whereas biliary obstruction is a consequence of bile duct or pancreatic masses. Certain masses such as hepatic adenomas may rupture and produce life-threatening hemorrhage. Abscesses may not respond to antibiotic therapy and may have lethal outcomes if not appropriately drained. Similarly, many malignant tumors are fatal, especially if dissemination has already occurred when diagnosed.

CHAPTER 15

Approach to the Patient with Ileostomy or Ileal Pouch

STANDARD END ILEOSTOMY

Technique

Proctocolectomy with end ileostomy (Brooke ileostomy) is performed for patients who require excision of the entire colon and rectum for ulcerative colitis, familial adenomatous polyposis, or multiple colonic malignancies. The technique was the gold standard for ulcerative colitis until the 1980s when the ileal pouch–anal canal anastomosis became widely available. The Brooke ileostomy is constructed from the terminal ileum and is positioned in the right lower quadrant of the abdomen (Table 15-1). The fecal effluent is collected in an external appliance that the patient wears continuously. If properly constructed, Brooke ileostomies are remarkably safe and reliable. Currently, the operation is reserved for older patients and obese individuals in whom construction of an ileal pouch–anal canal anastomosis would be technically difficult. Ileostomies also are the procedure of choice for individuals

TABLE 15-1
Characteristics of Ileostomy and Ileal Pouch Operations

PROCEDURE	CONTINENCE RETAINED	STOMA PRESENT	INTUBATIONS REQUIRED	DISADVANTAGES
Brooke ileostomy	No	Yes	No	Appliance needed
Kock pouch	Yes	Yes	Yes	Valve malfunction, pouchitis
Ileal pouch–anal canal	Yes	No	No	Incontinence, pouchitis

with intrinsic anal dysfunction or with Crohn's disease where concern exists for perianal complications.

Preoperatively, the nutritional and hemodynamic statuses are stabilized and the patient is given detailed education by a stoma therapist. For individuals on chronic corticosteroids, stress doses may be needed during the perioperative and early postoperative period. In most cases, the ileostomy usually begins to discharge effluent by the third postoperative day. The normal ileostomy output averages 600 mL per day. High ileostomy outputs (>1 L per day) may mandate intravenous fluid replacement.

Complications

The Brooke ileostomy has low postoperative morbidity. Rare cases of infection, abscess, bleeding, or delayed healing of the perineal dissection can occur in the early postoperative period. Impotence is reported by 2% to 3% of male patients after surgery. Development of urinary or sexual dysfunction can be minimized if excision of the rectum and anus is done in the intersphincteric or submucosal plane away from the nerve bundles. Temporary dyspareunia in women may result from posterior displacement of the vagina. Stomal obstruction, retraction, prolapse, and bleeding can occur in 5% of patients in the late postoperative period, as can diarrhea and peristomal hernias. Surgery may be required to treat these complications. Other late complications include nephrolithiasis and gallstones. Uric acid kidney stones result from mild chronic dehydration and acidosis that predispose to precipitation of uric acid in the urine. Adequate fluid intake, with supplemental alkali in rare cases, prevents this complication. Gallstones result from bile salt depletion in individuals who have undergone significant ileal resection in addition to the colectomy. There is no defined prophylaxis for this complication.

Outcome

After the Brooke ileostomy, patients quickly regain good health and should expect good long-term stomal function. For some patients, the appliances are unsightly, uncomfortable, and mildly odorous, and noises may emanate from the stoma. Peristomal skin breakdown may result from stool or gas leakage around ill-fitting appliances. Because of these factors, 15% of patients note mild to moderate restriction of daily activities, and 9% report severe restrictions.

CONTINENT ILEOSTOMY

Technique

The continent ileostomy, or Kock pouch, is constructed from the distal 30 cm of the terminal ileum. Intussuscepting the terminal ileum backward into the pouch and anchoring the intussusceptum in place with staples creates a valve that prevents distal outflow from the pouch. This operation serves as an alternative to the Brooke ileostomy, in that continence is provided, and to the ileal pouch–anal canal anastomosis, in those individuals for whom the procedure is contraindicated or fails (see Table 15-1). Because it provides continence, the Kock pouch does not require an ileostomy appliance, and the stoma may be fashioned flush with the skin and placed nearer the pubis to make it less conspicuous. With the advent of ileal pouch–anal canal anastomoses, Kock pouches have fallen out of favor to some degree. Contraindications to this operation include very young or very old individuals, obese patients, and patients with persistent ileal Crohn's disease.

The patient empties the pouch at regular intervals by passing a catheter through the stoma and valve into the pouch and draining the effluent directly into a toilet. The catheter is removed, washed, and carried by the patient until it is needed again. In the first postoperative month, the pouch is drained continuously to ensure healing. The pouch is drained every 2 hours for an additional month. When mature, Kock pouches require emptying four times daily, with no requirement for nightly intubation. The pouch should be irrigated free of debris once daily with warm water or saline.

Complications

Complications specific to the Kock pouch include malfunction of the valve and pouchitis. Valve slippage results from partial disruption of the intussuscepted segment within the pouch and presents as difficulty with pouch intubation and pouch leakage. This complication usually mandates reoperation. Valve prolapse requires surgery to replace and reanchor the valve into the pouch and narrow the opening in the abdominal wall. Stomal stenosis results from local ischemia and is correctable by local construction of a new stoma. Pouchitis presents with frequent watery stools, cramps, malaise, fever, arthralgias, and uveitis and results from bacterial overgrowth with retained feces or to immune reactions to bacterial products. Endoscopy reveals mucosal edema, friability, and punctate erosions. Treatment of pouchitis commonly relies on oral antibiotics (e.g., metronidazole), although probiotic compounds that contain active bacterial cultures are used in some individuals. Multiple antibiotic courses may be needed because pouchitis frequently is chronic.

Outcome

Long-term follow-up studies of patients who have undergone the Kock procedure report continence rates of 70% to 89% with 95% of patients free from wearing an appliance. The Kock pouch tends to restrict physical and sexual activity to greater degrees than the ileal pouch–anal canal anastomosis, but produces fewer such restrictions than the Brooke ileostomy.

ILEAL POUCH–ANAL CANAL ANASTOMOSIS

Technique

Total proctocolectomy and rectal mucosal stripping with construction of an ileal pouch–anal canal anastomosis is the procedure of choice for most patients with ulcerative colitis, familial adenomatous polyposis, and multiple colorectal malignancies (see Table 15-1). Because mucosal stripping is performed endorectally, the nerve supply to the anus, bladder, and genitalia is usually not disrupted, thereby minimizing the risks of postoperative fecal or urinary incontinence and sexual dysfunction. Contraindications to ileal pouch–anal canal anastomosis include Crohn's disease (high risk of disease activation in the pouch), distal rectal cancer (cannot ensure adequate tumor-free margins), and poor preoperative anal function (Table 15-2). Obesity is a relative contraindication to the procedure because of the increased technical difficulty in pouch construction and placement. The ileal pouch–anal canal anastomosis can be considered in patients with indeterminate colitis, although the risk of complications is higher due to possible subsequent evolution to ileal Crohn's disease. The operation is not usually performed in an emergency setting (i.e., acute severe colitis, toxic megacolon, colonic perforation with peritonitis, and acute colonic obstruction). In these instances, a temporary Brooke ileostomy

---

TABLE 15-2
Indications and Contraindications for ileal pouch–anal canal Anastomosis

Indications
  Chronic ulcerative colitis
  Familial adenomatous polyposis
  Multiple colorectal malignancies

Contraindications
  Crohn's disease
  Distal rectal or anal malignancy
  Poor anal sphincter function
  Anal sphincter excised

Relative Contraindications
  Morbid obesity
  Emergency operation

---

is formed, the rectum is closed at its proximal end, and the ileal pouch–anal canal anastomosis is accomplished at a second operation 6 to 12 months later. Severe inanition and chronic high-dose steroids may impair wound healing. Age over 50 years is no longer a contraindication to ileal pouch–anal canal anastomosis.

The goal of the operation is to remove all diseased colonic tissue. In most instances, a 3- to 5-cm mucosally stripped region of rectal muscle anchors the ileal pouch and preserves anal innervation. J-shaped pouches constructed from the distal 30 to 35 cm of ileum are most prevalent, although S-, H-, and W-shaped pouches are also assembled. Pouch capacities are similar to that of the healthy rectum (300 mL) and can evacuate 65% to 85% of their contents within 15 seconds. A temporary diverting ileostomy may be placed at the time of initial surgery to ensure anastomotic healing; it can then be closed 3 months later. Patients younger than 30 years, with minimal inflammation, in good health, and who are not taking high-dose steroids may not require a diverting ileostomy. In the first postoperative month, patients are started on low-fiber diets and given loperamide to reduce stool frequency.

Complications

Despite the clear advantages of the ileal pouch–anal canal anastomosis over other surgeries, postoperative complications are common. Septic complications occur in approximately 7% of patients, and reoperation is needed in 24%. Complications requiring removal of the pouch and conversion to an ileostomy occur in 3%. Daytime and nighttime incontinence persist in 7% and 12% of patients, respectively. One quarter of patients develop pouchitis. Sclerosing cholangitis, cirrhosis, and indeterminate colitis are risk factors for pouchitis. Early postoperative complications include obstruction (13%), local infection (8%), urinary dysfunction (7%), transient impotence and retrograde ejaculation (3%), dyspareunia (11%), and dehydration.

Outcome

Functional results and quality of life after ileal pouch–anal canal anastomosis are good to excellent in 93% of cases. After pouch maturation, the mean number of stools is five during daytime and once at night, although older patients may have a higher defecation frequency. Patients with familial adenomatous polyposis have fewer bowel movements than those with colitis. Nutrient digestion and absorption are unimpaired by the ileal pouch–anal canal anastomosis. Vitamin B_{12} malabsorption has not been reported. Fecal output averages 650 mL per day, leading to mild compensatory reductions in urine output. Resting anal pressures are initially reduced initially by 10% and return to normal within 1 year; anal squeeze pressures are normal. Episodic decreases in anal tone occur during rapid eye movement sleep, as they do in healthy controls, which may predispose some patients to nocturnal fecal leakage. Anal canal sensation is intact; however, the rectoanal inhibitory reflex is usually lost without apparent effect on defecatory function. In pregnant patients, ileal pouch–anal canal anastomosis does not preclude normal vaginal delivery.

CHAPTER 16

Approach to the Patient with Jaundice

DIFFERENTIAL DIAGNOSIS

Jaundice, a yellow discoloration of the sclera, skin, and mucous membranes, results from the accumulation of bilirubin, a by-product of heme metabolism. It must be distinguished from yellow pigmentation caused by ingesting foods rich in carotene (carrots) or lycopene (tomatoes) or drugs such as quinacrine (atabrine) or busulfan. Of the 250 to 300 mg of bilirubin produced daily, 70% results from the reticuloendothelial breakdown of senescent erythrocytes. Bilirubin is cleared by the liver in a three-step process. Bilirubin is first transported into hepatocytes by specific membrane carriers. It is then conjugated to one or two molecules of glucuronide. Finally, the conjugated bilirubin moves to the canalicular membrane, where it is excreted into the bile canaliculus by another carrier protein. Once in the bile, most conjugated bilirubin is excreted in the feces, although a small amount is deconjugated by colonic bacteria and reabsorbed. Colonic bacteria also reduce bilirubin to urobilinogens that are reabsorbed and excreted in urine.

Normal bilirubin levels are 0.4 ± 0.2 mg/dL, and more than 95% is unconjugated. Hyperbilirubinemia is defined as a total bilirubin level higher than 1.5 mg/dL, an unconjugated level higher than 1.0 mg/dL, and a conjugated level higher than 0.3 mg/dL. Generally, the serum bilirubin level must exceed 2.5 to 3.0 mg/dL for jaundice to be visible. Hyperbilirubinemia is separated into two classes: unconjugated (>80% of total bilirubin) and conjugated (>30% of total bilirubin) (Table 16-1). With prolonged jaundice, circulating bilirubin may bind covalently to albumin, which prevents its elimination until the albumin is degraded. Therefore, with certain cholestatic disorders, measurable hyperbilirubinemia persists after the disease is resolved. Conjugated bilirubin is cleared by renal glomeruli; in renal failure, bilirubin levels may increase enormously.

TABLE 16-1
Causes of Conjugated Hyperbilirubinemia

Congenital Conjugated
Hyperbilirubinemias
  Rotor syndrome
  Dubin-Johnson syndrome

Intrahepatic Cholestasis
Familial and congenital
  Progressive familial intrahepatic
    cholestasis, type 1 to 3
  Benign recurrent intrahepatic
    cholestasis
  Cholestasis of pregnancy
  Choledochal cysts, Caroli disease
  Congenital biliary atresia
Hepatocellular conditions
  Alcohol-related disorders
  Viral hepatitis
  Autoimmune disease
  Cirrhosis
  Drug-related disorders
  Wilson disease
  Hereditary hemochromatosis
Infiltrative conditions
  Granulomatous
  Carcinoma
  Hematologic malignant disease
  Amyloidosis
Cholangiopathies
  Primary biliary cirrhosis
  Idiopathic adult ductopenia
Infections
  Bacterial
  Fungal
  Parasitic
  HIV-related
Miscellaneous causes
  Postoperative sepsis
  Pregnancy
  Total parenteral nutrition
  Cholestasis after liver
    transplantation

Extrahepatic Cholestasis
Inside bile ducts
  Calculi
  Parasites
Inside wall
  Stricture
  Cholangiocarcinoma
  Sclerosing cholangitis
  Choledochal cysts
Outside duct wall
  Tumor in porta hepatis
  Tumor in pancreas
  Pancreatitis, acute or chronic

Unconjugated Hyperbilirubinemia

Hemolysis and Ineffective Erythropoiesis

Hemolysis and ineffective erythropoiesis lead to overproduction of bilirubin that exceeds the conjugative capability of the liver. Hemolysis may result from sickle cell anemia, thalassemia, glucose-6-phosphate dehydrogenase deficiency, paroxysmal nocturnal hemoglobinuria, ABO blood group incompatibility, or medications. Severe hemolysis rarely elevates serum bilirubin levels above 5 mg/dL, although hepatocyte dysfunction or Gilbert syndrome can magnify the hyperbilirubinemia. Iron deficiency, vitamin B_{12} deficiency, lead toxicity, sideroblastic anemia, and dyserythropoietic porphyria produce unconjugated hyperbilirubinemia due to ineffective erythropoiesis. Resorption of large hematomas may also increase production of unconjugated bilirubin.

Neonatal Jaundice

Physiological neonatal jaundice is noticed in the first 5 days of life in term infants; unconjugated bilirubin levels peak near 6 mg/dL by day 3 and then decrease to normal within 14 days because of the increased activity of uridine diphosphate glucuronosyltransferase (UGT), the hepatic enzyme responsible for bilirubin conjugation. Higher levels of unconjugated bilirubin may persist up to 1 month in preterm infants. Nonphysiological causes in neonates include ABO blood group incompatibility between mother and infant, glucose-6-phosphate dehydrogenase deficiency, pyruvate kinase deficiency, and hypothyroidism. Lucey-Driscoll syndrome is transient unconjugated hyperbilirubinemia resulting from a UGT inhibitor in the mother's blood. Breast milk jaundice, which may produce bilirubin levels up to 20 mg/dL, results from an inhibitor of UGT activity in breast milk. Severe unconjugated hyperbilirubinemia produces kernicterus in infants, which manifests as lethargy, hypotonia, and seizures.

Uridine Diphosphate Glucuronosyltransferase Deficiencies

Gilbert syndrome, which is inherited in an autosomal dominant manner, is the most common cause of unconjugated hyperbilirubinemia; it affects 3% to 8% of the population. One half of the patients have mild associated hemolysis, and some have splenomegaly. Gilbert syndrome results from a partial defect of bilirubin conjugation (50% of normal). However, affected patients are asymptomatic and occasionally exhibit jaundice (bilirubin levels up to 6 mg/dL) with intercurrent illness, fasting, stress, fatigue, and ethanol use, or during the premenstrual period. Type I Crigler-Najjar syndrome is an autosomal recessive disorder characterized by the absence of UGT activity. Untreated patients develop profound unconjugated hyperbilirubinemia and die by 18 months. Treatment consists of phototherapy, plasmapheresis, or liver transplantation, which is curative. Type II Crigler-Najjar syndrome (Arias disease) is an autosomal dominant condition characterized by 10% of normal UGT activity, which often leads to jaundice by age 1. Treatment of type II Crigler-Najjar usually is unnecessary unless it affects the very young who are at risk for developing kernicterus.

Other Causes of Unconjugated Hyperbilirubinemia

Probenecid and rifampin decrease hepatic bilirubin uptake. Sulfonamides, aspirin, contrast dye, and some parenteral nutritional formulations displace bilirubin from albumin and thereby reduce its transport into the hepatocyte. Penicillin, quinine, and methyldopa induce hemolysis.

Conjugated Hyperbilirubinemia

Congenital Forms

Rotor syndrome is a rare, asymptomatic, autosomal recessive disorder that manifests as mild conjugated hyperbilirubinemia (2 to 5 mg/dL) in childhood. It is unclear whether the primary defect involves impaired hepatocyte secretion or impaired storage of bilirubin; although oral cholecystograms appear normal, biliary scintigraphy shows absent or delayed secretion. Dubin-Johnson syndrome is an asymptomatic autosomal recessive disorder from the impaired secretion of bilirubin, which produces serum bilirubin levels of 2 to 5 mg/dL. The results of scintigraphy and oral cholecystography are abnormal, whereas histological examination of the liver reveals darkly pigmented tissue. Patients with progressive familial intrahepatic cholestasis (PFIC) present with watery diarrhea, cholestasis, fat-soluble vitamin deficiency, jaundice, and occasionally pancreatitis caused by defective hepatic secretion of bile acids at the canalicular membrane. PFIC exists in different forms; all are autosomal recessive disorders, which have been mapped to several cloned transporters (FIC1, BSEP, MDR3). Choledochal cysts and Caroli disease are congenital malformations of the bile ducts and can manifest as jaundice or cholangitis, and eventually, cholangiocarcinoma. Choledochal cysts often are resectable, whereas Caroli disease (Type IV choledochal cyst) usually requires liver transplantation for cure because of its diffuse intrahepatic nature.

Familial Forms

Benign recurrent intrahepatic cholestasis (BRIC) presents with intense pruritus and elevated alkaline phosphatase levels, with mild increases in levels of aminotransferases and serum bilirubin (<10 mg/dL). Attacks, which begin from age 8 to 30, can last weeks to months, only to recur every several months to years. Liver biopsies reveal centrilobular cholestasis, which appears to be related to altered bile acid transport and enterohepatic circulation. BRIC is a milder form of PFIC-1 and similarly, is caused by mutations in the FIC1 gene. Cholestasis of pregnancy is an autosomal dominant trait that manifests itself in the third trimester as pruritus. This benign condition must be distinguished from acute fatty liver of pregnancy, toxemia, acute cholecystitis, and acute or chronic hepatitis.

Acquired Forms

Acquired disorders constitute the largest group of diseases that manifest conjugated hyperbilirubinemia. Many of these conditions are associated with cholestasis and can exhibit symptoms of pruritus, hypercholesterolemia, and steatorrhea. Intrahepatic cholestasis may result from liver disease (e.g., fulminant hepatitis, chronic hepatitis with significant hepatocellular dysfunction, and the recovery phase of acute hepatitis), infections, and medications. Hyperbilirubinemia occurs in alcoholic patients with acute fatty liver, alcoholic hepatitis, and cirrhosis. Of patients with alcoholic hepatitis, 10% to 20% present with a predominantly cholestatic condition, which may have a poor prognosis if bilirubin levels exceed 10 mg/dL or if encephalopathy, renal failure, or coagulopathy develop. Primary hepatic malignancy, lymphoma, and metastatic carcinoma cause hyperbilirubinemia late in their courses, whereas cholangiocarcinoma and other biliary obstructing lesions produce early jaundice. Bone marrow transplant patients may develop jaundice because of chemotherapy-induced venoocclusive disease and acute or chronic graft-versus-host disease. Postoperative jaundice may result from anesthesia, intrahepatic cholestasis, transfusions, hypotension, hypoxia, and hemolysis. Rheumatologic disorders (e.g., rheumatoid arthritis, systemic lupus erythematosus, and scleroderma) elevate alkaline phosphatase levels but rarely produce jaundice. Sjögren syndrome has an increased occurrence of antimitochondrial antibodies and is associated with primary biliary cirrhosis, which produces jaundice late in its course. Congestive heart failure, shock, and trauma may produce hyperbilirubinemia, whereas renal failure can exacerbate hyperbilirubinemia from any cause. Furthermore, obstructive jaundice increases the risk of renal insufficiency, especially in the post-operative period.

Infections can cause jaundice by bile duct obstruction (e.g., ascariasis), cholestasis (e.g., tuberculosis), or by sepsis and endotoxemia. Infections with *Legionella*, *Escherichia coli*, *Klebsiella*, *Pseudomonas*, *Proteus*, *Bacteroides*, and *Streptococcus* produce conjugated hyperbilirubinemia. Two thirds of patients with acquired immunodeficiency syndrome have elevated levels of aminotransferases or alkaline phosphatase because of hepatitis, infectious sclerosing cholangitis, papillary stenosis, acalculous cholecystitis, malignancy, or medication effects, and all of these disorders may elevate bilirubin levels.

Hepatotoxicity accounts for 3.5% of adverse drug effects. Oral contraceptives induce intrahepatic cholestasis that leads to jaundice in up to 4 of 10,000 patients. Nonsteroidal antiinflammatory drugs can cause hepatitis, cholestasis, granulomatous liver disease, and hypersensitivity reactions. Acetaminophen can produce dose-dependent hepatotoxicity, a condition that occurs at lower doses in individuals who consume significant quantities of alcohol. Alcohol induces expression of cytochrome P450 and leads to increased metabolism of acetaminophen to its hepatotoxic metabolite. Alcoholic patients also may have reduced glutathione stores secondary to chronic malnutrition. Isoniazid produces jaundice in 1% of patients. Chemotherapeutic agents delivered into the hepatic arterial circulation may cause a syndrome similar to sclerosing cholangitis. Numerous other medications affect the liver; when identified, the offending medication should be discontinued. Total parenteral nutrition causes hyperbilirubinemia as a result of intrahepatic cholestasis, infection, and the development of gallstones.

The common extrahepatic obstructive causes of jaundice include stones, blood, and malignant and benign strictures. Gallstone disease represents the most common cause of obstructive jaundice in the United States, although biliary parasitic infection is a common problem in certain areas of the world. The most common malignant causes include pancreatic carcinoma, cholangiocarcinoma, and lymphoma. Pancreatitis may produce swelling of the pancreatic head, leading to common bile duct obstruction. Primary sclerosing cholangitis (PSC) is most commonly associated with inflammatory bowel disease. With obstructive jaundice, alkaline phosphatase levels are elevated concurrently. For hyperbilirubinemia to develop, the bile ducts must be largely obstructed. Ductal dilation may not be detectable on radiographs for 72 hours or in chronic liver disease, such as PSC.

WORKUP

History

The primary aim in evaluating a jaundiced patient is to determine if the hyperbilirubinemia is unconjugated or conjugated and if the process is acute or chronic. If it is unconjugated, the roles of increased production, decreased uptake, or impaired conjugation must be assessed. For conjugated hyperbilirubinemia, the process must be localized to an intrahepatic or extrahepatic site. Fever, abrupt-onset jaundice, right upper quadrant pain, and tender hepatomegaly suggest acute disease. Shaking chills and high fever suggest cholangitis or a bacterial infection, whereas low-grade fevers and flulike symptoms are more common with viral hepatitis. Pain radiating to the back may indicate pancreatic disease. Pruritus is reported with obstructive jaundice of more than 3 to 4 weeks' duration, regardless of the cause. Weight loss, anorexia, nausea, and vomiting are seen nonspecifically in many hyperbilirubinemic disorders.

Related historical features may provide etiologic clues. Recent blood transfusions, intravenous drug abuse, and sexual exposure suggest possible viral hepatitis. Drugs, solvents, ethanol, or oral contraceptives produce jaundice by inducing cholestasis or hepatocellular damage. A history of gallstones, prior biliary surgery, and previous episodes of jaundice suggest bile duct disease. A family history of jaundice raises the possibility of a defect in bilirubin transport or conjugation or a heritable liver disease (e.g., Wilson disease, hemochromatosis, α_1-antitrypsin deficiency). Patients younger than age 30 are likely to present with acute parenchymal disease, whereas those older than age 65 are at risk for stones or malignancy. Conditions more common in men include alcoholic liver disease, pancreatic or hepatocellular carcinoma, and hemochromatosis. Disorders that are more prevalent in women include primary biliary cirrhosis, gallstones, and autoimmune hepatitis.

Physical Examination

The examination can assess the cause, severity, and chronicity of jaundice. Fever may occur with acute or chronic disease, although high fever warrants a search for a bacterial process. Cachexia, muscle wasting, palmar erythema, a Dupuytren contracture, testicular atrophy, parotid enlargement, xanthelasma, gynecomastia, and spider angiomas suggest chronic liver disease. A shrunken, nodular liver with splenomegaly signals cirrhosis, whereas masses or lymphadenopathy raise the possibility of malignancy. A liver span of more than 15 cm suggests fatty infiltration, congestion, malignancy, or other infiltrative diseases. A friction rub may be found in malignancy. Ascites is found with cirrhosis, malignancy, and severe acute hepatitis. A palpable, distended gallbladder suggests malignant biliary obstruction. Asterixis and changes in mental status are noted with advanced liver disease.

Additional Testing

Laboratory Studies

Laboratory tests can confirm suspicions raised by the history and physical examination (Fig. 16-1). The reticulocyte count, lactate dehydrogenase and haptoglobin levels, and examination of the peripheral blood smear can provide evidence of hemolysis. If hemolysis is documented, specific testing of the immune mechanisms and tests for vitamin B_{12} deficiency, lead intoxication, thalassemia, and sideroblastic anemia can be performed. In the absence of hemolysis, most patients with pure, unconjugated hyperbilirubinemia are diagnosed with Gilbert syndrome.

Initial tests for conjugated hyperbilirubinemia should distinguish hepatocellular causes from cholestatic causes and include determining the levels of aminotransferases, alkaline phosphatase, total protein, and albumin. If the alkaline phosphatase level is normal, then extrahepatic biliary obstruction is unlikely. Although neither aspartate nor alanine aminotransferase levels are specific for liver disease, levels higher than 300 IU/mL are uncommon in nonhepatobiliary disease. Aminotransferase elevations less than 300 IU/mL characterize alcoholic hepatitis and most drug-induced injury, whereas elevations more than 1000 IU/mL usually indicate acute hepatitis, certain drug responses (e.g., acetaminophen), or ischemic injury. An aspartate aminotransferase level significantly higher than that of alanine aminotransferase characterizes ethanol injury, whereas in viral hepatitis, the ratio is reversed. Measurement of leucine aminopeptidase, 5'-nucleotidase, and γ-glutamyltransferase levels can help to distinguish alkaline phosphatase elevations caused by hepatobiliary disease from those of bony sources. Specific liver diseases can be evaluated by blood testing (e.g., antimitochondrial antibody with primary biliary cirrhosis; hepatitis serologic findings with viral hepatitis; α_1-antitrypsin levels,

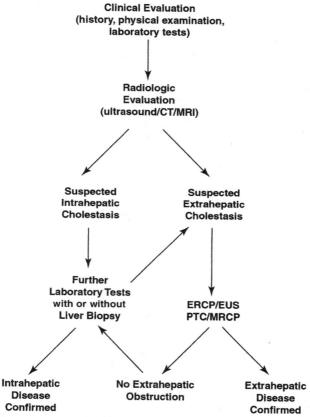

FIGURE 16-1. The evaluation of a jaundiced patient.

iron studies, and ceruloplasmin levels in hereditary liver disease; α-fetoprotein in malignancy; sedimentation rate, immunoglobulins, antinuclear and smooth muscle antibodies with autoimmune disease). Elevated globulin levels with hypoalbuminemia support the diagnosis of cirrhosis, as does failure of the prothrombin time to correct after administering vitamin K. Hypercholesterolemia often occurs with cholestasis.

Noninvasive Imaging Studies

Ultrasound, the initial test for detecting biliary obstruction, has an accuracy of 77% to 94%. With acute obstruction, biliary dilation may not be evident for 4 hours to 4 days. Partial or intermittent obstruction may not produce dilation. Ultrasound is inconsistent in defining the site of obstruction because the distal common bile duct is difficult to visualize. Furthermore, 24% to 40% of patients with choledocholithiasis have bile ducts of normal diameters. Computed tomography (CT) may be performed if ultrasound findings are equivocal or nondiagnostic. CT scans may provide better definition of intrahepatic and extrahepatic mass lesions. Fine needle aspiration of mass lesions is possible with both modalities. Magnetic resonance imaging (MRI) uses a nonnephrotoxic contrast agent and is a more sensitive method for detecting hepatic mass lesions. MR cholangiopancreatography (MRCP) has replaced invasive bile duct imaging with endoscopic retrograde cholangiopancreatography (ERCP) as a reliable diagnostic tool for many conditions. Radionuclide imaging with ^{99m}Tc-labeled iminodiacetic acid derivatives is the procedure of choice for detecting cystic duct obstruction resulting from acute cholecystitis. The inability to visualize the gallbladder after 6 hours is diagnostic of cystic duct obstruction, whereas common bile duct obstruction is reported if no contrast passes into the intestine within 60 minutes. False-positive test results (i.e., lack of gallbladder or duct filling) can occur with prolonged fasting, parenteral nutrition, and bilirubin levels higher than 5 mg/dL. Diisopropyl and p-isopropyl iminodiacetic acid tracers allow biliary duct visualization with greater degrees of jaundice.

Invasive Diagnostic Studies

Percutaneous transhepatic cholangiography (PTC) and ERCP use cholecystographic dye and radiography to visualize the biliary tree. ERCP is successful in localizing the site of biliary obstruction in 90% of cases and is particularly useful for patients with choledocholithiasis because of the therapeutic capability of endoscopic sphincterotomy. The complications of ERCP include pancreatitis, cholangitis, bleeding, and perforation. Unsuccessful ERCP may result from the inability to cannulate the ampulla of Vater or to reach the ampulla (e.g., the patient with a Roux-en-Y gastrojejunostomy). PTC localizes the site of biliary obstruction in 90% of patients with dilated ducts, but it is less useful if the ductal diameter is normal. Contraindications to PTC include thrombocytopenia, severe coagulopathy, and ascites. PTC complications include infection, bleeding, pneumothorax, and peritonitis. Both ERCP and PTC afford the capability of obtaining biopsy or brushing specimens of suggestive biliary strictures and provide the possibility of stent placement for benign and malignant biliary strictures.

If obstruction has been excluded or hepatocellular disease is suspected, a liver biopsy should be performed. Specific findings from liver biopsy include hepatitis, cirrhosis, granulomas, infection, malignancy, certain autoimmune diseases, venous congestion, infiltrative processes, and hereditary liver disease. For 15% of cases, a liver biopsy is not helpful in determining the cause of hyperbilirubinemia. Dilated ducts are a relative contraindication to liver biopsy. Liver biopsy can be done percutaneously with the aid of percussion, ultrasound, or CT or using a transvenous approach. The transjugular approach is recommended for patients with ascites, thrombocytopenia, or coagulopathy. Liver biopsy complications include bleeding, pneumothorax, infection, and puncture of the gallbladder, gut, or kidney.

PRINCIPLES OF MANAGEMENT

Management of a jaundiced patient depends on the underlying cause. In general, a patient with hereditary unconjugated hyperbilirubinemia does not need or does not respond to therapy, although phenobarbital may reduce bilirubin levels in type II Crigler-Najjar syndrome and Gilbert syndrome. Hemolysis may subside with discontinuation of an offending medication or with corticosteroid treatment of an underlying autoimmune process. Certain hepatocellular diseases may respond to specific therapies, for example, pegylated interferon and ribavirin for chronic active hepatitis C infection and therapeutic phlebotomy for hemochromatosis.

The goals for treating a patient with bile duct obstruction are to drain bile from above the blockage to provide relief of pruritus, to decrease the risk of complications, and to remove or bypass the cause of the obstruction. For an otherwise healthy patient with choledocholithiasis, laparoscopic cholecystectomy with common bile duct exploration and removal of the biliary stones is the standard of care, although some clinicians recommend preoperative or postoperative ERCP. For elderly or frail patients who cannot undergo surgery, ERCP with endoscopic sphincterotomy may represent the safest alternative. If a stone cannot be removed with standard endoscopic techniques, surgical extraction is indicated, and if surgery is associated with exceptional risk, endoscopic stenting or percutaneous transhepatic extraction is the alternative. If a malignant biliary obstruction cannot be drained endoscopically or radiographically, a surgical procedure (e.g., choledochojejunostomy or hepaticojejunostomy) may be necessary to bypass the obstructed segment.

COMPLICATIONS

The potential for complications depends on the cause and severity of the jaundice and on patient characteristics. Infants with unconjugated hyperbilirubinemia who have bilirubin levels higher than 20 mg/dL are at risk of kernicterus, in which bilirubin deposition in the thalamus, hypothalamus, and cerebellum produces irreversible impairment of motor and cortical function. Many hepatic diseases carry the risk of morbidity or death from the underlying disorder. Extrahepatic biliary obstruction may result in secondary biliary cirrhosis, bacterial cholangitis, or hepatic abscess formation; all are life threatening if the obstruction is not relieved. Pruritus, hepatic osteodystrophy, and fat-soluble vitamin deficiency are direct results of cholestasis and inadequate biliary secretion. Screening for fat-soluble vitamin deficiency and osteopenia and osteoporosis is recommended because effective therapy exists for these conditions.

CHAPTER 17

Approach to the Patient with Abnormal Liver Chemistry Values

DIFFERENTIAL DIAGNOSIS

Evaluating suspected liver disease requires understanding the diverse tests of liver function and serum markers of hepatobiliary disease. Abnormalities in liver chemistry levels may result from cholestasis, hepatocellular injury, and infiltrative diseases of the liver (Table 17-1). The approach to a patient with jaundice is discussed in Chapter 16. Hepatocellular disorders produce elevations in liver enzymes that are released by damaged hepatocytes. Infiltration from malignancy,

TABLE 17-1
Diagnosis of Selected Hepatobiliary Disorders

FORM OF LIVER INJURY	SUPPORTING LABORATORY DATA	ROLE OF LIVER BIOPSY
Hepatocellular		
Viral hepatitis	Viral serology	Usually required in hepatitis B and C
Drug-induced hepatitis	Eosinophil count	Rarely diagnostic
Autoimmune hepatitis	Immunoelectrophoresis Antinuclear antibody Anti–smooth-muscle antibody	Usually required
Wilson disease	Serum ceruloplasmin	Usually required
Hemochromatosis	Serum iron/total iron-binding capacity Serum ferritin	Usually required
α_1-Antitrypsin deficiency	Protein electrophoresis Serum α_1-antitrypsin level Pi typing	Usually required
Cholestatic		
Primary biliary cirrhosis	Antimitochondrial antibody Immunoelectrophoresis	Essential
Infiltrative		
Hepatocellular carcinoma	Serum α-fetoprotein	Essential

granulomas, amyloidosis, and other conditions results in elevations of enzymes that are localized to the bile canalicular membrane, usually without development of jaundice.

Cholestatic Disorders

Cholestasis may result from intrahepatic or extrahepatic processes. Intrahepatic causes of cholestasis include primary biliary cirrhosis (PBC), sepsis, medications, postoperative cholestasis, familial conditions (e.g., benign recurrent intrahepatic cholestasis, cholestasis of pregnancy), and congenital disorders (e.g., Rotor syndrome, Dubin-Johnson syndrome, Byler disease). Extrahepatic biliary obstruction is caused by choledocholithiasis, benign and malignant strictures, extrinsic compression, and sclerosing cholangitis.

Disorders with Hepatocellular Injury

Hepatocellular injury may result from a diverse group of diseases. Acute viral hepatitis in the United States most commonly results from infection with hepatitis A or B, or, less commonly, C viruses. Hepatitis D complicates the course of infection in chronic hepatitis B carriers. Hepatitis E occurs primarily in developing countries, where it is well recognized as a cause of fulminant hepatic failure, particularly in pregnant women. Other viral causes of hepatitis include cytomegalovirus, herpes simplex virus, Epstein-Barr virus, and varicella-zoster virus. Chronic infection with either hepatitis B or C viruses may also produce chronic hepatitis or cirrhosis.

Chronic ethanol consumption produces a broad range of liver diseases, including fatty liver, alcoholic hepatitis, and cirrhosis. Hereditary liver diseases that produce hepatocellular injury are Wilson disease, hemochromatosis, and α_1-antitrypsin deficiency. Congestive and ischemic disease in the liver is caused by congestive heart failure, constrictive pericarditis, hypotension, portal vein thrombosis or hepatic vein outflow obstruction from Budd-Chiari syndrome, inferior vena cava occlusion, or venoocclusive disease. Significant liver disease during pregnancy, such as acute fatty liver of pregnancy and hepatocellular damage secondary to toxemia, usually occurs in the third trimester. Medication-induced and toxin-induced causes of injury are very common and require a high index of suspicion and careful questioning.

Infiltrative Diseases

Malignant diseases, including primary tumors (e.g., hepatocellular carcinoma, cholangiocarcinoma), metastases, lymphoma, and leukemia, may produce infiltrative liver disease. Granulomatous liver infiltration may result from infections (e.g., tuberculosis, histoplasmosis), sarcoidosis, and numerous medications.

WORKUP

History

An accurate history is critical for a patient whose laboratory studies provide evidence of liver disease. The presenting symptoms provide important diagnostic clues. Pruritus is a common and early symptom in patients with cholestasis. Although classically associated with PBC and primary sclerosing cholangitis, pruritus also is reported in extrahepatic biliary obstruction and hepatocellular disease. Many conditions that produce abnormal liver chemistry levels are painless, but acute biliary obstruction from stones can produce intense right upper quadrant pain. Concurrent high fever raises concern for cholangitis. Acute hepatitis produces less well-defined right upper quadrant discomfort with profound fatigue, whereas hepatic tumors may cause subcostal aching.

A family history is useful in diagnosing and evaluating hereditary hemolytic states, benign recurrent intrahepatic cholestasis, hemochromatosis, Wilson disease, and α_1-antitrypsin deficiency. Exposure to ethanol and industrial and environmental toxins should be identified. A detailed medication history, including over-the-counter and herbal remedies, is critical. In particular, the use of episodic or intermittent medications, such as steroid tapers for asthma, or antibiotics, may require specific questioning. Alcoholic patients should be questioned about acetaminophen use because hepatotoxicity can occur in these persons with therapeutic dosing as a result of cytochrome P450 induction. Intravenous drug abuse, sexual contact, and blood transfusions are associated with a risk for viral hepatitis B or C, whereas sudden worsening of liver chemistry levels in a chronic hepatitis B carrier suggests possible hepatitis D superinfection. Waterborne outbreaks of viral hepatitis have been reported in Southeast Asia and India, underscoring the importance of obtaining a travel history. Risk factors for hepatitis A include recent ingestion of raw or undercooked oysters or clams, male homosexuality, or exposure through day care.

Other diseases associated with liver disorders should be ascertained. Right-sided congestive heart failure, hypotension, and shock are recognized causes of abnormal liver chemistry findings. Chronic pancreatitis may produce abnormal liver tests as a result of stenosis of the common bile duct. Primary sclerosing cholangitis affects 10% of patients with inflammatory bowel disease, in particular those with ulcerative colitis. Obesity, hyperlipidemia, diabetes, and corticosteroid use are risk factors for nonalcoholic fatty liver disease. Hematologic disorders (e.g., polycythemia rubra vera, myeloproliferative disorders, and paroxysmal nocturnal hemoglobinuria) associated with hypercoagulable states predispose to hepatic vein thrombosis. Hemoglobinopathies (e.g., sickle cell anemia, thalassemia) lead to pigment stone formation. Rashes, arthritis, renal disease, and vasculitis may develop with viral hepatitis. The presence of hypogonadism, heart disease, and diabetes suggests possible hemochromatosis. Concurrent lung disease may occur with α_1-antitrypsin deficiency, and central nervous system findings are associated with Wilson disease. Patients with leptospirosis will present with hepatic and renal abnormalities. Renal cell carcinoma manifests as abnormal liver chemistry levels in the absence of metastases. Recent surgery should be noted because anesthetic exposure, perioperative hypotension, and blood transfusions all may affect the liver. Recent biliary tract surgery raises concern for bile duct stricture. Cirrhosis is a late complication of jejunoileal, but not gastric, bypass surgery for morbid obesity.

Physical Examination

Physical findings are of discriminative value for a patient with abnormal liver chemistry findings. Fever suggests an infectious cause or hepatitis. Jaundice is visible when the serum bilirubin concentration exceeds 2.5 to 3.0 mg/dL. Spider angiomas, palmar erythema, parotid enlargement, gynecomastia, a Dupuytren contracture, and testicular atrophy are stigmata of chronic liver disease, usually cirrhosis, though many of these signs have low specificity. Hyperpigmentation is seen with hemochromatosis and PBC. Ichthyosis and koilonychia are manifestations of hemochromatosis. Xanthomas and xanthelasma appear in chronic cholestasis. Kayser-Fleischer rings and sunflower cataracts suggest Wilson disease. Conjunctival suffusion raises the possibility of leptospirosis. A liver span greater than 15 cm suggests passive congestion or liver infiltration. Splenomegaly is found with portal hypertension or infiltrative processes. Abdominal tenderness suggests an inflammatory process (e.g., cholecystitis, cholangitis, pancreatitis, hepatitis), whereas a palpable, nontender gallbladder (i.e, the Courvoisier sign) raises the possibility of an obstructive malignancy. A Murphy sign (i.e., inspiratory arrest during deep, right upper quadrant palpation) is highly suggestive of acute cholecystitis. A pulsatile liver suggests tricuspid insufficiency, and hepatic bruits or rubs raise the possibility of hepatocellular carcinoma. Occult or gross fecal blood on rectal examination suggests possible inflammatory bowel disease or neoplasm.

Additional Testing

Hepatic Function Tests

Measurements of hepatic function evaluate the liver's ability to excrete substances and assess its synthetic and metabolic capacity.

Bilirubin.   Serum bilirubin determination measures capabilities for hepatic conjugation and organic anion excretion. Hyperbilirubinemia can occur from increases in the unconjugated or conjugated bilirubin fractions. Increased production of bilirubin because of hemolysis and defective conjugation produces unconjugated hyperbilirubinemia, whereas hepatocellular disorders and extrahepatic obstruction cause conjugated hyperbilirubinemia. A third form of bilirubin, seen with prolonged cholestasis, is covalently bound to albumin. The presence of this albumin-bound bilirubin explains the slow resolution of jaundice in convalescing patients with resolving liver disease. The urine bilirubin level is elevated in conjugated, not unconjugated, hyperbilirubinemia.

Albumin.   Total serum albumin is a useful measure of hepatic synthetic function. With a half-life of 20 days, albumin is a better index of disease severity in chronic rather than acute liver injury. Hypoalbuminemia may result from increased catabolism of albumin, decreased synthesis, dilution with plasma volume expansion, and increased protein loss from the gut or urinary tract. Prealbumin has a shorter half-life (1.9 days) than albumin and therefore has been proposed as a useful measure of hepatic synthetic capacity after acute injury (e.g., acetaminophen overdose).

Clotting factors.   Prothrombin time detects the activity of vitamin K–dependent coagulation factors (II, VII, IX, and X). Synthesis of these factors requires adequate intestinal vitamin K absorption and intact hepatic synthesis. Therefore, prolonged prothrombin times result from hepatocellular disorders that impair synthetic functions and from cholestatic syndromes that interfere with lipid absorption. Parenteral vitamin K administration distinguishes these possibilities. Improvement in prothrombin time by 30% within 24 hours of vitamin K administration indicates that the synthetic function is intact and suggests vitamin K deficiency. Prolonged prothrombin time is a poor prognostic finding; it signifies severe hepatocellular necrosis in acute hepatitis and the loss of functional hepatocytes in chronic liver disease. Individual clotting proteins have been proposed as useful clinical guides in severe acute hepatitis. Factor VII is the best indicator of liver disease severity and prognosis.

Miscellaneous tests of hepatic function.   Serum bile acid determination has been advocated for assessing suspected liver disease, although poor diagnostic sensitivity in mild disease has prevented widespread application. However, the finding of normal levels of fasting serum bile acids in a patient with unconjugated hyperbilirubinemia supports a diagnosis of Gilbert syndrome in questionable cases. Plasma clearance of sulfobromophthalein, an organic anion, may help distinguish between Dubin-Johnson syndrome and Rotor syndrome. Serum globulin determinations can also give useful diagnostic information. Levels in excess of 3 g/dL are observed primarily in autoimmune liver disease, whereas selective increases in levels of immunoglobulin A (IgA) and IgM are noted in alcoholic cirrhosis and PBC, respectively. Elevated serum ammonia levels may be noted with severe acute or chronic liver disease and can correlate roughly with hepatic encephalopathy. Acute viral and alcoholic hepatitis decrease the alpha and pre-beta bands in serum protein electrophoresis because of the reduced activity of lecithin-cholesterol acyltransferase, whereas the beta band may be broad because of altered triglyceride lipase activity that results in elevated low-density lipoproteins. Breath tests of antipyrine clearance and aminopyrine demethylation measure impaired hepatic drug metabolism.

Serum Markers of Hepatobiliary Dysfunction or Necrosis

Aminotransferases.   Aspartate aminotransferase (AST, SGOT) and alanine aminotransferase (ALT, SGPT) are markers of hepatocellular injury. Because AST is also found in muscle, kidney, heart, and brain, ALT elevations are more specific for liver processes. The highest elevations occur in viral, toxin-induced, and ischemic hepatitis, whereas smaller (<300 IU/mL) elevations are observed in alcoholic hepatitis and other hepatocellular disorders. An AST/ALT ratio greater than 2 suggests alcoholic liver disease, whereas a ratio less than 1 characterizes viral infection and biliary obstruction. When evaluating a patient with liver disease, decreases in AST and ALT levels usually suggest resolving injury, although decreasing aminotransferase levels may also be an ominous indicator of overwhelming hepatocyte death in fulminant liver failure, especially when associated with progressive increases in prothrombin time.

Alkaline phosphatase. Alkaline phosphatase originates in the bile canalicular membranes. Elevations of this enzyme are prominent in cholestasis and infiltrative liver disease; smaller increases are observed in other liver diseases. Alkaline phosphatase activity also occurs in bone, placenta, intestine, kidney, and some malignancies. Low levels of alkaline phosphatase may be observed in acute hemolysis complicating Wilson disease, as well as in hypothyroidism, pernicious anemia, and zinc deficiency.

Miscellaneous markers of hepatobiliary dysfunction. Serum levels of γ-glutamyl-transferase (GGT), 5′-nucleotidase, and leucine aminopeptidase (LAP) are elevated in cholestatic syndromes and may help distinguish hepatobiliary from bony sources of alkaline phosphatase elevations. Levels of GGT are also elevated with pancreatic disease, myocardial infarction, uremia, lung disease, rheumatoid arthritis, nonalcoholic fatty liver disease, and diabetes. Alcohol, anticonvulsants, and warfarin induce hepatic microsomal enzymes, producing striking increases in GGT level. Levels of LAP may be elevated in normal pregnancy. The hepatic mitochondrial enzyme glutamate dehydrogenase is elevated in alcoholic patients and in patients with liver disease secondary to congestive heart failure. The lactate dehydrogenase concentration is frequently obtained as a "liver function test"; however, it has limited specificity for liver processes.

Disease-Specific Markers

Viral serology. The hepatitis A IgM antibody (anti-HAV IgM) is initially detectable at the onset of clinical illness and persists for 120 days. Anti-HAV IgG is a convalescent marker that may persist for life. Hepatitis B surface antigen (HBsAg) precedes aminotransferase elevations and symptom development and persists for 1 to 2 months in self-limited infections. The antibody to core antigen (anti-HBc) is detected 2 weeks after the appearance of HBsAg and initially is of the IgM class. The antibody to HBsAg (anti-HBs) appears sometime after the disappearance of HBsAg and may persist for life. During the period between the disappearance of HBsAg and the appearance of anti-HBs, anti-HBc IgM may be the only marker of recent hepatitis B infection. Measurement of hepatitis B e antigen and antibody, as well as a polymerase chain reaction assay for serum hepatitis B DNA levels, can be used to quantify the degree of active viral replication in some patients with chronic hepatitis B infection. Enzyme-linked immunosorbent assays (ELISAs) are screening tests for detecting exposure to hepatitis C. Recombinant immunoblot assays can be used as supplements to ELISAs if a false-positive result with the ELISA is suspected. Both tests may produce negative findings for up to 6 months after acute infection; therefore, if hepatitis C is a diagnostic possibility, hepatitis C viremia should be determined by a polymerase chain reaction assay of hepatitis C RNA. Quantitative measurement of hepatitis C RNA levels as well as genotype should also be determined prior to therapy, and RNA levels should be followed serially during hepatitis C therapy. Hepatitis D infection occurs only in patients with HBsAg positivity and can be measured by hepatitis D viral RNA and anti-hepatitis D antibodies, although these tests are not readily available. Persistence of anti-HDV IgM predicts progression to chronic hepatitis D infection. Acute hepatitis E can be detected by ELISA for antihepatitis E. A subset of patients in whom the tests for the above viral markers have negative results will exhibit positive serologic findings for cytomegalovirus, herpes simplex, coxsackievirus, or Epstein-Barr virus.

Immunologic tests.   Markers that may be detected in autoimmune liver disease include antinuclear antibody (ANA, homogeneous pattern in a titer of $\geq$1:160) and the anti–smooth muscle antibodies (ASMAs). ASMAs are detected in 70% of patients with autoimmune chronic active hepatitis but may also be present in 50% of patients with PBC. The presence of anti-liver/kidney microsomal antibodies (anti-LKM1) with reduced titers of antiactin antibodies or ANAs identifies a subset of patients with autoimmune chronic active hepatitis, a disease that follows an aggressive course in young women. Antimitochondrial antibodies (AMAs) are present in 90% of patients with PBC and 25% of patients with chronic active hepatitis or drug-induced liver disease. Antibodies to the Ro antigen and to anticentromeric antibodies are observed with PBC, especially in patients with sicca syndrome or scleroderma.

Copper storage variables.   Ceruloplasmin is a copper transport protein in the plasma that circulates in low concentrations in Wilson disease; low levels (<20 mg/dL) are measured in 90% of homozygotes and 10% of heterozygotes. Reduced levels may also occur with severely depressed synthetic function caused by other end-stage liver diseases. Alternate diagnostic tests for Wilson disease include urinary copper, which exceeds 100 mg per 24 hours in nearly all patients, and free serum copper, which is markedly elevated. Urinary copper also is elevated in patients with cholestasis or cirrhosis. Although the gene for Wilson disease has been identified (ATP7B), the lack of a dominant mutation has prevented the development of genetic tests for the disease.

Iron storage variables.   Serum iron level and total iron-binding capacity (transferrin) are useful measures in diagnosing hemochromatosis. Transferrin is normally 20% to 45% saturated. A transferrin saturation higher than 45% will identify more than 98% of patients with hemochromatosis. Elevations in serum iron with normal transferrin saturation occur in alcoholic liver disease. Serum ferritin more closely correlates with hepatic and total body iron stores, although ferritin may be elevated in inflammatory disease because it is an acute phase reactant. The identification of a single recessive mutation in the HFE gene (C282Y), which is responsible for the majority of hemochromatosis, has eliminated the need for a liver biopsy in diagnosing many cases. A liver biopsy may be required for older patients with high ferritin levels to quantify tissue iron and to determine the extent of fibrosis, which will guide the need for screening for hepatocellular carcinoma.

α_1-Antitrypsin. α_1-Antitrypsin is a hepatic glycoprotein that migrates in the α_1-globulin fraction in serum protein electrophoresis. Homozygotes for the Pi ZZ variant of this protein (normal is Pi MM) exhibit decreased serum α_1-antitrypsin activity, which predisposes to development of chronic liver and pulmonary disease. Hepatocytes that cannot excrete the Z protein accumulate periodic acid–Schiff (PAS)-positive, diastase-resistant globules, as seen in liver biopsy specimens. Phenotyping is more accurate for diagnosis than determination of serum levels of the protein. Whether heterozygotes (Pi MZ) can develop liver disease in the absence of other hepatic insults remains controversial.

α-Fetoprotein. α-Fetoprotein (AFP) is present in the serum of 70% to 90% of patients with hepatocellular carcinoma, although small resectable tumors may not produce AFP. Elevated AFP levels also occur with germ cell tumors, other gastrointestinal malignancies, PBC, and acute and chronic hepatitis. To exclude these disorders reliably, a level higher than 400 mg/mL is said to be specific for hepatocellular carcinoma; however, this level excludes nearly one third of patients with hepatocellular carcinoma. Radiologic imaging should be performed in all patients with chronic liver disease who have elevated levels of AFP.

Percutaneous Liver Biopsy

As a general rule, direct forms of liver injury tend to cause predominant centrizonal necrosis; immunologically mediated forms of hepatocyte injury are localized to the periportal region; and cholestatic injury is recognized by the accumulation of canalicular bile and feathery degeneration of hepatocytes in the absence of a significant inflammatory infiltrate. Clinical applications of liver biopsy include evaluating persistently abnormal liver chemistry levels, establishing the diagnosis in unexplained hepatomegaly, and evaluating suspected systemic disease or carcinoma involving the liver. Contraindications to liver biopsy are an uncooperative or unstable patient, ascites, right-sided empyema, and suspected hemangioma or echinococcal cyst. Impaired coagulation function is a relative contraindication. For patients with ascites or an increased risk of bleeding, a transjugular approach is an alternative to the percutaneous approach.

Coordinated Diagnostic Approach

Liver disease is classified into four groups: cholestatic, hepatocellular, immunologic, and infiltrative. Screening the patient by determining levels of AST and ALT activity, serum alkaline phosphatase, serum total and direct bilirubin, serum protein and albumin, and prothrombin time can direct the subsequent evaluation into one of these four groups.

Cholestatic liver disease usually results in increased serum bilirubin and alkaline phosphatase levels with normal to mildly elevated aminotransferase levels, although transient, profound, aminotransferase elevations may occur in early biliary obstruction (Fig. 17-1). In extrahepatic cholestasis, the serum bilirubin level increases by 1.5 mg/dL per day and reaches a maximum of 35 mg/dL in the absence of renal dysfunction or hemolysis. In partial biliary obstruction, the bilirubin level may remain normal in the face of an elevated alkaline phosphatase concentration. The most direct approach to evaluating suspected cholestasis is performing ultrasound to assess bile duct size. If malignancy or pancreatic disease is suspected, a computed tomography (CT) scan may provide better anatomic definition of the desired structures. If biliary dilation is detected, endoscopic retrograde cholangiopancreatography (ERCP) or percutaneous transhepatic cholangiography (PTC) can further define and potentially be used to treat the abnormality (see Chapter 16). In some cases of extrahepatic obstruction, bile duct size will be normal; in these cases, ERCP or PTC may still be indicated because of a high clinical suspicion. In questionable cases, percutaneous liver biopsy may provide a definitive diagnosis. However, intrahepatic cholestasis cannot always be distinguished from extrahepatic cholestasis on liver biopsy specimens.

Hepatocellular injury is suggested by aminotransferase levels higher than 400 IU/mL; levels less than 300 IU/mL are nonspecific and are observed with cholestasis as well as with hepatocellular disease. Alkaline phosphatase and bilirubin elevations are variable in hepatocellular disease, depending on the cause and severity of the clinical condition. Prolongation of prothrombin time and decreases in serum albumin levels indicate significant hepatic synthetic dysfunction. In acute malaise, anorexia, nausea, jaundice, tender hepatomegaly, and elevated levels of aminotransferases, serum should be screened for viral markers to exclude hepatitis A, B, or C infection, depending on the patient risk factors. With disease duration of more than 6 months, additional studies (e.g., serum protein electrophoresis, ferritin or

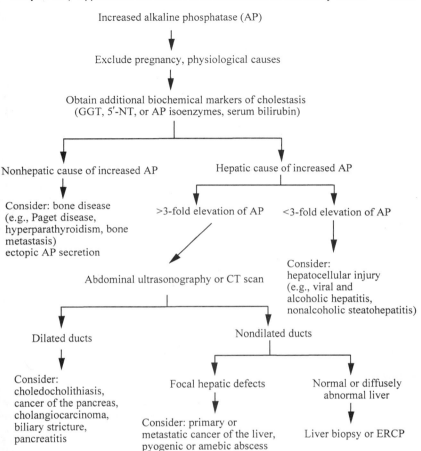

FIGURE 17-1. Evaluation of a patient with elevated serum alkaline phosphatase (AP) levels (CT, computed tomography; ERCP, endoscopic retrograde cholangiopancreatography; GGT, serum γ-glutamyltransferase; 5′ = NT, 5′ = nucleotidase).

iron studies, and measurement of serum ceruloplasmin) should be added to the viral serologic studies to exclude hereditary liver disease. Eosinophilia suggests possible drug hypersensitivity. For a patient with prominent systemic symptoms that suggest autoimmune disease, the clinician should determine the sedimentation rate; perform serum protein electrophoresis; measure quantitative immunoglobulins in the blood; and measure the presence of ANA, AMA, and ASMA. A hepatocellular pattern is observed with ischemic and congestive liver disease, but measures to improve hepatic blood flow in these conditions can produce brisk reductions in aminotransferases to near normal levels within 48 to 72 hours. With congestive liver disease, the prothrombin time may be prolonged out of proportion to other signs of liver disease. Hepatic vein thrombosis (Budd-Chiari syndrome) may be suggested by increased caudate lobe size on CT scanning and usually is confirmed by Doppler ultrasound, CT, or magnetic resonance imaging that shows hepatic vein outflow obstruction and narrowing of the inferior vena cava. Most acute elevations in aminotransferase levels do not require further evaluation unless they are severe or progressive. If aminotransferase levels remain high longer than 6 months without an identifiable cause, a liver biopsy is indicated for diagnosis and to offer prognostic information about possible progression to cirrhosis. Many persons with persistently high aminotransferase levels are obese or use ethanol, and the usual finding on liver biopsy is fatty liver disease in the absence of serologic diagnosis. However, the unexpected finding of chronic active hepatitis in a subset of these patients provides support for biopsy even in asymptomatic individuals.

Isolated elevation of alkaline phosphatase levels of hepatic origin (confirmed by LAP, 5′-nucleotidase, or GGT) suggests an infiltrative process. These patients should undergo diagnostic imaging as described previously, however, to rule out extrahepatic cholestasis. An increase of more than threefold in the alkaline phosphatase level in a patient with known cirrhosis raises concern for hepatocellular carcinoma. In these patients, levels of α-fetoprotein should be measured, and ultrasound or CT performed to exclude mass lesions. An elevated alkaline phosphatase level, detectable titers of AMA, and an elevated serum IgM level in a middle-aged woman are consistent with PBC. If imaging studies are nondiagnostic, liver biopsy is essential to exclude neoplasm, infection, cholestasis, or granuloma.

Patients who have undergone liver transplantation are frequently evaluated for abnormal liver function tests. Acute cellular rejection, hepatic artery thrombosis, opportunistic infection, drug-induced liver disease, or recurrence of the primary liver disease present at various times after transplantation. Liver biopsy and Doppler ultrasound of the liver usually are usually required to establish a diagnosis and to guide management.

PRINCIPLES OF MANAGEMENT

Managing patients with abnormal liver chemistry levels depends on obtaining an accurate diagnosis. For extrahepatic obstruction, the goal of treatment is to relieve or bypass the obstruction (see Chapter 16). In drug-induced intrahepatic cholestasis, removal of the offending medication is indicated, although normalization of liver chemistry levels is not always prompt. Management of PBC depends on the stage of disease. The synthetic bile acid, ursodiol, usually is given in the early stages of the disease with modest success; advanced liver failure in PBC usually warrants liver transplantation. Cholestyramine, rifampin, phenobarbital, or ondansetron are given for pruritus in cholestatic disorders.

Specific therapies for many hepatocellular disorders have been well described. Hemochromatosis is managed with phlebotomy, or alternatively, deferoxamine. Wilson disease is initially treated with D-penicillamine; maintenance regimens may include oral zinc to reduce intestinal copper absorption. Patients with severe acute hepatitis may require hospitalization for supportive care. An encephalopathic patient may need mechanical ventilation, intracranial pressure monitoring, and possible emergency liver transplantation to avert a fatal outcome. Pegylated interferon-α, which usually is given with the oral agent ribavirin, may eliminate the virus or slow the progression of chronic active hepatitis C. Interferon-α and oral nucleosides and nucleotides are used to treat hepatitis B. Chronic autoimmune active hepatitis is usually responsive to corticosteroids, although most patients require long-term immunosuppressives with a maintenance regimen of an antimetabolite immunosuppressive, such as azathioprine. Congestive and ischemic hepatopathy improves with control of the underlying hemodynamic state. Anticoagulants may be used in the early stages of Budd-Chiari syndrome or venoocclusive disease, although these often do not prevent clinical deterioration and many patients require portosystemic shunts (e.g., transjugular intrahepatic portosystemic shunt, TIPS). Drug-induced hepatocellular injury is managed by medication withdrawal, although some agents have the potential for fatal hepatic necrosis (e.g., acetaminophen). With recent acetaminophen ingestion, administering N-acetylcysteine is indicated.

There is no effective treatment for many of the causes of infiltrative liver disease. Hepatic tuberculosis and candidiasis are exceptions because they respond to antimicrobial therapy. Although advanced hepatocellular carcinoma usually has a poor prognosis, early stage (I–II) tumors may be cured with resection or transplantation. Young patients with the fibrolamellar variant of hepatocellular carcinoma have a better prognosis. Multiple metastatic carcinomas usually are unresectable and have dismal prognoses, although prolonged survival has been reported after excision of the primary tumor and three or fewer solitary hepatic metastases.

COMPLICATIONS

Patients with chronic cholestasis or hepatocellular injury may progress to end-stage liver disease, depending on the cause. With hepatocyte loss, coagulopathy and hypoproteinemia develop, increasing the risks for hemorrhage, edema, ascites, and infection. Portal hypertension may lead to ascites, hydrothorax, and hemorrhage from esophageal or gastric varices or portal gastropathy. Other complications of end-stage liver failure include hepatic encephalopathy and hepatorenal syndrome. Infiltrative fungal infections of the liver may progress to abscess formation and death. Infiltrative malignancy usually is fatal.

Hepatitis B and C may be transmitted to contacts of the infected patient, usually by transfer of body fluids (e.g., blood), although sexual transmission of hepatitis B (and to a much lesser degree, hepatitis C) is possible. Patients who report body fluid contact with an HBsAg-positive individual should receive hepatitis B immune globulin, and, in most instances, they will benefit from a vaccination against hepatitis B. Immune serum globulin is recommended for individuals potentially exposed to hepatitis A. There is no established role for immune serum globulin in hepatitis C prophylaxis.

CHAPTER 18

Approach to the Patient with Ascites

DIFFERENTIAL DIAGNOSIS

Ascites is the pathological accumulation of fluid within the peritoneal cavity. It is important to establish a cause for its development and to initiate a rational treatment regimen to avoid some of the complications of ascites. Most cases of ascites in the United States result from liver disease, although disorders involving other organ systems may produce abdominal fluid accumulation in certain situations (Table 18-1).

Hepatic Disease

Portal hypertension is a prerequisite for ascites formation in patients with liver disease. In general, ascites is a complication of chronic liver diseases (e.g., cirrhosis), but some acute diseases (e.g., acute alcoholic hepatitis or fulminant hepatic failure) may result in ascites. In this setting, a high (>1.1 g/dL) serum-ascites albumin gradient indicates acute portal hypertension and a mechanism of fluid formation similar to that in chronic liver disease. Ascites may complicate Budd-Chiari syndrome because of venous outflow obstruction. Three theories have been proposed to explain fluid accumulation. The underfill theory postulates that an imbalance of Starling forces produces intravascular fluid loss into the peritoneum, with resultant hormonally mediated renal sodium retention. The overfill theory proposes that primary renal sodium retention produces intravascular hypervolemia that overflows into the peritoneum. The more recent peripheral arterial vasodilation theory proposes that portal hypertension leads to vasodilation and reduced effective arterial blood volume, which increases renal sodium retention and promotes fluid accumulation. In the vasodilation theory, the underfill mechanism is operative in early, compensated cirrhosis, whereas the overflow mechanism operates in advanced disease.

Renal Disease

Nephrotic syndrome is a rare cause of ascites in adults. It results from protein loss in the urine, leading to decreased intravascular volume and increased renal sodium retention. Nephrogenous ascites is a poorly understood condition that develops with hemodialysis; its optimal treatment is undefined and its prognosis is poor. Continuous, ambulatory, peritoneal dialysis is an iatrogenic form of ascites that takes advantage of the rich vascularity of the parietal peritoneum to eliminate endogenous toxins and control fluid balance. Urine may accumulate in the peritoneum in newborns or as a result of trauma or renal transplantation in adults.

TABLE 18-1
Causes of Ascites

CAUSE	NUMBER	% OF TOTAL
Chronic parenchymal liver disease (cirrhosis and alcoholic hepatitis)	758	84.1
"Mixed" (portal hypertension plus another cause, e.g., cirrhosis and peritoneal carcinomatosis)	42	4.7
Heart failure	24	2.7
Malignancy without another cause	23	2.6
Tuberculosis without another cause	6	0.7
Fulminant hepatic failure	6	0.7
Pancreatic	4	0.4
Nephrogenous ("dialysis ascites")	2	0.2
Miscellaneous*	36	3.9

*Includes biliary ascites and chylous ascites resulting from lymphatic tears, lymphoma, and cirrhosis.

Reprinted with permission from Runyon BA, Montano AA, Akriviadis EA, et al. The serum-ascites albumin gradient is superior to the exudate-transudate concept in the differential diagnosis of ascites. *Ann Intern Med* 1992;117:215.

Cardiac Disease

Ascites is an uncommon complication of both high-output and low-output heart failure. High-output failure is associated with decreased peripheral resistance; low-output disease is defined by reduced cardiac output. Both lead to decreased effective arterial blood volume and subsequently, to renal sodium retention. Pericardial disease is a rare cardiac cause of ascites.

Pancreatic Disease

Pancreatic ascites develops as a complication of severe acute pancreatitis, pancreatic duct rupture in acute or chronic pancreatitis, or leakage from a pancreatic pseudocyst. Many patients with pancreatic ascites have underlying cirrhosis. Pancreatic ascites may be complicated by infection or left-sided pleural effusion.

Biliary Disease

Most cases of biliary ascites result from gallbladder rupture, which usually is a complication of gangrene of the gallbladder in elderly men. Bile also can accumulate in the peritoneal cavity after biliary surgery or biliary or intestinal perforation.

Malignancy

Malignancy-related ascites signifies advanced disease in most cases and has a dismal prognosis. Exceptions are ovarian carcinoma and lymphoma, which may respond to debulking surgery and chemotherapy, respectively. The mechanism of ascites formation depends on the location of the tumor. Peritoneal carcinomatosis produces exudation of proteinaceous fluid into the peritoneal cavity, whereas liver metastases or primary hepatic malignancy is likely to induce ascites by producing portal hypertension, either from vascular occlusion by the tumor or arteriovenous fistulae within the tumor. Chylous ascites can result from lymph node involvement with tumor.

Infectious Disease

In the United States, tuberculous peritonitis is a disease of Asian, Mexican, and Central American immigrants, and it is a complication of the acquired immunodeficiency syndrome. One half of patients with tuberculous peritonitis have underlying cirrhosis, usually secondary to ethanol abuse. Patients with liver disease tolerate antituberculous drug toxicity less well than patients with normal hepatic function. Exudation of proteinaceous fluid from the tubercles lining the peritoneum induces ascites formation. *Coccidioides* organisms cause infectious ascites formation by a similar mechanism. For sexually active women who have a fever and inflammatory ascites, chlamydia-induced, and the less common gonococcus-induced, Fitz-Hugh-Curtis syndrome should be considered.

Chylous Ascites

Chylous ascites is a result of the obstruction of or damage to chyle-containing lymphatic channels. The most common causes are lymphatic malignancies (e.g., lymphomas, other malignancies), surgical tears, and infectious causes.

Other Causes of Ascites Formation

Serositis with ascites formation may complicate systemic lupus erythematosus. Meigs syndrome—ascites and pleural effusion due to benign ovarian neoplasms—is a rare cause of ascites formation. Most cases of ascites caused by ovarian disease are from peritoneal carcinomatosis. Ascites with myxedema is secondary to hypothyroidism-related cardiac failure. Mixed ascites occurs in about 5% of cases when the patient has two or more separate causes of ascites formation, such as cirrhosis and infection or malignancy. A clue to the presence of a second cause is an inappropriately high white cell count in otherwise transudative ascites.

WORKUP

History

The history can help to elucidate the cause of ascites formation. Increasing abdominal girth from ascites may be part of the initial presentation of patients with alcoholic liver disease; however, the laxity of the abdominal wall and the severity of underlying liver disease suggest that the condition can be present for some time before it is recognized. Patients who consume ethanol only intermittently may report cyclic ascites, whereas patients with nonalcoholic disease usually have persistent ascites. Other risk factors for viral liver disease should be ascertained (i.e., drug abuse, sexual exposure, blood transfusions, and tattoos). A positive family history of liver disease raises the possibility of a heritable condition (e.g., Wilson disease, hemochromatosis, or α_1-antitrypsin deficiency) that might also present with symptoms referable to other organ systems (diabetes, cardiac disease, joint problems, and hyperpigmentation with hemochromatosis; neurological disease with

Wilson disease; pulmonary complaints with α_1-antitrypsin deficiency). Patients with cirrhotic ascites may report other complications of liver disease, including jaundice, pedal edema, gastrointestinal hemorrhage, or encephalopathy. The patient with long-standing, stable cirrhosis who abruptly develops ascites should be evaluated for possible hepatocellular carcinoma.

Information concerning possible nonhepatic disease should be obtained. Weight loss or a prior history of cancer suggests possible malignant ascites, which may be painful and produce rapid increases in abdominal girth. A history of heart disease raises the possibility of cardiac causes of ascites. Some alcoholics with ascites have alcoholic cardiomyopathy rather than liver dysfunction. Obesity, diabetes, and hyperlipidemia are risk factors for nonalcoholic fatty liver disease, which can cause cirrhosis on its own or can act synergistically with other insults (e.g., alcohol, hepatitis C). Tuberculous peritonitis usually presents with fever and abdominal discomfort. Patients with nephrotic syndrome usually have anasarca. Patients with rheumatologic disease may have serositis. Patients with ascites associated with lethargy, cold intolerance, and voice and skin changes should be evaluated for hypothyroidism.

Physical Examination

Ascites should be distinguished from panniculus, massive hepatomegaly, gaseous overdistention, intra-abdominal masses, and pregnancy. Percussion of the flanks can be used to determine rapidly if a patient has ascites. The absence of flank dullness excludes ascites with 90% accuracy. If dullness is found, the patient should be rolled into a partial decubitus position to test whether there is a shift in the air-fluid interface determined by percussion (shifting dullness). The fluid wave has less value in detecting ascites. The puddle sign detects as little as 120 mL of ascitic fluid, but it requires the patient to assume a hands-knees position for several minutes and is a less useful test than flank dullness.

The physical examination can help to determine the cause of ascites. Palmar erythema, abdominal wall collateral veins, spider angiomas, splenomegaly, and jaundice are consistent with liver disease. Large veins on the flanks and back indicate blockage of the inferior vena cava that is caused by webs or malignancy. Masses or lymphadenopathy (e.g., Sister Mary Joseph nodule, Virchow node) suggest underlying malignancy. Distended neck veins, cardiomegaly, and auscultation of an S_3 or pericardial rub suggest cardiac causes of ascites, whereas anasarca may be observed with nephrotic syndrome.

Additional Testing
Blood and Urine Studies
Laboratory blood studies can provide clues to the cause of ascites. Abnormal levels of aminotransferases, alkaline phosphatase, and bilirubin are seen with liver disease. Prolonged prothrombin time and hypoalbuminemia are also observed with hepatic synthetic dysfunction, although low albumin levels are noted with renal disease, protein-losing enteropathy, and malnutrition. Hematologic abnormalities, especially thrombocytopenia, suggest liver disease. Renal disease may be suggested by electrolyte abnormalities or elevations in blood urea nitrogen and creatinine. Urinalysis may reveal protein loss with nephrotic syndrome or bilirubinuria with jaundice. Specific tests (e.g., α-fetoprotein) or serologic tests (e.g., antinuclear antibody) may be ordered for suspected hepatocellular carcinoma or immune-mediated disease, respectively.

Ascitic Fluid Analysis

Abdominal paracentesis is the most important means of diagnosing the cause of ascites formation. It is appropriate to sample ascitic fluid in all patients with new-onset ascites, as well as in all those admitted to the hospital with ascites, because there is a 10% to 27% prevalence of ascitic fluid infection in the latter group. Paracentesis is performed in an area of dullness either in the midline between the umbilicus and symphysis pubis, because this area is avascular, or in one of the lower quadrants. Needles should not be inserted close to abdominal wall scars with either approach because of the high risk for bowel perforation; puncture sites too near the liver or spleen should be avoided as well. In 3% of cases, ultrasound guidance may be needed. The needle is inserted using a Z-track insertion technique to minimize postprocedure leakage, and 25 mL or more of ascitic fluid is removed for analysis.

Analysis of ascitic fluid should begin with gross inspection. Most ascitic fluid from portal hypertension is yellow and clear. Cloudiness raises the possibility of infectious processes, whereas a milky appearance is seen with chylous ascites. A minimum density of 10,000 erythrocytes per μL is required to provide a red tint to the fluid, which raises the possibility of malignancy if the paracentesis is atraumatic. Pancreatic ascitic fluid is tea colored or black. The ascitic fluid cell count is the most useful test. The upper limit of the neutrophil cell count is 250 cells per μL, even in patients who have undergone diuresis. If paracentesis is traumatic, only 1 neutrophil per 250 erythrocytes and 1 lymphocyte per 750 erythrocytes can be attributed to blood contamination. With spontaneous bacterial peritonitis (SBP), the neutrophil count exceeds 250 cells per μL and represents more than 50% of the total white cell count in the ascitic fluid. Chylous ascites may produce increases in ascitic lymphocyte counts. If infection is suspected, ascitic fluid should be inoculated into blood culture bottles at the bedside and sent for bacterial culture. Gram stain is insensitive for detecting bacterial infection, and results should not be considered reliable if negative because 10,000 organisms per milliliter are needed for a positive Gram stain, whereas spontaneous peritonitis may occur with only 1 organism per milliliter. Similarly, the direct smear has only 0% to 2% sensitivity for detecting tuberculosis. Ascites fluid culture for tuberculosis is only 40% sensitive and the sensitivity of peritoneal biopsy is 64% to 83%. If tuberculosis is strongly suspected, laparoscopic rather than blind biopsy of the peritoneum is indicated, because it requires direct visualization of the peritoneal surface with a laparoscope and is almost 100% sensitive. Certain infections can reduce ascitic fluid glucose levels (usually related to perforation of the gastrointestinal tract), but because glucose concentrations usually are normal with SBP, this measure has limited utility. Similarly, testing of ascitic fluid pH and lactate levels has been proposed to evaluate for infected fluid; however, their sensitivities are low.

The serum-ascites albumin gradient provides important information about the cause of ascites. Calculating the gradient involves subtracting the albumin concentration in the ascitic fluid from the serum value. A patient can be diagnosed with portal hypertension with 97% accuracy if the serum albumin minus ascitic albumin concentration is 1.1 g/dL or higher. Causes of high-gradient ascites include cirrhosis, alcoholic hepatitis, cardiac ascites, massive liver metastases, Budd-Chiari syndrome, portal vein thrombosis, venoocclusive disease, acute fatty liver of pregnancy, myxedema, and some mixed ascites. Conversely, a gradient less than 1.1 g/dL signifies ascites that is not caused by portal hypertension. Low-albumin gradient ascites may result from peritoneal carcinomatosis, tuberculosis, pancreatic or biliary disease, nephrotic syndrome, or connective tissue disease. Previous means of assessing the cause included measuring total ascitic fluid protein and ascitic fluid-to-serum lactate dehydrogenase ratios. Although sometimes still used to distinguish "exudative" from "transudative," the accuracy of these measures is only 55% to 60%.

Detecting malignancy in ascitic fluid can be a diagnostic challenge. Although nearly 100% of patients with peritoneal carcinomatosis have positive results on cytologic analysis of the peritoneal fluid, patients with liver metastases, lymphoma, and hepatocellular carcinoma usually have negative cytologic results. Peritoneal biopsy is rarely needed for peritoneal carcinomatosis. The value of ascitic fluid levels of carcinoembryonic antigen and humoral tests of malignancy in detecting malignant ascites is undefined.

Other ascitic fluid tests may be ordered, depending on the clinical scenario. In uncomplicated cirrhotic ascites, the ascitic fluid amylase level is low with an ascitic fluid-to-serum ratio of 0.4. With pancreatic ascites, the levels may exceed 2000 IU/L and amylase ratios may increase to 6. With milky ascitic fluid, a triglyceride level is obtained. Chylous ascites triglyceride levels exceed 200 mg/dL versus 20 mg/dL in cirrhotic ascites. Brown ascitic fluid and a bilirubin level higher in the ascitic fluid than in the serum suggest a biliary or bowel perforation.

Structural Testing

Radiography, endoscopy, and scintigraphy can be used to assess the cause of ascites. Computed tomography or Doppler ultrasound can show evidence of cirrhosis and can detect mass lesions of the liver, pancreas, or ovaries. These techniques can also evaluate portal or hepatic vein thrombosis. Upper endoscopy may show varices or portal gastropathy, which is indicative of portal hypertension. Liver-spleen scintigraphy may show colloid shifting in cirrhosis. Chest radiography may show apical disease consistent with tuberculosis. Abdominal radiography also is useful in assessing complications of ascites. Plain abdominal radiographs can be assessed for free subdiaphragmatic air, followed by water-soluble contrast studies to exclude bowel perforation as a cause of peritonitis.

PRINCIPLES OF MANAGEMENT

Ascites Unrelated to Portal Hypertension

In patients with peritoneal carcinomatosis, peripheral edema responds to diuretic administration, but the ascites does not. The mainstay for treating these patients is periodic therapeutic paracentesis. Peritoneovenous shunts may be used in selected cases; however, in most instances, the short life expectancy does not warrant this aggressive intervention. Nephrotic ascites will respond to sodium restriction and diuretics. Tuberculous peritonitis requires specific antituberculosis agents. Pancreatic ascites may resolve spontaneously, respond to octreotide therapy, or require endoscopic stenting or surgery if a ductal leak is present. Postoperative lymphatic leaks may require surgical intervention or peritoneovenous shunting. Nephrogenous ascites may respond to vigorous dialysis.

Ascites Related to Portal Hypertension

For patients with ascites secondary to portal hypertension, restricting dietary sodium to a daily level of 2 g is essential (Fig. 18-1). Fluids do not need to be restricted unless the serum sodium is less than 120 mEq/L. If single-agent diuretic therapy is planned, a daily dose of 100 mg spironolactone is the best choice. For patients who experience spironolactone side effects (e.g., painful gynecomastia), 10 mg/d of amiloride may be given. The physician should expect a slow response to spironolactone because of its long half-life; weight loss may not be evident for 2 weeks. It is often reasonable to add a loop diuretic (e.g., furosemide) at 40 mg/d

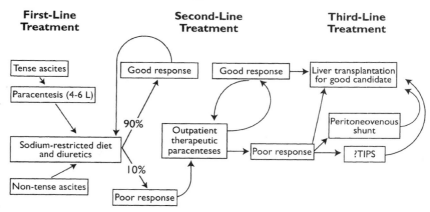

FIGURE 18-1.   Algorithm for treating patients with cirrhosis and ascites (TIPS, transjugular intrahepatic portosystemic shunt). Reprinted with permission from Runyon BA. Care of patients with ascites. *N Engl J Med* 1994;330:337.

to maximize natriuresis. Doses may be increased slowly to maximums of 400 mg/d of spironolactone and 160 mg/d of furosemide. If diuresis is still suboptimal, metolazone or hydrochlorothiazide may be added, although the hyponatremic and hypovolemic effects of such triple drug regimens mandate close physician follow-up, often on an inpatient basis. There should be no limit to the amount of weight that can be diuresed daily if pedal edema is present. Once the dependent edema has resolved, diuretics should be adjusted to achieve a daily weight loss of 0.5 kg. Urine sodium levels may be used to direct diuretic therapy. Patients with urine sodium excretion less than potassium excretion are likely to require higher diuretic doses. If urine sodium excretion exceeds potassium excretion, the total daily sodium excretion is likely to be adequate (i.e., >78 mmol/d) in 95% of circumstances. Development of encephalopathy, a serum sodium level less than 120 mEq/L that does not respond to fluid restriction, or serum creatinine higher than 2 mg/dL are relative indicators for discontinuing diuretic therapy. Because concurrent use of nonsteroidal antiinflammatory drugs promotes renal failure, inhibits the efficacy of diuretics, and may cause gastrointestinal hemorrhage, their use is discouraged.

Various nonmedical means to treat refractory ascites are available. Large-volume paracentesis, with removal of 5 L of fluid, can be performed in 20 minutes. Total paracentesis, with withdrawal of 20 L or more of fluid, can be performed safely. The issue of concurrent administration of intravenous albumin is controversial. Some clinicians advocate albumin infusion to prevent paracentesis-induced changes in electrolytes and creatinine. Other physicians avoid albumin infusion in view of its cost, particularly because differences in long-term survival have not been demonstrated with such measures. Transjugular intrahepatic portosystemic shunts (TIPSs) are effective in many patients with diuretic-resistant ascites. Peritoneovenous shunts (e.g., Denver and LeVeen) drain ascitic fluid into the central venous circulation; however, they have not achieved widespread use because of a lack of efficacy, shunt occlusion, and side effects (e.g., pulmonary edema, variceal hemorrhage, diffuse intravascular coagulation, and thromboembolism). Surgical portocaval shunt procedures were used in the past, but frequent postoperative complications (e.g., encephalopathy) have tempered enthusiasm for the techniques. Liver transplantation cures both refractory ascites and underlying cirrhosis and should be considered for patients without contraindications.

COMPLICATIONS

Infection

SBP is defined as ascitic fluid infection with pure growth of a single organism and an ascitic fluid neutrophil count higher than 250 cells per μL without evidence of a surgically remediable intra-abdominal cause. SBP occurs only in the setting of liver disease, for all practical purposes, although it has been reported with nephrotic syndrome. Ascites is a prerequisite for SBP; however, it may not be detectable on physical examination. Infection usually occurs with maximal fluid accumulation. *Escherichia coli*, *Klebsiella pneumoniae*, and *Pneumococcus* organisms are the most common isolates in SBP; anaerobes are the causative organism in 1% of cases. Eighty-seven percent of patients with SBP present with symptoms, most commonly fever, abdominal pain, and changes in mental status, although the clinical manifestations may be subtle. Antibiotics should be initiated when an ascitic fluid neutrophil count higher than 250 cells per μL is documented before obtaining formal culture results. The most accepted antibiotic for SBP is cefotaxime, the third-generation cephalosporin to which 98% of offending bacteria are sensitive, though ceftriaxone, amoxicillin-clavulanic acid, and fluoroquinolones have been used in trials with seemingly equivalent results. When susceptibility testing is available, a drug with a narrower spectrum may be substituted. A randomized trial comparing 5 to 10 days of therapy showed no difference, supporting a shorter antibiotic course. The treatment course generally is 5 to 7 days. A repeat paracentesis that demonstrates a reduction in neutrophil counts 48 hours after initiating antibiotic treatment indicates that the antibiotic choice was appropriate. If the correct antibiotics are given in a timely manner, the mortality rate of SBP should not exceed 5%; however, many patients succumb to other complications of the underlying liver disease. Oral quinolones and trimethoprim-sulfamethoxazole are given as prophylactic agents after an initial episode of SBP because of a reported 1-year recurrence rate of 69% in the absence of prophylaxis.

SBP is not the only infectious complication of ascites. Monomicrobial bacterascites is defined as the presence of a positive result from ascitic fluid culture of a single organism with a concurrent fluid neutrophil count lower than 250 cells per μL. One series of patients with bacterascites demonstrated a predominance of gram-positive organisms, whereas another showed flora similar to SBP. Because of the high mortality rate of untreated bacterascites (22% to 43%), antibiotic treatment is warranted for many patients. Alternatively, paracentesis may be repeated for cell count and culture. Culture-negative neutrocytic ascites is defined as ascitic fluid with a neutrophil count higher than or equal to 250 cells per μL with negative fluid culture results in patients who have received no prior antibiotics. Spontaneously resolving SBP is the likely explanation of culture-negative neutrocytic ascites; however, empirical antibiotics generally are given. A decline in ascitic neutrophil counts on repeat paracentesis indicates an appropriate response to therapy. If there is no response to antibiotics, cytologic analysis and culture of the ascitic fluid for tuberculosis may be indicated. Secondary bacterial peritonitis manifests as a polymicrobial infection with a very high ascitic fluid neutrophil count from an identified intra-abdominal source such as appendicitis, diverticulitis, or intra-abdominal abscess. In contrast to SBP, secondary peritonitis usually requires surgical intervention. Gut perforation is suspected with two of the following three criteria: ascitic protein concentration higher than 1 g/dL, glucose level lower than 50 mg/dL, and lactate dehydrogenase level higher than 225 mU/mL. Water-soluble contrast enemas are used in older patients to exclude a perforated colonic diverticulum, whereas young patients should have an upper gastrointestinal study using water-soluble dye because of the probability of a perforated ulcer. In patients with secondary peritonitis but no perforation, repeat paracentesis 48 hours after initiating antibiotic treatment will usually demonstrate increasing neutrophil counts. Polymicrobial bacterascites with an ascitic neutrophil count less than or equal to 250 cells per μL is diagnostic of inadvertent gut perforation by the paracentesis needle. It is usually treated with broad-spectrum antibiotics that include coverage for anaerobes. Alternatively, the decision to treat may be deferred until the results of a repeat paracentesis are obtained.

Tense Ascites

Some patients develop tense ascites with abdominal discomfort or dyspnea with as little as 2 L of ascitic fluid, whereas others may accumulate 20 L or more before becoming tense. Therapy for tense ascites relies on large-volume paracentesis, which may have the added benefit of increasing the venous return to the heart with resultant improvement in cardiac output and stroke volume.

Abdominal Wall Hernias

Umbilical and inguinal hernias are common in patients with ascites. These hernias may produce skin ulceration or rupture (Flood syndrome), or they may become incarcerated. More than one half of these patients will need surgery. If the patient is a candidate for liver transplantation, hernia repair should be delayed until the time of transplant. A more aggressive surgical approach is needed for ulceration, rupture, or incarceration because of the risk for systemic infection, but surgery should be performed after preoperative paracentesis or TIPS to control the ascites. The mortality of rupture is significant (11% to 43%), and it increases in patients with jaundice or coagulopathy.

Hepatic Hydrothorax

Pleural effusions (usually right-sided) are prevalent in patients with cirrhotic ascites. Left-sided effusions are more common with tuberculosis or pancreatic disease. Hepatic hydrothorax is postulated to result from a defect in the diaphragm, which preferentially permits fluid passage into the thorax when negative pressure is generated by normal inspiration. Infection of this fluid is unusual, except in a patient with concurrent SBP. Treatment of hepatic hydrothorax is often challenging because it often does not respond to diuretics. TIPS have been successful, whereas pleurodesis and peritoneovenous shunts often lead to complications.

Hepatorenal Syndrome

Hepatorenal syndrome is the final stage of functional renal impairment in patients with cirrhosis and portal hypertension; it occurs almost exclusively in patients with refractory ascites. It is characterized by peripheral vasodilation and a creatinine clearance less than 40 mL/min (or serum creatinine level higher than 1.5 mg/dL) with normal intravascular volume and the absence of intrinsic renal disease or other renal insults. Urine sodium content is not necessarily less than 10 mmol/L.

Treatment initially involves withdrawing diuretics and nephrotoxins, followed by infusing saline or albumin. Vasoactive agents, octreotide, midodrine, and vasopressin, as well as TIPS have been used with some encouraging results in largely uncontrolled studies. Liver transplantation is the only definitive cure and should be undertaken for all appropriate candidates.

CHAPTER 19

Approach to Gastrointestinal Problems in the Elderly

ALTERATIONS IN PHYSIOLOGY AND PHARMACOLOGY IN ELDERLY PATIENTS

In elderly individuals, age-related physiological changes must be distinguished from problems that result from disease. The clinician should avoid ascribing a constellation of symptoms and signs to the aging process when a correctable condition is present. Certain pathological disorders primarily affect older persons and should be considered more seriously in this population than in younger patients. Vascular diseases (e.g., mesenteric ischemia) preferentially affect older persons who have well-documented atherosclerosis. Atrophic gastritis and its consequences rarely appear in young persons. Aging leads to a decline in helper and killer T-cell function, but produces little impairment of B-cell, plasma cell, or antigen-presenting cell function, indicating that some but not all immune responses may be suppressed in the elderly. Gut-associated immunity may be impaired in older individuals as evidenced by reductions in intraepithelial lymphocytes.

Aging affects the pharmacodynamics and pharmacokinetics of some prescription drugs and alters their potency, duration of action, and side-effect profiles. Benzodiazepines exhibit greater effects in the elderly, whereas α-adrenoceptor agonists and antagonists are less effective. Changes in body composition may modify distribution and clearance of drugs in older patients. On average, fat comprises 40% of total body weight in an elderly person versus 25% in a young individual, thereby changing the distribution of lipid-soluble and water-soluble medications. Renal creatinine clearance falls progressively after age 60, and at 80 years, may be only one third that of a young person. Likewise, hepatic blood flow decreases with age. Thus, excretion of drugs that are cleared by the kidney or liver may be delayed in an older patient. Drug side effects may be additive according to selected age-related phenomena. Corticosteroids can produce dangerous bone demineralization in an elderly patient with osteoporosis, or they may accelerate cataract development.

Aging may produce striking alterations in disease presentation. Central nervous system disease, depression, or a fear of complex medical care may diminish symptom reporting. Acute abdominal pain may be muted by age in some conditions (e.g., appendicitis), providing false reassurance that the patient does not have a serious problem. Chemical peritonitis from ulcer perforation may be absent if the patient is achlorhydric. Pain localization may be atypical in persons older than 60 years. In general, most laboratory tests do not change with age. Most endoscopic or radiologic studies are well tolerated in the elderly, although sedative requirements usually are significantly reduced. Abdominal surgery should not be avoided purely because of patient age, as operative risk correlates more closely with the severity of associated diseases.

DISORDERS OF SWALLOWING AND FOOD INTAKE

Differential Diagnosis

Disorders of swallowing and food intake are prevalent in the elderly and result from anorexia, forgetfulness, depression, physical inability to prepare or consume food, dental problems (including ill-fitting dentures), diseases that impair bolus transfer to the esophagus, and diseases of esophageal transfer. The muscles of the mouth and pharynx may weaken with age, and lip closure may be impaired. Neuromuscular disease (e.g., Parkinson disease, cerebrovascular accidents, polymyositis, dermatomyositis, and myasthenia gravis) may cause pharyngeal muscle dyscoordination. Altered pharyngeal sensation and proprioception may change taste acuity and alter discrimination of bolus size and consistency. Taken together, these age-related changes promote slowed tongue function, food spills, prolonged swallowing, and drooling. Although the number and sensitivity of taste buds decrease with age, taste disturbances more commonly result from the effects of medication, inadequate oral hygiene, or denture problems. Certain pharyngeal disorders (e.g., Zenker diverticulum) occur primarily in elderly individuals.

Physiological changes in esophageal function may also affect the elderly. Dyssynchrony of deglutition and respiration occurs, the duration of swallowing is prolonged, the upper esophageal sphincter pressure is less, and upper esophageal sphincter relaxation is altered with aging. Radiographic evidence of corkscrew esophagus or presbyesophagus and manometric measurement of tertiary contractions are more prevalent in the elderly but have little or no pathophysiological consequence. Acid reflux episodes are more frequent in older persons, although lower esophageal sphincter pressure may be normal. Esophageal transit, measured using scintigraphy, commonly is delayed in older persons. Esophageal disorders that should be given special consideration include pill-induced esophagitis, achalasia, and esophageal carcinoma. Pill esophagitis is especially a risk for older individuals who take medications at bedtime because salivation and swallowing are reduced during sleep (Table 19-1). Secondary forms of achalasia must be more carefully considered in older patients than in younger persons.

Principles of Management

Management of swallowing dysfunction in an elderly patient is not significantly different from that in a younger individual. Barium swallow radiography and upper endoscopy are used to diagnose neoplasia, esophagitis, pill-induced injury, and ulcer disease. Esophageal manometry is useful for characterizing specific motor patterns that occur with achalasia. pH testing for 24 hours quantifies the degree of gastroesophageal reflux of acid. In general, drug therapy is similar for elderly and young patients. For the older person with oropharyngeal dyscoordination, special

---

TABLE 19-1
Medications Associated with Esophageal Injury

Doxycycline hydrate
Tetracycline hydrochloride
Clindamycin
Emepronium bromide
Potassium chloride
Ferrous sulfate or succinate
Alprenolol hydrochloride
Quinidine
Aspirin
Sustained release theophylline
Alendronate

---

instruction in swallowing techniques from a qualified speech pathologist may be indicated.

ULCER DISEASE AND ATROPHIC GASTRITIS

Differential Diagnosis

The incidence of gastroduodenal ulcer disease is greater in the elderly than in younger individuals because of the increased use of nonsteroidal antiinflammatory drugs (NSAIDs), smoking, poor nutrition, and other factors. Gastric acid secretion does not decrease with age in most elderly persons. Similarly, gastric emptying, intrinsic factor secretion, and other physiological functions are unaffected by patient age. Conversely, duodenal bicarbonate secretion may decrease in the elderly. Gastric ulcers occur in more proximal sites in older patients, often near the cardia. Ulcers located within hiatal hernias may produce atypical chest pain. Giant gastric ulcers (>2.5 cm in diameter) occur more frequently in the elderly and may be difficult to distinguish from malignancy. *Helicobacter pylori* infection of the gastric mucosa is more prevalent in the elderly and is likely to contribute to the increased incidence of ulcer disease and gastric malignancies in this age group.

Acid secretion is reduced in 25% to 30% of older individuals. Achlorhydria, caused by chronic atrophic gastritis, is largely a disorder of the elderly and confers a threefold to fourfold increased incidence of gastric cancer. Atrophic gastritis also predisposes to development of gastric polyps. Chronic reductions in gastric acid secretion also increase the risk for small intestinal bacterial overgrowth as well as acute infection with *Salmonella* species, *Vibrio cholera*, *Giardia* species, and perhaps *Clostridium difficile*. Other consequences of achlorhydria include iron, calcium, and vitamin B_{12} malabsorption.

Principles of Management

The symptoms of ulcer disease may be subtle or atypical in elderly patients. Many older individuals report anorexia or vague discomfort that does not radiate, or even substernal chest pain that mimics angina. One third of patients experience no pain at all. Ulcer hemorrhages are more common in older patients and include more frequent rebleeding after initial control of bleeding, more severe hypotension as a result of blood loss, and significant cardiorespiratory compromise with fluid resuscitation. The mortality rate for ulcer perforation is high in the elderly.

Because of the increased morbidity and mortality of ulcer disease in the elderly, the evaluation must be appropriately aggressive. Early endoscopy is performed in most patients, unless contraindicated by intercurrent illness. Uncomplicated ulcers without evidence of bleeding are managed similarly to those in younger patients, with acid-suppressing drugs such as histamine H_2 receptor antagonists or proton pump inhibitors, which are safe for most elderly individuals. *H pylori* infection should be eradicated if found. For those individuals who present with complicated ulcer disease (i.e., hemorrhage or perforation), confirmation of *H pylori* infection is advised. When NSAIDs are causative, they should be withdrawn if possible. If NSAIDs are not restarted, long-term maintenance acid-suppressive therapy is not required. If the patient needs to remain on chronic NSAID therapy, administering a long-term proton pump inhibitor may reduce the risk of rebleeding. Newer cyclooxygenase-2 inhibitors appear to reduce the risk of hemorrhage. The prostaglandin E_1 analog misoprostol has been advocated as prophylaxis against NSAID-induced ulcers; however, its significant side-effect profile (e.g., diarrhea and abdominal pain) may limit its use. If surgery is required for ulcer complications, it should be performed electively whenever possible because of the hazards of emergency surgery in the elderly. Long-term postgastrectomy complications (e.g., diarrhea) may be difficult to manage in the elderly.

The role of endoscopic surveillance in elderly patients with atrophic gastritis or pernicious anemia is controversial. In older individuals, endoscopic biopsies to exclude malignant degeneration need not be performed more often than every 3 to 5 years. Other complications such as nutrient malabsorption and bacterial overgrowth may be managed specifically.

MALABSORPTIVE DISORDERS

Differential Diagnosis

Intestinal absorption and proximal intestinal histology do not change with advancing age. Fecal fat excretion is not increased in the elderly, nor is D-xylose absorption altered. Pancreatic size diminishes in some older persons; however, this is not associated with reductions in pancreatic enzyme output or clinical evidence of malabsorption. Calcium absorption falls in some elderly patients because of reduced renal production of 1,25-dihydroxycholecalciferol or impaired intestinal responsiveness to 1,25-dihydroxycholecalciferol. Lower total body calcium also may result from reduced milk intake in older patients with age-related lactase deficiency.

Among older patients with malabsorption, 44% have pancreatic disease, and 25% have celiac sprue. A specific form of chronic pancreatitis in elderly women is characterized by mild pain, hypergammaglobulinemia, weight loss, pancreatic calcifications, and fever. One third of patients with newly diagnosed celiac sprue are older than 60 years. Many older individuals with celiac disease present with mild symptoms, rather than diarrhea and weight loss. Complications of celiac disease (e.g., osteomalacia, hypoprothrombinemia, and lymphoma) are more common in the elderly. Small intestinal bacterial overgrowth is another common cause of malabsorption in older persons and results from strictures, diverticula, achlorhydria, and small bowel dysmotility. Mesenteric vascular disease is a rare cause of malabsorption in the elderly. Covert ethanol abuse is high in older populations; thus alcohol-related suppression of intestinal mucosal absorption may contribute to impaired absorption in these individuals.

Principles of Management

Evaluation of an elderly patient with malabsorption should focus on risk factors for specific diseases. Prior surgery or Crohn's disease suggests possible small intestinal bacterial overgrowth from intestinal strictures or fistula formation. A long history of ethanol abuse raises the possibility of chronic pancreatitis or small intestinal absorptive dysfunction. In patients with no obvious cause, screening laboratory studies and abdominal radiography may detect anemia, mineral and vitamin deficiencies, and pancreatic calcifications. Further evaluation with celiac disease serologies, breath testing for bacterial overgrowth, barium radiography, and small bowel biopsy may detect intestinal causes of malabsorption. If pancreatic disease is suspected, specific structural and functional tests may characterize the cause of exocrine dysfunction. Therapy should be directed to a specific pathogenic condition. In addition, appropriate replacement of minerals and vitamins may be needed.

CONSTIPATION

Differential Diagnosis

Constipation is a prevalent complaint of elderly individuals and may be described as painful, difficult, or incomplete stool evacuation, rather than infrequent defecation. The symptom is especially common in less mobile patients in nursing homes or other chronic care facilities. Colonic transit testing usually is normal; however delayed rectal evacuation is found in elderly patients secondary to reduced rectal wall elasticity, decreased sensitivity to rectal distention, and abnormalities in colonic ganglia cells.

Several factors contribute to the development of constipation in the elderly (Table 19-2). Endocrine disorders such as hypothyroidism and hyperparathyroidism may be causative. A number of medications including antihypertensives, antidepressants, antispasmodics, and opiates can lead to constipation. Volvulus of the cecum and sigmoid colon are common in elderly individuals, especially in institutionalized patients with underlying cognitive deficiencies. Structural causes of constipation in the elderly include colon cancer as well as benign strictures secondary to diverticulitis, inflammatory bowel disease, prior surgery, or medications. Megacolon caused by long-standing fecal retention develops in patients who are institutionalized, who are taking psychotropic medications, or who have Parkinson disease or organic mental syndromes. Acute pseudoobstruction occurs in patients with electrolyte disturbances, infection, or hemodynamic instability.

TABLE 19-2
Constipation in the Elderly: Causes and Contributing Factors

Obstruction (e.g., malignancy, benign stricture)
Neuromuscular disease (e.g., parkinsonism, laxative colon)
Endocrine disease (e.g., hypothyroidism, hyperparathyroidism, diabetes)
Psychiatric disease (e.g., depression)
Dietary alterations (e.g., decreased food or fluid intake, inadequate bulk in diet)
Decreased defecatory sensation
Medications (e.g., laxative abuse, sedatives, tranquilizers, antihypertensives,
  ganglionic blockers, opiates, calcium-containing antacids)

Principles of Management

The elderly patient with new-onset constipation should be carefully examined to exclude systemic disorders and colonic obstruction. Serum calcium and thyroid stimulating hormone levels can screen for hyperparathyroidism and hypothyroidism. Colonoscopy is indicated to exclude colonic malignancy or benign strictures. Therapy begins by increasing fiber and fluid intake. Osmotic laxatives such as milk of magnesia may be slowly introduced if fiber therapy is inadequate. Poorly absorbed sugars (e.g., lactulose, sorbitol) or isotonic solutions that contain polyethylene glycol may benefit selected elderly patients. For patients with specific symptoms of obstructive defecation, pelvic floor testing with biofeedback retraining of rectosphincteric dyssynergia may be considered.

DIARRHEA

Differential Diagnosis

Diarrhea is a less common complaint in the elderly than constipation. New-onset diarrhea may result from the side effects of medication; intake of laxatives; small intestinal bacterial overgrowth; diabetic enteric neuropathy; as a paradoxical response to fecal impaction; or rarely as a result of infection with *Escherichia coli*, *C difficile*, *Campylobacter jejuni*, or other organisms. Chronic diarrhea secondary to inflammatory bowel disease (IBD) is more common in elderly patients than generally recognized. Many older patients with Crohn's disease are women with predominant involvement of the colon, often in a left-sided distribution similar to diverticular disease. Similarly, left-sided ulcerative colitis occurs more commonly in elderly individuals. IBD recurrences present less frequently, surgery is less often needed, and extraintestinal complications are less common than in the young. However, the mortality rate of IBD in the elderly is two to three times that in younger persons in part because delays in diagnosis necessitate risky emergency surgery. Other chronic conditions that produce symptoms similar to IBD include ischemic colitis, postradiation colitis, and diverticulitis. Fecal incontinence may be misreported as diarrhea. Etiologies of incontinence include rectal prolapse, previous obstetrical trauma, fecal impaction, neuropathy, prior anal surgery, and radiation therapy.

Principles of Management

The management of diarrhea in the elderly depends on its cause. Offending medications should be withdrawn. Fecal disimpaction may provide relief in some patients. Stool samples should be obtained for *C difficile* toxin assay if there is a history of recent antibiotic use. For suspected infection, stool samples for culture and for examination for ova and parasites are obtained as indicated. If laxative abuse is suspected, stool and urine samples can be sent for laxative screening.

Structural testing may be indicated if inflammatory causes of diarrhea are suspected. Abdominal radiography may show thumbprinting with mesenteric ischemia. Flexible sigmoidoscopy or colonoscopy may show evidence of mucosal injury in ulcerative colitis, Crohn's disease, ischemia, and radiation colitis. Biopsy specimens may help to distinguish the various possibilities. However, in some cases, the diagnosis is clinical and is based on the presence of other concurrent diseases and the anatomic distribution of colitis. Angiography or magnetic resonance angiography may be useful in some patients, but individuals with colonic ischemia as a consequence of a low-flow state may have normal mesenteric vessels. Diverticulitis may mimic the presentation of Crohn's disease. Computed tomography may show sigmoid thickening and fluid collections with diverticulitis or Crohn's disease.

Medication of IBD in elderly patients should be approached with care. Responses to treatment may be less complete than in younger individuals. Opiates and anticholinergics should be used sparingly because of sedating side effects, cardiac complications, and the risk of inducing megacolon. In general, sulfasalazine and mesalamine, as well as immunosuppressives such as azathioprine and 6-mercaptopurine are well tolerated. Metronidazole can prolong prothrombin time in patients who take warfarin. Steroid complications, including osteopenia, hyperglycemia, cataracts, glaucoma, and behavioral changes, increase in elderly populations. Thus, steroids should be withdrawn as quickly as possible from older patients, and long-term immunosuppressive therapy should be started early if clinically indicated.

Treatment of elderly patients with fecal incontinence must be individualized. Rectal prolapse or fecal impaction may respond best to treatment of underlying constipation. Biofeedback retraining of the external anal sphincter may be successful in some elderly patients, although bed-bound patients are unlikely to benefit from this technique. Surgical options including sphincter reconstruction, sacral nerve stimulation, and artificial sphincter implantations are available in cases that do not respond to more conservative measures.

HEPATOBILIARY DISORDERS

Differential Diagnosis

Liver structure and function change little with age, and liver chemistry abnormalities attributable to advanced age have not been reported. Elevations in alkaline phosphatase levels, which occur in 27% of elderly patients, are caused by bone disease in 50%, and liver disease in 25%. Hyperbilirubinemia may reflect the effects of congestive heart failure, whereas elevations of aminotransferases suggest hepatocellular injury. Hepatitis in elderly patients may be milder but often produces more severe complications. Drug-induced hepatotoxicity should be considered in elderly patients with new liver chemistry abnormalities.

The prevalence of gallstones increases with age, reaching 35% by age 80 years. Juxtapapillary duodenal diverticula are common in elderly patients and are associated with gallstone formation in 65% to 85% of patients. Postcholecystectomy bile duct stones are most common in the elderly. Clinical manifestations of gallstone disease in older individuals include biliary colic, cholecystitis, cholangitis, and pancreatitis. Cholecystitis may present as a vague discomfort or altered mental status in an elderly patient, whereas cholangitis may produce hypotension. Gallbladder empyema has a high mortality but also may produce only mild symptoms. Gallstone pancreatitis is potentially fatal. Clinical scoring systems to predict disease severity are less accurate in patients older than 75 years, and computed tomography may provide better prognostic information. Acalculous cholecystitis is difficult to diagnose and has a high mortality rate. Obstructive jaundice from choledocholithiasis is common in the elderly and may mimic the presentation of pancreatic carcinoma.

Principles of Management

The treatment of an elderly patient with suspected hepatic disease differs little from that of a younger patient. Isolated elevations of alkaline phosphatase should be evaluated for bony or hepatic causes. Potentially hepatotoxic drugs should be withdrawn if possible. Infectious, immune, or heritable causes of liver dysfunction should be evaluated with specific tests if clinically suspected. Liver biopsy should be considered if the information obtained will modify therapy for the older patient. Use of antiviral therapies for hepatitis B or C is not well established in the elderly.

Elderly patients with suspected biliary disease should be aggressively managed because of the potential for complications or death. If infection is suspected, blood cultures are obtained and antibiotics are instituted early. Ultrasound may detect bile duct dilation, pericholecystic fluid, or gallbladder wall thickening. Computed tomography may also define infection or pancreatitis. Bile duct stones may be detected by endoscopic ultrasound, magnetic resonance cholangiopancreatography, or endoscopic retrograde cholangiopancreatography (ERCP). ERCP also affords the capability to perform sphincterotomy and stone extraction in patients with gallstone pancreatitis, cholangitis, or obstructive jaundice. In an elderly patient with symptomatic common bile duct stones who is not a surgical candidate, ERCP with sphincterotomy represents a viable alternative to cholecystectomy. For patients without contraindication to surgery, elective cholecystectomy by the laparoscopic approach should be performed because of the 10% to 20% mortality of emergency biliary surgery. Percutaneous transhepatic cholangiography provides an alternative approach to the biliary tree, especially in some cases of cholangiocarcinoma. Asymptomatic gallstones do not warrant surgical intervention.

CHAPTER 20

Approach to Gastrointestinal and Liver Diseases in the Female Patient

PHYSIOLOGY OF PREGNANCY

Alterations in Physiology and Drug Metabolism in Normal Pregnancy

Profound physiological changes occur during pregnancy, and many are advantageous to the mother and fetus. The increases in blood volume and red cell mass in pregnancy facilitate oxygen delivery to the fetus and protect the mother from excess blood loss during delivery. Many of the pregnancy-related changes stem from hormonal and anatomic factors. Although peak levels of serum human chorionic gonadotropin (hCG) correlate temporally with the nausea of pregnancy, direct evidence supporting a pathogenic role for the hormone is lacking. Progesterone, which is synthesized initially by the ovary and then by the placenta, maintains the myometrium in a relaxed state, has inhibitory effects on contractile function in other smooth muscle structures, and modulates immune maintenance of fetal tissue. Estrogens (e.g., estradiol, estrone, estriol), which also are synthesized by the placenta, may have weak relaxant effects on smooth muscle, although research suggests that estrogen is a less potent smooth muscle relaxant than progesterone. Levels of progesterone and estrogens increase with advancing gestation.

Pregnancy induces changes in the absorption, distribution, and elimination of drugs. Slowed gastric emptying delays peak drug levels, whereas prolonged intestinal transit increases drug absorption or metabolism. Decreased acid secretion may alter drug solubility. Increases in the maternal and fetal plasma volumes increase the volume of drug distribution, whereas the decrease in plasma albumin associated with increased total volume increases unbound plasma drug levels. A 50% increase in glomerular filtration rate accelerates drug elimination.

Placental and fetal factors determine the effect of medications on the developing fetus. Drugs enter the fetal circulation by diffusion and by facilitated or active transport. The placenta contains enzymes for drug oxidation, reduction, hydrolysis, and conjugation. Fetal albumin levels initially are very low, causing high blood levels of drugs that are normally bound to albumin. Serum albumin rises progressively with increasing gestation. Drugs are responsible for 1% to 5% of fetal malformations, usually through unknown mechanisms. Most of the common gastrointestinal medications carry pregnancy category B or C designation, except for azathioprine, 6-mercaptopurine, methotrexate, and the combination of bismuth/metronidazole/tetracycline for treating *Helicobacter pylori* infection, which carry a designation of D (i.e., evidence of human fetal risk).

GASTROINTESTINAL SYMPTOMS IN PREGNANCY

Nausea and Vomiting and Hyperemesis Gravidarum

Pathophysiology

Nausea and vomiting occur in 50% to 90% of pregnancies, usually in the first trimester. However, they do not have deleterious effects on pregnancy outcome, birth weight, or the number of congenital malformations and may be associated with a lower risk for stillbirth and miscarriage. Intractable vomiting, which produces dehydration, electrolyte disturbances, and nutritional deficiencies, is termed hyperemesis gravidarum. It is a complication of 3.5 of every 1000 deliveries.

Estrogen and progesterone have been proposed as mediators of nausea in the first trimester of pregnancy because of the strong correlation between nausea and oral contraceptive use. Also, nausea of pregnancy occurs more often in nulliparous, nonsmoking, and obese women, all of whom exhibit high circulating estrogen levels. The nausea of pregnancy is associated with rhythm disturbances of gastric electrical activity, effects mimicked by exogenous estrogen and progesterone in nonpregnant women, raising the possibility that gastric pacemaker disruption induces symptoms. However, hCG is the hormone that exhibits the greatest temporal association with the nausea of pregnancy. An increase in the serum thyroxine level during the first trimester has been documented in as many as 70% of pregnancies complicated by hyperemesis gravidarum. Because of the inherent thyroid-stimulating effects of hCG, it has been suggested that high hCG levels in the first trimester are responsible for hyperthyroxinemia; however, the role of thyroxine in producing nausea is unknown. *H pylori* infection is more common in patients with hyperemesis gravidarum than in controls; antibiotic treatment provides symptom relief.

Principles of Management

Nausea and vomiting typically begin in the sixth week of gestation and subside in the second trimester, although 60% of patients with hyperemesis gravidarum may experience symptoms beyond 20 weeks. Managing mild nausea in pregnancy involves ingesting multiple small meals and avoiding situations known to aggravate symptoms; medications are rarely necessary. With a failure to gain weight or symptom onset in the second or third trimester, the clinician should consider hyperemesis gravidarum, preeclampsia, urinary infection, appendicitis, and intrahepatic cholestasis. In addition to fluid, electrolyte, and nutrient deficits, hyperemesis gravidarum may produce Mallory-Weiss tears, pulmonary aspiration, retinal hemorrhage, and neurological abnormalities. Hospitalization for fluid and electrolyte replacement often is necessary for hyperemesis gravidarum. Intravenous hyperalimentation is used in extreme cases. Phenothiazines and antihistamines are used with some success, although their safety in pregnancy has not been confirmed.

Gastroesophageal Reflux Disease

Pathophysiology

Heartburn is a common symptom of pregnancy. It affects about 60% to 70% of pregnant women, and its incidence increases in successive trimesters. Decreases in lower esophageal sphincter (LES) pressure and mechanical effects of the gravid uterus have been proposed as contributors to gastroesophageal reflux in pregnancy. In late pregnancy, LES pressure is reduced in patients with heartburn. However, even in early pregnancy, LES responses to contractile agents are blunted, which indicates impairment of LES competence before symptoms develop. The LES pressure response is probably mediated by circulating hormones because both estrogen and progesterone relax LES smooth muscle. Theories about mechanical factors are based on the positive correlation between reflux symptoms and the size of the gravid uterus. The effects of pregnancy on other mechanisms of gastroesophageal reflux (e.g., transient LES relaxations) are unknown.

Principles of Management

A compatible history given by a pregnant patient usually is sufficient to diagnose gastroesophageal reflux, and further diagnostic testing is not indicated. Endoscopy is safe during pregnancy but should be performed only if complications such as stricture or hemorrhage are suspected. As first-line treatment, antireflux programs use standard behavior modifications, such as small meals, no food before bedtime, and avoidance of caffeine, ethanol, and tobacco. Antacids and sucralfate are safe in the second and third trimesters. The safety of histamine H_2 receptor antagonists and proton pump inhibitors in pregnancy is not well established, although a prospective study showed no increased risk for premature birth or teratogenicity when H_2 blockers were used in the first trimester. Likewise, prokinetic agents (e.g., metoclopramide) are used to treat severe gastroesophageal reflux, but their safe use in pregnancy has not been studied in controlled trials.

Constipation

Pathophysiology

Constipation is prevalent in pregnancy and usually results from colonic hypomotility. Increases in colonic transit times correlate with increases in progesterone levels.

Animal studies document reduced contractile efficiency of colonic smooth muscle after exposure to progesterone. Other factors include rectosigmoid compression by the gravid uterus, increased colonic water and electrolyte absorption, and intake of prenatal vitamin supplements.

Principles of Management

Constipation during pregnancy rarely mandates extensive evaluation. Increases in dietary fiber and fluid intake often are effective. If constipation persists, a fiber supplement (e.g., psyllium) can be safely recommended. Bisacodyl and docusate stool softeners have been used without apparent adverse effects.

Acute Abdominal Pain

Differential Diagnosis

The differential diagnosis of acute abdominal pain in pregnancy includes the same nonobstetric causes that are seen in nonpregnant patients (Table 20-1), as well as several that are specific to pregnant women. Appendicitis is the most common gastrointestinal condition requiring surgery during pregnancy. Cephalad displacement of the appendix by the enlarging uterus may occur. Guarding, rigidity, and fever are less common with pregnancy, and the physiological leukocytosis of pregnancy reduces the diagnostic utility of a complete blood count. Pyuria and hematuria may be caused by local compression and irritation of the ureter. Local perforation may not be immediately evident because the uterus may act as a medial wall to contain the abscess. Alternatively, abscess formation may stimulate premature uterine contractions and delivery. Most cases of acute pancreatitis are associated with cholelithiasis or with an underlying lipoprotein disorder leading to hypertriglyceridemia. Other causes include hyperparathyroidism and ethanol abuse. Acute pancreatitis in pregnancy carries a high risk for maternal and fetal mortality. The early use of total parental nutrition is warranted to prevent a catabolic state in a pregnant female and to maintain nutrition in the fetus and the mother. Hepatic rupture may occur in preeclampsia with associated disseminated intravascular coagulation, usually near term or immediately postpartum. Spontaneous splenic rupture and

TABLE 20-1
Causes of Acute Abdomen in Pregnancy

Nonobstetric Causes
    Acute appendicitis
    Acute cholecystitis
    Acute pancreatitis
    Hepatic rupture
    Intestinal obstruction
    Adnexal torsion
    Sickle cell crisis

Obstetric Causes
    Ectopic pregnancy
    Abruptio placentae
    Red degeneration of a uterine myoma
    Uterine rupture

rupture of splenic arterial aneurysms are rare causes of acute abdominal pain and are usually associated with significant intraperitoneal hemorrhage. Intestinal obstruction usually results from adhesions from prior surgery and is most common in the third trimester, presumably because of pressure on preexisting adhesions from the expanding uterus. An ovarian cyst in a twisted adnexa can produce an acute abdomen during pregnancy. Its presentation may mimic that of acute appendicitis. Sickle cell crisis may produce acute abdominal pain and is associated with high maternal and fetal mortality rates.

The most common obstetric cause of acute abdomen in the first trimester is ectopic pregnancy. Abruptio placentae is an important cause of acute pain in late pregnancy. Classically, patients present with pain, uterine tenderness, and vaginal bleeding, which are caused by separation of the placenta from its uterine attachment. Abruptio placentae may be self-limited, or it may cause fetal demise or severe maternal complications, including blood loss, disseminated intravascular coagulation, and renal cortical necrosis. Red degeneration of a uterine myoma is caused by hemorrhagic infarction of a uterine fibroid and is characterized by focal acute pain. Uterine rupture generally occurs late in pregnancy—spontaneously or during labor—in patients who have undergone prior cesarean section. It usually results in fetal demise and intra-abdominal hemorrhage. Acute granulomatous peritonitis may result from premature rupture of fetal membranes or meconium spillage into the peritoneal cavity during cesarean section.

Principles of Management

Acute abdominal pain during pregnancy should be aggressively evaluated and treated according to the underlying cause, because many of the causative conditions have potentially fatal outcomes for both the fetus and the mother. Early surgery is indicated in appendicitis because mortality rates increase with the development of peritonitis. Emergency surgery nearly always is required for ectopic pregnancy, hepatic rupture, splenic or splenic artery rupture, uterine rupture, and adnexal torsion, whereas elective surgery usually is performed for intestinal obstruction. Medical therapy is appropriate for acute pancreatitis and sickle cell anemia. Treatment of abruptio placentae consists of blood replacement and expeditious delivery.

GASTROINTESTINAL AND LIVER DISEASES IN PREGNANCY

Peptic Ulcer Disease

Pathophysiology

Peptic ulcer disease is rare during pregnancy; its prevalence may not be different from that in age-matched, nonpregnant controls. In fact, pregnant patients with known peptic ulcer disease may experience symptom relief because of reduced gastric acid production. This remains controversial, however, because many studies show no change in acid secretion during pregnancy. Complications of peptic ulcer disease are exceedingly rare in pregnancy but may occur late in the third trimester or in the postpartum period when serum gastrin levels increase.

Principles of Management

The diagnosis of peptic ulcer disease during pregnancy is based on typical symptomatology and nonspecific tenderness on abdominal examination. Because invasive tests usually are avoided, the true incidence of this condition in pregnant women is unknown. More aggressive evaluation should be reserved for patients with hemorrhage or suspected obstruction. Endoscopy is preferred to upper gastrointestinal barium radiography to avoid radiation exposure. Suspected perforation should be aggressively diagnosed and treated. As with gastroesophageal reflux, antacids are the safest choice, although H_2 receptor antagonists often are used. In a pregnant patient with ulcer disease induced by *H pylori*, antibiotics should be chosen carefully to avoid harming the fetus (e.g., metronidazole has teratogenic effects).

Gallstone Disease

Pathophysiology

Because of multiple factors, cholesterol cholelithiasis is more prevalent in women than in men, especially in women with prior pregnancies. Gallbladder size increases during pregnancy and ejection efficiency declines. A decrease in the total bile salt pool during the second and third trimesters leads to an increase in the fractional concentration of cholesterol, creating favorable conditions for gallstone formation. It is unknown whether complications of cholelithiasis occur more frequently in pregnant than in nonpregnant women.

Principles of Management

The signs and symptoms of acute cholecystitis are similar to those in nonpregnant women. The diagnosis is based on typical symptoms, laboratory findings, and ultrasound demonstration of gallstones with or without gallbladder wall thickening or pericholecystic fluid. Ultrasound results may be difficult to interpret in late pregnancy because of gallbladder displacement. Oral cholecystography and biliary scintigraphy should be avoided. Many patients with acute cholecystitis are managed medically with analgesics, fluid resuscitation, and antibiotics. Although early studies suggested that there was an increased risk for fetal demise with surgical intervention in the first trimester, more recent data have shown that cholecystectomy is safe at any stage of pregnancy. Gallstone pancreatitis has high morbidity and mortality in pregnancy; therefore, early cholecystectomy and common bile duct exploration is recommended. Endoscopic retrograde cholangiopancreatography has been used in pregnancy, but data concerning its safety are sparse.

Inflammatory Bowel Disease

Pathophysiology

Infertility correlates with the activity of inflammatory bowel disease (IBD) and is inversely proportional to nutritional status. Pregnancy has variable effects on the activity of IBD. Patients with quiescent ulcerative colitis at the onset of pregnancy are likely to remain quiescent, whereas those with active disease are apt to experience a worsening of symptoms. The course of ulcerative colitis during a single pregnancy does not predict disease patterns in future pregnancies. Exacerbations, when they occur, usually present in the first trimester. Crohn's disease behaves in a similar fashion during pregnancy. Ulcerative colitis has little effect on the rates of congenital abnormalities and fetal loss, although severe colitis may increase the risk of spontaneous abortion and stillbirth. Active Crohn's disease confers a twofold-increased risk of spontaneous abortion, stillbirth, and premature delivery, although quiescent disease has little effect.

Principles of Management

Medical therapy for IBD during pregnancy can be accomplished without harm to the fetus. Sulfasalazine has not been associated with an increase in prematurity, low birth weight, or spontaneous abortion. The experience with 5-aminosalicylates in pregnancy is limited, although no complications have been reported. Patients who take sulfasalazine should receive supplemental folate because of sulfasalazine-induced inhibition of transport and metabolism of folate. Corticosteroids do not increase the risk for low birth weight, spontaneous abortion, or fetal abnormalities. Metronidazole and immunosuppressive agents have teratogenic effects in animals; therefore, their use in pregnancy is not advisable. Immunosuppressives should be discontinued at least 6 months before considering pregnancy.

Viral Hepatitis

Acute viral hepatitis in pregnancy is rare; it occurs in less than 1% of gestations. The clinical manifestations and laboratory findings of hepatitis A, B, and C are similar to those in nonpregnant women. Onset most often occurs in the third trimester. In contrast, hepatitis E in pregnant women can be more severe and is associated with a mortality rate higher than that in nonpregnant women. All forms of hepatitis are associated with increased rates of fetal loss and premature birth. Hepatitis B can be transmitted vertically during pregnancy or childbirth. Exposed infants are treated with hepatitis B immune serum globulin and hepatitis B vaccine, and similarly, infants exposed to hepatitis A are treated with immune globulin and hepatitis A vaccine at delivery. Because of the high incidence of chronic hepatitis B in exposed infants, universal screening for hepatitis B surface antigen in all pregnant women is recommended during the third trimester.

Intrahepatic Cholestasis of Pregnancy

Intrahepatic cholestasis of pregnancy, a benign cholestatic disorder that occurs in less than 1% of pregnancies in the United States, accounts for 30% to 50% of all causes of jaundice in pregnancy. The syndrome is similar to the cholestasis associated with estrogen supplements. Moreover, women with a prior history of intrahepatic cholestasis of pregnancy often manifest cholestasis when challenged with oral contraceptives in the nonpregnant state. The etiology remains unknown, but familial clustering suggests the presence of a genetically acquired sensitivity to the cholestatic effects of estrogens. Patients usually present with pruritus and mild jaundice in the third trimester. Liver chemistry levels demonstrate a cholestatic pattern. A biopsy specimen from the liver reveals bland cholestasis with no inflammatory reaction. A biopsy is occasionally needed to differentiate the syndrome from acute fatty liver of pregnancy or other more morbid disorders. Supportive treatment with ursodiol or cholestyramine may relieve the pruritus; cholestasis and pruritus resolve within 24 to 48 hours of delivery.

Acute Fatty Liver of Pregnancy

Pathophysiology

Acute fatty liver of pregnancy is a rare but serious disorder that occurs in less than one case per million pregnancies, and most often in first pregnancies, twin pregnancies, and pregnancies in which the fetus is male. There is no known genetic component, although it tends to recur in subsequent pregnancies. Histological findings include infiltration of the hepatocytes with microvesicular fat and abnormal mitochondria. Nonspecific symptoms of nausea, fatigue, malaise, vomiting, and abdominal distress usually manifest near 35 weeks of gestation. Right upper quadrant tenderness is typical and jaundice is rare. Hepatic encephalopathy and bleeding may occur. Complications of fulminant liver failure, including cerebral edema, hemorrhage, renal failure, and infection, may occur and portend a poor prognosis. Aspartate aminotransferase, alanine aminotransferase, bilirubin, and alkaline phosphatase levels are universally elevated, with a mixed hepatocellular and cholestatic profile.

Principles of Management

Therapy for acute fatty liver of pregnancy is supportive and prompt termination of the pregnancy is generally recommended. Delivery is often complicated by severe postpartum hemorrhage. Renal dysfunction is treated with dialysis. The signs and symptoms gradually resolve over weeks and liver function returns to normal in most patients, although maternal and fetal mortality rates are high.

Preeclampsia-Associated Liver Disease and HELLP Syndrome

Pathophysiology

Preeclampsia is a complication of 5% to 10% of all pregnancies. It is characterized by hypertension, proteinuria, and edema, with progression to seizures; seizures define true eclampsia. Liver involvement occurs in 10% of women with preeclampsia and is more common with eclampsia. Two pathophysiological liver conditions have been described. The first, a disorder of hepatocyte necrosis associated with thrombocytopenia, is termed HELLP syndrome (hemolysis, elevated liver enzymes, and low platelets). The second is acute liver hemorrhage and rupture; large hematomas form beneath the capsule and may rupture, resulting in the sudden onset of right upper quadrant pain and shock. Hepatic necrosis often is associated with necrosis in other organs, including the brain and kidney. Preeclampsia and HELLP syndrome are associated with intrauterine growth retardation, sudden fetal death, and perinatal instability.

Principles of Management

Close monitoring, supportive measures and rapid delivery are warranted in most cases. Hypertension is treated with magnesium sulfate. Patients with postpartum HELLP syndrome may benefit from corticosteroids. Liver necrosis generally heals rapidly after delivery; however, women remain at increased risk of recurrent preeclampsia and HELLP syndrome in subsequent pregnancies. Patients with hepatic rupture and contained hemorrhage are treated conservatively; emergent laparotomy and angiographic embolization are reserved for treating rupture of the Glisson capsule.

GYNECOLOGIC DISEASE AS A CAUSE OF LOWER ABDOMINAL PAIN

Acute and chronic abdominal and pelvic pain in women may result from various gynecologic causes (Table 20-2).

Acute Presentations

Differential Diagnosis

Pelvic inflammatory disease.   Acute pelvic inflammatory disease (PID) results from the ascent of bacteria into the uterus and fallopian tubes. Salpingitis (i.e., tubal infection) is the most characteristic manifestation, although peritonitis,

---

TABLE 20-2
Gynecologic Causes of Abdominal and Pelvic Pain in Women of
Reproductive Age

Acute Presentation
   Pelvic inflammatory disease
   Ectopic pregnancy
   Mittelschmerz
   Ruptured ovarian cyst
     Corpus luteum
     Ovarian endometrioma
   Adnexal torsion

Chronic Presentation
   Endometriosis
   Ovarian carcinoma
   Dysmenorrhea

---

intra-abdominal abscess formation, or sepsis may result. Risk factors for developing PID include sexual activity with multiple partners, the presence of an intrauterine device, and prior pelvic instrumentation. Oral contraceptives decrease the risk because of increased cervical mucus viscosity. Cervicitis resulting from sexually transmitted *Chlamydia trachomatis* or *Neisseria gonorrhoeae* commonly precedes PID development, whereas PID associated with an intrauterine device is caused by normal vaginal flora. Patients classically present with the triad of fever, lower abdominal pain, and vaginal discharge, although there is a wide spectrum of presentations.

Ectopic pregnancy.   Ectopic pregnancy is the leading cause of maternal mortality and should especially be considered in a patient with acute lower abdominal pain and a history of prior PID, previous pelvic surgery, progestin-only oral contraceptive, intrauterine device use, previous ectopic pregnancies, and use of advanced reproductive technologies. Tubal ectopic pregnancies are most common, but extrauterine implantation may also occur in the ovaries, cervix, and abdominal cavity. Although virtually all patients have abdominal or adnexal tenderness, only one half have adnexal masses palpable on pelvic examination. A ruptured ectopic pregnancy may produce hypotension or pain referral to the left shoulder.

Midcycle ovulatory pain.   Pain from intraperitoneal bleeding associated with physiological rupture of an ovarian follicle can range from mild discomfort to severe pain that prompts emergency evaluation. Ovulatory pain (i.e., mittelschmerz) is sudden, sharp, unilaterally localized, and lasts several hours.

Ruptured ovarian cysts.   Acute abdominal pain may result from hemorrhage into a corpus luteum cyst with subsequent rupture or rupture of an ovarian endometrioma. Hemorrhage into the cystic cavity usually occurs late in the menstrual period, often immediately before menstruation. Clinical presentations typically include lower quadrant pain, delayed menses, abnormal uterine bleeding, and an enlarged, tender adnexal mass. Leakage from an ovarian endometrioma may evoke intense chemical peritonitis, resulting in development of low-grade fever and rectal irritation.

Ovarian torsion.   Ovarian or adnexal torsion is most commonly associated with ovarian neoplasms. Patients typically present with sharp pain that is brief, irregular, and repetitive if torsion is intermittent. Symptoms may occur when a patient rises out of a chair or stoops over. With ovarian necrosis, pain may become dull and less precise and over 4 to 6 hours, generalized peritonitis may develop. Rarely, the process may wall off with omentum or bowel and produce low-grade chronic pain.

Principles of Management

All female patients with acute lower quadrant abdominal pain should be examined for possible gynecologic causes. Therefore, careful pelvic examination is required. Patients with salpingitis have marked tenderness on bimanual examination, although unilateral tenderness is rare. A Gram stain of cervical secretions may suggest gonococcal cervicitis. However, secretions should be rigorously tested for *N gonorrhoeae* and *C trachomatis* by culture, fluorescent antibody smear, or enzyme-linked immunoassay techniques.

Blood testing should include pregnancy testing, a white blood cell count, hemoglobin concentration, and in some cases, a sedimentation rate. However, only 45% of patients with salpingitis exhibit leukocyte counts in excess of 8000 cells per μL and 25% have a sedimentation rate less than 5 mm/h. All pregnant women are tested for possible ectopic pregnancy.

Other diagnostic studies may be useful. Pelvic and vaginal ultrasound studies have limited use in PID unless a palpable adnexal mass is noted, whereas vaginal ultrasound may facilitate early diagnosis of ectopic pregnancy, ovarian cysts, or ovarian torsion. Culdocentesis may recover purulent fluid in PID or blood in ectopic pregnancy or with ovarian cyst rupture. Diagnostic laparoscopy may distinguish PID, ectopic pregnancy, ovarian lesions, and appendicitis.

The management of acute pain secondary to gynecologic disease depends on its cause. Most patients with PID respond to parenteral cefoxitin plus oral doxycycline or intravenous clindamycin plus gentamicin. If an intrauterine device is present, it should be removed. Surgery is indicated in PID for a patient with sepsis or a ruptured abscess. Transvaginal or transabdominal drainage may be needed in rare cases that are unresponsive to antibiotics. Surgery is the mainstay of therapy for suspected or documented ectopic pregnancy. In stable patients, laparoscopic salpingectomy or salpingostomy may be possible, but emergency laparotomy is needed if hemodynamic compromise is present. Patients should be followed postoperatively with determination of hCG levels to exclude the possibility of residual trophoblastic tissue. Selected patients with smaller, unruptured ectopic pregnancies may be treated medically with methotrexate. Midcycle ovulatory pain usually resolves, but patients may need oral contraceptives for ovarian suppression. Patients with ovarian cysts and torsions often require surgical intervention.

Chronic Presentations

Differential Diagnosis

Dysmenorrhea.   Dysmenorrhea is defined as pelvic pain in association with menstruation and may range from mild discomfort to severe, debilitating symptoms. Primary dysmenorrhea may result from elevated uterine prostaglandin production, which can enhance uterine contractility and sensitize intrauterine pain fibers to mechanical and chemical stimuli. Secondary dysmenorrhea may result from endometrial polyps, submucous myomas, intrauterine devices, endometriosis, adenomyosis, and cervical stenosis. Dysmenorrhea is described as sharp, crampy, lower midabdominal pain that may radiate to the back or thigh. The pain usually starts before the onset of vaginal bleeding and peaks on the first day of menstruation.

Endometriosis.　Endometriosis is characterized by the ectopic growth of hormonally responsive endometrium outside the uterus, usually close to the fallopian tubes, ovaries, cul-de-sac, and uterosacral ligament. It represents an important cause of lower abdominal pain in women of reproductive age. Endometriosis involving the gastrointestinal tract is localized most frequently to the rectosigmoid colon, with less likely attachment to the rectovaginal septum, small intestine, cecum, appendix, and other sites. Hemoperitoneum may be present during menstruation. Extra-abdominal sites of implantation include the central and peripheral nervous systems and the lungs. Patients typically present with pain and cramping with or slightly before the onset of menstruation. Gastrointestinal involvement may produce rectal pain, pain on defecation, or constipation. Patients with colonic endometriosis may present with cyclic rectal bleeding or colonic obstruction with severe disease. Rare symptoms include intussusception, obstruction of the small intestine, hemorrhagic ascites, protein-losing enteropathy, and bowel perforation.

Ovarian malignancies.　Ovarian cancer is most prevalent in perimenopausal and postmenopausal women and most commonly occurs in patients with histories of late childbearing, early menarche, late menopause, and infertility. Hereditary ovarian cancer, which accounts for 3% to 5% of cases, often occurs in conjunction with hereditary syndromes such as hereditary nonpolyposis colorectal cancer (HNPCC). Oral contraceptives reduce the risk of ovarian cancer. Ovarian cancer spreads by contiguous invasion and intraperitoneal seeding and is confined to the ovary at the time of diagnosis in less than 30% of patients. Sites of metastasis include the fallopian tubes, uterus, bladder, and rectum. Diffuse involvement of the intestinal serosa may produce severe gastrointestinal dysfunction. Bowel encasement may further produce intestinal obstruction. Malignant ascites is present in 35% of women at the time of diagnosis and the diagnosis should be considered in any postmenopausal woman presenting with ascites. Rarely, the disease may metastasize to lymph nodes, lung, or liver.

Principles of Management

Physical examination can provide clues to the cause of chronic lower abdominal pain of gynecologic etiology. Patients with primary dysmenorrhea usually have a normal examination, whereas those with secondary dysmenorrhea may exhibit uterine masses, cervical stenosis, or endometriosis. Patients with endometriosis may have nodular thickening and tenderness along the uterosacral ligaments, on the posterior uterus, and in the cul-de-sac, which are all more conspicuous at the time of menstruation. Physical findings in ovarian cancer include ascites, abdominal or pelvic masses, signs of intestinal obstruction, and pleural rubs or effusions. In a postmenopausal woman, the presence of a palpable ovary, even in the absence of symptoms or other findings, should raise concern about ovarian malignancy.

Diagnostic testing usually is not necessary for primary dysmenorrhea, although ultrasound may occasionally be useful for some patients with secondary dysmenorrhea. Ultrasound may also detect ovarian endometriomas. Endoscopic ultrasound may be useful in defining mucosal lesions in patients with hematochezia and can determine the depth of invasion of endometrial tissue. Laparoscopy allows confirmation of endometriosis with the appropriate clinical presentation, whereas endoscopy or barium radiography may detect lumenal manifestations. Ultrasound is useful in differentiating ovarian neoplasms from ovarian cysts and may document ascites, liver metastasis, lymphadenopathy, and ureteral dilation. Computed tomography may provide further definition of the spread of malignant disease. The tumor marker CA-125 is 80% to 90% accurate in differentiating malignant ovarian tumors from benign disease in postmenopausal women when levels exceed 65 U/mL. α-Fetoprotein elevations may suggest ovarian endodermal sinus tumors, whereas hCG levels may rise with choriocarcinoma and embryonal carcinoma. Surgical staging and peritoneal fluid sampling are required before determining appropriate treatment of a patient with ovarian cancer.

Management of chronic abdominal pain in women depends on the cause. Patients with primary dysmenorrhea may respond to nonsteroidal antiinflammatory drugs or, in severe cases, oral contraceptives. Surgical resection may be necessary for some causes of secondary dysmenorrhea. Endometriosis may be pharmacologically treated with oral contraceptives, progestational agents, danazol, or gonadotropin-releasing hormone analogs (e.g., leuprolide). Laparoscopic laser treatments may benefit patients with severe pain caused by endometriosis, whereas total hysterectomy with bilateral salpingo-oophorectomy may be recommended for severely affected patients who do not desire further pregnancy or when pregnancy is not possible because of disease involvement. With ovarian malignancies confined to a single ovary, primary treatment is unilateral salpingo-oophorectomy. Surgical debulking and chemotherapy are used as palliative therapy for extensive disease.

CHAPTER 21

Approach to the Patient Requiring Nutritional Support

Most people can ingest the necessary fluids, nutrients, vitamins, and minerals to maintain health. Certain patients cannot satisfy their nutritional requirements with oral intake alone because of disease or surgical procedures. It is possible to supplement or provide complete fluid and nutrition needs of these patients with enteral or intravenous solutions. In healthy adults, 30 to 35 mL of fluid are required for each kilogram of body weight. An additional 360 mL per day is required for each degree centigrade of fever. In anabolic conditions, 300 to 400 mL more water is needed. Fluids may need to be restricted with volume overload or hyponatremia. Electrolyte requirements are affected by renal and gastrointestinal disease. Potassium and phosphate supplementation is required for diarrhea or vomiting and to compensate for intracellular shifts during intravenous nutrition. Sodium is restricted for heart failure, renal disease, and portal hypertension, whereas potassium, phosphate, and magnesium are reduced with renal failure. Levels of magnesium, iron, copper, selenium, and zinc should be monitored and supplemented as indicated.

Healthy adults require 20 to 25 kcal per kilogram of body weight to satisfy daily caloric requirements. With the stress of disease or surgery, this need increases to 30 to 40 kcal per kilogram per day. For nonstressed patients, the recommended dietary protein allowance is 0.8 g per kilogram daily. This increases to 1.5 to 2.0 g per kilogram daily for catabolic patients. There are nine amino acids that cannot be synthesized by human tissues and must be part of any protein-calorie supplement. Sufficient carbohydrates and fats must be provided to ensure that oral or intravenous proteins or amino acids are used for protein synthesis and not for energy from gluconeogenesis. For patients requiring long-term nutritional support, multivitamin supplementation may be necessary to prevent deficiency syndromes.

DIFFERENTIAL DIAGNOSIS

Causes of Nutrient Deficiency

A variety of clinical conditions mandate nutritional support (Table 21-1). Many patients have diminished nutritional intake as a consequence of oral and upper gastrointestinal problems such as poorly fitting dentures, esophagitis, ulcer disease, or neoplasm of the head and neck. Medications can induce dyspepsia or suppress appetite. Similarly, anorexia is common in depression. Neurological disease, as with a stroke, can produce dysphagia or aspiration that prevents adequate oral intake. Volitional food consumption is impossible with obtundation from any cause. Decreased intake is most likely to affect nutrients that have small body stores, such as folate, water-soluble vitamins, and protein. All of these patient subsets exhibit normal gut absorptive function and can be supplemented with oral or enteral formulas.

Other clinical conditions without impairment of food intake are associated with nutrient deficiencies. Malabsorptive conditions may produce profound nutrient deficiency, especially those that impair the effective small intestinal mucosal absorptive surface area (e.g., celiac disease, short bowel syndrome, Whipple disease). Affected patients also lose endogenous stores of minerals, vitamins, and proteins that are not reabsorbed from gastric, pancreaticobiliary, and small intestinal secretions. When steatorrhea is present, divalent cations (calcium, magnesium, zinc) are lost because they combine with unabsorbed fatty acids to form nonabsorbable soaps. Drugs may induce malabsorption by several mechanisms. Cholestyramine binds fats and fat-soluble vitamins, whereas neomycin precipitates bile salts. Sulfasalazine inhibits folate absorption, and colchicine inhibits enterocyte release of fat-soluble vitamins. In addition to suppressing appetite, chronic ingestion of large amounts of ethanol is toxic to intestinal enterocytes causing decreased transport of glucose, amino acids, folate, and thiamine. Protein-calorie malnutrition occurs in conditions with increased catabolism, such as Crohn's disease or high-dose corticosteroid use. Likewise, increased caloric and fluid needs are observed with pregnancy, lactation, sepsis, trauma, and burns. Additional deficiencies in Crohn's disease include those of calcium, vitamin D, iron, vitamin B_{12}, zinc, and potassium. Other causes of intestinal failure that result in malabsorption include radiation enteritis, intestinal pseudoobstruction with bacterial overgrowth, chronic adhesive peritonitis, and mucosal diseases without effective treatment (collagenous sprue). Advanced liver disease may alter the plasma amino acid profile. Increased fluid and electrolyte losses occur in the absence of malabsorption in patients with diarrhea, vomiting, enterocutaneous fistulae, gastric suctioning, and renal wasting.

Mineral Deficiency States

Major mineral deficiencies elicit a range of clinical manifestations. Sodium deficiency results from increased losses caused by vomiting, diarrhea, diuresis, salt-wasting renal disease, fistulae, or adrenal insufficiency. Among hospitalized patients, hyponatremia commonly results from excess free water caused by cardiac,

TABLE 21-1
Physical Signs of Deficiencies of Specific Nutrients

Hair

Thin, sparse (protein, zinc, biotin)
Flag sign (transverse pigmentation) (protein, copper)
Easy pluckability (protein)

Nails

Spoon-shaped (i.e., koilonychia) (iron)
No luster, transverse ridging (protein, energy)

Skin

Dry, scaling (i.e., xerosis) (vitamin A, zinc)
Seborrheic dermatitis (essential fatty acids, zinc, pyridoxine, biotin)
Flaky paint dermatosis (protein)
Follicular hyperkeratosis (vitamin A, vitamin C, essential fatty acids)
Nasolabial seborrhea (niacin, pyridoxine, riboflavin)
Petechiae, purpura (vitamin C, vitamin K, vitamin A)
Pigmentation, desquamation (niacin)
Pallor (folate, iron, cobalamin, copper, biotin)

Eyes

Angular palpebritis (riboflavin)
Blepharitis (B vitamins)
Corneal vascularization (riboflavin)
Dull, dry conjunctiva (vitamin A)
Bitot spot (vitamin A)
Keratomalacia (vitamin A)
Fundal capillary microaneurysms (vitamin C)
Ophthalmoplegia (Wernicke encephalopathy) (thiamine)

Mouth

Angular stomatitis (B vitamins, iron, protein)
Cheilosis (riboflavin, niacin, pyridoxine, protein)
Atrophic lingual papillae (niacin, iron, riboflavin, folate, cobalamin)
Glossitis (niacin, pyridoxine, riboflavin, folate, cobalamin)
Decreased taste and smell (vitamin A, zinc)
Swollen, bleeding gums (vitamin C)

Glands

Parotid enlargement (protein)
Sicca syndrome (vitamin C)
Thyroid enlargement (iodine)

Heart

Enlargement, tachycardia, high-output failure (i.e., beriberi) (thiamine)
Small heart, decreased output (protein, energy)
Cardiomyopathy (selenium)
Cardiac arrhythmias (magnesium, potassium)

Extremities

Edema (protein, thiamine)
Muscle weakness (protein, energy, selenium)
Bone and joint tenderness (vitamin C, vitamin A)
Osteopenia, bone pain (vitamin D, calcium, phosphorus, vitamin C)

(continued)

TABLE 21-1
(Continued)

Neurological
Confabulation, disorientation (i.e., Korsakoff psychosis) (thiamine)
Decreased position and vibration sense, ataxia (cobalamin, thiamine)
Decreased tendon reflexes (thiamine)
Weakness, paresthesias (cobalamin, pyridoxine, thiamine)
Mental disorders (cobalamin, niacin, thiamine, magnesium)

Other
Delayed wound healing (vitamin C, protein, zinc, essential fatty acids)
Hypogonadism, delayed puberty (zinc)
Glucose intolerance (chromium)

---

renal, or hepatic insufficiency. Severe sodium depletion with dehydration produces nausea and vomiting, exhaustion, cramps, seizures, and cardiorespiratory collapse. Pseudohyponatremia results from excess lipid, glucose, blood urea nitrogen, mannitol, or glycerin in the serum. Potassium depletion results from gastrointestinal or urinary losses (diuretics, alkalosis, mineralocorticoid excess, renal tubular acidosis). Hypokalemia also results from potassium shifts from the extracellular to the intracellular compartment during alkalosis, after insulin or glucose administration, or periodic paralysis. Symptoms of potassium depletion include confusion, lethargy, weakness, cramps, myalgias, cardiac arrhythmias, glucose intolerance, nausea, vomiting, diarrhea, ileus, and gastroparesis. Hypocalcemia is caused by vitamin D deficiency, failed vitamin D synthesis or action, hypoparathyroidism, hypomagnesemia, acute pancreatitis, osteoblastic malignancies, malabsorption, and medications (e.g., aminoglycosides, cisplatin, calcitonin, furosemide, phosphates, and anticonvulsants). Manifestations of hypocalcemia include a positive Chvostek or Trousseau sign, tetany, hyperreflexia, paresthesias, seizures, mental status changes, increased intracranial pressure, bradycardia, heart block, and choreoathetotic movements. Chronic calcium deficiency causes rickets in children and osteomalacia in adults. Eighty percent to 85% of phosphorus stores are in bone. Hypophosphatemia occurs in 2% to 3% of hospitalized patients because of decreased intestinal absorption (antacids, malabsorption, vitamin D deficiency, hypoparathyroidism), increased renal excretion (proximal tubule disease, alkalosis, diuretics, hyperparathyroidism, burns, corticosteroids), and intracellular shifts (respiratory alkalosis, carbohydrate administration). Severe hypophosphatemia produces hemolysis, encephalopathy, seizures, paresthesias, muscle weakness, rhabdomyolysis, decreased glucose utilization, and reduced oxygen delivery. Similarly, 70% of magnesium stores are in bone. Magnesium absorption decreases in malabsorption syndromes. Excessive urinary loss results from hypercalcemia, volume expansion, tubular dysfunction, alcoholism, diabetes, hyperparathyroidism, hypophosphatemia, and medications (e.g., diuretics, aminoglycosides, cyclosporin, amphotericin, cisplatin, digoxin). Shifts into the intracellular space result from refeeding, treating diabetic ketoacidosis, pancreatitis, and correcting acidosis in renal failure. Patients with hypomagnesemia present with tremors, myoclonic jerks, ataxia, tetany, psychiatric disturbances, coma, ventricular arrhythmias, hypotension, or cardiac arrest.

Trace mineral deficiencies also are prevalent. Iron deficiency results from gastrointestinal bleeding, excessive menstrual loss, and malabsorption (e.g., celiac sprue, achlorhydria). Clinical manifestations of iron deficiency stem from anemia and include weakness, lightheadedness, decreased exercise tolerance, and tachycardia. Zinc deficiency results from malabsorption, cirrhosis, alcoholism, nephrotic syndrome, sickle cell anemia, pregnancy, pica, pancreatic insufficiency, use of penicillamine, and chronic diarrhea of any cause. Clinical manifestations of zinc deficiency include growth retardation, scaling skin, alopecia, diarrhea, apathy, night blindness, poor wound healing, and dysgeusia. Copper deficiency in adults is rare and occurs with parenteral nutrition without copper supplements and during penicillamine therapy. Clinical manifestations of copper deficiency include microcytic anemia, leukopenia, neutropenia, and skeletal abnormalities. Selenium deficiency occurs with small bowel causes of malabsorption, fistulae, alcoholism, cirrhosis, acquired immunodeficiency syndrome, cancer, and with parenteral nutritional formulas without supplemental selenium. Symptoms of selenium deficiency include myositis, weakness, and cardiomyopathy. Only 2% of dietary chromium is absorbed. Chromium deficiency occurs with short bowel syndrome and in patients who receive poorly supplemented parenteral nutritional formulas. Clinical manifestations include hyperglycemia, insulin insensitivity, encephalopathy, peripheral neuropathy, and weight loss. Iodine deficiency usually is caused by inadequate intake and results in hypothyroidism and thyroid hyperplasia and hypertrophy. Iodine supplements are rarely needed in parenteral nutritional solutions, presumably because sufficient iodine is present as a contaminant or is absorbed from the skin.

Several minerals are considered essential, but deficiency syndromes have not been reported. Fluoride is essential for growth, reproduction, and iron absorption. Molybdenum is needed to metabolize purines and sulfur-containing compounds. Manganese is a cofactor for pyruvate carboxylase and manganese superoxide dismutase. Vanadium, nickel, cobalt, tin, and silicon also are considered essential in mammals. Cadmium, lead, boron, aluminum, arsenic, mercury, strontium, and lithium eventually may prove to be essential.

Vitamin Deficiency States

In general, deficiencies of fat-soluble vitamins (A, D, E, and K) take years to develop because large stores are present in adipose tissue. Vitamin D is made endogenously in sun-exposed skin. Vitamins that undergo enterohepatic circulation (e.g., A and D) may be lost in malabsorptive conditions. Blood values for fat-soluble vitamins are difficult to interpret because of adipose stores and plasma-binding proteins. Vitamin A or its carotenoid precursors are present in animal products (e.g., liver, kidney, dairy products, eggs) and in green and yellow vegetables. Vitamin A deficiency results from decreased intake and fat malabsorption, although impaired carotenoid conversion in mucosal disease, inability to store the vitamin in liver disease, and increased urinary losses (e.g., as from tuberculosis, cancer, pneumonia, urinary tract infection) may contribute. Vitamin A deficiency produces night blindness, xerophthalmia, follicular hyperkeratosis, altered taste and smell, increased cerebrospinal fluid pressure, and increased infections. Vitamin D from fish liver oils, eggs, liver, and dairy products is absorbed by the small intestine. Cholecalciferol (vitamin D_3) is synthesized on ultraviolet exposure of the skin. Vitamin D deficiency results from inadequate exposure to the sun, steatorrhea, severe liver or kidney disease, Crohn's disease, or small bowel resection. Manifestations of deficiency include hypocalcemia, hypophosphatemia, bone demineralization, osteomalacia in adults, rickets in children, and bony fractures. Vitamin E is a fat-soluble antioxidant and a free-radical scavenger found in plants and vegetable oils. Deficiency is rare in humans but may occur with malabsorption in abetalipoproteinemia, cystic fibrosis, cirrhosis, malabsorption, and from ingesting excess mineral oil. Vitamin E deficiency elicits hemolysis and a progressive neurological syndrome (areflexia, gait disturbance, decreased vibratory and proprioceptive sensation, and gaze paresis). Vitamin K is abundant in the diet and is synthesized by intestinal bacteria. Deficiency results from malabsorption of fat, diminished liver function or bile secretion, or antibiotic inhibition of bacterial production. Vitamin K deficiency prolongs prothrombin time and increases the risk of hemorrhage.

In contrast to fat-soluble vitamins, water-soluble vitamins are not stored in large quantities in the body. Blood levels of water-soluble vitamins reflect body stores and fall before clinical manifestations of vitamin deficiency develop. Thiamine (vitamin B_1) is readily available in the diet, and deficiency presents in alcoholics or in patients with malabsorption, severe malnutrition, prolonged fever, or on chronic hemodialysis. Thiamine deficiency causes beriberi, which is characterized by easy fatigability, weakness, paresthesias, and high-output congestive heart failure. Other manifestations include peripheral neuropathy, cerebellar dysfunction, subacute necrotizing encephalomyelopathy, and Wernicke encephalopathy (with mental changes, ataxia, nystagmus, paresis of upward gaze). Thiamine deficiency may also play a role in Korsakoff syndrome. Riboflavin (vitamin B_2) is present in milk, eggs, and leafy green vegetables. Deficiency occurs in conjunction with other B vitamin deficiencies in alcoholism and malabsorption. Riboflavin deficiency produces angular stomatitis, cheilosis, glossitis, seborrhea-like dermatitis, pruritus, photophobia, and visual impairment. Niacin (vitamin B_3) and its precursor, tryptophan, are found in animal proteins, beans, nuts, whole grains, and enriched breads and cereals. Niacin deficiency occurs rarely as a complication of alcoholism, malabsorption, carcinoid syndrome, or Hartnup disease. Niacin deficiency causes pellagra, which presents with a scaly, hyperpigmented dermatitis localized to sun-exposed surfaces, diarrhea, and central nervous system dysfunction (irritability and headache progressing to psychosis, hallucinations, and seizures). Pyridoxine (vitamin B_6) is present in animal protein and whole grain cereals. Pyridoxine deficiency most commonly occurs during treatment with pyridoxine antagonists (isoniazid, hydralazine, and penicillamine) but also occurs in alcoholics and malabsorption. Pyridoxine deficiency produces peripheral neuropathy, seborrheic dermatitis, glossitis, angular stomatitis, cheilosis, seizures, and sideroblastic anemia. Folate is abundant in vegetables, legumes, kidney, liver, and nuts. Folate deficiency is caused by poor intake or altered small bowel mucosal function in alcoholics, by malabsorption, and during use of sulfasalazine or anticonvulsants. Folate deficiency elicits macrocytic anemia, thrombocytopenia, leukopenia, glossitis, diarrhea, fatigue, and possibly neurological findings. Cobalamin (vitamin B_{12}) is found in animal tissues. Cobalamin deficiency occurs in some vegetarians and also is caused by pernicious anemia, gastrectomy, ileal disease or resection, or bacterial overgrowth, in which bacteria bind dietary cobalamin so that it cannot be absorbed. Clinical findings of deficiency include macrocytic anemia, anorexia, loss of taste, glossitis, diarrhea, dyspepsia, hair loss, impotence, and neurological disease (i.e., peripheral neuropathy, loss of vibratory sensation, incoordination, muscle weakness and atrophy, irritability, and memory loss). Ascorbic acid (vitamin C) is present in fruits (especially citrus) and vegetables. Scurvy develops after 2 to 3 months of a diet deficient in ascorbic acid. Other causes of deficiency include alcoholism, malabsorption, and Crohn's disease. Vitamin C deficiency produces weakness, irritability, aching joints and muscles, and weight loss, which progress to perifollicular hyperkeratotic papules, petechiae, and swollen, hemorrhagic gums. Biotin deficiency occurs in persons whose diet is high in egg whites, which contain a biotin-binding glycoprotein, and in patients who take hyperalimentation solutions without biotin supplements. Biotin deficiency produces anorexia, nausea, dermatitis, alopecia, mental depression, and organic aciduria.

Essential Fatty Acid Deficiency

Essential fatty acids are long-chain compounds that cannot be synthesized by mammals (i.e., linoleic, linolenic, and arachidonic acids). Because humans synthesize arachidonic acid from exogenous linoleic acid, only linoleic acid (and to a lesser degree, linolenic) is required in the diet. Vegetable oils are rich dietary sources. Parenteral nutritional lipid emulsions consist of soybean or safflower oil, which are predominantly linoleic acid. Essential fatty acid deficiency, caused by fat-free hyperalimentation, appears within 3 to 6 weeks as scaly dermatitis, alopecia, coarse hair, hepatomegaly, thrombocytopenia, diarrhea, and growth retardation.

Protein-Calorie Malnutrition

From 20% to 60% of inpatients may have protein-calorie malnutrition. Healthy adults die of starvation after 60 to 90 days if no proteins or calories are provided, which may decrease to 14 days in hypermetabolic conditions. Protein-calorie malnutrition produces weakness, impaired immune responses, skin breakdown, infection, apathy, and irritability. If malnutrition is severe, full recovery of cardiac and skeletal muscle function may not occur.

WORKUP

History and Physical Examination

Patients with diseases such as Crohn's disease or pancreatitis exhibit historical features and physical findings characteristic of the illnesses. Persons with protein-calorie malnutrition have weight loss and clinical evidence of deficiencies of essential nutrients, vitamins, and minerals. Loss of greater than 15% of body weight usually indicates significant malnutrition. Development of dependent edema may cause the clinician to underestimate the amount of muscle mass lost. Affected patients may report fatigue resulting from anemia, neuropathy secondary to vitamin B_{12} deficiency, impaired night vision with vitamin A deficiency, or easy bruising resulting from decreased vitamin K levels. The physical examination may detect muscle wasting, edema, as well as signs specific for nutritional deficiencies. Pallor indicates anemia, whereas cheilosis and stomatitis are observed with B vitamin deficiencies.

Additional Testing

Laboratory tests are important in assessing nutritional status and also are used during nutritional replenishment to test for the adequacy of supplementation and for complications of nutritional support. Low albumin, prealbumin, and transferrin levels are observed with malnutrition. Electrolyte abnormalities such as hypokalemia and alkalosis are consequences of chronic vomiting or diarrhea, whereas prerenal azotemia or renal failure may result from chronic fluid loss. Electrolytes (including magnesium, calcium, and phosphate), renal function, and albumin are monitored during enteral or parenteral supplementation. Because many regimens produce hyperglycemia or liver injury, serum glucose levels and liver chemistries are monitored during nutritional support.

PRINCIPLES OF MANAGEMENT

Implementation of Nutritional Support

The goal of nutritional support is to decrease morbidity and mortality by providing nutrients or modifying nutrient metabolism. A calorie count by the dietary staff may provide an assessment of nutrient intake. Allowance must be made for fecal losses in patients with malabsorption. Next, nutrient expenditure must be determined. The resting energy expenditure may double in highly catabolic conditions (e.g., burns). Finally, the degree of protein and calorie malnutrition is estimated using objective variables, including serum albumin, creatinine-height index, serum transferrin, total circulating lymphocyte counts, delayed cutaneous hypersensitivity skin testing, serum transthyretin, body mass index, and skinfold thickness. However, none of these measures is reliable by itself and there is no gold standard for determining nutritional status. Scales based on weight, dietary intake, symptoms, and functional capacity have been devised to correlate nutritional status with clinical outcome after surgery. General rules of nutritional supplementation have been proposed. For patients who are not eating, enteral feeding is provided within 7 to 10 days for well-nourished, noncatabolic patients; in 1 to 5 days for catabolic or malnourished patients; and in 1 to 3 days for catabolic and malnourished patients. If parenteral nutrition is required, this should be initiated in 14 to 21 days, 1 to 10 days, and 1 to 7 days for each category of patients, respectively.

When initiating a nutritional program, energy and protein goals must be set. For patients who are not critically ill, optimal calorie support is obtained if energy equal to 100% to 120% of the total daily energy expenditure is received. A crude calculation of the energy goal for a given patient is to estimate the basal energy expenditure (20 kcal per kg per day) and multiply by a stress factor for the severity of illness, which ranges from 1.0 for mild disease to 2.0 for severe burns. An additional 0% to 20% of the basal energy expenditure is added for activity level, and if weight gain is desired, an additional 500 to 1000 kcal per day is included. A positive nitrogen balance is desired to incorporate amino acids into new protein. To achieve this goal, ingesting 25 to 35 kcal/g of protein is required. Individuals with renal or liver failure may require less protein, whereas highly catabolic patients, such as those with burns, may require more.

Oral Rehydration Therapy

Prolonged vomiting or diarrhea can result in loss of excessive amounts of fluid and electrolytes. Oral rehydration therapy enhances sodium and water absorption by stimulating intestinal sodium/glucose cotransport. Various solutions are currently available and include a glucose component (70 to 150 mmol/L) with variable concentrations of sodium and other electrolytes. In some severe diarrheal conditions, making the solution hypotonic by replacing the glucose with rice solids or other polymeric forms can decrease stool output. In a patient with short bowel syndrome, sodium concentrations greater than 90 mEq/L produce a net sodium and fluid balance.

Enteral Nutrition

Enteral nutrition may be administered by several routes. Oral supplementation can be provided by increasing meal portions, adding high-caloric foods, or giving commercial nutritional supplements. Whole foods may include a standard diet or diets modified in consistency (liquid, pureed, or soft) or content (low residue, low fat, low sodium, low protein, high fiber). Nasogastric or nasoenteric formulas may be provided for patients who require short-term nutritional support (<6 weeks) and who cannot eat. If nutritional support is required for more than 6 weeks, a gastrostomy or jejunostomy is indicated and may be placed endoscopically, radiographically, or surgically. Gastrostomy feedings generally are delivered in bolus fashion four to six times daily, although they may be given continuously if there is esophageal reflux of feedings or if gastric emptying is delayed. Jejunostomy feedings are indicated for patients undergoing gastric surgery, who have duodenal obstruction or in whom pulmonary aspiration is a significant risk. Jejunostomy feedings require continuous infusion to prevent diarrhea and abdominal pain and to ensure adequate nutrient absorption. Standard formulas are appropriate for most patients, although high-protein formulas may be needed for those with extensive trauma or healing wounds. Formulas containing fiber can be given if diarrhea is a problem. Disease-specific preparations are available for patients with renal, hepatic, or pulmonary disease. Renal formulas are low in protein, high in essential amino acids, and low in electrolytes, whereas hepatic formulas are low in sodium, low in aromatic amino acids, and high in branched-chain amino acids. Pulmonary preparations are high in fat and low in carbohydrates because metabolism of carbohydrate generates carbon dioxide. Elemental formulas contain nitrogen as free amino acids and have very little fat. Such preparations are best for those with pancreatic insufficiency or for individuals who require an extremely low-fat diet.

Parenteral Nutrition

Intravenous nutritional supplementation is provided by a peripheral (peripheral parenteral nutrition [PPN]) or central (total parenteral nutrition [TPN]) vein. PPN is reserved for patients whose nutritional status is nearly normal and in whom the goal of nutritional supplementation is to maintain lean body mass for a relatively short period of time. Such patients include those undergoing elective surgery who will not be given oral nutrition for 3 to 7 days. PPN also benefits inpatients, who ingest inadequate nutrients or calories, by preventing a negative nitrogen balance during their hospitalization. The limiting factor for PPN is phlebitis induced by hypertonic solutions. Successful PPN mandates solutions with osmolarity less than 900 mOsm and glucose concentrations less than 10%. To meet the nutritional needs of most patients, combinations of hypertonic glucose, amino acids, and lipid emulsions are given with vitamins, minerals, and trace elements. These solutions provide the best nutritional support, if half of the caloric needs are met by the lipid infusion.

For patients who require long-term intravenous nutritional support (>10 days), TPN is preferred. TPN requires the central venous placement of a large-bore catheter, which permits rapid dilution of the hypertonic TPN formulation to prevent phlebitis or hemolysis. Temporary central venous access may be provided by peripherally inserted central catheter (PICC) lines or catheters aseptically placed into the subclavian or internal jugular veins. In patients who need TPN beyond their inpatient stay, permanent catheters (e.g., Hickman, Broviac) are surgically or radiographically placed for home TPN administration. TPN solutions are tailored to the specific needs of the patient. Standard TPN formulations provide 510 to 1020 kcal/L depending on the glucose concentration. Emulsified lipids are given 2 to 3 times weekly to prevent essential fatty acid deficiency in patients requiring TPN for more than 1 week. Commercially available multiple vitamin supplements are included that contain all the water-soluble and fat-soluble vitamins except vitamin K, which must be given separately. Mineral and trace elements usually are included in standard TPN solutions but also may be given as additives. Iodine may be included if TPN is to be given long term. Iron is not routinely included because it is incompatible with the lipid emulsion. Medications including acid-suppressive agents can be included in TPN formulations, as clinically indicated. Patients with renal disease can receive TPN formulations rich in essential amino acids and with little or no nonessential amino acids to minimize the nitrogen load. Formulas for hepatic encephalopathy are high in branched-chain amino acids (leucine, isovaline, valine), which are oxidized outside the liver and block hepatic and muscle protein breakdown.

TPN has been beneficial in several clinical settings. The most unequivocal indication for home TPN is intestinal failure from any cause. TPN is also the primary therapeutic modality that leads to closure of enterocutaneous fistulae in 30% to 50% of patients. If spontaneous closure does not occur after 30 to 60 days, continuation of TPN is unlikely to be successful. TPN is commonly used in managing inflammatory bowel disease, although bowel rest with TPN does not represent primary therapy nor does it decrease the need for surgery in patients with colitis. TPN corrects disease-associated vitamin, mineral, and nutrient deficiencies in severe Crohn's ileitis. TPN is indicated for patients with complicated acute pancreatitis, if enteral feeding exacerbates abdominal pain or if ascites, fistulae, or pseudocysts are present. Lipid emulsions are given cautiously and should be reduced if serum triglyceride levels exceed 400 mg/dL.

COMPLICATIONS

Enteral Nutrition

The major complications of enteral feedings are pulmonary aspiration, nausea and vomiting, abdominal pain, diarrhea, metabolic abnormalities, and infection (pneumonia, gut infections). Aspiration is rare if feedings are delivered distal to the ligament of Treitz. During gastric feedings, the upper body should be elevated at least 30 degrees above the horizontal. Residual volumes of 200 mL after nasogastric feeding or 100 mL after gastrostomy feeding predispose to aspiration. Diarrhea results from excessive infusion rates, concurrent use of antibiotics and antacids, sorbitol-containing elixir, inadequate fiber supplementation, too much lipid with fat malabsorption, hypertonic formulations, vitamin or mineral deficiency, or hypoalbuminemia. If no remediable cause of diarrhea is found, loperamide elixir, diphenoxylate with atropine, or tincture of opium may be given. Complications of gastrostomies and jejunostomies include wound infections, leakage, tube migration, ileus, fever, peritonitis, and necrotizing fasciitis.

Parenteral Nutrition

Potential complications of intravenous nutrition include mechanical, infectious, and metabolic problems. Pneumothorax, hemorrhage, brachial plexus injury, air or guidewire embolism, cardiac tamponade, and death may result from inserting a central venous catheter. Catheters can become occluded by blood, fibrin, intravenous lipid, or precipitated drugs. Vascular catheters are responsible for one third of nosocomial bacteremias and one half of candidemias. Skin flora are the most common pathogens and include *Staphylococcus aureus*, *Staphylococcus epidermidis*, *Klebsiella pneumoniae*, *Pseudomonas aeruginosia*, *Enterobacter species*, and *Candida albicans*. Early metabolic complications of TPN include electrolyte abnormalities, hyperglycemia or hypoglycemia, hyperlipidemia, acid-base disturbances, hypercapnia, and fluid overload (Table 21-2). Lipid emulsions can cause pulmonary

TABLE 21-2
Metabolic Complications Associated with Total Parenteral Nutrition

Early

  Electrolyte Abnormalities
    Sodium
    Potassium
    Calcium
    Magnesium
    Phosphate
  Refeeding syndrome
  Hyperglycemia
  Hypoglycemia
  Elevated urea nitrogen
  Adverse reactions to lipid emulsions
    Hyperlipidemia
    Poor lipid clearance
    Thrombocytopenia
  Hypercapnia
  Hyperammonemia
  Fluid Overload
  Hyperosmolar nonketotic hyperglycemic coma
  Acidosis
  Alkalosis

Delayed

  Lipid Overload Syndrome
  Essential fatty acid deficiency
  Metabolic bone disease
  Liver dysfunction
  Gallbladder disease
  Mineral Deficiency or Excess
    Zinc
    Copper
    Chromium
    Selenium
    Molybdenum
    Iron
    Manganese

dysfunction, impaired function of the immune system, pancreatitis, delayed platelet aggregation, and hypersensitivity reactions. Delayed metabolic consequences include liver dysfunction, bone demineralization, essential fatty acid deficiency, and mineral deficiency or excess. Liver abnormalities occur frequently with long-term TPN, including calculous and acalculous cholecystitis, hepatic steatosis, steatohepatitis, fibrosis, and cirrhosis. TPN-induced liver abnormalities may be minimized by not exceeding the caloric needs of the patient, especially the glucose component.

CHAPTER 22

Approach to the Patient with Alcohol or Drug Dependency

Alcohol and drug dependency are prevalent in the United States. There are about 14 million alcohol abusers, tens of millions who have tried cocaine or marijuana, about a million who have tried anabolic steroids, and more than 700,000 heroin addicts. The results of urine tests to detect drug use are positive in 3% to 16% of preemployment screens. Patients with chronic pain syndromes are at risk for addiction to prescription medications. Most drugs produce tolerance with continued use, causing the abuser to gradually increase the dose. Tolerance is often but not invariably accompanied by physical dependence, which is an adaptive state that manifests itself by intense physical disturbances when drug use is suspended, or by psychic dependence, a condition in which the agent produces satisfaction or a psychic drive that requires periodic drug use to maintain it. If drug discontinuation affects neural systems, the withdrawal syndrome will be physiologically violent (e.g., seizures), whereas withdrawal from psychic dependence may produce depression and drug craving. Many classes of agents with different physiological and psychological effects produce drug dependency.

ETHANOL

Clinical Features and Diagnosis

The risk of alcoholism involves a genetic component that is highly sensitive to environmental factors. The lifetime risk is 20% to 25% for men and 5% for women. Symptoms of intoxication include somnolence, dysarthria, ataxia, nystagmus, and impaired judgment. The alcohol dependence syndrome has several features: narrowing of the drinking pattern such that there is little variability from day to day; an awareness of the compulsion to drink; tolerance to the intoxicating effects of ethanol; physical dependence; early drinking to relieve "morning after" symptoms; the inability of negative consequences (e.g., family, social, professional, health) to deter drinking; and rapid reinstatement of the syndrome with recurrent drinking (Table 22-1). These issues should be raised with the patient and family members. The CAGE test is a simple, nonthreatening series of four questions that has 93% sensitivity and 76% specificity with two or more positive responses. There is no biochemical test to quantitate drinking behavior; however, elevations in mean corpuscular volume, uric acid, triglycerides, and γ-glutamyltransferase may support the suspicions of the family or clinician, and newer tests such as the assays to measure carbohydrate-deficient transferrin and acetaldehyde-protein adducts show promise as useful screening tests. Within 6 to 12 hours of ingestion, alcohol can be detected by analyzing breath, blood, or urine. In general, ethanol is cleared at a rate of 100 mg/kg per hour, but this may vary up to threefold according to individual metabolism.

TABLE 22-1
Alcohol Dependence Syndrome

Narrowing of the drinking repertoire
With increased severity of dependence, there is little variability of drinking pattern between drinking days and occasions.

Salience of drinking behavior
Negative social, family, and/or health consequences will not deter drinking behavior. Highest priority is given to securing alcohol.

Subjective awareness of a compulsion to drink
Severely dependent alcoholics are aware of an impaired capacity for moderate drinking. In the past, this characteristic was called "loss of control" drinking; in some cultures, it is characterized by an inability to abstain.

Tolerance
With increased severity of dependence and prior to the development of severe liver damage, alcoholics are less sensitive to the effects of alcohol.

Physical dependence

Relief avoidance drinking
With increased severity of dependence, drinking occurs earlier in the day (e.g., upon awakening) to avoid the discomfort of "morning-after" symptoms.

Rapid reinstatement of the syndrome with recurrent drinking

Reprinted with permission from Meyer RE, Kranzler HR, Alcoholism: clinical implications of recent research. *J Clin Psychiatry* 1998;49(Suppl):8.

Principles of Management

Ethanol detoxification, with intensive counseling, behavior modification, and support group enrollment, may be undertaken on an outpatient basis in the absence of major medical illness or withdrawal symptoms; otherwise, hospitalization should be considered. In the 1 to 2 days of abstinence, tremor and tachycardia occur, which may progress to hallucinations in 10% to 20% of cases. Seizures and delirium tremens, which is characterized by hallucinations and severe sympathetic overactivity (e.g., tachycardia, fever, dilated pupils, hypertension, diaphoresis), develop later in a minority of patients. Benzodiazepines and barbiturates are effective in preventing ethanol withdrawal symptoms. The response to a detoxification program depends on the underlying support system. Those with stable support have abstinence rates of 60% for up to 18 months, compared with 30% for unemployed individuals in lower socioeconomic strata. Monitoring alcohol consumption with the biomarker carbohydrate-deficient transferrin may be useful. The use of medications to maintain sobriety yields mixed results. Serotonin reuptake inhibitors (e.g., fluoxetine, zimeldine) have been somewhat effective, as have opiate antagonists (e.g., naltrexone). Alcohol-sensitizing drugs (e.g., disulfiram) inhibit aldehyde dehydrogenase and lead to nausea, tachycardia, flushing, and hypotension as a result of acetaldehyde accumulation. However, the largest controlled trial showed no difference in abstinence rates with disulfiram and placebo (about 20%), and further, disulfiram is associated with hepatotoxicity. Other drugs, including the serotonin type 3 receptor antagonist ondansetron and other opioid antagonists (e.g., nalmefene), may be useful in early-onset alcoholism.

SEDATIVE-HYPNOTICS

Clinical Features and Diagnosis

Barbiturates and benzodiazepines are used for sedation, muscle relaxation, seizure control, anxiety, and panic disorders. High doses produce emotional lability, dysarthria, ataxia, and rarely, delirium, disorientation, and altered perception, all of which may be increased by concurrent ethanol use. Dependence on barbiturates occurs in 1 month, whereas benzodiazepine dependence requires about 20 weeks of use. Users of benzodiazepines develop tolerance to the sedative effects of the drugs but not to their anxiolytic effects. Barbiturates and benzodiazepines are reliably detected by urine drug screening tests for several days after the last use (Table 22-2).

Principles of Management

Abrupt withdrawal from barbiturates and benzodiazepines produces tremor, dysphoria, insomnia, hyperreflexia, anxiety, and, rarely, seizures. Barbiturate withdrawal may be as dangerous as delirium tremens. Seizures may occur in patients who are dependent on benzodiazepines if flumazenil, a benzodiazepine antagonist, is administered. Safe withdrawal is accomplished by gradual dose reductions of 10% per day.

OPIATES

Clinical Features and Diagnosis

Heroin is the choice of most narcotic addicts, but prescription drugs such as codeine, methadone, meperidine, and oxycodone are also widely abused. Fentanyl is abused most frequently by medical personnel and carries a significant risk of overdose due to its potency. Methylphenyltetrahydropyridine is a synthetic derivative of meperidine that caused an outbreak of toxic parkinsonism in the 1970s by destroying substantia nigra neurons of users. No tolerance to the miotic or constipating effects of opiates develops, so these manifestations may provide clues to narcotic abuse. Urine tests for opiates may produce positive results for 2 to 5 days after the last use. Although ingesting large quantities of poppy seeds can give a false-positive result, the cough suppressant dextromethorphan usually does not give a positive test result. Fentanyl is difficult to detect in the blood of users because it is highly potent in very low doses.

Principles of Management

Fully developed symptoms of opiate withdrawal result from overactivity of the sympathetic nervous system and include lacrimation, rhinorrhea, dilated pupils, piloerection, diaphoresis, yawning, hypertension, tachycardia, and fever. In contrast, hallucinations, tremor, and delirium are not typical of opiate withdrawal and suggest other drug use. Withdrawal symptoms can be blocked by clonidine, which inhibits the activity of neurons in the locus ceruleus that are hyperactive secondary to the suspension of opiates. Methadone may be used to wean a patient from shorter-acting opiates. Relapse may be prevented by chronic use of methadone or oral naltrexone, but naltrexone is potentially hepatotoxic. Newer drugs that are being studied include levomethadyl acetate and buprenorphine, a partial opioid agonist.

TABLE 22-2
Guidelines for Using Urinary Screening Tests for Drug Abuse

Document quality of specimen: check temperature, color, pH, and specific gravity of urine to detect adulteration; check for presence of blood.
Document chain of custody.

Be aware of approximate duration of positive urine screening test results after drug use:
   Alcohol: 6–12 hours.
   Barbiturates and benzodiazepines: several days.
   Opiates: 2–5 days.
   Cocaine: 2–4 days.
   Amphetamines: 2–4 days.
   Marijuana: up to 30 days.
   PCP: up to 8 days.

Be alert to false positives:
   Barbiturates and benzodiazepines: ibuprofen.
   Opiates: poppy seeds (morphine), dextromethorphan.
   Amphetamines: ephedrine, phenylpropanolamine, pseudoephedrine, other sympathomimetics.
   Marijuana: ibuprofen, naproxen, fenprofen (older screening tests), passive smoke.

Be alert to false negatives:
   Adulteration of sample: addition of acids, bases, benzalkonium chloride (Visine), soap.
   Dilution of urine (includes use of diuretics for this purpose).
   Short time elapsed after ingestion.
   Intentional acidification of urine to speed elimination of amphetamine or PCP before test; alkalinization of urine to slow excretion during the testing period.
   Ibuprofen may interfere with the derivatization step in GC-MS confirmation for marijuana.
   Screening tests generally not available for LSD, mescaline, psilocybine, designer drugs.

GC-MS, gas chromatography–mass spectrometry; LSD, lysergic acid diethylamide; PCP, phencyclidine.

Compiled from Osterloh JD, Becker CE. Chemical dependency and drug testing in the workplace. *West J Med* 1990;152:506; Hubball J. The use of chromatography in forensic science. *Adv Chromatogr* 1992;32:131; Coffman NB, Fernandes J. Drugs of abuse testing. *J Am Osteopath Assoc* 1991;91:385.

COCAINE AND OTHER STIMULANTS

Clinical Features and Diagnosis

Cocaine may be sniffed or snorted, injected, or, in its base form (i.e., freebase, crack), smoked. It induces tolerance but only relatively mild withdrawal. Nonetheless, it has the highest abuse potential of drugs currently used. Amphetamines are active orally or intravenously and include many derivatives (e.g., methamphetamine or "crystal", 3-4 methylenedioxymethamphetamine [MDMA] or "ecstasy"). The sympathetic effects of cocaine and amphetamines include pupillary dilation, tachycardia, hypertension, cardiac arrhythmias, myocardial infarction, aortic dissection, myocarditis, intestinal ischemia, disseminated intravascular coagulation, rhabdomyolysis, ulcer perforation, and seizures. Use during pregnancy causes microcephaly, growth retardation, intrauterine cerebral infarction, and cerebral hemorrhage in the fetus. Amphetamines can produce hallucinations and delirium. If taken intravenously, they can cause necrotizing angiitis. Intravenous use also carries the risk of acquiring hepatitis B or C viruses and the human immunodeficiency virus. Cocaine metabolites can be detected by drug screening up to 48 hours after use. Detecting amphetamines is complicated by cross-reactions with over-the-counter sympathomimetics (e.g., ephedrine, pseudoephedrine).

Principles of Management

Withdrawal from stimulants produces depression, fatigue, disturbed sleep with increased dreaming, and intense drug craving. Treatment is usually on an outpatient basis and consists of complete abstinence, which is documented by mandatory urine testing. Cocaine craving is treated by intensive counseling, as well as by administering the tricyclic antidepressants, imipramine and desipramine, which may reduce dysphoria and improve sobriety. Extinction therapy, in which the user watches videotapes of cocaine use or handles drug paraphernalia without using the drug, has been used for some patients. Acupuncture, phenytoin, and amantadine have had some reported success.

CANNABIS

The active ingredient of marijuana, 9-tetrahydrocannabinol, causes euphoria, relaxation, subjective intensification of perception, altered sense of time, and impaired psychomotor function, as well as vasodilation (tachycardia, conjunctival injection) and appetite stimulation. Anxiety attacks or paranoia occur in 5% of episodes of cannabis use. Prolonged use may cause an "amotivational" syndrome of passivity, preoccupation with drug use, decreased drive, and memory loss. Cannabis withdrawal produces restlessness, insomnia, and nausea. Urine tests may produce positive results up to 30 days after the last use of the drug. Treatment is based on counseling and should include suspicion of other illicit drug use.

PHENCYCLIDINE

Phencyclidine (PCP or angel dust) may be taken by any route, including smoking. It produces euphoria at low doses and sympathetic activation, hyperactivity, and hallucinations at higher doses. The hallucinations are frequently auditory, thus producing behavior that mimics paranoid schizophrenia. Physical findings of drug use include vertical and horizontal nystagmus, sympathetic overactivity, numbness, increased pain thresholds, ataxia, and dysarthria. PCP may be detected by urine testing for up to 8 days after use; however, false-positive results occur with over-the-counter decongestants. Ketamine, a veterinary and pediatric anesthesia drug, has a similar pharmacological and clinical profile.

HALLUCINOGENS

Lysergic acid diethylamide (LSD) and hallucinogenic amphetamines are sympathomimetics that produce hypertension, pupillary dilation, tachycardia, hyperreflexia, and disordered perception. Users may experience loss of control, flashbacks (i.e., reexperiencing of drug-induced perceptions), and "bad trips" (i.e., terrifying hallucinations). Tolerance develops after three to four doses, but there is little physical dependence or craving. Screening urine tests are not widely available for detecting LSD.

OTHER DRUGS

Inhalants, including solvents (e.g., toluene, benzene), nitrous oxide, and trichloroethylene, are frequently the first drugs of abuse for children. These drugs produce acute effects similar to alcohol but they have been associated with sudden death and significant long-term neurological, hepatic, and renal toxicity. Flunitrazepam (Rohypnol) and γ-hydroxybutyrate, along with ketamine and MDMA, have been used by teens and young adults at rave parties and they have been associated with date rape. All of these so-called "club drugs" are central nervous system depressants. They can be taken orally and are odorless, colorless, and tasteless.

TOBACCO

Clinical Features

Tobacco is highly addictive because the nicotine is absorbed through the oral mucosa and lungs. Nicotine produces manifestations of increased sympathetic activity (e.g., tachycardia, mental arousal) and muscle relaxation. Tolerance to nicotine occurs rapidly (within hours) and a withdrawal syndrome that consists of restlessness, irritability, anxiety, impatience, and impaired concentration is common. Tobacco may also increase the metabolism of imipramine, lidocaine, oxazepam, propranolol, and theophylline.

Principles of Management

Several nicotine delivery systems have been developed to reduce the severity of tobacco withdrawal, including nicotine polacrilex in nicotine gum, transdermal nicotine patches, nasal sprays, and inhalers. When used in conjunction with counseling, these agents demonstrate efficacy superior to that of placebos. Nicotine preparations should be given cautiously to patients with angina, cardiac arrhythmias, or a recent myocardial infarction.

ANABOLIC STEROIDS

Clinical Features and Diagnosis

Anabolic steroids usually are used by athletes in 4-week to 12-week cycles to augment training, especially in power sports such as weight lifting and football. Several drugs, often containing recombinant growth hormone, are frequently used together in a practice referred to as stacking. Among high school students, 6% of males and 1% of females admit to steroid use. Hepatic complications of anabolic steroid abuse include reversible elevations in liver chemistry values, jaundice, liver cell hyperplasia, hepatic adenoma, hepatocellular carcinoma, angiosarcoma, and fatal peliosis hepatis. Other adverse effects include increases in low-density lipoproteins, with concurrent decreases in high-density lipoproteins, prostate hypertrophy, prostate carcinoma, testicular atrophy, decreased sperm counts, gynecomastia, premature epiphyseal closure in adolescents, irreversible masculinization of women, mood changes, psychosis, and aggressive behavior.

Principles of Management

Anabolic steroid abuse may be suspected from prominent muscular development in a patient, as well as from the development of adverse side effects. Needle tracks may be visible on the thighs or buttocks. Anabolic steroid use may be detected by gas chromatography–mass spectrometry and by measuring serum gonadotropins. Testosterone is found by detecting increased ratios of testosterone to epitestosterone in urine. Treatment of a patient who abuses steroids involves strict suspension of drug use. No significant withdrawal syndrome occurs after discontinuing anabolic steroids.

CHAPTER 23

Advice to Travelers

TRAVEL-RELATED ISSUES

Pretravel Preparations

A thorough travel itinerary should be prepared at least 6 weeks before traveling abroad because prophylaxis against infectious disease often requires multiple vaccinations. Some countries require evidence of yellow fever vaccination before allowing entry of persons who recently traveled to areas where the disease is endemic. No countries officially require cholera vaccination as a condition of entry, although some customs officials may still make this demand. Some diseases, such as traveler's diarrhea, present soon after arrival, whereas the risk of contracting other diseases, such as hepatitis, increases with length of stay. Other conditions are seasonal, such as Japanese encephalitis, which most often occurs in the summer. One's personal risk for illness is increased by venturing off the usual tourist routes, by camping or staying in primitive housing, or from animal exposure. The risk of disease increases for persons with impaired immune function, chronic obstructive pulmonary disease, diabetes, glucose-6-phosphate deficiency, malabsorption, achlorhydria secondary to gastric surgery or possibly medications, and extremes of age.

Air and Sea Travel

Disruption of the sleep-wakeful cycle ("jet lag") often occurs with air travel. Use of a short-duration benzodiazepine (e.g., triazolam) or other agents such as zoldipem (Ambien) during a long air flight or immediately after arrival may assist in sleep cycle adjustment. Reduced pressure in the aircraft cabin produces dehydration, which, when coupled with immobility, increases the risk of thromboembolic disease. In high-risk persons, low-dose aspirin may be advisable to prevent this complication. The reduced air pressure in an aircraft at high altitude may exacerbate symptoms of patients with obstructive lung disease.

Sea travel often is complicated by motion sickness. Over-the-counter diphenhydramine or dimenhydrinate may be used to prevent motion sickness. Severe cases may require promethazine or prochlorperazine in suppository form or use of a scopolamine patch.

Water Supplies

Unpurified water may contain bacterial, viral, or parasitic pathogens. Carbonated beverages usually are safe, but bottled water cannot be relied on. Water should be boiled or disinfected by halogen treatment or filtration. Effective halogen regimens per liter of water include 0.1 mL of 5% chlorine bleach or 0.2 mL of 2% tincture of iodine. The water must stand for at least 30 minutes at room temperature before use.

Medical Care Overseas

The United States embassy or consulate may recommend local physicians, hospitals, or emergency services. All medications for prophylaxis and treatment should be carried by the traveler because overseas medications may have different names and strengths. Many countries do not regulate the quality of over-the-counter medications. Such medications may contain dangerous components and should be avoided.

DISEASES FOR WHICH IMMUNIZATION IS AVAILABLE

The vaccination schedule should consider interactions of vaccines with each other and with immune serum globulin (ISG). If possible, doses of live-virus vaccines should be separated by 30 days or be given simultaneously at separate sites. Yellow fever and cholera vaccines should be given at least 3 weeks apart. Some live vaccines should not be given sooner than 6 weeks after receiving ISG to maximize the immune response, whereas ISG should not be given for 2 weeks after measles, mumps, and rubella vaccination to avoid impairing the immune response. Malaria prophylaxis with chloroquine may depress immune function; therefore, vaccination should be performed 2 weeks before initiating the drug.

Vaccines That May Be Required
Yellow Fever
Yellow fever is limited to sub-Saharan Africa, tropical South America, and Panama. It is prevalent especially in forested areas and is transmitted by mosquitoes. Fulminant disease may affect the liver, kidneys, and heart; fatality rates approach 40%, so vaccination is mandatory. The attenuated live-virus vaccine is highly effective (>90%) beginning 10 days after vaccination. Boosting is recommended at 10-year intervals. Vaccination is not recommended for immunocompromised patients, for infants younger than 6 months, for pregnant women, or for patients with egg allergies.

Cholera

The risk of cholera is extremely low (i.e., 1 in 500,000) for travelers to Asia and Africa, so with good hygiene and dietary discretion it is not a significant problem in regions with periodic pandemics (e.g., Central and South America). Transmission may occur through inadequately cooked fish or seafood or contaminated water. Antibiotics (e.g., tetracycline) effectively reduce the severity of the disease. The sale of the only licensed cholera vaccine has been discontinued in the United States.

Recommended Immunizations for Travelers

Hepatitis A

Hepatitis A virus (HAV) is prevalent in Africa, Asia, and Central and South America, especially in rural or unsanitary urban areas. Transmission is by the fecal-oral route through contaminated food, beverages, ice, or person-to-person contact. Prevention of hepatitis A infection is based on avoiding contaminated food and administering the hepatitis A vaccine composed of inactivated whole virus (1 dose at least 4 weeks before departure and one booster dose 6 to 12 months later). Protection has been estimated to last for 10 years. Travelers to endemic areas who have not received the vaccine should consider passive immunization with ISG: a dose of 0.02 mL/kg for short trips (<3 months) and 0.06 mL/kg for longer trips (≥5 months). Because 20% to 35% of adults in the United States are immune to HAV, determination of anti-HAV antibody titers may obviate the need for ISG.

Hepatitis B

The risk of hepatitis B virus (HBV) infection is increased in Asia, the South Pacific, and sub-Saharan Africa. Risk factors include drug abuse, sexual activity, blood transfusions, and medical exposures, although casual transmission may occur in highly endemic areas. HBV vaccines (recombinant viral surface antigens) are administered in three doses over 6 months to health care workers, long-term (>6 months) residents, persons who are sexually active with the local populace, persons who receive local medical care, and frequent travelers.

Typhoid Fever

Typhoid is prevalent in Africa, Asia, and South and Central America. Vaccination is recommended for those who travel to these areas, especially for persons planning on remaining in high-risk regions for more than 2 weeks. An oral live-attenuated vaccine made from *Salmonella typhi* strain Ty21a and the Vi capsular polysaccharide vaccine are 50% to 80% effective for prophylaxis. Children younger than 6 years, immunosuppressed individuals, and patients with febrile or gastrointestinal illness should not be vaccinated with the live strain. Booster doses are recommended every 5 years for the oral vaccine and every 2 years for the capsular vaccine.

Rabies

Canine rabies is widespread in urban and rural areas of Asia, Africa, and Latin America. Mongooses in the Caribbean and vampire bats in Latin America may also transmit the disease. The human diploid cell rabies vaccine (HDCV) is recommended for those planning visits of 30 days or longer. Three doses of HDCV are given over 21 to 28 days, and boosters are required every 2 years. HDCV does not eliminate the need for postexposure immunization of persons who have sustained bites, but it reduces the number of postexposure HDCV injections from five to two and eliminates the need for rabies immune globulin. Alternatives to HDCV include rabies vaccine adsorbed or purified chick embryo cell vaccine.

Meningococcal Disease

Epidemics of meningococcal disease are common in sub-Saharan Africa during the dry season from December to June and may also occur in New Delhi, Nepal, and Saudi Arabia. A tetravalent capsular polysaccharide vaccine is 75% to 100% effective for serogroups A and C, but it is much less effective in children, especially those younger than 2 years.

Plague

Although plague is endemic in rodents, it can infect humans in the western United States, South America, Africa, the Middle East, and Central and Southeast Asia. Antibiotics may be taken by a person who was exposed. The plague vaccine is not available in the United States.

Viral Encephalitis

Japanese encephalitis is a mosquito-borne illness endemic in Central and Southeast Asia, especially where rice culture and pig farming are common. An inactivated vaccine is available. Tick-borne encephalitis occurs in Russia and Central and Eastern Europe, where risks are increased in forested areas and by ingesting unpasteurized dairy products from infected animals. Although effective vaccines are available, vaccination is not necessary for most travelers.

RECOMMENDED VACCINES FOR BOTH TRAVELERS AND NONTRAVELERS

Polio is prevalent in the developing world, and it is recommended that previously immunized adult travelers receive a booster dose of the parenteral enhanced inactivated polio vaccine. Measles, mumps, and rubella are also common in the developing world. For those born after 1956 without measles immunity, a dose of the live, attenuated measles vaccine is recommended before travel. The schedule for tetanus and diphtheria boosters should be accelerated to 5-year intervals for travelers who will be at risk for dirty wounds. All of these vaccines should also be part of a routine immunization schedule for nontravelers.

DISEASES FOR WHICH CHEMOPROPHYLAXIS IS RECOMMENDED

Malaria

Most cases of severe malaria are caused by the parasite *Plasmodium falciparum*. Travelers should understand that no antimalarial is completely effective. Therefore, they should minimize the risk of mosquito bites by wearing long-sleeved clothing and using insect repellents containing DEET (*N,N*-diethyl-m-toluamide) on the skin. Mosquito nets should be used while sleeping. In those areas in which the organisms are sensitive, the drug of choice remains chloroquine at 300 mg/wk from 2 weeks before until 4 weeks after travel. Chloroquine resistance is increasing in Africa, Southeast Asia, India, South America, and Oceania, and multidrug-resistant strains have appeared in some areas. Mefloquine is available for chloroquine-resistant malaria and is the drug of choice for most regions of the world, except for certain Caribbean areas, parts of Central America, and the Middle East. Mefloquine is given at 250 mg weekly, from 2 weeks before entry until 4 weeks after departure from the malarious region. Drug side effects include gastrointestinal upset, dizziness, and, rarely, seizures and convulsions. Mefloquine should not be taken by children who weigh less than 15 kg, by travelers who take β-blockers or drugs that alter cardiac conduction, or by travelers with epilepsy or psychiatric disease. Doxycycline at 100 mg/d for 1 to 2 days before and 4 weeks after travel is an alternative drug for chloroquine-resistant malaria. Mefloquine-intolerant and doxycycline-intolerant travelers can take atovaquone/proguanil (Malarone, 250 mg atovaquone/100 mg proguanil) once a day, starting 1 to 2 days before travel and continuing for 7 days after leaving endemic areas.

Leptospirosis

Leptospirosis is transmitted by water contaminated by the urine of infected animals. In rare instances (e.g., military jungle maneuvers), doxycycline at 200 mg/wk may have prophylactic efficacy.

DISEASES REQUIRING TREATMENT DURING TRAVEL

Traveler's Diarrhea

Traveler's diarrhea attack rates in travelers to Latin America, Africa, the Middle East, or Asia are 30% to 70%. The usual onset of symptoms occurs within 2 to 3 days of arrival. Diarrhea usually persists for 3 to 4 days and rarely longer than 1 week. Causes of traveler's diarrhea include enterotoxigenic *Escherichia coli*, shigellae, salmonellae, *Campylobacter jejuni*, *Yersinia enterocolitica*, *Giardia lamblia*, *Entamoeba histolytica*, *Cryptosporidia*, and *Cyclospora*. Prophylaxis lies in dietary discretion by avoiding tap water, ice, and food items washed with water, including fresh vegetables and salads. Bismuth subsalicylate taken four times daily in liquid (60 mL) or solid (two 300-mg tablets) form decreases the incidence of traveler's diarrhea by 50%. Routine use of prophylactic antibiotics is not recommended for most travelers because of concerns for possible side effects and the existence of antibiotic-resistant organisms. However, certain high-risk travelers who cannot tolerate dehydration or travelers on brief trips who cannot miss scheduled appointments may be given prophylactic doxycycline, trimethoprim-sulfamethoxazole, ciprofloxacin, or norfloxacin, which can reduce the incidence of traveler's diarrhea by 90%. In areas where resistance to quinolones is present in *Campylobacter* species, azithromycin (500 mg daily) is a macrolide that may be effective.

Patients affected with traveler's diarrhea should begin treatment at the onset of symptoms. Maintaining hydration with glucose and salt solutions is essential. Packets of oral rehydration salts that contain glucose, sodium chloride, potassium chloride, and sodium citrate have been developed by the World Health Organization. Opiates (e.g., loperamide and diphenoxylate with atropine) may be used for mild to moderate traveler's diarrhea for up to 3 days, although they should be avoided in patients with bloody diarrhea or high fever. Bismuth subsalicylate taken every 30 minutes can reduce diarrhea, but it is not as effective as opiates. Prompt initiation of a 3-day course of twice-daily antibiotics (e.g., ciprofloxacin or norfloxacin) can shorten the duration of symptoms of severe traveler's diarrhea. Resistance to other antibiotic classes such as the sulfonamides has increased, thus these drugs are not recommended as first-line agents. The nonabsorbable antibiotic rifaximin was recently approved for treating traveler's diarrhea caused by noninvasive *E coli* strains. Synergistic therapeutic effects may be obtained by combining an antibiotic with an antidiarrheal agent.

Altitude Illness

Rapid ascent to altitudes above 8000 feet can produce insomnia, headache, nausea, vomiting, and pulmonary or cerebral edema, which are related to the degree of exertion and the altitude attained. Sleep may increase the symptoms as a result of decreased vascular integrity associated with hypoventilation-induced hypoxia. Altitude illness is best prevented by slowing the ascent. Acetazolamide, which induces metabolic acidosis with compensatory respiratory alkalosis, and dexamethasone decrease the incidence of altitude illness. For pulmonary or cerebral edema, oxygen is administered at 6 to 12 L/min and immediate descent is recommended. Dexamethasone, acetazolamide, or nifedipine may reduce symptoms but should not be used to delay descent.

Typhus

Treating the rare condition typhus with tetracycline or chloramphenicol is curative.

DISEASES WITHOUT IMMUNOPROPHYLAXIS OR TREATMENT

Hepatitis E

Hepatitis E is endemic in India, Pakistan, China, Mongolia, Hong Kong, North Africa, and Mexico. It has an incubation period of 45 days. Hepatitis E infection has a 15% to 20% mortality in pregnant women. ISG from sources in the United States does not protect against infection.

Human Immunodeficiency Virus

Human immunodeficiency virus (HIV) infection rates are high in Africa, India, and Southeast Asia. Risk factors for HIV infection include intravenous drug abuse, use of infected blood products, and sexual contact. Live viral vaccines should not be given to HIV-infected patients who have symptoms or CD4 counts lower than 200 cells per μL.

DISEASES IN THE RETURNING TRAVELER

Asymptomatic Illness

Travelers who experienced a febrile or diarrheal illness overseas may require a screening evaluation on their return, including complete blood count, liver chemistry determinations, tuberculin testing, fecal ova and parasites examination, and specific serologic tests for indigenous diseases, even if they are asymptomatic. The presence of eosinophilia suggests possible filariasis, liver flukes, or intestinal helminth infection.

Symptomatic Illness

Travelers who return with a febrile illness should be evaluated for possible malaria, amoebic liver abscess, enteric fever, hepatitis, and tuberculosis. Persistent diarrhea is the most common symptom evaluated by gastroenterologists in returning travelers. If diarrhea lasts longer than 2 weeks, *Salmonella*, *Shigella*, or *Campylobacter* organisms should be considered; northern travel raises the possibility of *Y enterocolitica*; and antibiotic use suggests possible *Clostridium difficile* infection. Persistent *E coli* infections are not detectable by standard cultures. If no agent can be identified, an empiric course of therapy with ciprofloxacin should be considered. In more prolonged diarrhea, evaluation for ova and parasites should be initiated by obtaining three fresh stool samples. Some cases of giardiasis may require duodenal aspiration or biopsy or a stool antigen test to detect small intestinal organisms. Therapy for proven or suspected *Giardia* infection includes quinacrine or metronidazole. Persons infected with *E histolytica* present with bloody diarrhea, mucus, and hematophagous trophozoites in the stool. Chronic nondysenteric diarrhea may be associated with *E histolytica* cyst passage, but the use of antiamoebic therapy in this setting is controversial. *Isospora belli* is a rare cause of chronic diarrhea and is treated with trimethoprim-sulfamethoxazole. *Cryptosporidium* infection usually produces self-limited diarrhea in immunocompetent individuals. *Cyclospora* species produce chronic diarrhea, fatigue, and weight loss in travelers from Nepal. Intestinal helminths (e.g., *Ascaris*, hookworm, *Trichuris*) and *Strongyloides* should be treated specifically. *Schistosoma mansoni* is diagnosed by serologic testing and rectal biopsy. Tropical sprue is considered in a traveler with diarrhea and malabsorption. The D-xylose test result is abnormal and jejunal fluid is culture-positive for several aerobic organisms, including *Klebsiella*, *Enterobacter*, and *E coli*. After confirmation by a biopsy of the small intestine, tropical sprue is treated with tetracycline and folate. Some patients report persistent diarrhea and malabsorption and exhibit flattened intestinal villi. Although this posttravel syndrome may be prolonged, the prognosis is good for ultimate recovery.

CHAPTER 24

Nosocomial Infections and Risks to Health Care Providers

HOSPITAL EPIDEMIOLOGY

Acquisition of Nosocomial Infections

Bacteria are the most common causes of nosocomial infections, but viruses, fungi, mycobacteria, and parasites also are transmitted in the health care setting. Most nosocomial infections arise from endogenous sources within patients. The likelihood of transmission is determined by organism pathogenicity, virulence, invasiveness, and the inoculating dose. Certain infections, such as those caused by *Legionella pneumophila*, may arise from exogenous reservoirs such as cooling towers or shower heads. Organisms may be spread by contact (e.g., methicillin-resistant staphylococci or vancomycin-resistant enterococci on people's hands), droplets (e.g., rubella), a common vehicle (e.g., contaminated catheters or endoscopes), or be airborne (e.g., aspergillosis). Increasingly, nosocomial pathogens are identified as resistant bacteria and fungi.

Nosocomial infections occur in 3% to 5% of hospitalized patients; nosocomial pneumonias are most common. The mortality rate of nosocomial infections is 20% to 50%. Risk factors for hospital-acquired pneumonias include age older than 70 years, chronic lung disease, decreased mental status, chest surgery, acid suppression, frequent change of ventilator circuits, and fall and winter seasons. Nosocomial pneumonia is usually caused by more than one organism. Gram-negative rods are involved in more than 60% of cases. Surgical wound infections are the second most common nosocomial infection and usually are caused by *Staphylococcus aureus*. Increases in postoperative antibiotic-resistant gram-positive bacteria, gram-negative bacteria, coagulase-negative staphylococci, and yeasts have been noted. Risk factors for surgical wound infections include the length of the preoperative stay, the length of the operation, the use of drains, remote infections, age, the timing of antibiotics, and illness severity. Other nosocomial infections include primary bloodstream infections relating to catheters and invasive procedures and urinary infections that most commonly occur in women or in patients with urinary catheters.

Infection Control

The most basic component of all isolation programs is hand washing before and after every patient contact, although compliance with this recommendation has been poor. Beyond this, there are six isolation categories whose implementation depends on the severity and cause of patient illness. Strict isolation is recommended for highly contagious diseases spread by air and contact (e.g., varicella) and requires a private room with negative-pressure ventilation and masks, gowns, and gloves for health care workers. Contact isolation is recommended for diseases spread by contact (e.g., staphylococcal, enterococcal, herpes simplex, and group A streptococcal skin infections) and requires masks, gowns, and gloves. Respiratory isolation is needed for airborne pathogens (e.g., measles and meningococcus), and a private room and masks are required. Tuberculosis (TB) isolation requires a private room, negative-pressure ventilation, and disposable particulate respirator masks. Enteric precautions are needed for diseases transmitted by pathogens in feces (e.g., hepatitis A [HAV], *Salmonella* species, or *Shigella* species), whereas precautions against drainage and secretion prevent transmission of pathogens from purulent secretions. Recommendations for these two categories include gloves and gowns. Universal precautions dictate that all blood and body fluid samples should be handled by gloved personnel. Protective eye or face shields and gowns should be worn if splashing or spraying of fluids is possible. Health care workers with weeping skin lesions should refrain from patient or equipment contact. Often, a patient's diagnosis will not be known. In these cases, the Body Substance Isolation protocol recommends barrier precautions, gloves, gowns, masks, and eyewear to prevent contact between health care workers and all moist body substances.

Health care workers should be immunized against measles, mumps, rubella, diphtheria, pertussis, tetanus, and hepatitis B (HBV) and should receive influenza vaccine annually. If a health care worker is exposed to a potential pathogen, first aid should be given, including washing the wound. The exposure should be categorized as high-risk or low-risk for human immunodeficiency virus (HIV), hepatitis C (HCV), and HBV transmission. High-risk exposures include needlestick or scalpel injuries with patient blood contact; low-risk exposures include needlesticks from subcutaneous or piggyback injections. For high-risk exposure, HBV, HCV, and HIV serologic testing of the patient and health care worker are performed at the time of exposure. Additional HIV testing of the health care worker is performed at 6 weeks, 12 weeks, 6 months, and 12 months. HCV testing algorithms are in flux but either include antibody testing at 6 months or HCV RNA testing at 1 to 3 months followed by antibody testing at 6 months. Prophylaxis with oral drugs is recommended for potential HIV transmission and with hepatitis B immunoglobulin (HBIg) for potential HBV transmission in unvaccinated individuals; there are no current recommendations for prophylaxis against HCV transmission.

TUBERCULOSIS

Nosocomial transmission of TB has occurred from patients with draining ulcers, those with osteomyelitis, and those undergoing bronchoscopy for unexplained pulmonary infiltrates. In addition, outbreaks of multidrug-resistant TB have been reported in HIV wards. Measures to prevent the spread of TB have been widely implemented by hospitals, but many nosocomial TB outbreaks result from breaches in standard infection control procedures and from improperly functioning isolation rooms. Health care workers should be screened annually for TB exposure by a tuberculin skin test. Workers in high-risk situations should undergo screening every 3 to 6 months. Workers with positive skin test results should be evaluated regularly for active TB by chest radiography. In patients without active TB who are younger than 35 years, isoniazid prophylaxis (300 mg daily) is given for 6 to 12 months (Table 24-1). This regimen is also recommended for workers of any age who are HIV-positive, who have had TB skin test conversion within the past 2 years, who have findings on chest radiographs consistent with old TB, who have a medical risk factor for acquiring TB, or who associate with TB-infected individuals.

TABLE 24-1
Indications for Isoniazid Prophylaxis

Any age
    A positive tuberculin skin test and any one of the following:
        Human immunodeficiency virus seropositivity
        Recent conversion of the tuberculin skin test (<2 yr)
        Abnormal findings on a chest radiograph compatible with old or healed tuberculosis
        Presence of a medical risk factor increasing the chance of developing active
            tuberculosis (e.g., diabetes, renal failure, immunosuppression, malignancy,
            silicosis, weight loss, intravenous drug abuse)
        Close contact with someone with active tuberculosis

<35 years of age
    A positive tuberculin skin test, regardless of duration of skin-test positivity

BLOOD-BORNE PATHOGENS

Human Immunodeficiency Virus

Percutaneous injuries (84%) are the predominant mode for transmitting HIV to health care workers, followed by mucocutaneous exposure to blood that contains HIV (13%), and combined mucocutaneous and percutaneous blood exposure (3%). Percutaneous injuries occur in 7% of operating room cases and occur most commonly from suture needles, from manually holding the tissue, or from instruments held by coworkers. In this group, despite frequent exposure and deviations from universal precautions, the risk of HIV transmission to a health care worker is small. In a survey of 3400 orthopedists, 3.2% reported previous injury with sharp objects from HIV-positive patients, yet none developed HIV seropositivity.

Several interventions are recommended to reduce HIV transmission, including refraining from recapping needles, use of puncture-resistant containers for disposal of sharp objects, and increased glove use (or even double gloving). For workers who sustain percutaneous exposure to known HIV-positive blood, HIV tests should be performed immediately and at 6 weeks, 12 weeks, 6 months, and 12 months. Given the low rate of seroconversion, the degree of efficacy of chemoprophylaxis is unproven, but offering drug treatment to exposed health care workers has evolved into standard practice. Several different regimens are used usually for 4 to 6 weeks, beginning within 4 to 6 hours of exposure. These drugs can be discontinued after 24 to 48 hours if the patient's HIV serology test results are negative. Antiretroviral therapy is not recommended after exposure to blood splashes, exposure to nonbloody fluid, or penetrating injuries from nonbloody instruments.

Hepatotropic Viruses

Hepatitis A

HAV is an enteric RNA virus that produces a brief viremic period followed by viral replication and fecal shedding. The process lasts about 28 days, with fecal shedding over the final 10 to 14 days. HAV is primarily spread through contaminated food or water, although parenteral transmission is reported rarely. Acute HAV infection is documented by detecting immunoglobulin M (IgM) antibodies to HAV (anti-HAV IgM), whereas detecting immunoglobulin G (IgG) antibodies to HAV (anti-HAV IgG) indicates prior exposure with recovery. Risk factors for HAV infection include homosexuality, drug abuse, travel to endemic areas, and contact with children in day care or with others who have hepatitis A. If universal precautions are followed, the risks for health care workers are small. In the rare instance of needle exposure, 0.02 mL/kg immune serum globulin (ISG) is given within 10 days of exposure. HAV vaccine (1 injection with a booster at 6 to 12 months) should be offered to health care providers who are at high risk.

Hepatitis B

HBV is a DNA virus that is spread horizontally by parenteral and sexual exposure, vertically by perinatal exposure, and in settings of close personal contact such as households and institutions. Acute HBV infection is diagnosed by detecting IgM antibodies to hepatitis B core antigen (anti-HBc IgM), whereas chronic HBV infection is defined by the persistence of hepatitis B surface antigen (HBsAg) positivity. Furthermore, active replication is indicated by high serum levels of hepatitis B e antigen (HBeAg) and HBV DNA. Antibodies to HBeAg (anti-HBe) should not be considered protective against infection as long as HBsAg is present, but their presence is usually associated with a lower level of viral replication. Anti-HBc IgM is a specific marker of acute infection, although rare cases of chronic hepatitis with high levels of viral replication exhibit this antibody. Persons who have received HBV vaccine are positive only for antibodies to HBsAg (anti-HBs) and are protected against new HBV infection in 95% of cases.

Risk factors for acquiring HBV include drug abuse, sexual contact with multiple partners, household contact and sexual contact with HBV carriers, infants of HBV-infected mothers, exposure in institutions for the developmentally disabled, exposure to blood products through one's employment, transfusion of certain plasma products prior to uniform blood screening, hemodialysis, and residence in areas of high HIV endemicity. The risk of needlestick transmission after exposure to HBsAg-positive blood is 7% to 30%. High HBV replicative status (HBeAg positive, high levels of HBV DNA) confers an increased risk of transmission. Prophylaxis with hepatitis B immune globulin (HBIG, 0.06 mL/kg) and revaccination is appropriate for the exposed worker who has not been vaccinated or who has inadequate titers of anti-HBs (Table 24-2). Booster injections are not currently recommended for HBV. However, for immunocompromised patients, a booster dose is indicated if anti-HBs titers are less than 10 mIU/mL.

Hepatitis D virus (HDV, delta virus) is an RNA virus that infects and replicates only in the presence of HBsAg positivity. During acute infection, HDV antigen (Ag) and IgM antibodies to HDV (anti-HDV IgM) are present, whereas chronic infection is marked by the presence of HDV Ag and the absence of anti-HDV IgM. The primary recommendation for avoiding HDV infection is adequate HBV vaccination. In exposed workers, HBIG therapy and HBV vaccination decrease the risk of HDV infection.

Hepatitis C

Hepatitis C virus (HCV) is an RNA virus transmitted by parenteral and other routes. HCV can be acquired via sexual transmission, but the risk is low. The presence of HIV infection may act as a cofactor for transmitting both HIV and HCV. Similarly, vertical maternal-to-fetal HCV transmission is rare unless the mother is also HIV positive. Both of these phenomena probably result from higher rates of HCV replication in HIV-positive women compared with those who are seronegative for HIV. HCV RNA is not present in saliva, urine, sweat, or semen. Current testing for HCV infection involves enzyme-linked immunosorbent assay (ELISA) or radioimmunoblot assay for HCV antibodies, but these tests measure only exposure and not necessarily active infection. Furthermore, anti-HCV positivity does not develop for 12 to 24 weeks after infection. Polymerase chain reaction (PCR) and branched-chain DNA tests for HCV RNA are available to document active viral replication.

Risk factors for HCV infection include drug abuse, blood transfusions or organ transplantation prior to 1991, hemodialysis, employment in a health care environment, and tattoos. Health care workers are at risk from needlesticks, with approximately a 3% transmission rate. Prophylaxis with immune globulin or antiviral therapy has not been shown to be beneficial. Initiation of early antiviral therapy for those with PCR documentation of active HCV replication may produce high clearance rates, although good data for this practice are limited. Infected health care workers should observe universal precautions to prevent transmission to patients.

TABLE 24-2
Prophylaxis for Hepatitis B After Parenteral Exposure

EXPOSED PERSON	HBsAg-POSITIVE SOURCE	HBsAg-NEGATIVE SOURCE	SOURCE HBsAg UNKNOWN
Unvaccinated	HBIG × 1[a] and initiate HB vaccine[b]	Initiate HB vaccine[b]	Initiate HB vaccine[b]
Previously vaccinated, known responder	Test exposed person for anti-HBs: (1) if adequate,[c] no treatment; (2) if inadequate, HB vaccine booster dose	No treatment	No treatment
Previously vaccinated, known nonresponder	HBIG × 2 or HBIG × 1 + 1 dose of HB vaccine	No treatment	If known high-risk source, treat as if source HBsAg-positive
Previously vaccinated, response unknown	Test exposed person for anti-HBs: (1) if adequate,[c] no treatment; (2) if inadequate, HBIG × 1 + HB vaccine booster dose	No treatment	Test exposed person for anti-HBs: (1) if adequate,[c] no treatment; (2) if inadequate, HB vaccine booster dose

HBsAg, hepatitis B surface antigen; HBIG, hepatitis B immunoglobulin; HB, hepatitis B.
[a] HBIG; 0.06 mL/kg intramuscular given immediately after exposure.
[b] HB vaccine; first dose within 1 wk, second dose in 1 mo, third dose in 6 mo.
[c] Adequate anti-HBs is >10 mIU by radioimmunoassay or positive by enzyme immunoassay.

Non-A, Non-B, Non-C Hepatitis

The diagnosis of non-A, non-B, non-C hepatitis is reserved for persons with presumed viral hepatitis and negative serologic tests. Precautions and work restrictions for this condition are similar to those for HCV.

Cytomegalovirus

Cytomegalovirus (CMV) is a ubiquitous DNA virus to which many adults in the United States (30%–100%) have evidence of prior exposure. Health care providers generally are not at high risk for CMV infection unless they are immunocompromised. In previously unexposed pregnant women, new CMV infection is teratogenic. Serologic tests (CMV IgM) as well as tests for CMV antigenemia and CMV DNA by PCR are available, but diagnosis of CMV disease usually requires clinical evidence of invasive infection such as viral isolation from tissue or cytologic specimens. Universal precautions and good hand washing should be protective for health care workers. No work restrictions have been issued for infected care providers.

GASTROINTESTINAL PATHOGENS

Enteric Viruses

The rotavirus is an RNA virus that produces 30% to 50% of the cases of pediatric gastroenteritis as well as rare cases of diarrhea in adults. Infection most commonly occurs during the winter in children younger than 3 years and is associated with shedding of large amounts of virus in the stool for up to 3 weeks. Adherence to universal precautions, good hand washing, and meticulous housekeeping of the infected patient's room and linens help to prevent transmission.

Enteric Bacteria

Clostridium difficile

Clostridium difficile is responsible for 70% to 90% of antibiotic-associated colitis and 15% to 25% of antibiotic-associated diarrhea. This pathogen also may be transmitted by person-to-person contact; carriage by and infection of hospital personnel have been documented. Adherence to universal precautions, hand washing, and use of gloves can prevent transmission.

Escherichia coli

Several groups of pathogenic *Escherichia coli* are known: enteropathogenic, enterotoxigenic, enteroinvasive, enteroadherent, and enterohemorrhagic. Transmission is by the fecal-oral route in areas of poor sanitation and commonly occurs in the summer. The diagnosis depends on a high index of suspicion; however, many laboratories now routinely culture specimens for this organism if diarrhea is bloody. Universal precautions and hand washing should prevent most transmission.

Salmonella Species

Salmonellae are gram-negative bacilli that cause gastroenteritis, most commonly in the summer and fall, in persons younger than 20 years and older than 70 years, often coincident with outbreaks of food poisoning. The major routes of transmission include person-to-person, via contaminated food (e.g., eggs), and via contaminated common sources (e.g., medications). Infections with *Salmonella* species are prevalent in health care facilities, with an attack rate 10-fold higher than that of other epidemics and 7% to 9% mortality. The incubation period is typically 1 to

2 weeks but may be as long as 2 months. Diagnosis of infection is based on culture of organisms from the blood or stool. The presence of *Salmonella* in the stool for more than 1 year defines the chronic carrier state. Health care workers are at risk for person-to-person transmission, which can be minimized by adherence to universal precautions and good hand washing. Chronic carriers should be given 4 to 6 weeks of antibiotics to eradicate the infection. Chronic carriers with biliary tract disease should receive a 10-day to 14-day course of antibiotics plus a cholecystectomy. Health care workers should not have patient contact during the period of fecal shedding.

Shigella Species

Shigellae are gram-negative bacilli that produce gastroenteritis, especially in children between 1 and 4 years of age, most often during the summer and fall. Transmission occurs by the fecal-oral route, and outbreaks may be food-borne or may occur in day-care facilities. The diagnosis of shigellosis is made by stool culture. Transmission is prevented by observing universal precautions. Health care workers who are infected may have temporary limitations on their patient interactions, but fecal shedding is almost always complete within 1 month. Although usually self-limited, treatment of shigellosis with a quinolone or trimethoprim-sulfamethoxazole is recommended to prevent transmission.

Campylobacter Species

Campylobacter jejuni is responsible for 5% to 7% of cases of gastroenteritis in the United States and can occur in all age groups during the summer and fall. Transmission is by the fecal-oral route, sexual contact, raw milk, poultry, and contaminated water. Special stool culture techniques are necessary to detect *C jejuni*. Universal precautions should be observed. Occasionally, the infection may persist for 3 weeks. It is prudent to treat infected health care workers with erythromycin or a quinolone to reduce fecal excretion of the organism.

Vibrio Species

Vibrio cholerae is an enterotoxigenic pathogen that causes cholera, an acute diarrheal illness that is rare in the United States. Infection results from inadequately cooked or raw shellfish and usually occurs in the summer. In contrast, *Vibrio parahaemolyticus* is an enteroinvasive pathogen. These infections are rare in health care providers and can be prevented by universal precautions. Antimicrobial therapy with tetracycline or trimethoprim-sulfamethoxazole may be considered for infected workers.

Aeromonas Species

Clinical illness from *Aeromonas* organisms is more severe in children than in adults and is acquired from water, farm animals, and vegetables. Hand washing and universal precautions can prevent most transmission. Tetracycline or trimethoprim-sulfamethoxazole treatment can be considered for infected health care providers, although most individuals experience self-limited disease.

Yersinia enterocolitica

Transmission of *Yersinia enterocolitica* occurs by contaminated food or by person-to-person spread, with an incubation period of 2 to 11 days. Health care providers may acquire this infection and should observe universal precautions and hand washing. Food handlers should not work when ill.

CHAPTER 25

Structural Anomalies and Miscellaneous Disorders of the Esophagus

ESOPHAGEAL EMBRYOLOGY AND ANATOMY

The esophagus is derived from the foregut and can be identified as a distinct structure by the fourth week of gestation. The muscular layers of the esophagus form in the sixth week and submucosal blood vessels develop by the seventh week. Epithelial tissue occludes the lumen in the seventh and eighth weeks, lumenal recanalization occurs by the tenth week, and from the fourth through the ninth month, stratified squamous epithelial tissue develops.

The adult esophagus is 18 to 26 cm long with a diameter of 2 to 3 cm. The cervical esophagus extends from the pharyngoesophageal junction to the suprasternal notch and is bounded anteriorly by the trachea, posteriorly by the spine, and laterally by the carotids and the thyroid. The thoracic esophagus is posterior to the trachea from T4 to T8 and crosses anterior to the aorta from T8 to T10. It passes through the diaphragmatic hiatus, which consists of the muscular crura, the median arcuate ligament, and collagen and elastic fibers of the phrenoesophageal membrane, at the level of T10, and terminates in the abdominal esophagus, which is about 0.5 to 2.5 cm long. The blood supply to the cervical esophagus is derived mainly from the inferior thyroid artery; the thoracic esophagus is supplied by the aorta, right intercostal, and bronchial arteries; the abdominal esophagus is supplied by the left gastric, short gastric, and left inferior phrenic arteries. Intraepithelial channels drain into a subepithelial superficial venous plexus, which then drains into deep intrinsic submucosal veins that communicate with the gastric venous system. In the thoracic esophagus, venous blood passes into the azygos, hemiazygos, and intercostal veins. There is a watershed zone between the portal and azygos systems at the gastroesophageal junction that is prone to the formation of varices in portal hypertension. These dilated veins or varices serve as collateral channels to return portal blood to the systemic circulation. Sympathetic innervation of the esophagus is provided by the superior cervical ganglion, sympathetic chain, major splanchnic nerve, thoracic aortic plexus, and celiac ganglion. The parasympathetic innervation is provided by the left and right vagus nerves, which intertwine with sympathetic fibers to form the esophageal plexus. Lymphatics drain into the deep cervical, internal jugular, tracheal, tracheobronchial, posterior mediastinal, and pericardial lymph nodes.

The esophageal wall is composed of the mucosa, submucosa, muscularis externa, and adventitia. The absence of a serosal layer explains the rapidity with which esophageal malignancies spread and metastasize. The mucosa consists of nonkeratinized squamous epithelium, the lamina propria, and the muscularis mucosae. The inner epithelial border is irregular because of projections of the lamina propria called *dermal papillae*. Foci of hyperplastic epithelial cells with intranuclear glycogen (glycogen acanthosis) can be seen as focal white elevations. Epithelial cytotoxic T cells and macrophages and lamina propria helper T cells and B lymphocytes comprise the gut-associated lymphoid tissue of the esophagus. Striated muscle tissue makes up the inferior pharyngeal constrictor, cricopharyngeus, and proximal 6 to 8 cm of the esophagus and is arranged into an inner circular and outer longitudinal layer. The distal esophagus is composed of circular and longitudinal smooth muscle layers. The physiological lower esophageal sphincter is immediately cephalad to the diaphragmatic hiatus. The myenteric (Auerbach) plexus lies between the circular and longitudinal muscle layers. A submucosal plexus (Meissner) is seen as an irregular network of nerve bundles near the inner layer of the muscularis externa. In the lower esophageal sphincter, the interstitial cells of Cajal initiate and coordinate contraction.

DEVELOPMENTAL ANOMALIES

Tracheoesophageal Fistula and Atresia

Etiology and Pathogenesis

Both the esophagus and trachea are derived from the foregut. A tracheoesophageal fistula (TEF) results from incomplete fusion of the tracheoesophageal septum, whereas esophageal atresia occurs when esophageal elongation outstrips proliferation of the foregut. There are five anatomic variations of TEF; the most common is a lower esophageal pouch fistula with proximal esophageal atresia. These disorders commonly are associated with prematurity and hydramnios as well as with other congenital abnormalities (e.g., imperforate anus, malrotation, duodenal atresia, and annular pancreas).

Clinical Features, Diagnosis, and Course

Symptoms generally manifest in infancy and include regurgitation, respiratory distress during feedings, pneumonia, and abdominal distention. A TEF is suggested by radiographic demonstration of a gasless abdomen or increased distention, depending on the anomaly. The diagnosis of TEF may be based on findings of air insufflation of the esophagus or contrast radiography. Early surgical repair is the recommended treatment for TEF or atresia. Long atretic segments may require colonic interposition. Long-term sequelae after surgical repair of TEF and atresia include esophageal dysmotility, gastroesophageal reflux, and respiratory complications.

Congenital Esophageal Stenosis and Duplication

Etiology and Pathogenesis

Congenital esophageal stenosis results from abnormal separation of the esophagus from the trachea during fetal development. It may not be diagnosed until late in childhood or adulthood. Duplication is believed to be the result of failed coalescence of embryonic lumenal vacuoles during the recanalization phase, with formation of cysts or parallel tubular channels within the esophageal wall that communicate with the lumen at one or both ends. Cystic duplications, after leiomyoma, are the second most common benign esophageal tumors; they form within the esophageal wall, most often in the distal esophagus. Gastric, bronchogenic, and neuroenteric cysts as well as cysts with squamous or respiratory epithelia may be found in the esophagus. Foregut duplication cysts are associated with cervical and thoracic vertebral anomalies.

Clinical Features, Diagnosis, and Management

Symptoms of esophageal stenosis include regurgitation, slow eating, or dysphagia to solids. Barium swallow radiographs show segmental stenosis with ring-like folds that can also be seen by endoscopic examination. Patients with tubular duplications present with symptoms of obstruction or gastroesophageal reflux. Barium swallow radiographs or endoscopy confirms the diagnosis. Proximal duplication cysts usually present in infancy with potentially fatal tracheobronchial compression. Distal esophageal cysts produce dysphagia, epigastric discomfort, chest pain, cough, dyspnea, or regurgitation. Chest radiography may demonstrate the duplication cyst as a mediastinal mass, which can be further defined by barium swallow radiography, ultrasound, or computed tomography. On endoscopic examination, a duplication cyst appears as a soft, compressible extrinsic mass. Endoscopic ultrasound reveals a cystic structure. Surgical resection is recommended for many patients with stenosis or duplication; however, selected patients with stenosis may respond to bougienage. Large duplication cysts may require marsupialization rather than resection. Malignant degeneration within tubular or cystic duplications occurs rarely.

Esophageal Rings and Webs

Etiology and Pathogenesis

Lower esophageal mucosal rings (i.e., Schatzki or "B" rings) are located at the squamocolumnar junction and consist of mucosa (squamous on the proximal side, columnar or squamous on the distal side), and submucosa. True mucosal rings are circumferential and symmetric and are associated with a hiatal hernia. In contrast, lower esophageal muscular rings ("A" rings) occur 1.5 cm proximal to the squamocolumnar junction and consist of an annular ring of hypertrophied or hypertonic muscle with normal overlying squamous mucosa. Muscular rings are broader than mucosal rings (4–5 mm compared to ≤3 mm) and are associated with esophageal dysmotility, gastroesophageal reflux, and hiatal hernias. Esophageal webs are thin, squamous, mucosal membranes that occur in the upper and middle esophagus and increase in prevalence with advancing age. Webs that involve the anterior wall of the postcricoid esophagus may be associated with iron deficiency anemia (Plummer-Vinson or Paterson-Kelly syndrome) and have a propensity for developing pharyngeal and esophageal carcinoma. Single or multiple midesophageal webs are believed to be congenital.

Clinical Features, Diagnosis, and Management

Most esophageal mucosal rings are asymptomatic, but if the remaining lumen is less than 20 mm in diameter, they may produce intermittent dysphagia. Rings less than 13 mm in diameter are often associated with persistent solid-food dysphagia. Barium swallow radiography is the diagnostic test of choice for esophageal rings. Their detection is enhanced by a Valsalva maneuver during the swallow or by using a barium tablet or marshmallow. Endoscopy also may diagnose Schatzki rings.

Muscular rings occasionally produce dysphagia. Barium swallow radiography may demonstrate broad, smooth, symmetric narrowing that varies in caliber. Esophageal manometry illustrates lower esophageal sphincter hypertension that correlates with the level of the ring. Most symptomatic patients with mucosal or muscular rings can be treated with sequential bougienage to a lumenal diameter of 17 to 20 mm, although some mucosal rings may require endoscopic cautery incision. Patients with both upper and midesophageal webs present with infrequent intermittent dysphagia that may be treated with bougienage, transendoscopic incision, or surgery.

Miscellaneous Developmental Esophageal Anomalies

Bronchopulmonary Foregut Malformations

Bronchopulmonary foregut malformations develop when respiratory cell rests or a portion of the lung bud arises from the esophagus, allowing communication between the respiratory and gastrointestinal systems. Infants may present with respiratory distress or congestive heart failure, whereas older children and adults develop pneumonia, bronchiectasis, hemoptysis, gastrointestinal bleeding, and dysphagia. Associated congenital defects are present in 40% of children. Barium swallow radiography, angiography, and bronchography are useful for diagnosis; surgical resection is the treatment for this condition.

Vascular Compression of the Esophagus

Dysphagia lusoria is a term used to describe symptomatic compression of the esophagus by an aortic arch anomaly, usually an aberrant right subclavian artery. Patients may initially present with dysphagia in infancy, childhood, or adulthood. The physical examination may reveal a reduced right radial pulse. Barium swallow radiography shows an oblique filling defect above the aortic arch. The condition is corrected surgically, although adults with mild dysphagia can be treated with dietary modification. Other vascular anomalies include esophageal compression by an anomalous vertebral artery and right aortic arch, double aortic arch, right aortic arch with patent ductus arteriosus, cervical aortic arch, and aberrant left pulmonary artery.

Heterotopic Gastric Mucosa

Inlet patch refers to heterotopic gastric mucosa in the proximal esophagus below the cricopharyngeus, although the condition may present at any esophageal site. The endoscopic appearance is that of patches of red-orange mucosa. Most cases are asymptomatic, although the acid-secretory capabilities of these patches may produce esophagitis. Other complications include cervical webs or rings, TEF, and adenocarcinoma.

DIVERTICULA

Etiology and Pathogenesis

Pharyngoesophageal, or Zenker, diverticula form by protrusion of the posterior hypopharyngeal mucosa between the inferior pharyngeal constrictor and the cricopharyngeus proximal to the esophagus. Zenker diverticula may result from high hypopharyngeal pressures during swallowing caused by a nonrelaxing cricopharyngeus. Diverticula also develop in the middle or distal esophagus and usually are secondary to esophageal dysmotility or esophageal strictures. In children, esophageal diverticula may develop proximal to a stricture induced by ingesting a foreign body. Esophageal intramural pseudodiverticulosis is a rare condition in which multiple, small pseudodiverticula in the esophageal wall arise from the submucosal glands that dilate secondary to stasis and inflammation. Esophageal strictures are seen in 70% to 90% of these patients; esophageal candidiasis and prior corrosive injury have been reported as risk factors.

Clinical Features, Diagnosis, and Management

Patients with Zenker diverticula generally present after age 50 with symptoms, including solid and liquid dysphagia, regurgitation of undigested food, cough, halitosis, a neck mass, weight loss, or aspiration pneumonia. Barium swallow radiography with lateral views helps to confirm the diagnosis. Surgery, consisting of diverticulectomy with or without cricopharyngeal myotomy, is the recommended treatment. Endoscopic division of the septum between the diverticulum and proximal esophagus has also been successful. Complications of Zenker diverticula include development of squamous cell carcinoma, spindle cell carcinoma, and benign tumors.

Esophageal diverticula and pseudodiverticula can be diagnosed using barium swallow radiographs or upper endoscopic studies. Symptoms from these conditions include dysphagia, regurgitation, and substernal chest pain. The symptoms often stem from the primary stricture rather than the diverticula; thus, if treatment of the stricture is successful, surgical diverticulectomy is rarely needed. Dilation of strictures, antireflux therapy, and calcium channel antagonists may be useful in selected cases.

ESOPHAGEAL HIATAL HERNIAS

Etiology and Pathogenesis

A hiatal hernia is defined as the cephalad displacement of the esophagogastric junction into the thorax by a distance of 2 cm or more. Hiatal hernias usually appear in later life and may be secondary to esophageal contraction from reflux-induced injury, increased intra-abdominal pressure (such as straining during defecation while on a low-fiber diet), or chronic intra-abdominal trauma due to obesity or lifting heavy weights. It is postulated that elongation of the phrenoesophageal membrane, the structure that anchors the esophagogastric junction, causes formation of the hernia. The condition is more common in persons with peptic ulcer disease, scleroderma, kyphosis, and ankylosing spondylitis. There is a controversial association between hiatal hernia, lower esophageal sphincter function, and gastroesophageal reflux. Most patients with hiatal hernias are asymptomatic; conversely, most patients with symptomatic gastroesophageal reflux have hiatal hernias.

Clinical Features, Diagnosis, and Management

Most patients with hiatal hernias do not require treatment; however, some patients will present with gastroesophageal reflux disease, stricture formation, occult or gross hemorrhage, or rarely incarceration with pain. Barium swallow radiography will define the hernia, but endoscopy is indicated in potentially complicated cases for hemorrhage control, stricture dilation, or diagnosis of Barrett esophagus. Proper medical therapy with acid-suppressing agents or prokinetic drugs controls reflux-induced symptoms in more than 90% of cases. Although surgical therapy to correct hiatal hernia is widely used, long-term outcomes indicate that most patients who undergo fundoplication eventually require reinstitution of medical therapy to control the symptoms of gastroesophageal reflux.

CAUSTIC ESOPHAGEAL INJURY

Etiology and Pathogenesis

The ingestion of caustic substances, either accidental or from a suicide attempt, may produce esophageal damage within seconds. First-degree burns produce mucosal hyperemia and edema but no scars. Second-degree burns extend into the muscle layers and produce exudation, mucosal loss, and ulcerations that may progress to scarring over weeks to months. Third-degree burns are transmural, with erosion into the mediastinal, pleural, or peritoneal cavities. Fistula formation and death due to overwhelming sepsis and complications are not rare.

In most instances, alkaline substances produce greater esophageal injury than acidic agents. Alkaline agents such as lye, detergents, Clinitest tablets (containing copper sulfate, sodium hydroxide, and sodium carbonate), and disc batteries (containing potassium or sodium hydroxide) produce liquefaction necrosis of the esophagus, depending on the concentration and duration of contact. Blood vessel thrombosis, edema, cell necrosis, and neutrophilic infiltration are followed by bacterial colonization. Ammonia and bleach generally do not cause severe esophageal damage. Acids in toilet bowl cleaners (e.g., sulfuric, hydrochloric, or phosphoric acid), swimming pool additives, antirust compounds, and soldering fluxes produce coagulation necrosis of the mucosa that may limit penetration of acid into the esophageal wall.

Clinical Features, Diagnosis, and Management

Symptoms of caustic ingestion include burning of the lips, tongue, or pharynx; dysphagia; odynophagia; drooling; vomiting; and dyspnea. Hematemesis and abdominal pain suggest possible gastric injury, whereas hoarseness, wheezing, and stridor suggest airway involvement. Patients with third-degree burns may present with shock, mediastinitis, or peritoneal findings. Initial diagnostic studies should include chest and abdominal radiography to detect pneumonitis, pleural effusions, mediastinal and subdiaphragmatic air. Upper gastrointestinal endoscopy generally is used to assess the extent of damage. Barium swallow radiography should not be performed because of the irritating effects of barium in the setting of perforation and because of the inability to visualize the mucosa subsequently with endoscopy. Computed tomography may further define the extent of damage or detect the development of an abscess. Endoscopic ultrasound may be used to stage the depth of injury to the esophagus.

The first step in treating patients who have ingested caustic substances is to stabilize the airway. If respiratory distress is present, endotracheal intubation is indicated. Emesis should not be induced and oral intake is prohibited. Intravenous fluids should be provided. The use of antibiotics is reasonable in patients with second- and third-degree burns. The role of corticosteroids is controversial because prospective trials are lacking; however, retrospective data indicate that steroid treatment reduces the rate of stricture formation. If used, corticosteroids (e.g., dexamethasone, 1 mg/kg per day) should be reserved for patients at high risk of stricture formation, such as those who present with circumferential burns. Sucralfate was shown to be beneficial in one uncontrolled trial, and antisecretory agents are advocated because concomitant reflux may contribute to stricture formation. Patients with impending or frank perforation require surgery, which may include esophagectomy and colonic interposition. If, after ingestion of a disc battery, radiographs localize the foreign body to the esophagus, immediate endoscopic removal is indicated to minimize the burn area and decrease the risk of perforation.

Complications of caustic ingestion include esophageal stricture, carcinoma, and gastric damage. Esophageal stenosis may develop as early as 2 weeks postingestion, and most commonly occurs after full-thickness circumferential burns. Careful esophageal dilation is recommended 2 to 4 weeks after caustic ingestion if dysphagia is present. After lye ingestion, the risk of squamous cell esophageal carcinoma increases 1000-fold, with a latent period of several decades; therefore, surveillance endoscopy may be indicated in this patient subset. Gastric outlet obstruction may develop 2 to 6 weeks after the ingestion of acid substances. Squamous metaplasia and gastric carcinoma have been reported, but the causative role of ingested caustics is uncertain.

MEDICATION-INDUCED ESOPHAGEAL INJURY

Etiology and Pathogenesis

Multiple factors determine whether any particular medication has damaged the esophagus. Round tablets take longer to pass through the esophagus than oval pills. Large volumes of water assist transit of gelatin-coated pills or capsules. Ingestion of medications while supine increases the transit time through the esophagus. In young patients, antibiotics are the most common cause of pill-induced damage, whereas potassium, NSAIDs, and bisphosphonates are more common causes in the elderly. Most cases occur in patients without prior esophageal disease. Pills tend to lodge at the level of the left atrium and aortic arch.

Clinical Features, Diagnosis, and Management

Odynophagia and dysphagia are the typical symptoms of pill-induced esophageal damage that usually occurs within hours of ingestion but occasionally days or weeks later. Substernal pain and hematemesis are sometimes reported. Barium swallow radiography may show ulceration or stricturing. The diagnosis is confirmed by upper endoscopy, which often shows a discrete ulcer or ulcers with exudation in the middle esophagus. Biopsy specimens show inflammation and reactive hyperplasia. Therapy focuses on removing the offending medication and educating the patient about ingesting medication with plenty of fluid and at least 15 to 30 minutes before lying down. Viscous lidocaine, antacids, and analgesics may be used to relieve discomfort. Esophageal dilation may be necessary for chronic stricture formation.

ESOPHAGEAL FOREIGN BODIES

Etiology and Pathogenesis

Adults with dentures, patients with psychiatric illness, prisoners, and young children are at risk of ingesting foreign bodies. Children most commonly ingest coins, whereas the most common esophageal foreign bodies in adults are meat or bones.

These items tend to lodge in the cervical esophagus, at the level of the aortic arch, above the lower esophageal sphincter, or proximal to a preexisting stricture. Food impaction often occurs in a Schatzki ring.

Clinical Features, Diagnosis, and Management

Dysphagia is the most common presenting complaint, followed by odynophagia, choking, drooling, coughing, dyspnea, or wheezing. Chest radiography may detect a radiopaque object or suggest soft-tissue swelling with a radiolucent foreign body. Contrast studies are contraindicated in high-grade obstruction, due to the risk of aspiration pneumonitis (water-soluble contrast) and because the agents (barium) obscure the view of endoscopy, which may be required for definitive therapy. Esophageal relaxation with nitroglycerin or glucagon (1 mg intravenously) may allow spontaneous passage of the food bolus into the stomach. Most foreign bodies pass through the gut uneventfully, but some objects require endoscopic or surgical extraction. If the foreign body has been present for a long time, surgery may be required for extraction, repair of perforation, drainage of an abscess, or closure of a fistula. Endoscopy can be used to remove a broad range of objects; in most cases, an overtube should be used to prevent tracheal aspiration. A variety of devices, including baskets, snares, forceps, and friction-fit adapters on the end of the endoscope, are used to remove the foreign object. Alternatively, if lumenal visualization is adequate, the endoscopist may gently push the foreign body into the stomach. After the esophagus is cleared, acid suppression is begun; esophageal dilation is deferred until a later date. Surgery rarely is necessary to clear a food impaction. Note that food impactions usually are associated with underlying esophageal disease.

SYSTEMIC DISEASES THAT AFFECT THE ESOPHAGUS

There are a number of systemic diseases that affect the esophagus. The diseases and associated esophageal findings are listed in Table 25-1.

Sarcoidosis

Sarcoidosis rarely manifests as granulomatous esophagitis. Patients with sarcoidosis may exhibit dysphagia as a result of long strictures or esophageal dysmotility. More commonly, dysphagia in these patients results from gastroesophageal reflux, esophageal infection, or extrinsic compression by enlarged lymph nodes.

Crohn's Disease

Crohn's disease of the esophagus is extremely rare. Inflammation usually parallels the activity of the disease in other regions of the gastrointestinal tract. Occasionally, dysphagia is the presenting symptom of Crohn's disease. Symptoms of esophageal involvement include odynophagia, dysphagia, pyrosis, and substernal chest pain. Fistulous tracts to the bronchi, mediastinum, or stomach may develop. The esophagus may have a cobblestone appearance by barium radiography. Upper endoscopy is more useful in excluding other disorders because diagnostic granulomas are rare. Endoscopic ultrasound may be able to detect the transmural nature of this disease.

TABLE 25-1
Effects of Systemic Diseases on the Esophagus

Disease	Esophageal Findings
Sarcoidosis	Long strictures
Crohn's disease	Aphthous ulcers, linear ulcers, impaired motility, strictures, sinus tracts
Behçet disease	Superficial ulcers, diffuse esophagitis, perforated ulcers, severe stenosis
Graft-versus-host disease	Esophageal mucosal desquamation, webs, strictures, gastroesophageal reflux
Pemphigus vulgaris	Erythema, hemorrhagic bullae, esophageal mucosal desquamation
Bullous pemphigoid	Intraepidermal bullae, esophagitis dissecans superficialis
Benign mucous membrane pemphigoid	Bullae, webs, long strictures
Epidermolysis bullosa dystrophica	Bullae, blebs, ulceration with deep scarring, long strictures, spontaneous dissection

Corticosteroids usually are helpful, but surgical resection and esophagogastrostomy may be necessary if medications and bougienage are unsuccessful.

Behçet Disease

Manifestations of Behçet disease include oral and genital aphthous ulcerations and ocular inflammation. Odynophagia, dysphagia, chest and epigastric pain, and hematemesis are consequences of esophageal involvement (erosions, diffuse esophagitis, perforated ulcers with mediastinal abscess, and severe esophageal stenosis, usually in the middle to distal esophagus). Endoscopic biopsy specimens show ulceration with nonspecific inflammation and neutrophilic infiltration. Some success has been reported in treating Behçet disease with whole blood and plasma transfusions, corticosteroids, and cyclosporine.

Graft-Versus-Host Disease

Up to 40% of bone marrow transplant survivors develop graft-versus-host disease (GVHD). GVHD esophagitis presents with odynophagia, dysphagia, pyrosis, and substernal chest pain. Infectious esophagitis complicating chronic immunosuppression is important in the differential diagnosis. Upper endoscopy in a GVHD patient typically reveals erythematous, friable, and desquamative esophagitis. Strictures and webs may be seen by endoscopy and are also detectable by barium swallow radiography. Manometry may show aperistalsis of the esophageal body. Esophageal histological examination in acute GVHD reveals an increase in the number of lamina propria lymphocytes, whereas chronic GVHD is characterized by a band-like lymphocytic infiltrate and destruction of the basal layer. Paradoxically, treatment is directed at increasing immunosuppression. Adjuvant therapy consists of acid suppression to prevent secondary damage from gastroesophageal reflux. Esophageal strictures usually respond to bougienage. In rare cases, parenteral nutrition or gastrostomic feedings are necessary.

Pemphigus Vulgaris

Pemphigus vulgaris is a chronic disease that usually presents in the fourth to sixth decade of life with flaccid bullae of the skin and oral mucous membranes and occasionally of the esophagus. The disease is more common in women and among people of Jewish and Mediterranean descent. Pemphigus autoantibody against keratinocytes causes loss of cell-cell adhesion and leads to marked susceptibility to the separation of the superficial epithelium from the basal layer after only minimal trauma. Esophageal complaints include dysphagia, odynophagia, epigastric pain, and pyrosis. Upper endoscopic examination may show esophageal erosions, white plaques, flaccid hemorrhagic bullae, and sheets of desquamating mucosa. Biopsy specimens show acantholysis with IgG and complement (C3) deposits in intracellular spaces. Esophageal pemphigus vulgaris may require high-dose corticosteroids, azathioprine, cyclophosphamide, cyclosporine, methotrexate, or plasmapheresis.

Bullous Pemphigoid

Bullous pemphigoid is a benign vesiculobullous disease of older patients that infrequently has symptomatic esophageal manifestations. Bullae form as a result of antibodies directed against the squamous epithelial basement membrane, with deposition of IgG and C3 above the basement membrane. Although usually asymptomatic, patients with esophageal bullous pemphigoid may develop cicatrix formation and present with odynophagia, dysphagia, or even emesis of an esophageal cast (i.e., esophagitis dissecans superficialis). The presence of serum antibasement membrane antibody is diagnostic, but the test is insensitive (only 70% are positive), and thus biopsy and immunohistochemistry may be required to confirm the diagnosis. Prednisone with or without cyclophosphamide is the most effective therapy, although azathioprine, cyclosporine, or methotrexate are also used.

Benign Mucous Membrane Pemphigoid

Benign mucous membrane pemphigoid is a chronic blistering disease of the conjunctiva and mouth, usually beginning in the fourth decade of life. It may also involve the esophagus, manifesting as dysphagia, odynophagia, cough, and aspiration pneumonia. Barium swallow radiography may show bullae, webs, or strictures. Bullae are rarely seen endoscopically; biopsy specimens show chronic subepithelial inflammation with a lack of acanthosis. Immunofluorescence reveals IgG and C3 deposits intracellularly and on the basement membrane. Long strictures may temporarily respond to esophageal dilation; however, endoscopy may be hazardous, producing esophageal sloughing. Administration of corticosteroids and dapsone has been beneficial. Colonic interposition may be needed to treat severe esophageal strictures.

Epidermolysis Bullosa Dystrophica

Epidermolysis bullosa dystrophica is a hereditary vesiculobullous disease of squamous epithelium. Esophageal involvement is prominent in the autosomal recessive form of the disease but is rarely significant in the dominant forms. Histopathologically, there is separation of the basal lamina from the underlying dermis resulting from a loss of anchoring fibrils between the two layers. The underlying cause appears to be defective assembly or transport of type VII collagen. Cutaneous bullae present early in life, leading to a recurrent scarring-healing pattern known as mummification. Esophageal bullae ulcerate, bleed, and then heal with scarring and stricture formation. Upper esophageal webs may contribute to dysphagia. Spontaneous dissection of the esophageal wall may occur, creating a double-barrel deformity, and esophageal rupture may occur spontaneously or with attempted dilation. Barium swallow radiography is the preferred diagnostic procedure. Upper endoscopy may induce further bulla formation; however, careful endoscopic dilation may be performed in selected cases. Patients should avoid hot or coarse foods, and if necessary, switch to a nutritionally complete liquid diet. A regimen of corticosteroids or phenytoin may be effective therapy, but esophagectomy with colonic interposition may be required.

TRAUMATIC ESOPHAGEAL INJURY

Etiology and Pathogenesis

Mallory-Weiss tears are linear, nonpenetrating lacerations in the gastric or esophageal mucosa near the esophagogastric junction. They are often induced by retching and vomiting, although 40% of patients deny this history. Tears may be multiple, and they occur in men more frequently than in women. Hiatal hernias are found in 42% to 80% of cases and may be a risk factor for developing Mallory-Weiss tears.

Esophageal intramural hematomas occur spontaneously in patients with coagulopathies or with retching or vomiting and are thought to result from sudden changes in intramural pressure. Other causes of hematoma include foreign body ingestion, pill-induced injury, and esophageal variceal sclerotherapy.

Esophageal perforation is a life-threatening injury that may result from severe retching (i.e., Boerhaave syndrome), a perforated Barrett ulcer, after thoracic or abdominal trauma, or from iatrogenic causes. Boerhaave syndrome usually develops in a region of anatomic weakness in the left posterolateral aspect of the esophagus just above the diaphragm. Iatrogenic causes of esophageal perforation include endoscopy, bougienage, passage of a nasogastric tube, sclerotherapy, and balloon tamponade for variceal hemorrhage. Blunt thoracoabdominal trauma from motor vehicle crashes or even from the Heimlich maneuver occasionally may produce upper esophageal perforation because of the rapid change in esophageal transmural pressure.

Clinical Features, Diagnosis, and Management

Patients with Mallory-Weiss tears present with upper gastrointestinal hemorrhage and usually, but not always, describe a history of retching or vomiting. Upper endoscopy is most useful for diagnosis and offers the capability of therapeutic intervention (e.g., injection therapy or cautery) if bleeding does not stop spontaneously. Other diagnostic modalities such as angiography are not useful. Surgery is rarely necessary for refractory hemorrhage. Patients with intramural hematomas most often present with chest discomfort or hematemesis. Upper gastrointestinal endoscopy reveals a mass with bluish discoloration protruding into the esophageal lumen. Computed tomography, magnetic resonance imaging, or endoscopic ultrasound rarely may be necessary to distinguish hematomas from benign or malignant esophageal masses. Intramural hematomas usually resolve spontaneously over 2 to 10 days. Coagulopathies should be corrected. Rarely, esophageal perforation may be a complication.

Cervical and upper esophageal perforations present with neck and chest pain, subcutaneous emphysema, dysphagia, odynophagia, nausea, vomiting, hematemesis, hoarseness, or aphonia, whereas distal perforations may produce abdominal pain. A Hamman crunch, a crackle in cadence with cardiac activity, may be noted on auscultation, indicating the presence of pneumomediastinum. Chest and abdominal radiographs may demonstrate subcutaneous emphysema, pneumothorax, pneumomediastinum, pleural effusion, or pneumoperitoneum. Contrast esophagography with water-soluble agents may be diagnostic. If no perforation is found, barium swallow radiography or upper endoscopy may provide better definition of the esophageal anatomy. Both of these techniques are potentially hazardous for patients with possible rupture, and they should be used cautiously. Cervical penetrating injuries are a special case requiring preoperative or intraoperative endoscopy. Thoracentesis may reveal pleural fluid with an acidic pH because of the gastric contents and with increased amylase owing to the salivary secretions. With small ruptures, medical management may be adequate; however, most patients require surgical intervention. If diagnosis is delayed, drainage of the infected areas may be needed. The course of treatment is likely to be prolonged in complicated cases and usually requires parenteral nutrition.

CHAPTER 26

Motor Disorders of the Esophagus

DISORDERS OF THE HYPOPHARYNX, UPPER ESOPHAGEAL SPHINCTER, AND CERVICAL ESOPHAGUS

Incidence and Epidemiology

Neurological or muscular diseases that involve the oropharynx can be associated with dysphagia. Structural diseases that involve the upper esophageal sphincter (UES, cricopharyngeus) also produce oropharyngeal dysphagia. Most patients with oropharyngeal dysphagia are older. Thirty percent to 40% of nursing home patients have eating or swallowing abnormalities and many cases of aspiration pneumonia stem from swallowing dysfunction. Certain neurological and myopathic conditions that may be more amenable to therapy may appear in younger patients.

Etiology and Pathogenesis

Hypopharyngeal Diverticula and Cricopharyngeal Bars

Acquired hypopharyngeal (Zenker) diverticula are common in men over age 60 and occur between the fibers of the inferior pharyngeal constrictor and the cricopharyngeus muscle. When such diverticula become filled with food or fluid, patients become symptomatic and present with dysphagia, halitosis, regurgitation, and aspiration. Hypopharyngeal diverticula may result from delayed or failed UES relaxation, premature UES contraction, or restrictive UES myopathy with poor compliance. Such impaired compliance also gives the radiographic appearance of a cricopharyngeal bar on barium swallow in some patients with oropharyngeal dysphagia.

Neurological Disorders

The most common causes of acute oropharyngeal dysphagia are cerebrovascular accidents. Symptoms usually appear abruptly and are associated with other neurological deficits. Most often, brainstem infarctions are the cause. Less commonly, hemispheric strokes may produce dysphagia as a result of brainstem distortion from adjacent cerebral edema. Degenerative neuronal changes with progressive bulbar palsy and pseudobulbar palsy produce tongue and pharyngeal paralysis. Polio and the postpolio syndrome alter pharyngeal function, as does amyotrophic lateral sclerosis. Patients with amyotrophic lateral sclerosis present with choking attacks and aspiration pneumonias secondary to dysfunction of the tongue as well as the pharyngeal and laryngeal musculature. Hypopharyngeal stasis, aspiration, and UES dysfunction are prevalent in Parkinson disease. Swallowing abnormalities, including difficult initiation, UES abnormalities, and incoordination, occur in more than one half of patients with multiple sclerosis. Rare neurological causes of oropharyngeal dysphagia include brainstem tumors, syringobulbia, tetanus, botulism, lead poisoning, alcoholic neuropathy, carcinoma, chemotherapy, and radiation therapy.

Primary Muscle Disorders

Polymyositis and dermatomyositis are characterized by proximal muscle weakness and atrophy that involve the esophagus in 60% to 70% of cases and produce poor pharyngeal and proximal esophageal contraction, barium pooling in the valleculae, and decreased UES tone. Myotonic and oculopharyngeal dystrophy are the two forms of muscular dystrophy that affect the swallowing mechanism. Myotonic dystrophy presents with myopathic facies, swan neck, myotonia, muscle wasting, frontal baldness, testicular atrophy, and cataracts. Radiographic studies demonstrate impaired pharyngeal emptying and abnormal esophageal body peristalsis. Oculopharyngeal dystrophy presents with ptosis and dysphagia but does not have other gastrointestinal manifestations. Myasthenia gravis affects striated esophageal musculature, producing dysphagia in two thirds of patients, which worsens as the patient eats a meal. Hyperthyroidism and hypothyroidism affect swallowing, as do sarcoidosis, systemic lupus erythematosus, and the stiff man syndrome.

Clinical Features

Neuromuscular diseases of the hypopharynx and upper esophagus produce a form of dysphagia in which the patient cannot initiate swallowing or propel the food bolus from the hypopharynx into the esophageal body. The patient can usually localize symptoms to the cervical region. Patients may also describe nasal regurgitation, tracheal aspiration, drooling, or the need to dislodge impacted food manually.

Gurgling, halitosis, and a neck mass suggest a Zenker diverticulum, whereas hoarseness may reflect nerve dysfunction or intrinsic vocal cord muscular disease. Dysarthria and nasal speech suggest muscle weakness of the soft palate and pharyngeal constrictors. Physical examination may demonstrate focal deficits with cerebrovascular accidents, a palpable neck mass with a hypopharyngeal diverticulum, ptosis and end-of-day weakness with myasthenia gravis, and paucity of movement with Parkinson disease.

Findings on Diagnostic Testing

Endoscopy and Barium Swallow Radiography

The initial test performed in the patient with unexplained oropharyngeal dysphagia usually is a structural test to exclude organic etiologies. Transoral or transnasal endoscopy detects tumors or webs. Barium studies define diverticula and other obstructive lesions when the results of endoscopy are inconclusive.

Videofluoroscopy

Videofluoroscopy records the complex and rapid sequence of events in the mouth, pharynx, and upper esophagus during a swallow. Preliminary lateral neck radiographs of soft tissue detect structural problems of the cervical spine, tongue, hyoid, mandible, pharynx, and larynx. Dynamic recordings of the barium swallow include lateral and posteroanterior views after ingesting thin and thick liquid barium and barium cookies. Motility disturbances manifest as delayed initiation and prolonged duration of swallowing or a disturbance in the sequence of muscle movements. Barium retention in the pharyngeal recesses is caused by altered mucosal sensitivity, decreased muscle tone, or alterations in recess shape or size. Pharyngeal stasis is another sign of altered motility. Misdirected swallows with laryngeal penetration or aspiration are striking abnormalities. Delayed UES opening and cricopharyngeal bars also may be noted.

Manometry

Intralumenal manometry obtains measurements from the oropharynx and proximal esophagus, including the strength of pharyngeal contraction, the completeness of UES relaxation, and the timing of these events. When coupled with videofluoroscopy, manometry provides complementary information on UES function.

Other Modalities

Scintigraphic studies can demonstrate hypopharyngeal stasis, regurgitation, and tracheal aspiration. Brain images can be obtained from computed tomographic or magnetic resonance imaging studies. Testing with the anticholinesterase agent edrophonium is useful in diagnosing myasthenia gravis.

Management and Course

The first step in managing a patient with oropharyngeal dysphagia is to recognize and correct reversible causes of symptoms, including Parkinson disease, myasthenia gravis, hyperthyroidism or hypothyroidism, and polymyositis. The treatment for hypopharyngeal diverticula is cricopharyngeal myotomy with or without diverticulectomy. Myotomy reduces resting UES tone and resistance to UES flow. Dilation with a large caliber bougie may be effective for a cricopharyngeal bar. The role of myotomy in this condition is less clear. The results of videofluoroscopy can be used to modify the properties of meals and the mechanics of food ingestion in some patients with neuromuscular etiologies of oropharyngeal dysphagia. In patients who cannot safely obtain adequate nutrition, enteral feedings through a nasoenteric tube or gastrostomy may be necessary.

ACHALASIA

Incidence and Epidemiology

Achalasia usually presents in persons aged 25 through 60 years. Childhood onset should raise concern of a congenital or systemic disease, whereas onset in an elderly person may indicate achalasia secondary to malignancy. The disorder shows no sex preference and has an annual estimated incidence of 1 per 100,000 in the United States.

Etiology and Pathogenesis

Achalasia is characterized by failure of the lower esophageal sphincter (LES) to relax completely with swallowing and aperistalsis of the smooth muscle esophagus. Neuroanatomic changes are well described in primary achalasia, including loss of myenteric ganglion cells in the esophageal body and LES, reductions in esophageal body nerve fibers, degeneration of the vagus nerve, and changes in the dorsal motor nucleus of the vagus. The esophageal ganglion cells that remain are surrounded by mononuclear inflammatory cells, most of which are CD3/CD8-positive lymphocytes. Damaged ganglion cells may contain intracytoplasmic hyaline or spherical eosinophilic inclusions (Lewy bodies). Esophageal muscle tissue from patients with achalasia contracts and relaxes in response to direct stimulants or inhibitors but does not respond to ganglionic agents, confirming local denervation of the involved tissues. Physiological and immunohistochemical studies demonstrate reductions in nerves containing the relaxant neurotransmitters nitric oxide and vasoactive intestinal polypeptide. Cholecystokinin, which normally acts to relax the LES via stimulation of ganglionic inhibitory pathways, causes paradoxical contraction by direct action on LES muscle in achalasia. Impairment of gastric acid secretion and pancreatic polypeptide release in response to sham feeding suggests an additional vagal neuropathy. The lower esophageal smooth muscle is thickened in achalasia, which is considered an adaptive phenomenon rather than a pathogenic factor.

Other disorders present similarly to primary achalasia. Malignancy-related pseudoachalasia accounts for 5% of manometrically defined achalasia. Most commonly, these tumors are adenocarcinomas of the gastroesophageal junction, but pancreatic carcinoma, small cell and squamous cell lung carcinoma, prostate carcinoma, and lymphoma may also cause the syndrome either by direct compression of the distal esophagus or by malignant cell infiltration of the esophageal myenteric plexus. Other tumors (e.g., Hodgkin disease, lung carcinoma, and hepatocellular carcinoma) produce achalasia by a paraneoplastic mechanism. Although most patients with pseudoachalasia are older, have short duration of symptoms, and report weight loss, these criteria do not have significant predictive value in determining the cause of the disease. Chagas disease is caused by the protozoan *Trypanosoma cruzi*, which is transmitted by the reduviid (kissing) bug, endemic in Brazil, Venezuela, and Argentina. After an acute septic phase, chronic destruction of ganglion cells in the gut, urinary tract, heart, and respiratory tract develops over years. The presence of megaureter, megaduodenum, megacolon, or megarectum is helpful in distinguishing Chagas disease from achalasia. Complement fixation and polymerase chain reaction tests are available to confirm the diagnosis. Other causes of secondary achalasia include infiltrative diseases (with amyloid, sphingolipids, eosinophils, or sarcoid), diabetes, intestinal pseudoobstruction, pancreatic pseudocysts, von Recklinghausen disease, multiple endocrine neoplasia type IIB, juvenile Sjögren syndrome, and familial adrenal insufficiency with alacrima.

Clinical Features

All patients with achalasia report solid-food dysphagia, and most also report liquid dysphagia. Symptoms may be intermittent and insidious in onset. The duration of symptoms when diagnosed averages 2 years. The patient may have learned special maneuvers such as throwing the shoulders back, lifting the neck, performing a Valsalva maneuver, and drinking carbonated beverages to promote passage of the esophageal bolus into the stomach. Other manifestations of achalasia include fullness or gurgling in the chest, regurgitation of undigested food eaten hours before, nocturnal regurgitation of food and saliva, choking, coughing, bronchitis, pneumonia, tracheal compression, and lung abscess. Postprandial or nocturnal chest pain is reported by one third of patients. It may be so severe as to cause decreased food intake and weight loss, but it tends to improve as the disease progresses. Heartburn may result from bacterial production of lactic acid in the esophagus.

Findings on Diagnostic Testing

Radiographic Studies

Chest radiography may reveal mediastinal widening with an outline of the esophagus, loss of the gastric air bubble, an esophageal air-fluid level, and changes in chronic pulmonary aspiration. Barium swallow radiography is the initial screening test for achalasia and may show impaired contrast transit within a dilated lumen, a loss of peristalsis, impaired LES relaxation, a characteristic tapering of the distal esophagus ("bird's beak"), and, rarely, an esophageal diverticulum proximal to the LES. The presence of mucosal irregularities warrants a search for malignancy.

Upper Gastrointestinal Endoscopy

Upper gastrointestinal endoscopy is necessary to exclude malignancy. Typically, endoscopy reveals esophageal dilation, atony, and erythema, friability, and ulcerations from chronic stasis. Esophagitis caused by an infection with *Candida* organisms is a common finding and should be treated before therapeutic intervention. The LES may be puckered, but passage of the endoscope into the stomach should not be difficult in the absence of malignancy. Careful retroflexion of the endoscope in the gastric fundus is mandatory, and biopsy specimens should be obtained from any suggestive areas.

Esophageal Manometry

The defining manometric features of achalasia are aperistalsis and incomplete LES relaxation (Table 26-1). Some patients exhibit higher amplitude (>60 mm Hg), simultaneous, repetitive esophageal body contractions with swallowing that define the variant known as vigorous achalasia. Incomplete LES relaxation with swallowing is usually (>80% of cases) but not always present in patients with achalasia because early in the course of disease, some patients exhibit complete LES relaxations of very short duration. Additionally, some individuals have only short segments of aperistalsis. Sixty percent of patients have elevated LES pressure (>35 mm Hg). Elevated intraesophageal pressures often are noted but are not required for diagnosis.

TABLE 26-1
Manometric Findings in Achalasia

Absence of peristalsis in esophageal body
Incomplete relaxation of lower esophageal sphincter
  (complete relaxation of short duration may be seen in early achalasia)
Elevated resting pressure of lower esophageal sphincter (common, not required)
Elevated intraesophageal pressure relative to gastric pressures (common, not required)

Scintigraphic Studies

Esophageal scintigraphic emptying studies may show retention of a semisolid meal but are rarely useful in the initial diagnosis of achalasia. Scintigraphy is sometimes performed after therapy to assess reductions in esophageal retention.

Management and Course

Achalasia is not curable, and no treatment can restore normal esophageal body peristalsis or complete LES relaxation. Treatment therefore rests with measures to reduce LES pressure sufficiently to enhance gravity-assisted esophageal emptying. The most feared complication of achalasia is squamous cell carcinoma, which results from chronic stasis and occurs in 2% to 7% of patients, usually those who have had unsatisfactory treatment or no treatment.

Medication Therapy

Nitrates and calcium channel antagonists are the most common medical therapies for achalasia. Sublingual isosorbide dinitrate reduces LES pressures by 66% for 90 minutes; however, no placebo-controlled trials have assessed the efficacy of this agent. Sublingual nifedipine lowers LES pressure by 30% to 40%, and a placebo-controlled study showed good to excellent clinical responses in 70% of patients in one study but lower responses in other studies. Sildenafil is another smooth muscle relaxant that transiently decreases LES pressure in achalasia. Medication therapy has significant limitations, such as duration of action and tachyphylaxis. However, elderly patients, patients who refuse more invasive therapy, patients who cannot give consent, and patients with very mild symptoms may benefit from these relaxant drugs.

Injection Therapy

Botulinum toxin, a potent inhibitor of neural acetylcholine release, reduces LES pressure and relieves symptoms for up to 6 months in patients with achalasia when directly injected into the LES during endoscopy. Because of incomplete symptom control and the requirements for costly repeat injections, botulinum toxin is best reserved for elderly or frail patients who are poor risks for more definitive therapy.

Pneumatic Dilation

Standard bougienage with a maximum dilator (20 mm) usually produces only transient symptomatic relief. In contrast, pneumatic dilation to >3 cm that forcefully disrupts the LES circular muscle produces long-lasting reductions in LES pressure. Most clinicians use preprocedure sedation despite the concerns about medication-induced LES relaxation minimizing the efficacy of dilation. Balloons are inflated for several seconds to 5 minutes at pressures ranging from 360 to 775 mm Hg, which produce responses in 32% to 98% of cases. A postdilation LES pressure of less than 10 mm Hg predicts a 100% remission rate at 2 years. Approximately 20% to 40% of patients require further dilation several years later. The most common complication of pneumatic dilation is perforation (1%–5% of cases). Some clinicians obtain a water-soluble radiographic swallow film followed by barium swallow radiography (if no perforation is detected) before sending the patient home. Postprocedure gastroesophageal reflux is rare. Epiphrenic diverticula and large hiatal hernias are considered relative contraindications to pneumatic dilation. Patients younger than 18 years usually respond better to surgery than to dilation.

Surgery
Surgical therapy of achalasia usually involves a longitudinal incision of the muscle layers from several centimeters above the LES to 1 cm below (i.e., Heller myotomy). Patients with vigorous achalasia may require more extended myotomy. Good to excellent responses to myotomy occur in 62% to 100% of patients. Thoracoscopic and laparoscopic procedures are associated with similar benefits and less morbidity than open approaches. Symptomatic gastroesophageal reflux may occur in 10% of cases, which may be further complicated by strictures, Barrett esophagus, and adenocarcinoma. Rarely, refractory cases mandate more aggressive operations, including esophageal resection with gastric pull-up or colonic interposition.

SPASTIC MOTOR DISORDERS OF THE DISTAL ESOPHAGUS

Incidence and Epidemiology

Disorders of spastic esophageal motor activity have been characterized in patients with noncardiac chest pain. The apparent prevalence is approximately 1 per 100,000 of population. Despite extensive literature on these disorders, it remains uncertain if these conditions have clinical significance. The heterogeneity among patients, the absence of specific pathological features, and the paucity of well-defined clinical implications caution against considering them akin to achalasia. Patients with spastic disorders present at any age with a mean age of onset of 40 years. A predominance of female patients is characteristic of most studies.

Specific spastic disorders of the esophagus have been characterized on the basis of manometric criteria (Table 26-2). The required manometric feature of diffuse esophageal spasm (DES) is the presence of simultaneous esophageal body contractions with greater than 30% of water swallows. Other findings that may be present include repetitive or prolonged contractions, high-amplitude contractions (>180 mm Hg), spontaneous contractions, and rarely incomplete LES relaxation. Other conditions that produce similar findings include diabetic neuropathy, rheumatologic disease, alcoholism, and pseudoobstruction. Some cases of DES progress to achalasia, suggesting that these disorders represent a spectrum of a single encompassing disease in some patients. Nutcracker esophagus, characterized by high-amplitude (>180 mm Hg) peristaltic contractions of prolonged duration (>6 seconds), is found in 27% to 48% of patients with noncardiac chest pain. However, the relevance of these manometric findings is questionable because they correlate poorly with symptoms and clinical responses to therapy. Hypertensive LES is defined by a pressure higher than 45 mm Hg with normal relaxation and esophageal body peristalsis. Radiographic and scintigraphic transit tests usually show no delay in bolus passage into the stomach, raising questions about the importance of

TABLE 26-2
Manometric Criteria for Spastic Esophageal Motor Disorders

Disorder	Required Findings	Associated Findings
Diffuse esophageal spasm	Simultaneous contractions with >30% of water swallows	Repetitive contractions Prolonged contractions High-amplitude contractions Spontaneous relaxations Incomplete LES relaxation Increased LES pressure
Nutcracker esophagus	High-amplitude contractions (>180 mm Hg on average)	Repetitive contractions Prolonged contractions Increased LES pressure
Hypertensive LES	Increased LES pressure (>40 mm Hg) Normal LES relaxation	
Nonspecific esophageal motor disorder	Findings insufficient for other diagnoses	Frequent aperistaltic contractions Retrograde contractions Repetitive contractions Low-amplitude contractions Prolonged contractions High-amplitude contractions Spontaneous relaxations Incomplete LES relaxation

this condition. Nonspecific esophageal motor disorders do not satisfy manometric criteria for any other condition and are of uncertain relevance. Manometric findings include frequent simultaneous contractions, retrograde contractions, low-amplitude contractions, prolonged contractions, and isolated incomplete LES relaxation.

Etiology and Pathogenesis

Spastic motor disorders of the esophagus rarely require surgery; so very little tissue is available for pathological evaluation. Most striking is the thickening of the lower esophageal muscle (≤2 cm) that is seen in some patients with DES. In contrast to achalasia, the loss of ganglion cells has not been demonstrated in the spastic disorders, although changes in vagus nerve integrity are found in DES. Other physiological studies suggest that a selective, intermittent impairment of esophageal myenteric plexus inhibitory interneuronal function is present in DES. Additionally, some patients with spastic disorders exhibit enhanced esophageal motor responses to cholinergic agonists, edrophonium, and ergonovine, which suggests dysfunction of excitatory neurons as well. A role for central nervous system dysfunction has been suggested by the demonstration of simultaneous, repetitive esophageal contractions with stress. In addition to these motor events, patients with noncardiac chest pain of esophageal origin may exhibit hypersensitivity to esophageal distention or acid perfusion, suggesting a pathogenic afferent neural defect.

Clinical Features

The major symptoms of spastic disorders are dysphagia and chest pain. Intermittent dysphagia for solids and liquids is present in 30% to 60% of patients with spastic disorders and may be exacerbated by large boluses of food, medications, or foods of extreme temperatures. Dysphagia is usually not severe enough to produce weight loss. Intermittent substernal chest discomfort with radiation to the back, neck, jaw, or arms lasting minutes to hours is reported by 80% to 90% of patients. Among patients with chest pain, there is a high prevalence of psychiatric illness (anxiety, depression) and irritable bowel syndrome. Features that suggest an esophageal rather than a cardiac cause include pain that is nonexertional, continues for hours, interrupts sleep, is meal related, and is relieved by antacids. Associated heartburn (20% of cases), dysphagia, or regurgitation may favor an esophageal cause. Heartburn may not reflect excessive acid reflux into the esophagus, but rather may result from hypersensitivity to normal amounts of esophageal acid.

Findings on Diagnostic Testing

Endoscopic and Radiographic Studies

Upper endoscopy is useful in evaluating patients with dysphagia or suspected esophageal pain to exclude structural lesions or esophagitis. Barium swallow radiography may define corkscrew esophagus, rosary bead esophagus, pseudodiverticula, or curling in some patients with DES. "Bird's beak" deformities are not observed.

Manometry and 24-Hour pH Monitoring

The manometric characteristics of each spastic disorder are described in *Incidence and Epidemiology*. Typically, abnormal motor events are intermittent and may not be associated with symptoms. In unequivocal cases, nonperistaltic, high-amplitude, prolonged contractions seen during esophageal manometry are associated with the patient's report of chest pain. These unequivocal cases probably result from a myenteric neuronal defect that places the affected individuals along the continuum of vigorous achalasia and achalasia. Nevertheless, current practice guidelines do not support pursuing these findings in evaluating most patients with unexplained chest pain. In one large study combining 24-hour pH monitoring of the esophagus, 43% of patients had chest pain associated with episodes of acid reflux, whereas manometry provided little diagnostic yield. Thus, pH testing is probably the most useful functional test in patients with unexplained chest pain of presumed esophageal origin.

Other Studies

Abnormal peristalsis and delayed transit may be detected by scintigraphic evaluation, especially in DES, although similar findings are noted in radiographic evaluation. False-negative results on studies are obtained with intermittent spastic disorders or disorders with preserved peristalsis (e.g., nutcracker esophagus). Esophageal balloon distention produces chest pain in 60% of patients, but in only 20% of controls. This technique may also induce dysphagia.

Management and Course

Spastic motor disorders of the esophagus are not life-threatening or progressive (in most cases). Treatment should attempt to reduce symptoms without exposing the patient to potential therapeutic complications. If symptoms suggest gastroesophageal acid reflux, structural testing, 24-hour pH monitoring, or aggressive antireflux treatment with proton pump inhibitors should be used. If reflux is not a consideration, the most important step is to reassure the patient that there is no serious heart condition or other disease. When reassurance fails, medical, mechanical, and surgical treatment options are available. Behavioral modification and biofeedback have shown some efficacy in selected refractory cases.

Medications
Small trials suggest that some DES patients experience relief with smooth muscle relaxants such as nitrates, calcium channel blockers, and hydralazine. One double-blind, placebo-controlled trial of the antidepressant trazodone reported improvements in global well-being as well as esophageal symptoms, possibly secondary to effects on visceral pain perception. Botulinum toxin injected at the gastroesophageal junction reduced symptoms in one investigation of patients with nonachalasic esophageal spasm.

Mechanical Dilation
Therapeutic bougienage probably does not produce symptomatic benefits greater than sham dilation. However, pneumatic dilation has reduced symptoms in some patients with DES and hypertensive LES, especially if dysphagia is prominent.

Surgery
For patients with dysphagia or intractable pain caused by spastic motor esophageal dysfunction, a Heller myotomy to include the LES and the spastic portions of the esophageal body may reduce symptoms in more than 50% of cases. However, the risk of the procedure coupled with the uncertain therapeutic response mandates a cautious approach to surgery.

ESOPHAGEAL MOTILITY DISORDERS ASSOCIATED WITH SYSTEMIC DISEASES

Scleroderma

The esophagus is involved in 75% to 85% of patients with scleroderma, regardless of whether the diffuse or CREST (calcinosis, Raynaud phenomenon, esophageal dysfunction, sclerodactyly, telangiectasia) variants are present. Scleroderma produces smooth muscle atrophy and fibrosis that leads to absent distal esophageal contractions and LES incompetence. Clinically, patients present with dysphagia and heartburn. Symptomatic individuals usually have Raynaud phenomenon. Erosive or ulcerative esophagitis may be present in 60% of cases, with some progression to Barrett esophagus and adenocarcinoma. Dysphagia results from dysmotility, peptic stricture, or *Candida* esophagitis. Barium swallow radiography shows a dilated, aperistaltic esophagus with marked gastroesophageal reflux and delayed esophageal clearance if the patient is supine. Wide-mouth esophageal diverticula may also be present. Manometry shows low to absent LES pressure, weak or absent distal peristalsis, and normal proximal esophageal peristalsis. Gastroesophageal reflux is aggressively treated with proton pump inhibitors. Frequent bougienage may be necessary for peptic strictures. If antireflux surgery is contemplated for intractable esophagitis, loose 270-degree fundoplications are necessary to minimize postoperative dysphagia.

Other Connective Tissue Diseases

Up to 35% of patients with systemic lupus erythematosus have esophageal manometric abnormalities (DES, reduced peristalsis and LES pressure), although symptoms are rare. Thirty percent of patients with rheumatoid arthritis exhibit minimal decreases in peristaltic amplitude. One half of patients with Sjögren syndrome report dysphagia, which usually results from diminished lacrimal and salivary secretions. Mixed connective tissue disease combines features of scleroderma, polymyositis, and systemic lupus erythematosus and is suggested by high titers of antibodies to nuclear ribonucleoprotein antigen. More than 60% of patients have esophageal involvement, including aperistalsis and reduced UES and LES pressures.

Other Disorders

More than 60% of diabetics with neuropathy exhibit disordered esophageal motility from autonomic degeneration, but most patients are asymptomatic. Manometric findings in diabetes include decreased peristaltic amplitude, reduced LES pressure with incomplete relaxation, double-peaked waves, and simultaneous and repetitive contractions. Graves disease produces acceleration of esophageal peristalsis, whereas thyrotoxic myopathy may present with DES. Dysphagia in patients with myxedema may result from decreased peristaltic amplitude and velocity and incomplete LES relaxation. Amyloidosis produces decreased LES pressure, reduced peristaltic amplitude, simultaneous contractions, or an achalasia-like pattern in 60% of patients, which may produce dysphagia. Acute ethanol ingestion reduces the amplitude of peristaltic contractions, lowers LES tone, and induces simultaneous contractions. Chronic alcoholics with neuropathy exhibit increased simultaneous contractions and reductions in primary and secondary peristalsis. Ethanol withdrawal produces LES hypertension and increases peristaltic amplitude. Advancing age may slightly decrease peristaltic amplitude but has no other specific effects on esophageal motor function.

CHAPTER 27

Reflux Esophagitis and Esophageal Infections

GASTROESOPHAGEAL REFLUX DISEASE

Incidence and Epidemiology

The passage of gastric contents retrograde into the esophagus is a normal physiological event. The development of symptoms, signs, or complications of this process is termed *gastroesophageal reflux disease* (GERD). In addition to the esophagus, other structures affected by GERD include the pharynx, larynx, and respiratory tract. A minority of patients with GERD have *reflux esophagitis*, a term used to describe mucosal damage and inflammation. GERD is extremely common and is reported at least once monthly by about 44% of adult Americans. Furthermore, 20% report weekly heartburn, and nearly 7% have erosive esophagitis. There is significant geographic variation in the worldwide prevalence of GERD. Rates are low in Africa and Asia. The prevalence is equal among men and women, but there is a male predominance for complications such as esophagitis and Barrett esophagus. Among patients with GERD, 5% present with ulceration, 4% to 20% with strictures, and 5% to 15% with Barrett esophagus. It is unclear whether one form of GERD progresses to another; alternatively, a spectrum of disease severity may exist within each form, with little crossover between erosive esophagitis, nonerosive disease, and Barrett esophagus. The opposing time trends of peptic ulcer and GERD in the United States suggest that *Helicobacter pylori* has had a protective effect against the development of GERD, and the increasing prevalence of GERD may reflect decreasing rates of chronic infection with *H pylori*.

Etiology and Pathogenesis

Factors associated with the development of GERD include the potency of the refluxate, anti-reflux barriers, lumenal acid clearance, esophageal tissue resistance, and gastric emptying.

Potency of the Refluxate

Gastric contents that contribute to the potency of the refluxate include hydrochloric acid, pepsin, bile salts, and pancreatic enzymes. Mucosal damage is increased if the pH of the refluxate is less than 2 or if pepsin or conjugated bile salts are present. Most patients with GERD secrete normal amounts of gastric acid. However, acid seems to be necessary to produce tissue injury in these patients because pepsin and bile salts are innocuous at neutral pH. Conversely, in patients with Zollinger-Ellison syndrome, increased acid production contributes to the development of esophagitis.

Antireflux Barriers

Anatomic barriers to reflux of gastric contents include the lower esophageal sphincter (LES), the intra-abdominal segment of the esophagus, the diaphragmatic crura, the phrenoesophageal ligament, the mucosal rosette, and the angle of His. The high-pressure barrier is provided mainly by the LES; however, the crura are important during coughing, sneezing, and bending. LES pressure may be affected by a variety of drugs (Table 27-1). A certain amount of physiological gastroesophageal reflux occurs by transient LES relaxations (TLESRs), which increase after a meal to permit venting gas from the stomach. In patients with GERD, there may be spontaneous reflux associated with increased TLESRs, reductions in LES pressure that permit retrograde reflux during increases in intra-abdominal pressure, or free reflux with an incompetent LES. The mechanisms of increased TLESRs in patients with GERD are unknown, although a small subset exhibits delayed gastric emptying with gastric distention. Increases in gastric distention with hypersecretory conditions such as Zollinger-Ellison syndrome may increase TLESRs and exacerbate acid-induced esophageal damage. LES pressures may be reduced in pregnancy, diabetes, and scleroderma. The role of hiatal hernias is controversial; although most patients with GERD have hiatal hernias, only a few patients with hiatal hernias have significant GERD.

TABLE 27-1
Substances that Modulate Lower Esophageal Sphincter Pressure

	Increase Pressure	Decrease Pressure
Hormones	Gastrin Motilin Substance P	Secretin Cholecystokinin Somatostatin Vasoactive intestinal polypeptide
Neural Agents	α-Adrenergic agonists β-Adrenergic antagonists Cholinergic agonists	α-Adrenergic antagonists β-Adrenergic agonists Cholinergic antagonists
Foods	Protein	Fat Chocolate Peppermint
Miscellaneous	Histamine Antacids Metoclopramide Domperidone Prostaglandin $F_{2(\alpha)}$ Cisapride	Theophylline Prostaglandins E_2 and I_2 Serotonin Meperidine Morphine Dopamine Calcium blockers Diazepam Barbiturates

Lumenal Acid Clearance

Important factors in esophageal lumenal clearance include gravity, peristalsis, and salivary and esophageal bicarbonate secretion. After a reflux episode, the bolus usually is returned to the stomach with one or two swallow-induced peristaltic contractions. The remaining esophageal contents should be neutralized by bicarbonate secreted by the salivary and esophageal glands. The duration, not the frequency, of esophageal acidification correlates best with esophagitis, highlighting the importance of acid clearance mechanisms. Nocturnal reflux has the greatest potential for esophageal damage because most lumenal acid clearance factors are inactive during sleep. Esophagitis itself may lead to peristaltic dysfunction, but it is also possible that primary motility disturbances predispose to GERD and esophageal damage. However, many patients with GERD do not have delayed esophageal transit or abnormal levels of salivary bicarbonate, and defects in contractile activity are minimal. In these patients, tissue resistance factors may be deficient, or the volume of refluxate may overwhelm the protective mechanisms of the esophagus.

Tissue Resistance

In healthy individuals, the esophageal mucosa is in contact with acid for about 1 to 2 hours per day. In contrast to the stomach and duodenum, the esophagus does not secrete a protective mucous layer and maintains only a minimal lumen-to-cell H^+ gradient. Protective structural components include cell membranes and intercellular junctions that limit H^+ diffusion into the esophageal tissue. Esophageal cells can buffer and extrude H^+ by the actions of intracellular phosphate and proteins, bicarbonate production by carbonic anhydrase, and ionic transporters that exchange intracellular H^+ and Cl^- for extracellular Na^+ and bicarbonate. Esophageal blood flow delivers oxygen, nutrients, and bicarbonate and removes H^+ and carbon dioxide in a dynamic fashion. The strongest evidence for defective tissue resistance factors comes from studies in which large subsets of patients with esophagitis showed no increase in esophageal acid contact time. Smoking and alcohol impair LES function and acid clearance. Nicotine inhibits sodium transport across the esophageal epithelium, whereas ethanol and aspirin increase the permeability to H^+.

Delayed Gastric Emptying

The importance of delayed gastric emptying in the development of GERD is controversial. Although early studies showed a delay in solid emptying in 50% of patients with GERD, more recent studies have reported only 6% to 38% prevalence of delayed gastric emptying.

Clinical Features

The most common symptom of GERD is heartburn, which is described as substernal burning that moves orad from the xiphoid. Heartburn generally occurs after meals and may be relieved by acid-neutralizing agents. The frequency and severity of heartburn correlate poorly with endoscopically defined esophagitis. Patients with GERD may also present with substernal chest discomfort that mimics cardiac-related angina pectoris. Studies that complicate this clinical picture show that acid regurgitation decreases coronary blood flow, thus increasing the risk of cardiac ischemia. Regurgitation of bitter or acid-tasting liquid is common. Water brash is the spontaneous appearance of salty fluid in the mouth from reflex salivary secretion in response to esophageal acid. Solid-food dysphagia in a patient with GERD may be caused by either peptic strictures or adenocarcinoma from Barrett metaplasia. Note that odynophagia is not a common symptom associated with erosive esophagitis.

Extraesophageal manifestations of GERD include otolaryngological and pulmonary complications. Acid damage to the oropharynx may produce sore throat, earache, gingivitis, poor dentition, and globus, whereas reflux damage to the larynx and respiratory tract causes hoarseness, wheezing, bronchitis, asthma, and pneumonia. Vagally mediated bronchospasm may be initiated by acidification of the esophagus alone; thus, tracheal penetration by the refluxate is not required for the development of asthma with GERD. Shared risk factors (e.g., tobacco smoking) also may increase the association of GERD and pulmonary disease.

Findings on Diagnostic Testing

A history of classic heartburn is sufficient for diagnosing GERD and provides an adequate rationale for initiating therapy. The proton pump inhibitor (PPI) test, which evaluates symptom response to proton pump inhibition, is likewise as sensitive and specific as more invasive tests for diagnosing GERD. Diagnostic studies should be considered for patients with atypical symptoms, symptoms unresponsive to therapy, or warning signs of GERD complications or malignancy (e.g., dysphagia, odynophagia, hematemesis, guaiac-positive stool, and anemia) (Table 27-2).

Radiographic Studies

If careful double-contrast techniques are used, barium swallow or upper gastrointestinal radiography can identify ulcers, strictures, and hiatal hernias. Although barium radiography may show free gastroesophageal reflux of the contrast agent, this finding has high specificity but low sensitivity for diagnosing GERD.

TABLE 27-2
Tests for Assessing Gastroesophageal Reflux

Tests for the presence of reflux
    Barium swallow radiography
    Acid reflux testing
    Esophageal pH monitoring
    Radionuclide ^{99m}Tc scintigraphy
    Esophageal impedance testing

Tests for assessing symptoms
    Bernstein acid perfusion test
    Esophageal pH monitoring
    Empiric trial of acid-suppressive medications

Tests for assessing esophageal damage
    Barium swallow radiography
    Upper gastrointestinal endoscopy with or without biopsy
    Esophageal potential difference measurement

Tests for assessing disease pathogenesis
    Acid clearance test
    Radionuclide ^{99m}Tc scintigraphy
    Esophageal manometry
    Gastric acid secretory studies

Upper Gastrointestinal Endoscopy

Upper gastrointestinal endoscopy is used to document reflux-induced mucosal injury and complications of GERD. Endoscopic findings in patients with GERD include normal mucosa, erythema, edema, friability, exudate, erosions, ulcers, strictures, and Barrett metaplasia. Histological hallmarks of esophagitis are increased height of the esophageal papillae and basal cell hyperplasia. Acute injury to the vascular bed, edema, and neutrophilic (and sometimes eosinophilic) infiltration indicate esophageal damage. Chronic inflammation is characterized by the presence of macrophages and granulation tissue. With severe injury, fibroblasts may deposit enough collagen to form a stricture. Long-standing acid damage also promotes aberrant repair of the mucosa by specialized columnar epithelium that contains goblet cells (i.e., Barrett metaplasia).

Scintigraphic Studies

Scintigraphy with ^{99m}Tc–sulfur colloid may provide complementary information in evaluating a patient with GERD. Gastroesophageal reflux may be detected by scanning the esophagus after instilling a tracer in the stomach; this procedure has a specificity of 90% and a sensitivity of 14% to 90%. Clearance of a swallowed tracer can estimate esophageal clearance of acid.

Esophageal Manometry

Esophageal manometry generally is reserved for patients being considered for surgery. Although GERD may be considered a condition of disordered motility, 30% to 50% of GERD patients have normal LES pressures (10 to 30 mm Hg). Manometric assessment of esophageal body peristalsis also is important preoperatively because documentation of abnormal peristalsis may influence the type of antireflux surgery chosen.

Provocative Tests

Provocative tests are sometimes requested as part of a manometric examination to establish the diagnosis of GERD. The *acid reflux test* involves measuring the esophageal pH 5 cm above the LES in the basal state after straight leg raising during a Valsalva and Muller maneuver and during abdominal compression. If these maneuvers do not produce a pH less than 4, testing is repeated after gastric perfusion of 300 mL of 0.1 N hydrochloric acid. Acid reflux testing has a sensitivity of 54% to 100% and a specificity of 70% to 95%. The *Bernstein test* determines whether symptoms are reproduced with esophageal acidification. It has a sensitivity of 7% to 27% and a specificity of 83% to 94% for diagnosing GERD. Initially, normal saline is infused into the middle esophagus for 5 to 15 minutes followed by infusion of 0.1 N hydrochloric acid. If symptoms are reproduced within 30 minutes of acid infusion, saline is reinfused to relieve symptoms and symptoms are again provoked by acid delivery. The appearance of symptoms with acid infusion in a patient who is blinded to the infusion sequence constitutes a positive test result. Complete symptom relief by saline infusion is not essential.

Ambulatory Esophageal pH Monitoring

Traditionally, continuous 24-hour pH monitoring is performed with a nasally inserted pH probe positioned 5 cm above the LES. The patient is given an event marker to use with a recording device that is triggered to correlate symptoms with changes in esophageal pH. Maximal sensitivity (93%) and specificity (93%) are obtained by quantitating the percentage of time during which the pH is less than 4, using threshold values of 10.5% in the upright position and 6% in the supine position. Esophageal pH monitoring also can be used to correlate atypical symptoms, such as chest pain with acid reflux. More recently, it has been possible to conduct ambulatory esophageal pH monitoring without the inconvenience and discomfort of transnasal catheters by using miniature probes attached to the esophageal mucosa that transmit a wireless signal to a receiver worn by the patient. This system affords the ability to study the patient under conditions of more normal eating and physical activity, and to record esophageal pH over several days.

Miscellaneous Tests

Intralumenal electrical impedance is a technique that measures the conductance of the esophageal contents. This test relies on the electrical properties of liquids (low impedance and high conductance) and gases (high impedance and low conductance) to differentiate between liquid and gas reflux (belching). More importantly, impedance allows detecting nonacidic reflux that would otherwise not be detectable by esophageal pH monitoring. This method permits characterizing esophageal reflux as either acid or nonacid in content. The electrical potential difference of squamous epithelium differs from that of columnar epithelium; thus impedance testing can be used to detect Barrett metaplasia in research settings. Tests of gastric secretory function may be performed in a patient who fails to respond to acid-suppressive drugs to exclude acid hypersecretion from conditions such as Zollinger-Ellison syndrome.

Management and Course

The course of GERD is highly variable; most patients require medical therapy continuously, but some respond to intermittent or on-demand strategies of medication and can discontinue medical therapy altogether. In patients with documented healing of erosive esophagitis over a 6.5-year follow-up period, 7.7% were subsequently diagnosed with Barrett esophagus, 2.5% developed strictures, and 2.2% developed ulcers.

Lifestyle Modification

The modification of lifestyle is an integral part of initially managing GERD (Table 27-3). The head of the bed should be elevated to enhance nocturnal esophageal acid clearance. Smoking and alcohol, which have deleterious effects on LES pressure, acid clearance, and epithelial function, should be avoided. Reducing meal size and limiting the intake of fat, carminatives, and chocolate limit gastric distention, lower TLESR incidence, and prevent LES pressure reductions. Caffeinated and decaffeinated coffee, tea, and carbonated beverages should be avoided because they stimulate acid production. Tomato juice and citrus products may exacerbate symptoms because of osmotic effects. Medications that reduce LES pressure should be limited whenever possible (e.g., anticholinergics, theophylline, diazepam, opiates, calcium channel antagonists, β-adrenergic agonists, α-adrenergic antagonists, and progesterone).

TABLE 27-3
Lifestyle Modifications for Patients with Gastroesophageal Reflux

---

Elevate the head of the bed 6 in.

Stop smoking

Stop excessive ethanol consumption

Reduce dietary fat

Reduce meal size

Avoid bedtime snacks

Reduce weight (if overweight)

Avoid specific foods
Chocolate
Carminatives (e.g., spearmint, peppermint)
Coffee (caffeinated, decaffeinated)
Tea
Cola beverages
Tomato juice
Citrus fruit juices

Avoid specific medications (if possible)
Anticholinergics
Theophylline
Benzodiazepines
Opiates
Calcium channel antagonists
β-Adrenergic agonists
Progesterone (some contraceptives)
α-Adrenergic antagonists

Medication Therapy

Antacids provide rapid, safe, and effective relief from GERD symptoms. High-dose regimens may heal erosive disease; however, the required doses often induce significant side effects (e.g., diarrhea with magnesium antacids and constipation with aluminum antacids) that make compliance difficult. Low-sodium antacids (e.g., magaldrate [Riopan]) are preferable for patients on salt-restricted diets. Gaviscon (aluminum hydroxide and magnesium carbonate), an antacid-alginate combination, decreases reflux by producing a viscous mechanical barrier, but it may also adversely affect bowel function. Sucralfate, the basic salt of aluminum hydroxide and sucrose octasulfate, acts topically to increase tissue resistance, buffer acid, and to bind pepsin and bile salts, but its efficacy in treating patients with GERD is limited.

H_2 receptor antagonists (e.g., cimetidine, ranitidine, famotidine, and nizatidine) are safe and effective for treating mild to moderate disease. Mild GERD can be treated with over-the-counter H_2 receptor antagonists, but they must often be given in doses double those used to treat duodenal ulcer. For erosive esophagitis, H_2 receptor antagonists are only marginally better than placebo, and when dose reduction is attempted, relapse is common. PPIs (e.g., omeprazole, lansoprazole, rabeprazole, pantoprazole and esomeprazole) are the drugs of choice for endoscopically proven erosive esophagitis and symptomatic GERD refractory to H_2 receptor antagonists. These agents, which are H^+,K^+-adenosine triphosphatase antagonists, produce superior acid suppression compared with H_2 receptor antagonists. There were initial concerns about the long-term safety of PPIs, because they produced twofold to fourfold increases in serum gastrin, which led to the development of enterochromaffin tumors (i.e., carcinoids in experimental animals). Other considerations included the promotion of bacterial colonization of the upper gut and the induction of certain hepatic and small intestine cytochrome P450 enzymes. However, long-term studies have not demonstrated significant adverse sequelae after several years of use and consequently, the Food and Drug Administration has approved chronic use of PPIs.

Prokinetic agents have been used as primary therapy or as adjunctive agents for patients with GERD. Cisapride, an agent that acts on serotonin 5-HT$_4$ receptors to facilitate myenteric acetylcholine release, promotes gastric emptying and increases LES pressure and was approved for treating GERD. However, cisapride has been withdrawn from the market because of increased risk of cardiac arrythmias. Metoclopramide and bethanechol have limited efficacy for patients with GERD.

Treatment Strategy

Most patients with heartburn self-medicate with over-the-counter antacids, H_2 receptor antagonists, or PPIs. Those who do not respond to therapy or those who initially respond but relapse may seek medical attention. In such individuals, the clinician should exclude the causes of heartburn, including functional dyspepsia, functional heartburn, and malignancy. The first step is to determine the presence of "alarm" symptoms or signs such as bleeding, anemia, dysphagia, or weight loss that may suggest the presence of upper gastrointestinal malignancy. Upper endoscopy is indicated if any of these factors is present. In the absence of alarm features, it is important to ensure that an adequate trial of acid suppression has been attempted because most other disorders respond variably to acid suppression. PPIs are the most potent class of medications to treat GERD; therefore, the use of these drugs is advocated. PPIs reduce symptoms of GERD most effectively if taken 30 to 60 minutes before ingesting a meal. Failure to respond to PPI therapy is an indication for upper endoscopy. Dyspepsia (discomfort in the upper abdomen) without heartburn or acid regurgitation should be managed differently from GERD and generally requires upper gastrointestinal endoscopy to examine the disorders under this differential diagnosis. Patients with heartburn or acid regurgitation (with or without accompanying dyspepsia) may be further evaluated using a PPI test in which double or triple dose medication is used to assess symptom response. If symptoms are not relieved, ambulatory esophageal pH monitoring may differentiate between those individuals with persistent acid reflux (requiring higher doses of acid suppression) and those without abnormal esophageal acid exposure. The latter group comprises patients with nonacid reflux, which can be diagnosed by esophageal impedance testing, and patients who have functional heartburn. Baclofen may be a reasonable therapy for nonacid reflux, whereas therapy aimed at decreasing esophageal sensation may be useful for functional heartburn (e.g., trazodone, tricyclics).

Surgical Treatment

The indications for antireflux surgery have narrowed. Failure of medical therapy is not a reason for referral to surgery because the outcome of surgical treatment in this group is poor. Patients who respond to medication, but wish to consider surgical intervention to avoid drugs, should be counseled about the high rate of relapse requiring reinstitution of drugs after surgery. Appropriate candidates include patients intolerant or allergic to medical therapy and patients with symptoms associated with nonacid reflux. The Nissen (360-degree wrap) and Belsey (270-degree wrap) fundoplications and the Hill gastropexy produce an initial 85% success rate in relieving symptoms and healing lesions. Postoperative dysphagia or gas-bloat syndrome (i.e., the inability to belch or vomit) affects 2% to 8%. The operative mortality for these procedures is 1%. Fundoplications reduce hiatal hernias and enhance LES competency, whereas a gastropexy anchors the gastroesophageal junction to the median arcuate ligament. The Belsey procedure is chosen for patients with impaired esophageal peristalsis to reduce the likelihood of postoperative dysphagia. The Hill operation is used for patients with prior gastric resection. The incidence of recurrent symptoms after surgical therapy, whether open or laparoscopic, remains high.

Endoscopic Therapy

Several emerging endoscopic technologies have been approved for treating GERD. Application of radiofrequency energy to the distal esophagus and proximal stomach (Stretta) has been subjected to sham-controlled clinical study. Although this procedure was shown to be associated with symptom control and quality of life parameters superior to those of sham-treated patients, the rate of GERD medication use between groups did not differ. Other endoscopic therapies include endolumenal plication (EndoCinch), full-thickness plication, and injection of a biopolymer into the muscle layer of the distal esophagus (Enteryx). Although nonblinded prospective cohort studies of each of these modalities show promising results, none of the endoscopic therapies has been evaluated to the extent required for widespread use at this time.

Management of GERD Complications

Strictures are characterized by progressive dysphagia over months to years. Although strictures may be defined radiographically, endoscopy is required in all cases to exclude malignancy. Esophageal bougienage dilation may be performed without (Maloney, Hurst) or with (Savary) endoscopic guidance or may be accomplished using balloon dilation.

Barrett esophagus is an acquired condition in which squamous epithelium is replaced by specialized columnar epithelium in response to chronic acid exposure.

The clinical consequence of intestinal metaplasia is that up to 10% of patients with this condition develop esophageal adenocarcinoma. Barrett metaplasia is present in 5% to 15% of patients with GERD who undergo endoscopy. Diagnosis of Barrett esophagus requires endoscopic biopsy directed at mucosa that is endoscopically identified as salmon-colored. If the color distinction is not clear, Lugol solution will preferentially stain the squamous mucosa blue-black. Endoscopic surveillance is currently recommended for patients with Barrett esophagus. Current guidelines indicate endoscopy with biopsy every 3 years for patients who have two consecutive surveillance endoscopies showing no dysplasia. The diagnosis of low-grade dysplasia prompts a shortened surveillance interval of 6 to 12 months. Unifocal high-grade dysplasia should be surveyed every 3 months; multifocal high-grade dysplasia is an indication for futher therapy, which may consist of photodynamic treatment; and appearance of an identifiable lesion associated with high-grade dysplasia may be treated with endoscopic mucosal resection. Currently, esophageal resection is reserved for development of adenocarcinoma.

Hemorrhage may occasionally develop from esophageal erosions and ulcers. It may be chronic, with production of iron-deficiency anemia, or acute. Perforation of an esophageal ulcer is a serious complication that may cause life-threatening mediastinitis.

Gastroesophageal Reflux Disease in Infants and Children

Symptoms of GERD in infants and children include regurgitation, irritability, difficulty feeding, rumination, failure to thrive, apnea, asthma, pneumonia, and near sudden infant death syndrome. Many children with GERD outgrow their disease as a result of LES maturation. Infants should be fed small volumes of thickened formula and given acid-suppressive agents in size-adjusted doses. For intractable symptoms or reflux that has produced severe airway disease, a Nissen fundoplication may be considered.

ALKALINE REFLUX ESOPHAGITIS

Alkaline reflux esophagitis develops from prolonged contact of esophageal epithelium with nonacidic gastric or intestinal contents, usually in patients who have undergone ulcer surgery with vagotomy or, less commonly, in patients with achlorhydria who have not undergone surgery. Factors responsible for mucosal damage include deconjugated bile salts and pancreatic enzymes. Medications that may be effective include bile salt–binding agents (e.g., cholestyramine, colestipol, sucralfate) and mucosal coating agents (e.g., antacids). When medications fail, a Roux-en-Y gastrojejunostomy may divert intestinal contents away from the esophagus. Alternatively, fundoplication may be performed in patients with intact stomachs or adequate gastric remnants.

FUNGAL INFECTIONS OF THE ESOPHAGUS

Etiology and Pathogenesis

Esophageal infections are rare in immunocompetent persons but are common in patients with acquired immunodeficiency syndrome (AIDS) and in organ transplant recipients. Immunocompetent patients who develop esophageal infections usually have impaired esophageal defenses, such as reduced peristalsis, altered flora, or local infection that spreads to the esophagus, as in mediastinal tuberculosis.

The most common esophageal fungal infection is caused by *Candida albicans*, but other *Candida* species (*C tropicalis*, *C parapsilosis*, and *C glabrata*) may also cause infection. These organisms are normal components of oral flora, but they may become pathogenic if the patient is immunosuppressed (e.g., by therapy with corticosteroids or cyclosporine or by the development of hematologic malignancy or AIDS). Grossly, *Candida* may produce esophageal involvement ranging from scattered white plaques to a dense pseudomembrane that consists of fungi, mucosal cells, and fibrin overlying friable, ulcerated mucosa. In severe cases, lumenal narrowing, pseudodiverticula, and fistulae may develop.

Esophageal aspergillosis, histoplasmosis, and blastomycosis are rare. Histoplasmosis and blastomycosis usually spread to the esophagus from paraesophageal lymph nodes. Infection with *Aspergillus* species causes large, deep ulcers, whereas esophageal histoplasmosis and blastomycosis are characterized by focal lesions and abscesses that may produce odynophagia if muscle layers are involved. Complications of these fungal infections include stricture and tracheoesophageal fistula formation.

Clinical Features

Patients with esophageal fungal infections present with dysphagia and odynophagia, which usually are worse with solid foods and may be severe enough to limit oral intake. Oral candidiasis may be associated with esophageal infection in AIDS, whereas chronic mucocutaneous candidiasis may have associated involvement of other mucous membranes, hair, nails, and skin as well as associated adrenal or parathyroid dysfunction. Infections with *Candida* can produce mild blood loss, but life-threatening hemorrhage is rare. Fistulization may lead to pulmonary infection.

Findings on Diagnostic Testing

Radiographic or endoscopic studies may confirm suspected fungal esophageal infection. Barium swallow radiography may reveal a shaggy mucosal appearance, or plaques, pseudomembranes, cobblestoning, nodules, strictures, fistulae, and mucosal bridges. Upper gastrointestinal endoscopy is more sensitive and specific for diagnosing fungal esophageal infection. Brushings of mucosal lesions should be examined immediately after 10% potassium hydroxide is added or after they are fixed in 95% ethanol before permanent staining. Biopsy specimens should be obtained for histological examination. The microscopic appearances of *Candida* and *Aspergillus* species are distinctive, and it usually is not necessary to culture the organism. Because *Histoplasma* organisms usually do not invade the esophageal mucosa, brushings and biopsy specimens may be nondiagnostic. Therefore, bronchoscopy, mediastinoscopy, or surgery may be necessary to characterize this infection.

Management and Course

The clinical picture of a patient with AIDS and oral candidiasis with symptoms of odynophagia and dysphagia may be sufficient to initiate empiric antifungal therapy without embarking on a diagnostic evaluation. Fluconazole and ketoconazole are effective oral imidazole antifungals that alter fungal cell membrane permeability. Ketoconazole is also effective against histoplasmosis and blastomycosis. Doses of ketoconazole may need to be increased to treat infection in patients with reduced gastric acid production, such as occurs with AIDS, use of acid-suppressive medication, post-gastric surgery, or atrophic gastritis. In contrast, fluconazole absorption is not pH dependent. The adverse effects of these agents include nausea, hepatotoxicity, adrenal insufficiency, decreased gonadal steroid production, and inhibition of cyclosporine metabolism. Intravenous miconazole is occasionally used, but it may produce anemia, thrombocytopenia, hyponatremia, hyperlipidemia, anaphylaxis, cardiac arrest, and acute psychosis.

Polyene antibiotics (e.g., nystatin and amphotericin) bind to fungal membrane sterols, causing cell death. Nystatin is useful for oral candidiasis, but it is less effective than imidazoles for esophageal disease. Intravenous amphotericin B is an agent of last resort for treating fungal esophageal infections because of its potential to cause severe side effects (e.g., fever, hypotension, mental status changes, wheezing, renal toxicity, nausea, hypokalemia, hypomagnesemia, and bone marrow suppression). Dose reduction or discontinuation is recommended if serum creatinine levels exceed 3 mg/dL. Amphotericin is the drug of choice for treating systemic aspergillosis and can be used to treat ketoconazole-resistant histoplasmosis and blastomycosis. Flucytosine is a fluorinated pyrimidine that interferes with fungal RNA translation and is frequently given in combination with amphotericin; its side effects include rash, hepatitis, diarrhea, and bone marrow suppression. Flucytosine should not be given alone because fungi develop resistance to this drug.

VIRAL INFECTIONS OF THE ESOPHAGUS

Etiology and Pathogenesis

Herpes simplex virus 1 (HSV-1), cytomegalovirus (CMV), and varicella-zoster virus (VZV) are the main viral causes of infectious esophagitis. HSV-1 occurs most often in patients with immunosuppression, although esophageal involvement in healthy individuals occurs. HSV-1 esophageal infection begins as discrete vesicles, which may combine to form larger hemorrhagic ulcerations. Biopsies of the squamous cells at the edge of the ulcers reveal characteristic multinucleation, ground-glass nuclei, and eosinophilic Cowdry type A inclusions surrounded by halos, with enveloped virions observable by electron microscopy. CMV esophageal infection most commonly complicates the course of AIDS and produces prominent esophageal ulcers, which may be numerous, round or serpiginous, and deep, in some cases reaching the muscularis. Inclusion bodies are seen in the cytoplasm of infected cells. Chicken pox may produce esophageal ulcerations that appear similar to HSV-1 lesions in association with thoracic dermatomal zoster reactivations. These esophageal ulcerations resolve with resolution of the skin lesions.

Clinical Features

HSV-1 esophageal infection produces severe odynophagia. In immunodeficient patients, this esophageal infection can also produce hemorrhage, perforation with tracheoesophageal fistula formation, or disseminate. Immunocompetent persons, however, usually experience only self-limited infection. CMV esophagitis produces either dysphagia or odynophagia and may be associated with involvement of other organ systems.

Findings on Diagnostic Testing

Radiography and endoscopy are used to diagnose viral esophageal infections. In barium swallow radiography, HSV-1 infection appears as focal ulcerations; however, a diffuse, shaggy appearance of the mucosa is common and indistinguishable from that observed in infections with *Candida*. Barium studies of CMV esophagitis reveal vertical linear ulcers with central umbilication. Confirmation of viral esophageal infection requires upper gastrointestinal endoscopy with biopsy. Infection with HSV-1 appears as discrete, punched-out ulcers (0.3 to 2.0 cm in diameter) with raised yellow rims (i.e., volcano ulcer), but may also appear as bullae or diffusely hemorrhagic mucosa. Biopsy specimens and brushings taken from the edges of ulcers reveal multinucleate squamous cells with characteristic Cowdry type A inclusions. Patients with CMV esophagitis present with small (0.3 to 0.5 cm in diameter), longitudinal, or giant ulcers (1.0 to 3.5 cm diameter) in the distal esophagus or polypoid masses. Examination of brushings or biopsy specimens, respectively, may reveal epithelial or endothelial CMV inclusions. Viral cultures of esophageal tissue for HSV-1 and CMV may be performed if the diagnosis is unclear.

Management and Course

Oral viscous lidocaine may be sufficient therapy for HSV-1 esophageal infection in immunocompetent persons. Intravenous acyclovir for 7 to 10 days has been shown to reduce symptoms, shorten viral shedding, and hasten healing in immunocompromised patients. VZV is susceptible to acyclovir, but there are few data regarding its use as therapy for esophagitis. An acyclovir derivative, ganciclovir, has been shown to be effective in treating CMV esophageal infection, but side effects include rash and neutropenia. Foscarnet, a pyrophosphate analog that inhibits viral DNA polymerase and reverse transcriptase, also is efficacious in treating CMV infections, but this drug can cause renal failure, anemia, and heart failure.

MYCOBACTERIAL, BACTERIAL, AND TREPONEMAL INFECTIONS OF THE ESOPHAGUS

Etiology and Pathogenesis

Esophageal tuberculosis (TB) usually affects the middle third of the esophagus. Less commonly, TB pharyngitis or laryngitis may spread to the upper esophagus. Multiple esophageal miliary mucosal granulomas may result from the hematogenous spread of infection. Primary esophageal TB is exceedingly rare.

Bacterial esophageal infection may be caused by gram-positive organisms, including *Streptococcus viridans*, staphylococci, and bacilli. Bacterial infection can occur after esophageal injury from nasogastric tubes, chemotherapy, radiation, or GERD. More rare causes include *Actinomyces israelii*, *Corynebacterium diphtheriae*, and *Lactobacillus acidophilus*. Endoscopic views of the esophagus may appear normal, or they may reveal erythema, plaques, pseudomembranes, blood vessel infiltration, and hemorrhage. Actinomycosis produces granulomatous esophagitis with drainage of sulfur granules from abscess cavities.

Tertiary syphilis of the esophagus produces submucosal gumma, mucosal ulcers, or diffuse inflammation with fibrosis in the upper esophagus. Syphilitic periarteritis is evident from histological examination.

Clinical Features

TB esophagitis causes odynophagia, and patients with strictures will note dysphagia. A history of choking or coughing with meals should suggest possible esophageal fistula formation. In neutropenic patients undergoing chemotherapy, bacterial esophagitis appears as odynophagia or dysphagia and may be associated with fever. Patients with syphilitic esophageal involvement present with dysphagia or with complications of fistulous disease; odynophagia is rare.

Findings on Diagnostic Testing

Upper gastrointestinal endoscopy with biopsy is essential for diagnosing bacterial or mycobacterial esophagitis because radiography is nonspecific. Endoscopic biopsy specimens obtained from around the edges of lesions may show granulomas or acid-fast bacilli on microscopic examination. Specimens should be subjected to a polymerase chain reaction (PCR) test for TB and may be cultured to confirm and determine antimycobacterial sensitivities. With syphilitic involvement, barium swallow radiography may show a long, ulcerated stricture in the upper esophagus. Biopsy may not be helpful in this disorder; therefore, the diagnosis will rest on clinical judgment or on other disease manifestations.

Management and Course

A diagnosis of esophageal TB infection mandates multidrug therapy. If fistulae do not close with medical treatment, surgery may be necessary, including possible colonic interposition. Bougienage may be performed for strictures. Bacterial esophagitis should be treated with appropriate antibiotics if the sensitivities of the infecting organisms are known, or with empirical high-dose penicillin. Penicillin cures esophageal syphilis infection; however, bougienage or surgery may be necessary to treat complicated disease.

CHAPTER 28

Esophageal Tumors

SQUAMOUS CELL CARCINOMA

Incidence and Epidemiology

Squamous cell carcinoma (SCC) is the most common malignant tumor of the esophagus worldwide. The geographic variation in the prevalence of SCC between and within countries shows the importance of environmental factors in its pathogenesis. Most notably, portions of Iran, China, and the former Soviet Union have exceptionally high rates, with as much as a 500-fold difference in incidence between regions of high and low risk.

In the United States, African Americans have a fivefold increased risk for SCC relative to whites: the annual rate for African American males is 15 per 100,000 compared to 3 per 100,000 for white males. Men have a threefold higher risk than women. The higher incidence in some ethnic groups may be linked to environmental and socioeconomic factors.

Etiology and Pathogenesis

Environmental risk factors have been clearly linked to the development of esophageal SCC. Alcohol and tobacco consumption increase the risk for SCC in a dose-dependent manner. This effect appears to be additive because the risk for patients who smoke and drink excessively is much higher than the risk for patients who use either substance alone. Deficiencies of vitamins A, C, E and B_{12}, folic acid, and riboflavin are risk factors for cancer. Populations that consume large quantities of green and yellow vegetables rich in beta-carotene and vitamin C are protected from the development of esophageal SCC. Trace elements, including selenium, molybdenum, and zinc, also protect against esophageal SCC.

Other risk factors for esophageal SCC have been elucidated. Achalasia is associated with a 10-fold to 30-fold increase in the rate of SCC, which can develop 17 to 20 years after the initial symptoms of achalasia. Synchronous or metachronous esophageal SCC develops at an annual rate of 3% to 7% in patients with SCC of the head and neck. Tylosis, a rare autosomal dominant condition characterized by hyperkeratosis of the palms and soles, is highly linked with esophageal SCC; 50% of patients will develop cancer by age 45 and 95% by age 65. Lye ingestion that causes an esophageal stricture has been associated with development of squamous cell tumors several decades after the exposure. Other factors associated with esophageal SCC include ionizing radiation, celiac sprue, human papillomavirus, Plummer-Vinson syndrome, esophageal diverticula, and drinking hot maté.

Clinical Features

Patients with esophageal SCC present with progressive dysphagia. Odynophagia and weight loss may occur, as well as nausea, vomiting, hematemesis, and back pain. Involvement of adjacent mediastinal strictures may be indicated by a chronic cough caused by a tracheoesophageal fistula, hoarseness caused by recurrent laryngeal nerve involvement, and, rarely, exsanguination due to invasion into the aorta.

A generalized loss of muscle mass and subcutaneous fat is often evident. In patients with early disease, the physical examination findings may be normal, but patients with metastatic disease may exhibit hepatomegaly, bony pain, and supraclavicular adenopathy.

Findings on Diagnostic Testing

Radiographic Studies

The diagnostic evaluation of patients with dysphagia should begin with esophageal imaging. Barium swallow radiography is very sensitive in detecting cancers large enough to cause symptoms, but its sensitivity for detecting early lesions is only 75%, which limits its usefulness as a screening test for patients at high risk. Fluoroscopic examination can often detect motility abnormalities or proximal diverticula that may not be appreciated in endoscopic studies. Because some malignancies produce a smooth symmetric stricture, barium radiographs cannot reliably distinguish tumors from benign peptic strictures.

Endoscopic Studies

Diagnostic confirmation of esophageal SCC requires upper gastrointestinal endoscopy. Early cancers can be detected as elevated plaques or small erythematous erosions. All mucosal abnormalities should undergo brushing and biopsy for cytological and histological examination, respectively. The sensitivity of biopsy alone is 70% to 90%, and by adding cytological examination, nearly all cancers are detected. Because a sampling error occasionally leads to false-negative biopsy and cytologic results, any lesion that highly suggests malignancy should be rebiopsied.

Staging

Esophageal cancer should be staged on the basis of the depth of invasion (T stage), the nodal status (N stage), and the presence of distant metastatic disease (M stage). Staging helps determine the therapeutic approach and assess the prognosis (Table 28-1). The tools for staging include computed tomography (CT) and endoscopic ultrasound. Although a sensitive means of documenting aortic invasion or pulmonary and hepatic metastases, CT has low accuracy in determining nodal involvement. Magnetic resonance imaging does not provide an advantage over CT. Endoscopic ultrasound is superior to CT for determining the T and N stages in all types of esophageal tumors, and it is useful for predicting resectability. Endoscopic ultrasound has accuracy rates of about 90% and 85% for establishing the T and N stages of a tumor, respectively.

ADENOCARCINOMA

Incidence and Epidemiology

The incidence of esophageal adenocarcinoma (EAC) is increasing more rapidly than any other cancer in the United States, which is likely due to the rising prevalence of gastroesophageal reflux disease and development of Barrett esophagus. EAC is mainly a disease of white males older than 40 years, with a male to female predominance of 3 to 5.5:1. Currently, the annual age-adjusted incidence of EAC among white males is 1.3 per 100,000.

Etiology and Pathogenesis

The presence of Barrett esophagus (intestinal metaplasia with specialized columnar epithelium) is the most important risk factor for developing EAC. Essentially all esophageal adenocarcinomas arise in areas of Barrett metaplasia. In addition, adenocarcinoma of the gastric cardia often arises from a short segment of Barrett epithelium. Given the similar epidemiologic and clinical associations of these two tumors, adenocarcinoma of the esophagus and gastric cardia are likely to share a common disease process. The mechanism by which gastric reflux of acid into the esophagus induces the metaplastic response is unknown, but medical or surgical treatment of gastroesophageal reflux does not effect regression of Barrett metaplasia. The risk for EAC among patients diagnosed with Barrett esophagus is 1 per 55 to 1 per 441 patient-years, or about a 0.5% annual rate of cancer development.

The mechanism regulating the transition from intestinal metaplasia to malignancy is unknown. Genomic instability is common in dysplastic Barrett

TABLE 28-1
TNM Staging System for Cancer of the Esophagus (American Joint Committee on Cancer criteria)

Primary Tumor (T)

TX	Primary tumor cannot be assessed
T0	No evidence of primary tumor
Tis	Carcinoma in situ
T1	Tumor invades lamina propria or submucosa
T2	Tumor invades muscularis propia
T3	Tumor invades adventitia
T4	Tumor invades adjacent structures

Lymph Node (N)

NX	Regional lymph nodes cannot be assessed
N0	No regional lymph node metastasis
N1	Regional lymph node metastasis

Distant Metastasis (M)

MX	Presence of distant metastasis cannot be assessed
M0	No distant metastasis
M1	Distant metastasis

Stage Grouping

0	Tis	N0	M0
I	T1	N0	M0
IIA	T2	N0	M0
	T3	N0	M0
IIB	T1	N1	M0
	T2	N1	M0
III	T3	N1	M0
	T4	N1	M0
IV	Any T	Any N	M1

mucosa. Aneuploid cell populations and deletions or alterations of tumor suppressor genes, particularly chromosomal regions 17p ($p53$), 5q (APC, MCC), 18q (DCC), and 13q ($RB1$), often are observed in the mucosa of patients who develop carcinoma. Abnormalities of cell proliferation, as evidenced by the expression of proliferating cell nuclear antigen (PCNA) and Ki-67, are noted in Barrett tissue and EAC. Microsatellite instability, a marker of defective mismatch repair, has also been detected in patients with Barrett esophagus and EAC.

Clinical Features

The clinical manifestations of EAC are similar to those of SCC, although chronic pyrosis, regurgitation, and chest pain caused by long-standing gastroesophageal reflux may be more common with EAC. Barrett metaplasia does not produce symptoms, and the endoscopic appearance of Barrett mucosa correlates poorly with the severity of reflux symptoms. As with SCC, symptoms attributable to adenocarcinoma occur in advanced stages when the tumor is large enough to interfere with swallowing.

Findings on Diagnostic Testing

Endoscopic Studies

Barrett metaplasia is diagnosed using upper gastrointestinal endoscopy along with biopsy. Endoscopic examination of Barrett metaplasia reveals circumferential or isolated islands (or tongues) of salmon-colored mucosa proximal to the esophagogastric junction. Biopsy specimens should be obtained from tissue that in endoscopic examination appears only to harbor Barrett metaplasia, as well as from any erosions, nodules, and strictures, because EAC may be present in Barrett esophagus in the absence of otherwise detectable structural lesions. The concurrent performance of brush cytological examination may increase the yield of random biopsies in detecting malignant tissue associated with Barrett metaplasia. Distinguishing between benign and malignant strictures can require extensive mucosal sampling with biopsies and brush cytology specimens.

Histological Evaluation

The interpretation of biopsy samples from patients with Barrett metaplasia requires the expertise of an experienced gastrointestinal pathologist. There is a high degree of interobserver variation in distinguishing low-grade dysplasia from no dysplasia, in addition to variability in interpreting high-grade dysplasia. It may be difficult or impossible to distinguish high-grade dysplasia from invasive carcinoma if biopsy samples fail to include the lamina propria; therefore, large or jumbo forceps should be used when sampling areas of Barrett metaplasia. Flow cytometry has been used to identify aneuploid or tetraploid cell populations and shows considerable promise in predicting the development of EAC. Other markers of cell proliferation such as PCNA, Ki-67, tritiated thymidine uptake, and ornithine decarboxylase may be predictive; however, the ability of these tests to impact clinical practice positively has not been established.

Radiographic Studies

Advanced tumors often are obvious in barium swallow radiographic studies, where they appear as apple core strictures or ulcerated mass lesions. Because Barrett metaplasia tends to concentrate in the distal esophagus, adenocarcinomas are more likely than squamous cell tumors to occur in the distal esophagus. Despite being useful for establishing the extent of advanced cancers, barium swallow radiography is clearly inferior to upper gastrointestinal endoscopy for detecting uncomplicated Barrett metaplasia and early adenocarcinoma.

Screening and Surveillance

Identification of the link between EAC and Barrett esophagus has led to the implementation of endoscopic screening and surveillance programs. Because medical and surgical antireflux therapy do not appear to lead to regression of Barrett metaplasia, surveillance programs usually are lifelong, although surveillance is indicated only for patients who are well enough and willing to undergo surgical resection if adenocarcinoma is detected. The strategy proposed by the American College of Gastroenterology includes screening patients with long-standing (5 years or more) symptoms of gastroesophageal reflux disease for the presence of Barrett esophagus using upper gastrointestinal endoscopy. If intestinal metaplasia is histologically confirmed, surveillance is performed at intervals dependent on the presence and degree of dysplasia. Current guidelines suggest taking systematic four-quadrant biopsy specimens every 2 cm along the length of Barrett metaplasia. In addition, any endoscopic abnormalities such as erosions, nodules, or strictures should be biopsied. Patients with no dysplasia and no endoscopic abnormalities should be reexamined in 1 year; if no dysplasia is confirmed, the surveillance interval may be extended to 3 years. Patients in whom low-grade dysplasia is diagnosed should have surveillance performed every 12 months. High-grade dysplasia must be confirmed on review by an experienced pathologist, and management depends on whether the findings are unifocal, multifocal, or are associated with a lesion (mass or ulcer). Unifocal high-grade dysplasia may be surveyed by repeated endoscopy with biopsy at 3-month intervals. Multifocal high-grade dysplasia should be treated with a form of ablation such as photodynamic therapy. Lesions associated with high-grade dysplasia should be removed by endoscopic mucosal resection techniques. If the capability for ablation or endoscopic mucosal resection does not exist at a particular institution, referral to a specialized center capable of performing these services or surgical resection should be considered. A diagnosis of EAC should prompt surgical evaluation. The decision to proceed with surgical resection should consider the risk of morbidity and mortality from malignancy against the operative risks and the desires of the patient.

Case-control studies report survival benefit from endoscopic surveillance of patients with Barrett esophagus. Prospective studies to confirm the efficacy of surveillance are lacking, however, and recent analyses have called into question the cost-effectiveness of surveying patients with Barrett esophagus in the absence of dysplasia or other markers that predict the development of EAC.

THERAPY FOR ESOPHAGEAL SQUAMOUS CELL CARCINOMA AND ADENOCARCINOMA

Therapeutic approaches for esophageal SCC and EAC are similar. Surgical resection is the primary therapy for patients with tumors that are confined to the esophagus. However, because of the advanced stage at which most esophageal cancers are diagnosed, surgical exploration is indicated in only 60% of patients, and only two-thirds of these can undergo resection. Overall, the 1- and 5-year survival rates are 18% and 5%, respectively. Although curative resection is unlikely for T3 or N1 lesions, palliative resection can provide 1 to 2 years of symptom-free survival. Locally advanced (T4) or metastatic (M1) disease is not amenable to curative resection, and the poor long-term survival of these patients makes surgical palliation an unfavorable option.

There are several accepted surgical approaches to treating esophageal cancer. The choice of procedure depends on tumor location, lymph node status, the patient's body habitus and performance status, and the preference of the surgeon and institution. Traditionally, a transthoracic esophagectomy with esophagogastric anastomosis is performed. An alternate procedure for lesions in the upper one third of the esophagus involves a subtotal esophagectomy with a gastric pull-up into the neck and requires a combined abdominal and cervical approach. Both procedures provide the adequate exposure and tissue resection margins necessary for a cancer operation. With the increase in incidence of EAC in the distal esophagus, transhiatal resection and primary anastomosis has become popular. Recent studies report surgical mortality rates of 2% to 13%. Complications include anastomotic leak or stricture, pulmonary disease (e.g., pneumonia, pulmonary emboli), recurrent laryngeal nerve injury, and cardiac disease (e.g., myocardial infarction, arrhythmia, and congestive heart failure).

The overall 5-year survival of patients who undergo resection is 12% to 27%. High rates of recurrence have prompted trials of perioperative chemotherapy and radiation therapy to improve systemic and regional control of the tumor.

Multiple studies have investigated the role of radiation alone, chemotherapy alone, and the combination of radiation with chemotherapy before or after surgical resection; however, most studies fail to provide definitive evidence that these interventions improve survival. Potential exceptions include neoadjuvant (preoperative) chemotherapy, which was shown in one trial to increase resectability and improve 2-year survival rates. Neoadjuvant chemoradiation has not been associated with statistically significant gains in survival; however, larger randomized trials are needed to clarify the potential role of combination therapy for esophageal cancer.

Palliative therapies may be used to treat local or metastatic disease. Radiotherapy has been shown to relieve obstruction but is associated with significant esophagitis. Endoscopic placement of self-expanding metal stents is quickly becoming the palliative therapy of choice to relieve esophageal obstruction. A silicone-coated stent placed across a tracheoesophageal fistula allows the patient to swallow saliva and food without aspirating. Unfortunately, a high rate of complications occurs with these stents, including intractable chest pain, stent migration, perforation, and bleeding. Endoscopic therapy using laser, argon plasma coagulation, or bipolar electrocautery may also help to relieve obstruction. Photodynamic therapy, which the Food and Drug Administration has approved for the palliation of esophageal cancer, consists of administering a photosensitizer, followed by local exposure of the tumor to light of a specific wavelength (630 nm). Tumor destruction occurs as a result of singlet oxygen production that leads to ischemia and necrosis. Systemic chemotherapy with fluorouracil and cisplatin has not achieved good results; however, newer agents such as paclitaxel, docetaxel, gemcitabine, irinotecan, and oxaliplatin have shown response rates up to 60%, including increased survival and quality of life.

OTHER MALIGNANT NEOPLASMS

Epithelial Tumors

A variant of SCC characterized by a prominent spindle cell component has been variably termed carcinosarcoma, pseudosarcoma, spindle cell carcinoma, and polypoid carcinoma. These lesions are large and polypoid and may be solitary or multiple. Men are affected more often than women, and most are middle-aged or elderly at the time of presentation. Another variant of SCC is termed verrucous carcinoma because the primary lesion grows slowly and invades local tissues with only rare metastases. Adenoid cystic carcinomas are rare tumors thought to arise from submucosal glands. Adenosquamous carcinomas or adenocanthomas combine features of the two common forms of esophageal cancer. Mucoepidermoid carcinoma, also composed of glandular and squamous elements likely arising from submucosal glands or ducts, has a poor prognosis. Melanoma of the esophagus may be primary or metastatic, although the esophagus is a less common site of metastatic gastrointestinal disease than the stomach, small intestine, or colon.

Neuroendocrine tumors of the esophagus include small cell carcinomas, carcinoids, and choriocarcinomas. Small cell carcinoma of the esophagus may be a primary esophageal tumor, or it may represent a metastatic lesion from the lung. Neoplasia may be associated with a paraneoplastic phenomenon, including inappropriate antidiuretic hormone secretion and hypercalcemia.

Nonepithelial Tumors

Malignant nonepithelial tumors of the esophagus include leiomyosarcomas, metastatic cancers, and lymphomas. Leiomyosarcomas may be polypoid or infiltrative and can be located anywhere in the esophagus. Metastatic lesions are most commonly due to melanoma, followed by breast cancer; less common etiologies include gastric, renal, liver, prostate, testicular, bone, skin, lung, and head and neck cancer. Primary esophageal lymphoma may be of the Hodgkin or non-Hodgkin type and are more common among immunocompromised patients.

BENIGN ESOPHAGEAL TUMORS

Squamous Cell Papillomas

Squamous cell papillomas are small, sessile, polypoid lesions discovered incidentally during endoscopic examination for unrelated symptoms. Papillomas usually are solitary and are located in the distal third of the esophagus. They may be associated with chronic irritation from gastroesophageal reflux disease or may result from infection with human papillomavirus. Cancer development has not been documented in these neoplasms.

Submucosal Neoplasms

Leiomyomas are the most common benign esophageal tumor. The male to female ratio is 2:1. Most are asymptomatic, but large tumors may cause dysphagia or chest pain. They occur most commonly in the distal esophagus. The diagnosis is made by barium swallow radiography or upper gastrointestinal endoscopy. Large benign leiomyomas may be difficult to distinguish from rare malignant leiomyosarcomas. Other submucosal lesions of the esophagus are rare and include lipomas, fibromas, fibrovascular polyps, granular cell tumors, hemangiomas, and lymphangiomas. As with leiomyomas, most of these lesions are found incidentally and are not considered morbid.

CHAPTER 29

Structural Disorders and Miscellaneous Disorders of the Stomach

GASTRIC EMBRYOLOGY AND ANATOMY

The stomach develops from the embryonic foregut. After the fourth week of gestation, it rotates 90 degrees clockwise around its longitudinal axis. The new left portion of the stomach elongates more rapidly than the right to form the greater and lesser curvatures, respectively. The cephalic aspect moves downward, and the caudal aspect moves upward and to the right, moving the stomach into its final position. The dorsal gastric mesentery forms the omental bursa (lesser peritoneal sac), and the ventral mesentery attaches the stomach to the liver. The embryonic endoderm forms the gastric epithelium and glands, whereas the mesoderm forms the connective tissue, muscle, and serosa of the stomach.

The size, shape, and position of the stomach vary greatly because of distensibility. When empty, the stomach volume is only a few hundred mL, whereas postprandially it may expand to 2 L. The stomach is separated into the cardia (the 1-cm to 2-cm segment distal to the esophagogastric junction), the fundus (the superior portion of the stomach above a horizontal plane that passes through the esophagogastric junction), the body (the large portion between the fundus and the antrum), the antrum (the distal one fourth to one third of the stomach), and the pylorus (the 1-cm to 2-cm channel that connects the stomach to the duodenum). Along the lesser curvature at the junction of the body and antrum is a bend that is accentuated during peristalsis (i.e., the angularis).

The blood supply to the stomach is derived from the celiac axis and superior mesenteric artery. The celiac arises from the aorta and branches into the splenic artery (which branches to form the short gastric and left gastroepiploic arteries), left gastric artery, and hepatic artery (which branches to form the right gastric, gastroduodenal, and right gastroepiploic arteries). The inferior pancreaticoduodenal branch of the superior mesenteric artery also feeds the distal stomach and pylorus, thus providing a dual arterial supply of blood to the stomach. The venous drainage of the stomach accompanies the arteries and leads either directly or indirectly into the portal vein.

The stomach receives autonomic innervation from spinal sympathetic nerves and the vagus nerve. Sympathetic nerves from T7 to T8 pass through the thoracic sympathetic chain to form the splanchnic nerves that terminate in the celiac ganglia. Postganglionic fibers from the celiac ganglia innervate the stomach wall. Afferent fibers from the stomach synapse with cell bodies in the dorsal root ganglia of the spinal cord. The motor component of the vagus nerve, which originates from the dorsal motor nucleus of the medulla, provides parasympathetic innervation to the stomach. The anterior vagus divides into the hepatic and anterior gastric branches; the posterior vagus divides into the celiac and posterior gastric branches. Vagal fibers from the gastric branches synapse within the myenteric (Auerbach) and submucosal (Meissner) plexuses.

The lymphatic drainage from the stomach is divided into four regions: (1) lymph from the upper stomach drains into the superior gastric lymph nodes; (2) the fundus and proximal body drain into the pancreaticolienal and splenic lymph nodes; (3) the distal greater curvature empties into the inferior gastric and subpyloric nodes; and (4) lymph from the pylorus drains into the superior gastric, hepatic, and subpyloric nodes.

Anatomically, the stomach is divided into four tissue layers: the mucosa, the submucosa, the muscularis propria, and the serosa. The mucosa is further divided into the epithelium, lamina propria, and muscularis mucosae. The epithelium comprises surface lining cells and regenerative cells and involutes to form long glands that are lined by specialized cells, including parietal (oxyntic) cells, mucous cells, chief cells, and endocrine cells. Gastric pits, or foveolae, are located at the junction between the glands and the gastric mucosal surface. Parietal cells contain the proton pump, or H^+, K^+-adenosine triphosphatase, which mediates acid secretion and is located on the microvillous membranes. Mucous neck cells release mucin, a neutral glycoprotein. Chief cells secrete proenzyme pepsinogens that are hydrolyzed to pepsin in the acidic environment of the stomach. Endocrine cells include enterochromaffin-like (or ECL) cells in the fundus that release histamine, G cells in the antrum that secrete gastrin, and D cells in the fundus and antrum that contain somatostatin.

The proliferative zone of the gastric mucosa is located in the base of the pits and in the upper portion of the glands. Cells migrate from this zone to renew the surface epithelium every 2 to 6 days. Renewal of glandular epithelium from the same zone is slower, taking weeks to months. The lamina propria contains connective tissue, smooth muscle, lymphatics, blood vessels, nerves, lymphocytes, plasma cells, mast cells, fibroblasts, macrophages, and eosinophils. The submucosa is a layer of connective tissue that provides a framework for the blood and nerve supply to the stomach. The muscularis propria consists of a uniform circular layer of smooth muscle surrounded by a longitudinal layer and a layer of oblique fibers most prominent in the upper stomach. The serosa is composed of areolar tissue and a single layer of squamous mesothelial cells.

DEVELOPMENTAL ABNORMALITIES OF THE STOMACH

Gastric Atresia

Etiology and Pathogenesis

Gastric atresia is a blind ending of the antrum or pylorus and may involve all layers of the gastric wall or be limited to the mucosa and submucosa. Atresia may result from failed recanalization of the gut lumen during embryogenesis. The condition may be familial with autosomal recessive transmission.

Clinical Features, Diagnosis, and Management

In utero, there may be a large volume of amniotic fluid. After birth, infants with gastric atresia present with nonbilious vomiting, upper abdominal distention, dehydration, and hypochloremic, hypokalemic metabolic alkalosis. Abdominal radiography will reveal an air-distended stomach with no intestinal gas. Treatment for an atretic segment that involves only the mucosa requires resection of the occluding membrane and pyloroplasty, whereas more extensive atresia requires resection with gastroduodenostomy.

Gastric Mucosal Membrane

Etiology and Pathogenesis

A congenital mucosal membrane in the antrum or pylorus may contain squamous or columnar epithelium and probably results from the same factors that cause gastric atresia.

Clinical Features, Diagnosis, and Management

Nausea and vomiting may not develop until late childhood or adulthood. Abdominal radiographs usually are normal, and the diagnosis usually is made from upper gastrointestinal (GI) barium radiographic studies, which show a bandlike defect that may simulate a second pylorus. Treatment involves endoscopic lysis of the membrane or surgical excision with or without pyloroplasty.

Gastric Duplication
Etiology and Pathogenesis
Gastric duplications contain mucosa, submucosa, and muscularis propria, and share a common wall with, but are separate from the stomach. Usually they are found as extragastric masses, but they occasionally communicate with the stomach or pancreas.

Clinical Features, Diagnosis, and Management
Symptoms of gastric duplication manifest within the first year of life and include vomiting, failure to thrive, and weight loss. Older children may complain of epigastric abdominal pain. There may be signs of an abdominal mass or obstruction and occult or gross bleeding if the duplication is in communication with the GI tract. Complications include perforation, hemoptysis due to fistula formation to the lung, or development of cancer in the duplication. Diagnosis may be made using upper GI barium radiography (which will reveal lumenal compression or contrast filling of the cyst), ultrasonography, computed tomography, or magnetic resonance imaging. Treatment is surgical excision.

Microgastria
Etiology and Pathogenesis
Microgastria results from the failure of the stomach to develop from the foregut and is usually associated with fatal cardiac abnormalities, limb and spinal deformities, micrognathia, and asplenia.

Clinical Features, Diagnosis, and Management
Symptoms of microgastria, which include vomiting, malnutrition, and anemia, manifest soon after birth. Death usually occurs within weeks to months. If the patient survives, a jejunal pouch can be surgically constructed.

Gastric Teratoma
Etiology, Clinical Features, Diagnosis, and Management
Gastric teratomas are rare tumors composed of all three primary embryonic germ layers. They are found almost exclusively in males. Patients present in childhood or adulthood with abdominal masses, bleeding, or obstructions. Plain abdominal films may show a calcific mass (reflecting the presence of teeth and bone), and a gastric mass may be seen on upper GI barium radiographs. Surgical resection is the preferred treatment; however, total gastrectomy with construction of a jejunal pouch may be needed for large tumors.

Gastric Diverticula
Etiology, Clinical Features, Diagnosis, and Management
Gastric diverticula are rare congenital diverticula containing all layers of the gastric wall (true diverticula). They usually are located on the posterior gastric wall near the gastroesophageal junction but may also occur in the antrum and pylorus. Their etiology is unknown, but they are associated with other GI diverticula and hiatal hernia. Ectopic pancreatic tissue may reside within the diverticula, which may

ulcerate and bleed. These lesions, however, usually are asymptomatic and are discovered incidentally. Heartburn, chest pain, or vomiting may occur on occasion. Diagnosis is made by endoscopy or barium contrast studies. No therapy is generally required, although severe symptoms or bleeding may warrant surgical excision.

Hypertrophic Pyloric Stenosis

Etiology and Pathogenesis

Neonatal hypertrophic pyloric stenosis is a congenital gastric outlet obstruction resulting from pyloric muscular edema and hypertrophy. There is a male predominance with a prevalence of 1 of 150 male and 1 of 750 female births. There is familial clustering, and it is more common in whites than in other races. It has been suggested that a lack of nitric oxide synthase may produce pylorospasm.

Adults manifest hypertrophic pyloric stenosis rarely, secondary to chronic peptic ulcer disease, severe gastritis, or cancer in the pyloric region.

Clinical Features, Diagnosis, and Management

Infants typically develop regurgitation and projectile, nonbilious vomiting in the third or fourth week of life. Complications include malnutrition, weakness, constipation, oliguria, and weight loss. On physical examination, the stomach is dilated, and gastric peristalsis may be visible. The hypertrophic pylorus may be palpable and appreciated as an olive-sized mass in the upper abdomen. Abdominal radiography shows a large gastric bubble with little intestinal gas; upper GI barium radiography may show a long, narrow, pyloric canal. Ultrasound demonstration of the hypertrophied pylorus may obviate the need for contrast radiography. After correcting fluid and electrolyte deficiencies, the surgical procedure of choice is longitudinal division of the anterior pyloric muscle from the serosa to the submucosa (Ramstedt pyloromyotomy). Long-term results are excellent.

Adults with pyloric stenosis present with nausea, vomiting, early satiety, weight loss, and epigastric pain. The diagnosis is made by upper GI barium radiography or upper endoscopy. Endoscopic dilation may successfully relieve symptoms; however, surgical therapy with pyloric resection may be advisable to exclude a small focus of cancer.

GASTRIC BEZOARS

Etiology and Pathogenesis

Bezoars are concretions of foreign material that are retained in the stomach, esophagus, and rectum. Bezoars are classified by their composition, which may be plant fibers (phytobezoars), hair (trichobezoars), medications (pharmacobezoars), or persimmons (disopyrobezoars). Risk factors for bezoar formation include reduced gastric motility, hypochlorhydria, inadequate mastication caused by missing teeth or poorly fitting dentures, prior gastric surgery (pyloroplasty, antrectomy, or partial gastrectomy), mixed connective tissue disease, hypothyroidism, and myotonic dystrophy. Foods implicated in phytobezoars include grapes, oranges, raisins, figs, cherries, coconuts, peaches, apples, bran, oats, celery, pumpkins, sauerkraut, peanuts, cabbage, and potato peels.

Trichobezoars are mucus-covered masses of hair that occur most commonly in women who swallow their hair. Men with beards also may be at risk. Drug intoxication may result from medication trapped within the mass of hair. Pharmacobezoars may be composed of aluminum-containing antacids, enteric-coated aspirin, calcium preparations, magnesium carbonate, sucralfate, nifedipine, sodium polystyrene sulfonate (Kayexalate), and lecithin. Disopyrobezoars form when tannin present in unripe persimmons interacts with gastric acid to create a bezoar nidus. Fungus balls, or yeast bezoars, may complicate gastric surgery, but they are often asymptomatic. Other nonfood substances that produce bezoars include furniture polish, cement, fruit pits, plastic, paper, string, cotton, and Styrofoam.

Clinical Features, Diagnosis, and Management

Some patients with bezoars are asymptomatic, whereas others complain of nausea, vomiting, anorexia, bloating, halitosis, early satiety, dyspepsia, weight loss, and feelings of epigastric fullness or pain. Complications of bezoars include gastric obstruction, anemia, hemorrhage, ulceration, and perforation. Diagnosis may be made using abdominal radiography that shows an ill-defined mass within the gastric air bubble; however, upper GI endoscopy is the most sensitive test for diagnosing a bezoar, and in addition, can identify the type.

Therapy for gastric bezoars includes enzymatic digestion, endoscopic mechanical disruption, medication, and surgery (Table 29-1). Phytobezoars may respond to enzymatic agents, including papain (protease), Adolph's meat tenderizer (1 teaspoon in 4 ounces of water before each meal), cellulase, and acetylcysteine (mucolytic). Insoluble bezoars may be removed endoscopically using endoscopic baskets, forceps, and snares. It is recommended that an overtube be placed to reduce the potential for pulmonary aspiration. Alternatively, endoscopically directed water pulses may fragment some bezoars (usually phytobezoars) so that they may be lavaged from the stomach or pass spontaneously into the intestine. Nd:YAG lasers have also been used to fragment enzyme-resistant bezoars. Prokinetic medications (e.g., metoclopramide, domperidone) may accelerate gastric emptying and help fragment loosely adherent bezoars. However, these agents are more likely to be useful as prophylactic agents after the bezoar has been fragmented, dissolved, or removed. Certain bezoars, such as trichobezoars, are not amenable

---

TABLE 29-1
Treatment of Gastric Bezoars

Treatment Type	Mechanism	Specific Therapy
Enzymatic	Proteolysis	Papain, pancrelipase, pancreatin, Adolph's meat tenderizer
	Cellulolytic	Cellulase
	Mucolytic	Acetylcysteine
Medication	Prokinetic	Metoclopramide
Endoscopic	Extraction	Snare, basket, forceps
	Fragmentation	High-pressure water pulses, Nd:YAG laser
Surgical	Removal	

to medical management and require surgical excision. Surgery also is necessary for complications such as perforation, gastric or small intestinal obstruction, or hemorrhage.

GASTRIC FOREIGN BODIES

Etiology and Pathogenesis

About 1500 people die each year in the United States from swallowing or aspirating foreign objects. Children often accidentally swallow coins, small household items, and toys. Adults may swallow dental prostheses and toothbrushes as a result of carelessness, rapid eating, or ethanol intoxication. Intentional ingestion usually occurs in psychotic, demented, or incarcerated individuals. Illicit drugs may be concealed within the body by swallowing plastic or rubber bags that contain the drugs.

Clinical Features, Diagnosis, and Management

Most (80% to 93%) ingested foreign bodies pass spontaneously. Symptoms may be caused by gastric penetration or perforation (leading to localized or generalized peritonitis), gastritis, mucosal tears or ulcers, abscess, hemorrhage, and fistulae. Removal of sharp or potentially toxic objects, in addition to objects more than 2 cm in diameter or more than 5 cm long, should be strongly considered because these dimensions predispose to duodenal obstruction. Button batteries lodged in the esophagus should be removed endoscopically; however, those that pass into the stomach generally do not require removal unless the battery is mercury-based, is larger than 15 mm in diameter, remains in the stomach for more than 48 hours, or if the patient has evidence of GI injury (hematochezia or abdominal pain). Most objects can be removed endoscopically with a snare, basket, or forceps with an overtube to prevent aspiration and additional injury. Surgery rather than endoscopy is indicated for large, jagged objects and packets of illicit drugs. Fluoroscopic removal of metallic foreign bodies using a magnet-tipped catheter is possible.

GASTRIC RUPTURE

Etiology and Pathogenesis

Spontaneous gastric rupture is rare, accounting for 0.1% in autopsy statistics. The stomach is normally resistant to rupture because it is distensible and able to decompress through the pylorus and gastroesophageal junction. Predisposing conditions that increase the risk of rupture include fundoplication; neoplasia of the esophagus, distal stomach, pancreas, or duodenum; peptic ulcer disease; or other causes of gastric outlet or inlet obstruction that limit the ability of the stomach to vent pressure either proximally or distally.

Causes of gastric rupture include emesis, blunt abdominal trauma, or conditions of gastric overdistention. Emesis-induced gastric rupture usually develops along the greater curvature in the fundus as a consequence of gastric herniation into the chest and may occur during labor or the postpartum period, with pyloric stenosis, and after ipecac administration. Traumatic causes of gastric rupture include coughing, seizures, lifting of heavy objects, upper GI endoscopy, and the Heimlich maneuver. Overdistention may cause gastric rupture as a result of nasal oxygen, mouth-to-mouth resuscitation, aerophagia, inadvertent gastric inflation during anesthesia, gas-producing food fermentation, gastric lavage, gastric variceal tamponade balloons, sodium bicarbonate ingestion, and scuba diving. The site of rupture with overdistention is the lesser curvature near the cardia or fundus in 60% of cases.

Clinical Features, Diagnosis, and Management

Symptoms and signs appear immediately after rupture and include severe pain, abdominal distention, dyspnea, shock, subcutaneous emphysema, and peritoneal signs. Chest and abdominal radiographs reveal pneumoperitoneum. The need for additional diagnostic information should be weighed with the emergent need for intervention. Mortality is 100% without surgery because of massive peritoneal soiling from the rupture. Even with surgery, mortality rates exceed 60% due to complications of peritonitis, air embolism, respiratory failure, mediastinitis, bleeding, and sepsis.

GASTRIC VOLVULUS

Etiology and Pathogenesis

Gastric volvulus is defined as an abnormal rotation of one part of the stomach around another. The volvulus is classified as either organoaxial (rotation around a line joining the pylorus and esophagogastric junction) or, less commonly, mesenteroaxial (rotation around a line from the center of the greater curvature to the porta hepatis). The condition affects both genders equally and has a peak incidence in the fifth decade, although 20% of cases occur in children. Predisposing factors include prior trauma, phrenic nerve injury, paraesophageal hernia, and abnormal ligament fixation. Complete volvulus may impair the gastric blood supply, leading to ischemia and infarction.

Clinical Features, Diagnosis, and Management

Gastric volvulus can manifest as an acute abdominal emergency or as a chronic recurrent gastric obstruction. Symptoms of an acute volvulus include substernal or epigastric pain that radiates to the neck and arms. Associated complaints may include retching with an inability to vomit and hematemesis. Physical examination may reveal a distended, tense upper abdomen, whereas the lower abdomen is soft. It may not be possible to pass a nasogastric tube beyond the obstructing volvulus, thus completing the clinical (Borchardt) triad that includes abdominal pain and violent retching. Complications of acute volvulus include infarction, perforation, and shock. The mortality from acute volvulus is 30% to 50%.

In contrast, chronic gastric volvulus presents with more vague symptoms of mild, continuous, or intermittent upper abdominal discomfort, postprandial bloating, dysphagia, or pyrosis. Large meals worsen the symptoms, whereas emesis may relieve them.

The diagnosis is often made incidentally by abdominal or chest radiography that shows a spherical stomach bubble with two air-fluid levels (fundus and antrum) in mesenteroaxial volvulus or a horizontal stomach with a single air-fluid level in organoaxial volvulus. Upper GI barium radiography may reveal gastric dilation, the site of the volvulus twist, and delayed passage of the contrast agent distal to the obstruction.

Acute volvulus in the absence of vascular compromise has been treated by endoscopic reduction; however, the risk of ischemia, perforation, and peritonitis is sufficient to recommend immediate surgery to reduce the volvulus in most cases. Anterior gastropexy should be performed and any anatomical defects, such as paraesophageal hernias, should be corrected. Excision or gastrectomy may be necessary if necrosis is present.

The requirement for surgery is less stringent in chronic volvulus, because some patients with minimal symptoms do well without surgical intervention.

CHAPTER 30

Disorders of Gastric Emptying

DISORDERS WITH DELAYED GASTRIC EMPTYING

Incidence and Epidemiology

Many conditions produce secondary symptomatic delays in gastric emptying, or gastroparesis, by disrupting the normal neuromuscular function of the stomach. These include diseases that are localized to the stomach, disorders that involve the gastrointestinal tract diffusely, and nongastrointestinal diseases. The epidemiology of these conditions parallels that of the underlying disease. Other patients present with idiopathic gastroparesis. Some of these individuals report a viral prodrome suggestive of an infectious etiology. Such idiopathic or viral cases of gastroparesis are common in young women. Many cases of functional dyspepsia have associated delayed gastric emptying and exhibit overlap with idiopathic gastroparesis.

Etiology and Pathogenesis

Disorders Involving the Stomach

Diabetic gastroparesis.   Patients with long-standing diabetes (usually type I for >10 years with other neuropathic complications) may experience periods of nausea, vomiting, early satiety, and fullness. In many cases, solid-phase gastric emptying is delayed significantly. However, some individuals with diabetes and nausea exhibit normal gastric emptying, which suggests that other factors participate in the genesis of symptoms. Such individuals are more appropriately considered to have diabetic gastropathy. Motor abnormalities that contribute to delays in gastric emptying include loss of antral contractions, increased pyloric activity (pylorospasm), increased fundus compliance, and increased intestinal motor activity (which acts as a brake on gastric evacuation). Most investigators believe that diabetic gastroparesis results from impaired intrinsic and extrinsic neural function of the stomach; however, impaired contractility at the smooth muscle level has been demonstrated in animal models. The degree of hyperglycemia can exacerbate delays in gastric emptying in diabetics.

Idiopathic gastroparesis.   Many patients (25%–30%) with gastroparesis have no predisposing factor for their disease. In most series, a large majority of affected patients are young women. In a subset of these individuals, fever, myalgias, nausea, and diarrhea precede the onset of gastroparesis, which suggests an underlying viral cause. Patients with a viral prodrome tend to have a better prognosis. Up to 70% experience remission during a 2-year period, whereas those without an apparent viral cause frequently experience enduring symptoms. The virus responsible in most cases is not identified. Rotavirus and certain parvovirus-like agents (e.g., Norwalk agent) produce acute gastroparesis, whereas herpes simplex virus, cytomegalovirus, Epstein-Barr virus, and varicella-zoster virus reportedly cause gastroparesis in immunocompromised individuals.

Postoperative gastroparesis.   A minority of patients (<5%) who have undergone vagotomy and drainage for peptic ulcer disease or malignancy experience nausea, vomiting, and early satiety secondary to postoperative stasis primarily of solid foods. Abnormalities in antral peristalsis and fundus tone have been demonstrated in this condition. Gastric stasis may also complicate gastroplasty or gastric bypass operations for morbid obesity, producing early satiety, anorexia, and weight reduction. Patients undergoing fundoplication for gastroesophageal reflux develop gastroparesis possibly by intraoperative vagus nerve damage. Alternatively, some cases of presumed postoperative gastroparesis may have had undetected defects in gastric emptying prior to surgery that were unmasked by the operation.

Functional dyspepsia.   Functional dyspepsia is a disorder that shows overlap with irritable bowel syndrome. Delayed gastric emptying is reported in 30% to 82% of cases of functional dyspepsia. Many affected patients also exhibit increased sensitivity to gastric balloon distention, suggesting that sensory nerve abnormalities may be involved in symptom induction. Nevertheless, motor dysfunction in functional dyspepsia is probably pathogenic for symptoms in some individuals because prokinetic agents can be effective therapy.

Medication-induced delays in gastric emptying.   Many prescription and over-the-counter medications delay gastric emptying (Table 30-1). Nonmedicinal compounds, including tobacco, marijuana, and intoxicating quantities of ethanol, also inhibit gastric motor function. Total parenteral nutrition has been associated with delayed gastric emptying, which may relate in part to the induction of hyperglycemia.

Miscellaneous gastric disorders.   Delayed gastric emptying is rarely observed with gastric ulcer; however, the pathogenic relevance of this association is uncertain. Nausea, vomiting, and intolerance to solid and liquid meals are common after abdominal irradiation. Patients with upper abdominal malignancy (usually pancreatic) develop symptomatic gastroparesis by unknown mechanisms. Ischemic gastroparesis secondary to atherosclerosis of the mesenteric vasculature produces symptoms most often in women. Delayed emptying of solids is found with atrophic gastritis, which may relate to the decrease in gastric secretions that are necessary to process ingested food. Hypertrophic pyloric stenosis is a common cause of delayed gastric emptying in infants but is rare in adults.

TABLE 30-1
Effects of Medications on Gastric Emptying

Delay gastric emptying
   Ethanol (high concentration)
   Aluminum hydroxide antacids
   Anticholinergics
   β-Adrenergic receptor agonists
   Calcitonin
   Calcium channel antagonists
   Dexfenfluramine
   Diphenhydramine
   Glucagon
   Interferon-α
   L-Dopa
   Octreotide
   Opiates
   Progesterone
   Proton pump inhibitors
   Sucralfate
   Tetrahydrocannabinol
   Tobacco/nicotine
   Tricyclic antidepressants

Accelerate gastric emptying
   β-Adrenergic receptor antagonists
   Clonidine
   Domperidone
   Erythromycin/other macrolides
   Nizatidine
   Metoclopramide
   Naloxone
   Tegaserod

Disorders with Diffuse Gastrointestinal Involvement

Rheumatologic disorders.   Scleroderma produces dysphagia, heartburn, nausea, vomiting, bloating, abdominal pain, and bowel disturbances as a result of diffuse dysmotility that involves the esophagus, stomach, small intestine, and colon. In most patients, gastroduodenal manometry demonstrates diffuse low-amplitude contractions that are consistent with myopathic involvement. However, a subset of patients with early disease exhibits high-amplitude, uncoordinated contractile activity, which indicates neuropathic disease. Polymyositis-dermatomyositis and systemic lupus erythematosus rarely produce gastroparesis.

Chronic idiopathic intestinal pseudoobstruction.   Patients with this disorder may have associated gastric dysmotility with prominent nausea, vomiting, bloating, and early satiety. The presence of bladder dysfunction or orthostatic hypotension suggests diffuse neuromuscular disease. Pseudoobstruction may be familial, it may occur after a viral prodrome, or it may be a paraneoplastic consequence of certain malignancies (usually small cell lung carcinoma).

Miscellaneous diffuse disorders. Delayed gastric emptying can occur in diffuse muscle disorders (e.g., myotonic dystrophy and progressive muscular dystrophy) or with amyloidosis. Chagas disease, resulting from an infection with *Trypanosoma cruzi*, can cause gastroparesis as part of a diffuse process that involves smooth muscle tissues. Some patients with idiopathic achalasia have delayed emptying, suggesting a process involving more than just the esophagus. Other infections that diffusely affect gut motor activity include those caused by herpes simplex virus, cytomegalovirus, varicella-zoster virus, Epstein-Barr virus, and *Clostridium botulinum*. Delayed emptying is found with variable frequency in different studies of patients with gastroesophageal reflux disease and individuals with chronic constipation. Up to 50% of patients with celiac disease exhibit delayed gastric emptying, which is reversed by ingesting a gluten-free diet.

Nongastrointestinal Disorders

Eating disorders. Delayed gastric emptying with reduced antral contractility is a common manifestation of anorexia nervosa, a disorder that has associated symptoms of bloating, nausea, early satiety, heartburn, and epigastric pain. Causes of gastroparesis with anorexia nervosa include central nervous system inhibition and malnutrition, but no specific gastric pathology has been demonstrated. Some patients with bulimia nervosa exhibit delayed solid emptying. Rumination syndrome usually is not associated with delayed emptying, although small reductions in postprandial antral motor activity have been documented.

Cyclic vomiting syndrome. Cyclic vomiting syndrome is a disorder of unknown etiology that is characterized by intermittent symptomatic periods that last for days followed by prolonged asymptomatic intervals that last for weeks to months. Some patients with cyclic vomiting syndrome exhibit delayed gastric emptying, which suggests underlying gastric motor dysfunction. Metabolic derangements, mitochondrial disorders, atopy, and migraine headaches are associated with distinct subsets, suggesting a heterogeneous pathogenesis.

Neurological disorders. Nausea and vomiting are commonly reported by patients with neurological disorders (e.g., cerebrovascular accidents, tumors, migraine headaches, seizures, Ménière disease, and labyrinthitis). Altered gastric motility or emptying has been demonstrated after cerebrovascular accidents, with migraines, and after high cervical spinal injury. Gastric stasis may occur with disorders of autonomic function (e.g., Shy-Drager syndrome, Parkinson disease, Guillain-Barré syndrome, and multiple sclerosis).

Endocrinologic and metabolic disorders. Nausea, vomiting, and anorexia are frequently reported by patients with end-stage renal disease, even after adequate dialysis, but only a minority of these patients exhibit abnormal gastric emptying. Gastroparesis or intestinal pseudoobstruction may develop as a consequence of hypothyroidism, hyperparathyroidism, and hypoparathyroidism.

Miscellaneous nongastrointestinal disorders. Some patients with gallbladder disease and those who have undergone cholecystectomies have dyspepsia and delayed gastric emptying; however, the causal relationship between the biliary process and the gastric dysmotility is not proven. Some patients with chronic pancreatitis exhibit delayed gastric emptying. Similarly, abnormal emptying is reported in many individuals with cirrhosis, which correlates with the severity of liver disease measured by the Child-Pugh status.

Clinical Features

Symptoms of gastroparesis include chronic or intermittent nausea, vomiting, bloating, early satiety, and postprandial abdominal pain. In mild cases, symptoms may be absent when the stomach is empty. As the disease progresses, bloating and nausea increase slowly for several days because of incomplete gastric evacuation of multiple ingested meals, only to be relieved by voluminous vomiting of foul-smelling food ingested hours to days before. In severe cases, intractable retching may develop even if no meal has been ingested in several hours. Other symptoms of gastroparesis include heartburn from delayed gastric acid clearance, hemorrhage secondary to Mallory-Weiss tears or stasis-induced mucosal irritation, and weight loss. Bezoar development may supervene and exacerbate symptoms of fullness and early satiety. Symptoms and signs of systemic diseases associated with gastroparesis or diffuse gastrointestinal dysmotility may be present, for example, neuropathic findings with diabetes and skin changes with scleroderma. Diabetics with gastroparesis may also exhibit alterations in insulin requirements with erratic blood glucose levels because of unpredictable intestinal nutrient delivery.

Findings on Diagnostic Testing

Laboratory Studies

Laboratory studies may assist in determining the severity and chronicity of the patient's disorder. Hypokalemia and contraction alkalosis result from severe vomiting, whereas anemia and hypoproteinemia are consistent with long-standing malnutrition. Specific serologic findings may suggest rheumatologic diseases such as systemic lupus erythematosus or scleroderma, whereas antineuronal antibody tests can screen for paraneoplastic dysmotility syndromes. Blood tests also can detect diabetes, uremia, or thyroid and parathyroid disease.

Radiographic and Endoscopic Studies

Patients with presumed gastroparesis should undergo structural evaluation to exclude mechanical obstruction as a cause of symptoms. Abdominal radiography can be used to screen for obstruction of the small intestine, which can be followed by barium radiography, if clinically indicated. Upper gastrointestinal endoscopy is appropriate if gastric outlet obstruction secondary to peptic ulcer disease or malignancy is suspected. In patients with gastroparesis, endoscopy may detect a bezoar. Endoscopic disruption of organized bezoars improves symptoms in some individuals.

Functional Testing

Gastric scintigraphic quantitation of gastric emptying is the standard for diagnosing gastroparesis. Liquid-phase gastric emptying scans that involve ingesting an aqueous-phase isotope such as ^{111}In-DTPA show first-order kinetics with an emptying half-time of of 8 to 28 minutes. Solid-phase gastric-emptying scintigraphic images using ^{99m}Tc–sulfur colloid mixed with a solid food such as scrambled eggs exhibit a biphasic emptying profile: an initial lag phase followed by a linear emptying phase, which persists until all digestible residues have been expelled by the stomach. In normal controls, 40% to 80% of a solid meal is emptied within 2 hours of ingestion and more than 95% is expelled at 4 hours. Gastroparesis is diagnosed when the emptying times exceed the normal range. Solid-phase scintigraphy is more sensitive for detecting gastroparesis than liquid-phase scans. The result of a gastric emptying scan should be used in patient management in conjunction with the clinical presentation because some profoundly symptomatic patients will exhibit normal emptying, whereas other asymptomatic individuals may show pronounced gastric retention. Recently, some centers have begun to use isotope breath tests which measure the gastric emptying of nonradioactive substances such as ^{13}C-octanoate bound to a solid food such as a muffin. These tests can be performed in an office but are not as well standardized as scintigraphy. Other methods of assessing gastric emptying, such as ultrasound, magnetic resonance imaging, gastric impedance, and applied potential tomography, do not have significant advantages over gastric scintigraphy.

Other tests of upper gut function are performed in selected cases in referral centers. Gastroduodenal manometry involves the peroral or transnasal placement of a catheter that monitors pressure changes during a 6- to 8-hour period. During the initial 4 to 5 hours, fasting motility is recorded. During this time, one or more cycles of the migrating motor complex should be seen. Motor activity is then measured for 1 to 2 hours after a meal to detect the development of the characteristic fed motor pattern. Manometry also affords the option of testing the acute motor effects of prokinetic drugs. Manometry is considered for patients with unexplained nausea who have not responded to prokinetic therapy when a small intestinal dysmotility syndrome such as intestinal pseudoobstruction is a diagnostic possibility. Some clinicians use manometry to exclude small bowel motor dysfunction prior to placing a jejunostomy or considering a gastric resection in a patient with refractory gastroparesis. Electrogastrography (EGG) noninvasively measures gastric electrical activity. In humans, a pacemaker area in the proximal gastric body generates rhythmic depolarizations at 3 cycles per minute (cpm). They are known as slow waves, which regulate contractile activity in the stomach. EGG detects disruptions in slow wave rhythm that are too rapid (tachygastria) or too slow (bradygastria), as well as abnormal electrical responses to meal ingestion in some patients with nausea and vomiting. Abnormal EGGs are demonstrated in approximately 70% of patients with delayed gastric emptying; thus the technique has been proposed as another means of testing gastric emptying. EGGs also may be abnormal in patients with normal emptying, suggesting that slow wave disturbances are associated with symptom development independent of any motor disruption. EGG may be performed on patients with unexplained nausea and symptoms refractory to medical treatment; however, its clinical utility is limited by the lack of therapies designed to correct abnormal gastric electrical activity.

Management and Course

Dietary and Nonmedicinal Therapies

Nonmedicinal therapies are included in the initial recommendations for the treatment of gastroparesis. Medications that inhibit gastrointestinal motility should be discontinued if possible. The diet can be modified to reduce prolonged gastric distention. Ingesting several small meals per day may produce fewer symptoms than two to three large meals. Because liquids empty more rapidly than solids, solid foods with large amounts of indigestible residue should be avoided. Because lipids are the most potent nutrient inhibitors of gastric emptying, a low-fat diet may also reduce symptoms. Hyperglycemia delays gastric emptying of solid foods in type I diabetes. Although no long-term studies have confirmed a beneficial effect of tight glycemic control on gastric function in diabetic patients, it is reasonable to strive for near euglycemic blood levels to maximize gastric motor function and possibly to prevent further neuronal damage to the upper gut.

TABLE 30-2
Drugs with Prokinetic Effects on the Stomach

Medication	Mechanisms of Action	Dosage
Metoclopramide	Dopamine receptor antagonism	5–20 mg qid
	$5\text{-}HT_4$ agonist facilitation of acetylcholine release from enteric nerves	
	$5\text{-}HT_3$ receptor antagonism	
Erythromycin	Motilin receptor agonism	50–250 mg qid
Domperidone	Peripheral dopamine receptor antagonism (does not cross blood-brain barrier)	10–30 mg qid
Tegaserod	$5\text{-}HT_4$ agonist facilitation of acetylcholine release from enteric nerves	2–6 mg bid

5-HT, serotonin.

Prokinetic Medication Therapy

Medication therapy for gastroparesis focuses on agents that promote gastric emptying (Table 30-2). Metoclopramide is a substituted benzamide that acts by serotonin ($5\text{-}HT_4$) receptor facilitation of cholinergic transmission in the gastric myenteric plexus, as well as by dopamine and serotonin ($5\text{-}HT_3$) receptor antagonism. Metoclopramide acutely enhances gastric emptying, but a sustained prokinetic effect is not always attained. Despite this, patients report prolonged symptom improvement, indicating that the antiemetic effects of metoclopramide may be as important as its prokinetic action. Drowsiness, dystonias, galactorrhea, agitation, and mood disturbances caused by the central nervous system antidopaminergic actions limit the use of metoclopramide. Some cases of irreversible tardive dyskinesia also have been observed with this drug. Erythromycin is a potent stimulant of gastric emptying through its action on gastroduodenal receptors for motilin, a hormone that regulates normal fasting upper gut motility. At low doses, erythromycin is an effective prokinetic agent, but at high doses it causes vomiting and pain as a result of intense motor spasms. There appears to be some desensitization to the beneficial effects of erythromycin with long-term use. Domperidone is a peripheral dopamine-receptor antagonist that does not cross the blood-brain barrier and, thus, does not cause many of the central nervous system side effects such as dystonias, agitation, or tardive dyskinesia that are seen with metoclopramide. The drug is not marketed in the United States but is available in most other countries. The $5\text{-}HT_4$ receptor agonist tegaserod accelerates gastric emptying in gastroparesis, but its clinical utility in this condition is unproven.

In some patients, oral administration of prokinetic drugs in pill form does not produce significant clinical benefit. Liquid suspensions of metoclopramide and erythromycin may provide superior responses in some patients because liquids are more quickly emptied into the duodenum where they can be absorbed. Both drugs may be given intravenously in inpatient settings for acute gastroparesis exacerbations. Metoclopramide also may be administered subcutaneously for refractory symptoms in an effort to preclude hospitalization.

Antiemetic Medication Therapy

Antiemetic drugs without prokinetic properties may serve useful adjunctive roles in managing gastroparesis. Antidopaminergic agents such as prochlorperazine may provide additional symptom control. 5-HT_3 receptor antagonists such as ondansetron and anticholinergics such as scopolamine are advocated by some clinicians, although there have been no studies proving their efficacy. Tricyclic antidepressants reduce nausea in many patients with diabetic gastropathy and have also been used in some diabetics with delayed gastric emptying.

Endoscopic, Radiographic, and Surgical Therapies

For patients resistant to diet and drug therapy, endoscopic and surgical treatments may be offered. Endoscopic injection of botulinum toxin into the pylorus reportedly improves gastric emptying and symptoms of gastroparesis, presumably by reducing resistance to outflow into the duodenum. Endoscopic, radiographic, or surgical placement of a gastrostomy tube can provide intermittent decompression if the stomach becomes filled with gas or fluid. Placement of a feeding jejunostomy allows the patient to continue receiving enteral nutrition when food ingestion is precluded by severe nausea and vomiting. In rare cases, home total parenteral nutrition can be given to maintain caloric and fluid sustenance. This option is best reserved for individuals with associated small bowel dysmotility. Surgical implantation of a gastric neurostimulator may produce striking reductions in nausea and vomiting in selected patients with diabetic or idiopathic gastroparesis. Pancreatic transplantation can stabilize the loss of neuronal function in a patient with severe diabetic complications; however, its benefits in diabetic gastroparesis are not established. Gastric resections usually are of limited benefit, although total gastrectomy reportedly reduces symptoms specifically in patients with severe gastroparesis caused by prior vagotomy and gastric drainage.

DISORDERS WITH RAPID GASTRIC EMPTYING

Incidence and Epidemiology

Abnormally rapid gastric emptying is clearly clinically relevant in only one subset of patients—those who have undergone vagotomy and gastric drainage for ulcer disease or malignancy. The clinical manifestation of this complication is the dumping syndrome, which occurs after 8% to 15% of surgeries. Other conditions are associated with accelerated emptying, but their clinical relevance is uncertain.

Etiology and Pathogenesis
Postsurgical Dumping Syndrome

Any surgical procedure involving vagotomy may produce the dumping syndrome. In general, the greater degrees of vagal interruption produce more severe symptoms. Characteristically, these operations produce accelerated emptying of liquids with variable effects on solid-phase gastric emptying. The acceleration of liquid emptying overwhelms the postprandial absorptive capabilities of the proximal intestine, leading to fluid shifts and massive release of vasoactive peptide hormones, including vasoactive intestinal polypeptide, serotonin, bradykinin, substance P, enteroglucagon, gastric inhibitory peptide, and neurotensin, which are responsible for the gastrointestinal and vasomotor symptoms of dumping syndrome. There may also be an excessive release of insulin that persists into the late postprandial period and produces hypoglycemia 1 to 4 hours after eating. Certain procedures (e.g., truncal vagotomy with antrectomy or pyloroplasty, and subtotal gastrectomy) accelerate the initial emptying of solids and impair gastric sieving. As a result, large quantities of larger-than-normal food particles are delivered to the intestine, where they are inefficiently digested and absorbed.

Other operations that restrict the accommodation of the proximal stomach to an ingested meal also may produce the dumping syndrome. This condition has been observed in some patients after fundoplication for gastroesophageal reflux disease. In these individuals, food is quickly propelled to the distal stomach where it is evacuated into the intestine more rapidly than normal.

Other Causes of Rapid Emptying

Gastric emptying of fatty liquid meals is accelerated in patients with pancreatic insufficiency and marked steatorrhea. Liquid emptying may be accelerated in some individuals with duodenal ulcer disease. Patients with Zollinger-Ellison syndrome exhibit rapid liquid and solid emptying, which is probably not caused by gastric hypersecretion. Many newly diagnosed diabetics have accelerated rather than delayed gastric emptying. Patients with hyperthyroidism may have accelerated emptying, as do some morbidly obese individuals. In most instances, these findings of accelerated emptying probably do not cause symptoms and are not clinically important.

Clinical Features

The early dumping syndrome that occurs 15 to 60 minutes after ingesting a meal is characterized by alimentary symptoms (abdominal pain, diarrhea, gas, bloating, borborygmi, and nausea) and vasomotor symptoms (flushing, palpitations, diaphoresis, lightheadedness, tachycardia, and even syncope). Physical examination of these patients may reveal orthostatic or even supine effects on pulse and blood pressure. When severe, the dumping syndrome can be debilitating, producing greater than 30% weight loss. The late dumping syndrome occurs 2 to 4 hours after eating. Symptoms include diaphoresis, palpitations, tremulousness, hunger, weakness, confusion, and syncope and are believed to result from reactive hypoglycemia.

Findings on Diagnostic Testing

The diagnosis of dumping syndrome is based on eliciting a characteristic constellation of symptoms in a patient who has undergone gastric surgery. Diagnostic testing usually is not necessary. A hematocrit or plasma osmolarity determination in the early postprandial period after a glucose challenge may show hemoconcentration. Measures of packed cell volume and gastric scintigraphy are occasionally obtained, but they rarely provide critical information.

Management and Course

Dietary Management

Dietary recommendations for patients with dumping syndrome include ingesting foods high in proteins and fats and low in carbohydrates with minimal fluid intake during the meal. Nonnutritive fluids should be taken before or after ingesting solids. After vagotomy, liquid emptying is more rapid while sitting; thus, some patients may benefit by assuming a supine position immediately after eating. Viscous guar and pectin have been recommended to thicken ingested liquids, but the efficacy of this practice is not proven.

Medication Therapy

The somatostatin analog octreotide reduces symptoms of early and late dumping syndrome. The effects of octreotide on gastric emptying are controversial, but it clearly blunts exaggerated postprandial hormone release. Although the acute benefits of octreotide on the dumping syndrome are well documented, there is less information on its long-term efficacy. Diarrhea has been reported with long-term use of octreotide in the dumping syndrome.

Surgical Therapy

Proposed surgical therapies for the dumping syndrome include pyloric reconstruction, placing a Roux-en-Y gastrojejunostomy, reversing a gastrojejunostomy, constructing an antiperistaltic loop between the stomach and intestine, and retrograde electrical pacing of the small intestine. Each treatment has its enthusiasts; however, treatment fails in many patients and postoperative gastroparesis develops in others. Thus, it is difficult to recommend surgical therapy for the majority of patients with dumping syndrome.

CHAPTER 31

Acid Peptic Disorders and Zollinger-Ellison Syndrome

ACID PEPTIC DISEASE

Incidence and Epidemiology

Despite decreasing prevalence in the United States, peptic ulcer disease (PUD) remains a significant medical problem with considerable morbidity, mortality, and resource expenditure. In 1995, there were 500,000 new cases and 4 million recurrences of PUD. The total direct cost of gastric and duodenal ulcers has been estimated at $3.3 billion dollars annually, plus an additional $6.2 billion in productivity (indirect) costs. The incidence of duodenal ulcer peaked from 1950 to 1970 and has declined since, probably because of the decreasing prevalence of *Helicobacter pylori*. Conversely, there has been a significant increase in hospitalizations of elderly patients with ulcer hemorrhage and perforation, which has been attributed to the increased use of NSAIDs. In addition to *H pylori* and NSAIDs, it appears that genetic factors play a role in ulcer pathogenesis, as there is a threefold increase in lifetime prevalence among first-degree relatives and a 50% concordance among monozygotic twins. Persons whose blood group is O and those who are nonsecretors of blood group antigens are at increased risk of PUD. Other causes of PUD include gastrinomas, systemic mastocytosis, and diseases that occur sporadically and, less commonly, as genetically linked syndromes (multiple endocrine neoplasia type 1 and familial mastocytosis).

Etiology and Pathogenesis

Helicobacter pylori

Helicobacter pylori is a curved, gram-negative rod that produces a characteristic highly active urease. Chronic *H pylori* infection causes most cases of histological gastritis and PUD and predisposes to development of gastric carcinoma. Evidence suggests that *H pylori* is transmitted by fecal-oral routes, based on increases in prevalence among family members, in chronic care facilities, among endoscopy personnel, and the demonstration of positive stool cultures for *H pylori* in affected individuals. Contaminated water also may be a source in some populations. In the United States, the prevalence of *H pylori* gastritis increases from 10% at age 20 to 50% at age 60; however, this finding is likely to be the result of a birth cohort phenomenon and does not indicate increased acquisition with advancing age. The age-adjusted prevalence rates are higher among Latin Americans and African Americans.

H pylori colonizes the fundus, body, and antrum of the stomach and is found in 70% to 95% of patients with active chronic gastritis, which is characterized by histological increases in mucosal neutrophils and round cells. Histological gastritis may occur only in the distal stomach, and when *H pylori* is eradicated, the lesion resolves. Patients who contract *H pylori* may progress from active superficial chronic gastritis to atrophic gastritis, which may then be associated with *H pylori* clearance. It has been postulated that gastric metaplasia in the duodenum secondary to acid production is necessary for developing duodenal ulcer disease.

H pylori infection affects 90% of patients with duodenal ulcers and 70% to 90% of those with gastric ulcers. The etiologic role of this organism is supported by numerous studies showing that *H pylori* eradication prevents ulcer recurrences. Treatment of *H pylori* also may produce more rapid ulcer healing and higher rates of ulcer healing. However, only 15% of those infected by *H pylori* develop PUD, which suggests that specific factors are required for ulceration to occur. The role of *H pylori* in complicated PUD is less defined; more recent data indicate that only 50% to 70% of patients with bleeding duodenal ulcers were infected with *H pylori*. The pathogenicity of *H pylori* appears to be related to abnormalities of acid secretion, mucosal bicarbonate production, mucosal immune response, cytotoxin production, and ammonia production, which injures the gastric mucosal barrier. Patients who are positive for *H pylori* have higher basal and meal-stimulated gastrin release, which decreases after *H pylori* is eradicated. Acid secretion is higher in *H pylori*–positive duodenal ulcer patients; however, it may not decrease after *H pylori* eradication. *H pylori* releases a chemotactic factor for neutrophils and monocytes and elaborates cytokines and reactive oxygen metabolites, which may contribute to mucosal damage.

H pylori may be a predisposing factor for developing gastric adenocarcinoma as well as for some gastric lymphomas. Chronic gastritis and *H pylori* infection are commonly associated with the development of adenocarcinoma, often in patients who acquired *H pylori* early in life. *H pylori* may be a risk factor for gastric lymphoma of mucosa-associated lymphoid tissue; regression of this low-grade lymphoma may occur after *H pylori* is eradicated. Cancers of the gastric cardia are not associated with *H pylori* and appear to be more linked to adenocarcinoma of the esophagus.

NSAIDs

Each year, 2% to 4% of persons who take NSAIDs develop serious complications, and up to 20,000 deaths per year are attributed to NSAID-related complications. Gastric erosions are diagnosed by endoscopy in 30% to 50% of patients on chronic

NSAID therapy, although these lesions are usually superficial and are not associated with subsequent ulcer development or symptoms. The relative risk of developing gastric ulcer among NSAID users compared to non–NSAID users is 4.0 and for duodenal ulcer is 1.7 to 3.2. Dyspepsia in patients who take NSAIDs is more common in the first few weeks of therapy and declines with time. Only 26% of patients with dyspepsia have ulcers; conversely, 40% of patients with NSAID-induced ulcers are asymptomatic. More worrisome is the finding that among patients who develop hemorrhage, 60% have no prior symptoms. Thus, the absence of dyspepsia in NSAID users does not eliminate the possibility of ulcer complications.

Risk factors associated with NSAID-induced ulcer complications include a previous history of complicated or uncomplicated PUD, a regimen of multiple or high-dose NSAIDs, advanced age, and concurrent anticoagulant or steroid use. The relative risk of NSAID-related complications is about 14-fold higher among persons with a past history of complicated ulcer disease compared to NSAID users without such as history. Complications also depend on medication doses. A 30-mg dose of aspirin is associated with an increased risk of GI bleeding, and the risk increases with higher doses. Persons who take 1200 mg/d have an eightfold increase in developing complicated ulcers compared to placebo-treated subjects. Concomitant use of corticosteroids and NSAIDs increases the risk of complications compared with using NSAIDs alone. The risk of gastrointestinal injury differs among specific NSAIDs and generally relates to the potency and duration of cyclooxygenase (COX)-1 isoenzyme inhibition. Nabumetone and etodolac inhibit systemic prostaglandin production but spare gastroduodenal prostaglandin synthesis, leading to lower rates of ulceration and fewer gastrointestinal side effects. COX-2 specific inhibitors have been compared with traditional NSAIDs in several large, randomized trials, where they showed a significantly lower incidence of gastrointestinal injury. One important caveat is that the protective effect of the COX-2 specific inhibitors is diminished if there is concomitant use of low-dose aspirin. In addition to gastric and duodenal ulcers, complications of NSAID use include the development of dyspepsia; ulceration and weblike strictures of the small intestine; acute colitis; exacerbations of inflammatory bowel disease; and ulcers, strictures, and perforation of the colon.

NSAIDs induce mucosal injury by direct damage and systemic effects. NSAIDs may directly damage epithelial cells, inhibit mucosal prostaglandin secretion, reduce mucus secretion, and interfere with cell turnover. COX inhibition causes reduced prostaglandin production, which leads to diminished mucus and bicarbonate secretion, decreased mucosal blood flow, persistence of gastric acid secretion, and enhanced neutrophil adherence to vascular endothelial linings. Platelet COX inhibition also increases the risk of hemorrhage from mucosal lesions.

Additional Factors Associated with Ulcer Disease

Tobacco smokers are twice as likely as nonsmokers to develop ulcers. Cigarette smoking may increase susceptibility to *H pylori* infection. Cigarette smokers have altered gastric motility and increased production of oxygen free radicals, platelet-activating factor, pituitary vasopressin, and gastric endothelin. Additional effects of smoking include reduced gastroduodenal prostaglandin production, decreased bicarbonate secretion, decreased mucosal blood flow, and increased duodenogastric reflux.

Although psychological factors may play a role in the pathogenesis of PUD, the causality of these elements is uncertain. In a study of 4500 patients conducted in

TABLE 31-1
Diseases Associated with Duodenal Ulcers

Evidence strongly supports an association
    Zollinger-Ellison syndrome
    Systemic mastocytosis
    Multiple endocrine neoplasia type I
    Chronic pulmonary disease
    Chronic renal failure
    Cirrhosis
    Kidney stones
    α_1-Antitrypsin deficiency

Evidence only suggests an association
    Crohn's disease
    Hyperparathyroidism without multiple endocrine neoplasia type I
    Coronary artery disease
    Polycythemia vera
    Chronic pancreatitis
    Cystic fibrosis

the United States, emotional stress was associated with a relative risk of 1.4 to 2.9 for developing ulcers.

Specific diseases are associated with increases in PUD (Table 31-1). The prevalence of PUD is increased threefold with chronic pulmonary disease, although the role of tobacco smoking in this association is uncertain. Patients with cystic fibrosis have an increased risk of PUD because of reduced bicarbonate secretion. α_1-Antitrypsin deficiency may lead to PUD because of a lack of protease inhibitors. Cirrhosis and renal failure predispose to development of PUD by unknown mechanisms.

Seasonal variations have been reported for PUD development, as have regional and geographic differences. The effect of corticosteroid use on ulcer development, in the absence of NSAID use, is controversial. Ethanol in amounts routinely ingested has no proven ulcerogenic effect on the gastroduodenal mucosa. There are no obvious dietary components that increase the risk of PUD, although foods that induce dyspepsia should be avoided.

Associated Factors in Pathogenesis

Mucosal defenses. The prevention of gastroduodenal mucosal damage involves preepithelial, epithelial, and subepithelial factors. The preepithelial factors include the mucus-bicarbonate barrier, which serves as a modest barrier to H^+ and pepsin; the mucoid cap, which is a mucus and fibrin structure that forms in response to injury; and surface-active phospholipids, which enhance cell membrane hydrophobicity and increase mucus viscosity. Epithelial factors include restitution, which involves repair of epithelium by movement of existing cells over the damaged area; epithelial cell metabolism (e.g., transmembrane, transcellular resistance); acid-base transporters; and mucus secretion. The principal subepithelial factor is mucosal blood flow, which delivers nutrients and bicarbonate to the epithelium. Impairment of one or more of these defense mechanisms by *H pylori*, NSAIDs, or ischemia leads to mucosal injury and ulceration.

Duodenal ulcer pathophysiology.   Abnormalities associated with duodenal ulcer formation include acid dysregulation and abnormalities in duodenal mucosal defense. About one third of patients with duodenal ulcers have abnormal responses to pentagastrin or histamine, whereas 60% have increased and abnormally prolonged acid responses to meal ingestion. When basal acid output (BAO) is expressed as a fraction of maximal acid output (MAO) stimulated by pentagastrin, only 10% to 20% of patients with duodenal ulcers are abnormal. Some clinicians postulate that increased nocturnal acid secretion may be more important than BAO in the pathogenesis of duodenal ulcer. Infection with *H pylori* increases basal and meal-stimulated gastrin concentrations, but it remains uncertain whether patients with duodenal ulcers exhibit normal or increased sensitivity to circulating gastrin. The adherent mucus gel layer in the duodenum is weaker in patients with duodenal ulcers than in healthy individuals, and bicarbonate production in the duodenal bulb is reduced.

Gastric ulcer pathophysiology.   Most (70%) gastric ulcers are associated with *H pylori* infection or NSAID use. Three types exist: type I ulcers occur in the gastric body but are not associated with other gastroduodenal disease; type II ulcers also occur in the body but are associated with duodenal scarring or ulcers; type III ulcers occur in the prepyloric area. The pathophysiology of type II and type III ulcers is similar to that of duodenal ulcers, whereas type I ulcers are associated with reduced or normal acid secretion. Antral gastritis is prominent early in the course of gastric ulcer disease and may progress to gastric atrophy. Pyloric sphincter dysfunction and abnormal gastric motility have been hypothesized to play a role in gastric ulcer formation. Basal and stimulated gastric acid secretion are normal in patients with gastric ulcers. Gastric ulcers also can form in achlorhydric conditions. Gastric ulcers tend to occur near the angularis, a region where the mucosa is supplied arterially, rather than by a rich submucosal plexus, which suggests an ischemic pathogenesis.

Clinical Features

Abdominal pain, the most common presenting symptom of PUD, occurs in 94% of patients. The pain usually is burning in quality, epigastric in location without radiation, and is relieved by food or antacids. The most discriminating symptom is pain that awakens the patient between midnight and 3 AM. This symptom affects two thirds of patients with duodenal ulcers and one third of those with gastric ulcers; however, this is not specific because one third of patients with nonulcer dyspepsia also report nocturnal pain. About 10% of patients with PUD, especially with NSAID-related disease, present with complications without a history of ulcer pain.

Complications of PUD include hemorrhage, perforation, penetration, and obstruction. Hemorrhage occurs in 15% of patients with PUD and is most common after age 60, probably because of NSAID use in this age group. Antecedent dyspepsia affects 80% to 90% of patients. If *H pylori* is the etiology of the ulcer, eradication of *H pylori* prevents recurrent ulcers and ulcer complications. Perforation occurs in 7% of patients and is increasing in incidence secondary to increased NSAID use. Duodenal ulcers perforate anteriorly, and gastric ulcers perforate along the anterior wall of the lesser curvature. Penetration differs from perforation in that the ulcer erodes into an adjacent organ instead of the peritoneal cavity. Gastric ulcers penetrate into the left lobe of the liver or the colon, causing a gastrocolic fistula, whereas duodenal ulcers penetrate into the pancreas, producing pancreatitis. Inflammation, edema, and scarring near the gastroduodenal junction can cause outlet obstruction, which occurs in 2% of patients with PUD, producing symptoms of heartburn, early satiety, weight loss, abdominal pain, and vomiting.

Findings on Diagnostic Testing

The differential diagnosis of dyspepsia includes a wide variety of gastrointestinal disorders, including PUD, functional dyspepsia, upper gastrointestinal neoplasia, pancreaticobiliary diseases, mesenteric ischemia, and Crohn's disease. There are two major approaches to managing dyspepsia: evaluate and base treatment on findings or treat empirically with medical therapy. There is growing acceptance for the latter approach, endorsed by the American College of Gastroenterology, if the patient is younger than age 45 to 50, has no warning signs (dysphagia, weight loss, bleeding, or anemia), and is otherwise at low risk of upper gastrointestinal malignancy or complications of disease. If the patient presents at an older age, with warning signs or failure to respond to empiric therapy, appropriate diagnostic evaluation should be pursued. The details of specific diagnostic tests and therapy are presented in the following sections.

Radiographic and Endoscopic Studies

Although air-contrast upper gastrointestinal barium radiography and upper gastrointestinal endoscopy show nearly equivalent sensitivity and specificity in diagnosing PUD, endoscopy has emerged as the preferred test because biopsy specimens can be obtained to document the presence of histological gastritis or *H pylori* infection and to exclude malignancy in gastric ulcers. Radiographic tests cannot definitely exclude malignant disease; therefore, endoscopic biopsy is required for gastric ulcers found by barium radiography. In patients with ulcers that are not secondary to NSAID use, four to eight biopsy specimens will yield a correct diagnosis in more than 95% of gastric malignancies. All suggestive gastric ulcers should be examined by repeat upper gastrointestinal endoscopy 8 weeks after initiating appropriate therapy. Although gastric ulcers that clearly develop in association with NSAID use do not always need biopsy, they should be observed until healed.

Helicobacter pylori Testing

A variety of invasive and noninvasive methods may be used to document *H pylori* infection. Some tests can document active infection whereas others cannot distinguish current from prior infection.

Invasive tests. Biopsy specimens obtained by endoscopy are examined using Giemsa, Warthin-Starry silver, or hematoxylin-eosin stains, which are the standard for diagnosing *H pylori*. Biopsy specimens may also be placed in gels containing urea and an indicator (e.g., CLO-test, Hpfast, PyloriTek, Pronto Dry) to detect the presence of *H pylori*–associated urease activity. Urease tests have 90% sensitivity with specificity of 95% to 100%. Rapid urease or biopsy examination will indicate the presence of active *H pylori* infection. Biopsy tests may give false-negative results in patients who are bleeding acutely or who have been given short courses of antibiotics. Polymerase chain reaction assays may be performed on biopsy specimens, but this technique has been largely limited to research that seeks to identify different *H pylori* strains.

Noninvasive tests. Enzyme-linked immunosorbent assays are available for detecting serum immunoglobulin G (IgG) antibodies to *H pylori*, with sensitivities of 80% to 95% and specificities of 75% to 95%. Titers may decrease over 6 to 12 months but frequently remain abnormal; therefore, serologic testing is a poor means of assessing active *H pylori* infection and is not recommended for documenting eradication after therapy. Breath tests may be performed using either ^{13}C-urea (nonradioactive isotope) or ^{14}C-urea (radioactive isotope) labels, which are orally administered. Exhaled isotopic carbon dioxide concentrations correlate with intragastric *H pylori* urease activity. Breath tests have 90% to 100% sensitivities and specificities for active *H pylori* infection; however, false-negative results can be produced by intake of proton pump inhibitors (PPIs), bismuth compounds, histamine receptor antagonists, and antibiotics. It is recommended that these drugs be held for 2 to 4 weeks prior to examination by breath tests. Fecal antigen detection is another noninvasive method to measure active *H pylori* infection. With this test, an enzymatic immunoassay (HpSA) detects the presence of *H pylori* antigen in stool specimens with high levels of sensitivity and specificity.

Initial Management of Dyspepsia

The initial treatment of patients who present with uninvestigated dyspepsia is controversial. The timing of structural evaluation of the upper gastrointestinal tract and *H pylori* testing is balanced by the practicality and economic advantage of empiric therapy. In patients younger than age 45 to 50 with mild or intermittent symptoms, empiric treatment with acid-suppressive drugs for 4 weeks is reasonable. If symptoms resolve and do not recur, no further evaluation is needed. Some clinicians advocate *H pylori* serologic testing in this population, and, if the test results are positive, treatment with triple or quadruple therapy, including antibiotics and acid suppression. Initial upper gastrointestinal endoscopy is recommended for patients older than age 50, for those with long-standing or recurrent symptoms, and for those with "alarm symptoms," such as weight loss, bleeding or anemia, or dysphagia, to assess for the presence of upper gastrointestinal malignancy. For endoscopically documented PUD, a biopsy specimen should be obtained for urease testing and histological study. Urea breath or stool antigen testing is reserved to confirm *H pylori* eradication. Decision analyses have been conducted to determine the most cost-effective approach to patients with dyspepsia, but to date, the results depend highly on the prevalence of *H pylori* in the population and the costs of diagnostic testing. No one diagnostic approach is consistently favored.

Management and Course

Most gastric and duodenal ulcers are treated medically with drugs that suppress acid secretion, neutralize gastric acid, have cytoprotective effects, and eradicate *H pylori*. Endoscopy is indicated for control of hemorrhage and possibly gastric outlet obstruction. Surgery is required for hemorrhage not controlled by endoscopic methods and for other complications such as perforation and obstruction.

Medical Therapy for Ulcers

Antacids. Over-the-counter antacids are often used by patients for symptomatic control of dyspepsia, although their role in primary management of PUD is limited. Antacids bind bile salts, inhibit pepsin activity, and have cytoprotective effects (e.g., increased prostaglandin release, mucus production, bicarbonate release), in addition to their acid-neutralizing effects. Adverse effects include sodium overload, hypercalcemia, metabolic alkalosis, or renal insufficiency, depending on the formulation. Antacids that contain magnesium may cause diarrhea, whereas aluminum compounds cause constipation and are associated with neurotoxicity in patients with renal failure.

Bismuth subsalicylate coats ulcer craters, possibly forming a protective layer against the effects of acid and pepsin. Bismuth has no effect on acid secretion, but it may decrease degradation of epidermal growth factor and inhibit the growth of *H pylori*. Toxicity of bismuth subsalicylate is extremely rare, although significant blood salicylate levels may occur. A drug combination containing ranitidine and a bismuth compound has been released for treating *H pylori* infection.

H₂ receptor antagonists. Four H_2 receptor antagonists are approved for clinical use: cimetidine, ranitidine, famotidine, and nizatidine. These agents inhibit basal, histamine-stimulated, pentagastrin-stimulated, and meal-stimulated acid secretion in a linear, dose-dependent manner with a maximal 90% inhibition of vagal-stimulated and gastrin-stimulated acid production and near-total inhibition of nocturnal and basal secretion. Equipotent oral doses are 40 mg famotidine, 300 mg ranitidine, 300 mg nizatidine, and 1200 to 1600 mg cimetidine. Once daily, bedtime dosing of H_2 receptor antagonists has been approved for treating PUD. Plasma concentrations of H_2 receptor antagonists are affected by renal insufficiency; doses should be halved when creatinine clearance is less than 15 to 30 mL/min (cimetidine, famotidine) or less than 50 mL/min (nizatidine, ranitidine). Side effects from these agents are rare but include cardiac rhythm disturbances with intravenous therapy, antiandrogenic effects resulting in gynecomastia and impotence (caused by cimetidine), hyperprolactinemia with galactorrhea, central neural effects (e.g., headache, lethargy, depression, memory loss), and hematologic effects (e.g., leukopenia, anemia, thrombocytopenia, and elevations in hepatic aminotransferases). Cimetidine (and less commonly ranitidine) binds to hepatic cytochrome P450 enzymes and strongly inhibits the metabolism of theophylline, phenytoin, lidocaine, quinidine, and warfarin.

Proton pump inhibitors. There are many PPIs currently available, including omeprazole, lansoprazole, rabeprazole, pantoprazole, and esomeprazole. These substituted benzimidazoles inhibit H^+, K^+-adenosine triphosphatase activity in the gastric parietal cell canalicular membrane, leading to nearly complete inhibition of basal and stimulated acid secretion. PPIs have far greater effects on daytime (meal-stimulated) acid secretion than H_2 receptor antagonists. The optimal time for drug intake is a half hour to 1 hour before meals because PPIs are maximally stimulated by food. PPI dosing is not modified by renal or hepatic disease. PPIs are well tolerated but have been associated with side effects, including headache, constipation, nausea, abdominal pain, and diarrhea. Omeprazole inhibits certain cytochrome P450 activities, which alters the metabolism of diazepam, phenytoin, and warfarin; but the drug has no effect on the metabolism of theophylline, lidocaine, and quinidine. Studies have shown that 3% to 6% of patients on chronic omeprazole develop profound hypergastrinemia (>400 pg/mL). The clinical consequence of hypergastrinemia is unknown; however, long-term omeprazole therapy has not been associated with gastric dysplasia, carcinoid tumors, or carcinoma, although enterochromaffin-like cell hyperplasia has been reported. Atrophic gastritis may accelerate in *H pylori*–infected individuals treated with PPIs, although eradication of the organism in patients requiring long-term PPI therapy has not been strongly advocated.

Cytoprotective agents. Sucralfate is a complex salt of sucrose that binds to tissue proteins and forms a protective barrier that decreases exposure of the epithelium to acid, bile salts, and pepsin. Sucralfate may also stabilize gastric mucus and have trophic effects on the mucosa. Adverse effects of sucralfate include constipation and, in renal failure, the possibility of aluminum toxicity. The drug also binds several drugs, limiting their absorption.

Misoprostol is a prostaglandin E_1 analog that inhibits gastric acid secretion, stimulates bicarbonate and mucus secretion, enhances mucosal blood flow, and inhibits cell turnover. The major limitation on its use relates to dose-related diarrhea that occurs in 10% to 30% of patients. The use of misoprostol is contraindicated in women who may be pregnant.

Treatment of *Helicobacter pylori*–Induced Peptic Ulcer Disease

Most peptic ulcers are caused by *H pylori* infection, and the presence of an *H pylori*–related duodenal or gastric ulcer is an indication for specific therapy to eradicate the organism (Table 31-2). Currently, eradication of *H pylori* to treat nonulcer (functional) dyspepsia is controversial. A variety of antibiotics are effective against *H pylori*, including ampicillin, amoxicillin, metronidazole, tetracyclines, quinolones, erythromycin, and clarithromycin. Bismuth compounds are also effective. Acid suppression with PPIs (and to a lesser extent, H_2 receptor antagonists) enhances eradication of the organism. Single-agent regimens are rarely effective in eradicating *H pylori*. Triple or quadruple therapy with antibiotics and acid suppression is advocated for treating *H pylori*. Numerous regimens have documented efficacy, but a 2-week course of bismuth subsalicylate (2 tablets, four times daily), metronidazole (250 mg, four times daily), and tetracycline (500 mg, four times daily), plus an antisecretory drug (e.g., an H_2 receptor antagonist or PPI) is an inexpensive and effective program that has eradication rates of 80% to 95% and is considered the standard of treatment. Alternative strategies include a high-dose PPI with clarithromycin and a second antibiotic (e.g., amoxicillin or metronidazole) for 2 weeks. Shorter courses have been proposed to enhance compliance,

---

TABLE 31-2
Eradication Rates of *Helicobacter Pylori* with Various Regimens

Regimen	Eradication Rate (%)
Bismuth	
Bismuth subsalicylate	5–10
Colloidal bismuth subcitrate	10–35
Single antibiotics	
Amoxicillin	15–25
Clarithromycin	50
Other antibiotics	0–5
Proton pump inhibitors	0–15
(omeprazole, lansoprazole)	
Dual therapy	
Bismuth/amoxicillin	30–60
Bismuth/metronidazole	30–75
Amoxicillin/metronidazole	55–95
Omeprazole/amoxicillin or clarithromycin	55–85
Triple therapy	
Bismuth/metronidazole/tetracycline or amoxicillin	80–95

but the eradication rates decrease significantly if treatment is less than 10 days. The management of *H pylori* that is refractory to two courses of triple therapy is controversial; some clinicians recommend therapy with four to five drugs given in very high doses. However, these aggressive programs may produce adverse effects (e.g., antibiotic-associated colitis in 25% of cases), raising questions about their risk-benefit profiles.

After treatment is concluded, no follow-up is needed in most cases unless the patient remains symptomatic. Urea breath or stool antigen testing 1 month after completing therapy should be considered to document *H pylori* eradication in patients with complicated disease, who have severe underlying medical illness, or who have recurrent symptoms. After successful eradication of *H pylori*, the recurrence rate of gastric and duodenal ulcers is less than 10%. In contrast, PUD recurs within 2 years in 50% to 100% of patients infected with *H pylori* if no eradication or chronic acid suppression is provided.

Treating and Preventing NSAID-Related Peptic Ulcer Disease

Whenever possible, a patient with an NSAID-induced ulcer should discontinue the inciting drug. In the absence of concomitant NSAID use, antisecretory therapy with H_2 receptor antagonists, PPIs, or cytoprotective agents leads to ulcer healing within 8 weeks in most cases. If NSAIDs must be continued for their analgesic or antiinflammatory effects, a number of regimens have demonstrated efficacy. H_2 receptor antagonists in conventional doses may heal duodenal ulcers, but gastric ulcers generally are resistant to healing if NSAIDs are continued. In randomized clinical trials, PPIs have effectively healed both duodenal and gastric ulcers in the presence of continued NSAID use (95% rate of healing within 8 weeks). Misoprostol has efficacy equal to PPIs in healing ulcers associated with NSAID use.

Strategies to prevent NSAID-associated ulcers should be considered for patients at high risk. Factors associated with the development of ulcer complications among patients using NSAIDs include a past history of complicated or uncomplicated ulcer, multiple or high-dose NSAIDs, advanced age, and use of anticoagulants or steroids. Misoprostol in 200-μg doses, four times per day, significantly reduces the 3-month incidence of gastric and duodenal ulcers. PPIs have also been demonstrated to reduce the incidence of recurrent ulcers and ulcer complications significantly in patients with NSAID-associated ulcers who must remain on NSAID therapy. COX-2 specific inhibitors are associated with rates of ulcers and ulcer complications significantly lower than those of conventional NSAIDs; however, unlike PPIs, their protective effect is limited to patients who are not taking aspirin.

Management of Refractory Ulcers

Duodenal ulcers are considered refractory if 8 weeks of therapy fail to heal the ulcer; refractory gastric ulcers are defined by lack of response to 12 weeks of treatment. Overall, 5% to 10% of ulcers are considered refractory. Causes of refractory ulcers include patient noncompliance, surreptitious NSAID use, tobacco use, untreated *H pylori* infection, gastric acid hypersecretion (gastrinoma), and malignancy. Rare causes of chronic ulceration are Crohn's disease, amyloidosis, sarcoidosis, eosinophilic gastroenteritis, and infections (e.g., tuberculosis, syphilis, and cytomegalovirus). Compliance with prescribed therapy should be evaluated, and any NSAID consumption should be examined. Endoscopic follow-up is indicated with performance of multiple biopsies to exclude malignancy and nonpeptic causes of ulcer. Serum gastrin should be measured to exclude Zollinger-Ellison syndrome. High doses of PPIs can heal 90% of refractory ulcers after 8 weeks, reducing the need for surgical intervention. However, surgery should be considered for diagnosing and treating patients who do not respond to this aggressive regimen.

ZOLLINGER-ELLISON SYNDROME

Incidence and Epidemiology

Zollinger-Ellison syndrome (ZES) is a disorder of acid hypersecretion secondary to a gastrin-secreting tumor or gastrinoma. The incidence of ZES among patients with PUD is estimated at 0.1% to 1%. Although most patients diagnosed with ZES are between ages 30 and 50, the age range of affected individuals is from 7 to 90 years, with a male-to-female dominance of 2:1 to 3:2. Gastrinomas may be sporadic or they may be genetically transmitted and associated with multiple endocrine neoplasia type I (MEN I). Sporadic gastrinomas often are malignant, whereas MEN I–associated gastrinomas follow a more benign course.

Etiology and Pathogenesis

ZES is characterized by severe PUD caused by gastric acid hypersecretion resulting from gastrin derived from non–beta-cell neoplasms. More than 80% of gastrinomas are localized in the gastrinoma triangle, which is bounded by the confluence of the cystic duct and common bile duct superiorly, the junction of the second and third duodenal portions inferiorly, and the junction of the pancreatic neck and body medially. Although classically considered a pancreatic tumor, 40% of gastrinomas arise within the duodenal wall. Primary tumors less commonly originate in the stomach, bones, ovaries, liver, and lymph nodes. More than 50% of gastrinomas are malignant, and 30% to 55% of patients present with multiple tumors or metastatic disease.

Gastrinoma cells are heterogeneous; generally well differentiated; and contain chromogranin, neuron-specific enolase, and tyrosine hydroxylase. Other peptides produced by gastrinomas include somatostatin, pancreatic polypeptide, adrenocorticotropic hormone, and vasoactive intestinal polypeptide (VIP). Cushing syndrome may occur in association with ZES.

Clinical Features

More than 90% of patients with ZES develop ulcers at some point, most commonly in the duodenal bulb (75%). These ulcers usually are less than 1 cm in diameter but occasionally may be giant lesions. Other sites include the distal duodenum (14%) and the jejunum (11%). Clues to the possible presence of ZES include PUD refractory to medications; recurrent ulcers after surgery; PUD with diarrhea; or PUD with obstruction, perforation, or hemorrhage. Two thirds of patients with ZES experience gastroesophageal reflux symptoms, which may be severe. Diarrhea is present in more than 50% of cases and can occur in the absence of ulcer symptoms. Diarrhea is ameliorated by nasogastric suction or potent acid suppression, which provides evidence for the causative role of acid hypersecretion. Features of diarrhea in ZES include high-output secretion (often several liters per day from the acid itself and from the effects of other peptides, such as VIP), maldigestion with steatorrhea secondary to acid inactivation of pancreatic enzymes, a sprue-like state caused by acid-induced villous damage, and reduced micelle formation caused by insoluble bile salts.

MEN I syndrome occurs in 25% of patients with gastrinoma. This autosomal dominant disorder affects the parathyroid (85%), pancreas (81%), pituitary (65%), and, less commonly, the adrenal cortex and thyroid. The major morbidity and mortality associated with MEN I are related to ZES, and ZES is the initial presentation of MEN I in one third of patients. Hypercalcemia due to hyperparathyroidism may exacerbate the hypergastrinemia and acid hypersecretion of ZES. Other findings include visual field defects resulting from pituitary tumor development and hyperprolactinemia. Gastric carcinoid tumors develop in 13% of patients with ZES and MEN I.

Findings on Diagnostic Testing

Serum Gastrin Determination

Fasting gastrin levels in healthy persons and in patients with other forms of PUD usually are lower than 150 pg/mL. A serum gastrin level of more than 1000 pg/mL in a person who demonstrates gastric acid secretion is virtually diagnostic of ZES. Rarely, pernicious anemia, in the setting of achlorhydria, may produce gastrin levels that exceed 1000 pg/mL. Almost all patients with ZES have gastrin levels higher than 150 pg/mL and some have levels that exceed 100,000 pg/mL. The differential diagnosis of hypergastrinemia includes retained gastric antrum after gastrojejunostomy, G-cell hyperplasia, renal insufficiency, resection of the small intestine, gastric outlet obstruction, rheumatoid arthritis, vitiligo, diabetes, and pheochromocytoma (Table 31-3).

Provocative Testing

The secretin stimulation test can distinguish among the possible causes of hypergastrinemia. After secretin injection (2 mg/kg intravenously), serum gastrin levels increase by 200 pg/mL within 15 minutes in more than 90% of patients with ZES, with few false-positive results (occasionally with achlorhydria). In contrast, patients with non–ZES associated PUD and G-cell hyperplasia exhibit decreases, no change, or only small increases in serum gastrin levels. The calcium infusion test (5 mg/kg per hour intravenously) produces an increase higher than 400 pg/mL in the serum gastrin level within 3 hours in more than 80% of patients with ZES. This test is prone to false-positive results, however, and adverse effects secondary to systemic

---

TABLE 31-3
Differential Diagnosis of Hypergastrinemia

Hypochlorhydria, and achlorhydria with or without pernicious anemia
Retained gastric antrum
G-cell hyperplasia
Renal insufficiency
Massive resection of the small intestine
Gastric outlet obstruction
Rheumatoid arthritis
Vitiligo
Diabetes mellitus
Pheochromocytoma

hypercalcemia may also occur. Thus, calcium testing is reserved for patients with negative findings in secretin stimulation tests who are still strongly suspected of having ZES. Gastrin levels in most patients with ZES increase less than 50% after meal ingestion, compared with increases exceeding 200% in patients with G-cell hyperplasia, but the sensitivity and specificity of the standard meal test are low.

Gastric Acid Secretion Testing

A BAO of 15 mEq/hr or more is found in more than 90% of patients with ZES. However, 12% of patients with common duodenal ulcers also exhibit increased BAO. A BAO-to-MAO ratio of more than 0.6 is highly suggestive of ZES, but a lower ratio does not exclude the diagnosis. Because secretin stimulation testing is not 100% specific, some clinicians advocate gastric acid secretion testing before secretin stimulation testing to confirm acid hypersecretion. If the specialized equipment for acid analysis is not available, a gastric pH higher than 3 essentially rules out a diagnosis of ZES.

Tumor Localization

Somatostatin receptor scintigraphy relies on the premise that many gastrinomas express somatostatin receptors. This method is better than computed tomography (CT), magnetic resonance imaging (MRI), and angiography for localizing primary and metastatic tumors, with a sensitivity and specificity greater than 75%. Endoscopic ultrasound provides a sensitive means of detecting primary gastrinomas that are located in the pancreas, with a sensitivity of 80% to 100%. Abdominal ultrasound has a much lower sensitivity. CT scanning has a sensitivity of 59% for extrahepatic gastrinoma; however, the sensitivity of CT for liver metastasis is higher (72%), with the added advantage that if metastatic disease is found, no further evaluation is needed. MRI can detect primary and metastatic disease with yields similar to CT scanning. Selective angiography is useful for detecting hepatic metastases with high specificity (84%–100%), although extrahepatic lesions are not well visualized. Selective portal venous sampling can detect step-ups in gastrin levels at the site of a primary or metastatic gastrinoma with high sensitivity (70%–90%), but this method is plagued by poor specificity.

In summary, somatostatin receptor scintigraphy in combination with CT or MRI is performed to exclude metastatic disease. If no metastasis is identified, endoscopic ultrasound may be useful for identifying a primary tumor located in the pancreas or duodenum. Intraoperative ultrasonography may also be used to evaluate patients for surgery in selected centers.

Management and Course

A primary gastrinoma in the absence of metastatic disease should be surgically resected. Cure of disease has been demonstrated in up to 30% of cases. Because of the trophic effects of the elevated gastrin levels, mild acid hypersecretion may persist for several years postoperatively. The 5-year survival of all patients with gastrinoma varies between 62% and 75%, with 10-year survival between 47% and 53%. Patients with MEN I have better prognoses, with a 10-year survival of 93% compared to 74% among non–MEN I gastrinoma patients. When curative surgical resection is not possible, a number of medical or chemotherapeutic options exist.

Medical Treatment

The primary aim of medical therapy in ZES is control of acid hypersecretion. The most potent agents in ZES are the PPIs, which inhibit acid secretion, reduce dyspepsia, and promote ulcer healing. The median doses of omeprazole or lansoprazole required to control acid hypersecretion are 60 to 90 mg/d; little tachyphylaxis or toxicity has been observed with long-term PPI therapy. Octreotide, which inhibits gastrin release and gastric acid secretion, also has efficacy in controlling symptoms of ZES.

CHAPTER 32

Surgery for Peptic Ulcer Disease and Postgastrectomy Syndromes

SURGERY FOR DUODENAL ULCER DISEASE

Effective antisecretory medications, the use of antibiotic regimens to eradicate *Helicobacter pylori* infection, and withdrawal of nonsteroidal antiinflammatory drugs have made surgery for duodenal ulcer disease a rare event, although certain disease complications require emergency or elective surgical intervention. Several surgical techniques have been developed to manage these complications acutely and prevent their recurrence.

Operative Techniques

Vagotomy and Drainage

Truncal vagotomy reduces basal acid secretion by 85%, stimulated acid output by 50%, and pepsin secretion by 80%. After vagotomy, the sensitivity of parietal cells to gastrin and histamine is also reduced. Vagal sectioning removes the tonic inhibitory effect of the vagus on pyloric motor activity; therefore, a drainage procedure must be performed with truncal vagotomy to prevent gastric retention. The commonly performed Heineke-Mikulicz pyloroplasty is a longitudinal incision of the pyloroduodenum, which is then closed transversely. Alternatively, a gastrojejunostomy is performed if severe duodenal disease or an inflammatory mass is present. Jaboulay gastroduodenostomy and Finney pyloroplasty to promote more rapid gastric emptying are rarely performed.

Highly Selective Vagotomy

Highly selective vagotomy has become the most widely accepted procedure for elective surgery of duodenal ulcer disease because it produces fewer long-term complications. With this operation, only the vagal branches that supply the proximal stomach are severed, leaving antropyloric innervation intact. Thus, gastric drainage is not necessary. Highly selective vagotomy reduces acid output by 50% to 70%. In some cases, an extended, highly selective vagotomy will include additional section of the gastroepiploic nerve pedicles, which reduces the risk of recurrent ulceration.

Vagotomy and Antrectomy

Antral resection with truncal vagotomy or selective vagotomy to preserve the celiac and hepatic vagal branches has the lowest ulcer recurrence rate. The gastric remnant is joined to the intestine in a Billroth I anastomosis, in which the duodenum is sewn directly to the stomach, or a Billroth II anastomosis, in which a blind duodenal afferent limb is constructed and gastric drainage is through a gastrojejunostomy. The choice between these anastomoses depends on the condition of the duodenum and the amount of stomach resected.

Laparoscopic Ulcer Surgery

Laparoscopy may be used to perform posterior truncal vagotomy with pylorotomy, posterior truncal and anterior highly selective vagotomy, and (rarely) truncal vagotomy with antrectomy.

SURGERY FOR BENIGN GASTRIC ULCERS

Various surgical procedures are used to treat benign ulcers at specific gastric sites. Antrectomy to include the ulcer is the standard procedure for disease involving the distal stomach. When possible, a Billroth I anastomosis is advocated. Vagotomy provides no benefit except in *H pylori*–negative patients with associated duodenal ulcer. Local excision may be possible for small lesser curvature or gastric body ulcers. Ulcers near the gastroesophageal junction present the greatest challenge. Some of these patients will require subtotal gastrectomy with construction of a large esophagogastrojejunostomy.

INDICATIONS FOR SURGERY OF PEPTIC ULCER DISEASE

Intractable Ulcer Disease

Intractable duodenal ulcer disease has become rare since the introduction of potent antisecretory agents, particularly proton pump inhibitors and eradication regimens for *H pylori*. It is defined by the persistence of severely symptomatic (e.g., pain, blood loss) and endoscopically proven persistent ulceration. The operations that are most useful in this setting are highly selective gastric vagotomy and truncal vagotomy with antrectomy (with resection of 30% to 40% of the stomach). Highly selective vagotomy has a very low incidence of postoperative dumping syndrome, diarrhea, maldigestion, anemia, and weight loss, but it has a higher rate of ulcer recurrence. If resection is needed, a Billroth I anastomosis is preferred, although a Billroth II procedure is indicated for severe scarring of the duodenal bulb. Vagotomy and pyloroplasty should be reserved for ill, elderly patients for whom an expedient operation is indicated. Refractory gastric ulcer disease should raise concern for underlying gastric carcinoma. In some instances, operative intervention will be considered to exclude this possibility. The role of surgery in giant duodenal and gastric ulcers >3 cm in diameter has been controversial. Most recent studies indicate that aggressive medical treatment will resolve most giant ulcers, although surgery may be necessary for ulcer complications in 16% of patients.

Ulcer Perforation, Penetration, and Fistulae

Perforation of an ulcer is followed by chemical peritonitis that, if untreated, progresses to bacterial peritonitis, sepsis, and death. Immediate abdominal exploration and repair of the perforation is standard treatment for the majority of patients. If the edges of a perforated duodenal ulcer are friable, a tongue of vascularized omentum may be sewn over the perforation. If the edges are not edematous or friable, the ulcer margins may be approximated before omental patching. Gastric ulcer perforations more commonly are repaired by gastric resection to include the ulcer. Addition of highly selective vagotomy to specific treatment of the perforation is of questionable value. Such definitive ulcer surgery should be performed if the perforation has existed for longer than 24 hours, if the abdomen is not contaminated, and if the patient is otherwise in good health. If bleeding occurs in association with perforation, suture ligature of the ulcer bed may be needed in addition to closure of the perforation and definitive ulcer surgery. Nonoperative management is contemplated in those without peritonitis or sepsis in whom a water-soluble contrast radiography study demonstrates a contained perforation. Reports suggest that surgery can be avoided in 70% of highly selected patients.

Duodenal ulcer penetration may cause intractable ulcer symptoms and is best managed by vagotomy with antrectomy, rather than highly selective vagotomy, because of the postulated increased virulence of the ulcer disease. Fistulae rarely develop between the duodenum and common bile duct or gallbladder. Vagotomy and antrectomy with Billroth II anastomosis treats the ulcer and excludes the fistula. However, if the duodenal stump cannot be closed, nonresectional therapy with vagotomy should be considered, leaving the fistula intact.

Hemorrhage

Approximately 5% of patients with transfusion-requiring hemorrhage from peptic ulcers require surgery. Prompt operative intervention after one to two unsuccessful attempts at endoscopic control is a reasonable management strategy. An ongoing need for blood transfusions also is a good general indicator for surgery. In general, gastric ulcers are three times as likely to rebleed after endoscopy as duodenal ulcers. For bleeding ulcers of the first portion of the duodenum, the duodenum and pylorus are longitudinally incised and the hemorrhage is controlled by direct suture. The role of adding vagotomy to the operation once bleeding is controlled is unclear because the likelihood of ulcer recurrence probably is less than the risk of postgastrectomic symptoms. A bleeding gastric ulcer may be exposed by a longitudinal gastrotomy. Bleeding is then managed by antrectomy to include the ulcer, ulcer excision alone, or oversewing of the ulcer, if the clinical condition is unstable.

Obstruction

Obstruction results from chronic scarring, acute edema, and spasm in the pyloroduodenal area. A 1-week course of intravenous hydration, electrolyte supplementation, intravenous hyperalimentation, intravenous antisecretory therapy, and nasogastric suction is undertaken. Surgery is indicated if these nonoperative measures fail. If Heineke-Mikulicz pyloroplasty is not feasible, Finney pyloroplasty,

TABLE 32-1
Ulcer Recurrence Rates After Different Operations

Operation	Recurrence Rate
Gastric resection	2%–5%
Vagotomy and drainage	10%–15%
Vagotomy and antrectomy	0%–2%
Highly selective vagotomy	10%–17%

Jaboulay gastroduodenostomy, or a gastrojejunstomy may be performed. Addition of highly selective vagotomy has fewer complications than either selective or truncal vagotomy.

POSTGASTRECTOMY COMPLICATIONS

Recurrent Ulcer After Surgery

Most cases of recurrent ulcer after ulcer surgery stem from untreated *H pylori* infection. Rates of recurrent ulcer also depend on the surgery performed (Table 32-1). Other causes include an inadequate operation, a poor selection of operating technique, a hypersecretory state, and use of ulcerogenic drugs such as NSAIDs. Most commonly, inadequate surgery results from incomplete vagotomy. Poor antral drainage may also promote ulcer recurrence because gastric retention can stimulate acid production. The retained gastric antrum syndrome may develop with anatomic isolation of gastrin-producing tissue in the afferent limb of a Billroth II anastomosis, a region that is not subject to inhibition of acid-regulated feedback. The incidence of unsuspected gastrinoma is 2% in patients with postoperative recurrent ulcer. Because of this, many surgeons advocate obtaining serum gastrin levels prior to surgery for a duodenal ulcer. A second rare cause of hypergastrinemia is G-cell hyperplasia, which is effectively treated by antrectomy. Ulcers recur in this condition if the initial operation is only a vagotomy without resection. Hypercalcemia and Cushing syndrome are rare causes of acid hypersecretion.

The diagnosis of recurrent ulcers is best made with upper gastrointestinal endoscopy. If gastrinoma is suspected, fasting gastrin levels are obtained and, if elevated, secretin stimulation is tested. Gastric acid secretion can be measured to assess completeness of vagotomy. Incomplete vagotomy is suggested by a basal acid output of higher than 5 mEq/h or by a significant increase in acid output after modified sham feeding (in which the patient chews meat and spits it out without swallowing). Retained gastric antrum syndrome is diagnosed by hypergastrinemia, negative findings on secretin stimulation testing, a dilated duodenal stump on upper gastrointestinal barium radiography, and positive findings on a technetium pertechnetate scan.

The therapy for a recurrent ulcer depends on its cause. When appropriate, eradication therapy for *H pylori* is given. Surgery is recommended for retained gastric antrum or a resectable gastrinoma. If acid-suppressing proton pump inhibitors do not heal recurrent ulcers that are secondary to other causes, surgical revision may be necessary. If vagotomy is incomplete, a repeat vagotomy is indicated. Antrectomy is performed for recurrent ulcer after pyloroplasty.

TABLE 32-2
Chronic Sequelae of Surgery for Peptic Ulcer Disease

Complication	Rate After Various Operations (%)			
	HSV	TV+D	V+A	SG
Dumping syndrome	5	10–15	10–20	10–20
Diarrhea	2–5	15–30	5–40	2–18
Anemia	0.5	3–15	7	10–40
Bone disease			20	30
Weight loss	2–10	5–20	10–30	20–40

HSV, highly selective vagotomy; TV+D, truncal vagotomy plus drainage; V+A, vagotomy plus antrectomy; SG, subtotal gastrectomy.

Postgastrectomy Syndromes

Ulcer surgery also is associated with a number of other chronic sequelae. The incidence rates of these complications depend on the surgery performed (Table 32-2).

Dumping Syndrome

Surgery that impairs distal vagal function and includes drainage or resection may allow rapid passage of hyperosmolar gastric contents into the intestine, producing fluid shifts and release of vasoactive hormones. The early dumping syndrome includes abdominal symptoms (diarrhea, pain, borborygmi, nausea and vomiting) and vasomotor symptoms (flushing, weakness, palpitations, diaphoresis, lightheadedness, and syncope). These symptoms occur in the first 15 to 60 minutes after eating. The late dumping syndrome, which is postulated to result from excessive postprandial insulin release, produces reactive hypoglycemia 2 to 4 hours after ingesting a meal. The dumping syndrome occurs less frequently after highly selective vagotomy, suggesting that preserving pyloric innervation is important. Treatment of the dumping syndrome relies on low-carbohydrate diets and separation of the solid and liquid components of a meal. Assuming a supine position after eating may delay gastric emptying of nutrients. Adding pectin or acarbose to delay carbohydrate absorption may have benefit in some cases. The somatostatin analog octreotide alleviates symptoms by inhibiting the release of vasoactive peptides and insulin and by slowing transit. Surgical procedures may be attempted, but they are often unsuccessful.

Other Functional Consequences of Ulcer Surgery

Chronic diarrhea after vagotomy has an uncertain pathogenesis, although accelerated intestinal transit, decreased absorption, increased bile acid excretion, and humoral factors may play roles. Kaolin-pectin may be helpful for mild cases, although loperamide or diphenoxylate/atropine are more commonly needed. Maldigestion may result from rapid gastric emptying and intestinal transit, inadequate food particle dispersion owing to reduced trituration, impaired pancreatic and gallbladder responses to food, intestinal bacterial overgrowth, and dyscoordination of intestinal nutrient and pancreaticobiliary delivery. Maldigestion is rarely a significant problem alone, but it may aggravate other postgastrectomy complications.

Severe gastroparesis, usually for solid foods, is a rare complication of gastric surgery. It is less common after highly selective vagotomy. Affected patients should avoid poorly digestible foods. The condition is treated with prokinetic agents, although refractory cases may require total gastrectomy to improve symptoms. Excessive duodenogastric reflux of bile, pancreatic enzymes, and intestinal secretions is thought to produce a characteristic syndrome of burning epigastric pain, with or without bilious vomiting, unresponsive to acid-suppressing medications, and aggravated by eating. The diagnosis is one of exclusion of recurrent ulcer. A pathogenic role for *H pylori* in symptom production is not proven. Surgical construction of a Roux-en-Y gastrojejunostomy to direct intestinal fluid distally produces symptom relief in only 30% to 60% of cases.

Metabolic Consequences of Ulcer Surgery

Chronic anemia frequently occurs secondary to iron, folate, or vitamin B_{12} deficiency. Iron deficiency results from impaired dissociation of ferric iron from food; thus, ferrous iron supplements should be given. In rare instances of vitamin B_{12} deficiency (usually after subtotal or total gastrectomy), monthly vitamin B_{12} injections are given.

Bone disease is more common after gastrectomy than after vagotomy and usually takes years to develop. Osteomalacia is caused by calcium and vitamin D malabsorption and is manifested by loss of bone radiodensity, reduced serum calcium levels, retention of infused calcium, and elevated parathyroid hormone levels.

Gastric Cancer

Gastric adenocarcinoma is a late complication of ulcer surgery, and may be a consequence of hypochlorhydria, alkaline reflux, reduced gastrin secretion, untreated *H pylori*, and nitrosation. The risk for gastric cancer reaches fourfold to fivefold that of the population 20 to 25 years after surgery. Some have advocated aggressive endoscopic surveillance with biopsy to rule out dysplasia. If dysplasia or cancer is found, surgery with completion of the gastrectomy or an esophagogastrectomy may be needed.

CHAPTER 33

Functional Dyspepsia

INCIDENCE AND EPIDEMIOLOGY

Dyspepsia is persistent or recurrent upper abdominal pain or discomfort characterized by postprandial fullness, early satiety, nausea, and bloating. Patients with dyspepsia and no definable structural or biochemical abnormality are classified as having functional dyspepsia, also known as nonulcer dyspepsia. Functional dyspepsia has been subclassified into different subgroups (ulcer-like, dysmotility-like, and unspecified) based on the dominant symptoms (Table 33-1). However, the utility of this categorization is unproven because the different groups overlap considerably and there is a lack of stability among the categories. Although less than half of patients with dyspepsia seek medical care, it is estimated that functional dyspepsia and related functional disorders of the gut account for 2% to 5% of consultations with family physicians. Functional dyspepsia is at least twice as common as peptic ulcer disease. Medical attention may be sought because of symptom severity, fear of malignancy, and underlying anxiety or other psychosocial factors.

ETIOLOGY AND PATHOGENESIS

Disturbed Gastric Motor Function

Approximately 40% of patients with functional dyspepsia in tertiary centers exhibit postprandial antral hypomotility or delayed gastric emptying. The rate may be lower in community settings. However, symptoms and delays in gastric emptying are weakly linked at best. After ingesting a meal, the gastric fundus normally relaxes to accommodate the ingested meal. Some patients with functional dyspepsia have an impaired accommodation reflex, which may underlie postprandial discomfort or fullness. Additional rhythm disturbances of the gastric slow wave have been reported with functional dyspepsia.

Disturbed Gastric Sensory Function

Many patients with functional dyspepsia exhibit reduced tolerance to balloon distention of the stomach and duodenum, which is not accompanied by changes in wall compliance. This finding suggests that functional dyspepsia in these individuals stems from exaggerated responsiveness of visceral afferent nerve pathways. The pathogenesis of visceral hypersensitivity in functional dyspepsia is poorly understood. The prevalence of back pain and headache in functional

TABLE 33-1
Rome II Criteria for Functional Dyspepsia

At least 12 weeks, which need not be consecutive, in the preceding 12 months of:
1. Persistent or recurrent dyspepsia (pain or discomfort centered in the upper abdomen);
2. No evidence of organic disease (including at least upper gastrointestinal endoscopy) that is likely to explain the symptoms; *and*
3. No evidence that dyspepsia is exclusively relieved by defecation or associated with the onset of a change in stool frequency or stool form (i.e., not irritable bowel syndrome)

Dyspepsia subgroups:
1. Ulcer-like dyspepsia: pain centered in the upper abdomen is the predominant (most bothersome) symptom.
2. Dysmotility-like dyspepsia: an unpleasant or troublesome nonpainful sensation (discomfort) centered in the upper abdomen is the predominant symptom; this may be characterized by or associated with fullness, early satiety, bloating, or nausea.
3. Unspecified dyspepsia: symptoms do not fulfill the criteria for ulcer-like or dysmotility-like dyspepsia.

dyspepsia suggests possible abnormalities in cerebral cortical processing of pain information.

Gastric Acid, Duodenitis, and Postinfectious Dyspepsia

Acid secretion is normal in most patients with functional dyspepsia. Moreover, most individuals exhibit normal sensitivity to acid perfusion of the stomach. Histological duodenitis is present in 14%–83% of individuals with functional dyspepsia. Many of them ultimately develop duodenal ulcers. However, erosive duodenitis is more appropriately considered within the spectrum of peptic ulcer disease, rather than functional dyspepsia. *Helicobacter pylori* infection is found in 40% of patients with functional dyspepsia; however, similar rates are found in matched asymptomatic populations. Furthermore, eradication of *H pylori* clearly alleviates symptoms in only a small subset of functional dyspeptics. A small subgroup of patients with functional dyspepsia develops symptoms after an acute attack of infectious gastroenteritis.

Psychological Factors

Patients with functional dyspepsia are more psychologically distressed than healthy controls and have increased anxiety, depression, neuroticism, and somatization. However, some have suggested that these emotional disturbances may be consequences rather than the cause of dyspeptic symptoms. Acute stress elicits gastric motor responses similar to those observed with functional dyspepsia. As in studies of irritable bowel syndrome, the prevalence of prior physical or sexual abuse is higher in functional dyspepsia.

Diet and Environmental Factors

Aspirin and nonsteroidal antiinflammatory drugs cause acute dyspepsia, but their roles in chronic dyspepsia are less well established. There is no evidence that smoking tobacco or ingesting ethanol cause functional dyspepsia. Similarly, it is unlikely that food intolerance is a major contributor to the pathogenesis of functional dyspepsia. Coffee stimulates gastric acid production and may elicit dyspeptic symptoms, but it is unknown if it acts via gastric irritation or induction of gastroesophageal reflux.

CLINICAL FEATURES

Ulcer-like functional dyspepsia is characterized by episodes of epigastric pain that is relieved by antacids or food, whereas dysmotility-like non ulcer dyspepsia presents with discomfort that is aggravated by food or associated with early satiety, fullness, nausea, retching, vomiting, or bloating. Patients with unspecified dyspepsia report symptoms that do not fulfill criteria for ulcer-like or dysmotility-like disease. In evaluating a patient with unexplained dyspepsia, the clinician should consider stopping medications that may produce dyspepsia, including iron, potassium, digoxin, theophylline, erythromycin, and ampicillin. Other conditions that evoke dyspepsia include chronic pancreatitis, intestinal angina, malignancies, Ménétrier disease, infiltrative diseases (e.g., Crohn's disease, sarcoidosis, eosinophilic gastroenteritis, tuberculosis, and syphilis), and abdominal wall pain from muscle strain, nerve entrapment, or myositis.

FINDINGS ON DIAGNOSTIC TESTING

It is important to exclude organic disease in a patient with unexplained dyspepsia. Patients younger than age 45 without weight loss, bleeding, dysphagia, or recurrent vomiting very rarely have gastric cancer. However, individuals with new onset dyspepsia who are older than age 45 should undergo upper endoscopy to detect this condition. Endoscopy also will exclude benign conditions such as ulcer disease and esophagitis. In young patients without alarm findings, empiric therapy with an acid-suppressing drug is a reasonable approach with optional endoscopy if symptoms persist. Alternatively, such patients may first undergo *H pylori* serology or ^{13}C or ^{14}C urea breath testing. If such testing is positive, endoscopy is performed. If serologic or breath testing is negative, empiric acid-reducing drugs are given. Such an approach reduces the rate of endoscopy utilization. Barium radiography is less useful than endoscopy; abdominal ultrasound has a low yield and is not ordered routinely. Although other tests (24-hour pH monitoring, gastric scintigraphic emptying scanning, biliary scanning, lactose tolerance testing) may find abnormalities in up to 50% of patients, the gain from these additional tests is small.

MANAGEMENT AND COURSE

A positive clinical diagnosis and confident reassurance by the clinician are key steps in managing patients with functional dyspepsia and may obviate the need for medication therapy in many patients. Patients should avoid aggravating medications and foods if possible. Postprandial symptoms may be reduced by eating low-fat meals or more frequent but smaller meals throughout the day.

Medication Therapy

There is no universally effective medication for treating functional dyspepsia. Many controlled trials in functional dyspepsia have yielded unimpressive results, in part, because of high placebo response rates (30%–70%) in this condition. A meta-analysis of H_2 receptor antagonists showed a response rate 20% greater than that of placebo. Several studies suggest that proton pump inhibitors provide superior relief compared to H_2 receptor antagonists. However, these trials may have included significant numbers of patients with gastroesophageal reflux. Eradicating *H pylori* has limited benefits. It cures no more than one of every 15 patients treated. Prokinetic drugs such as metoclopramide and domperidone may reduce symptoms in some patients, although side effects are prevalent with metoclopramide. Small studies suggest potential efficacy of tricyclic antidepressant medications such as amitriptyline. Simethicone may produce improvement if gas retention or aerophagia is present. In one study, the cytoprotective drug sucralfate reduced dyspeptic symptoms. Drugs in the dopamine receptor antagonist and serotonin 5-HT_3 receptor antagonist classes may decrease associated symptoms of nausea. Limited placebo-controlled trials have reported symptomatic improvements in functional dyspepsia with herbal medicines.

Psychological Therapies

Small trials have shown the benefits of cognitive psychotherapy and hypnotherapy in functional dyspepsia. However, studies of psychological treatment have been suboptimal and comparisons with drug therapy have not been performed.

CHAPTER 34

Gastritis, Duodenitis, and Associated Ulcerative Lesions

Gastritis is defined as inflammation of the gastric mucosa; the term denotes a histopathological condition, not a disease. It is paramount to understand that the mere presence of inflammation does not produce signs or symptoms and that complications of inflammation such as ulcer formation are generally required to produce symptoms. The Updated Sydney System is used to classify and grade gastritis, thus providing a basis for diagnosis and treatment (see Table 34-1).

TABLE 34-1
Classification of Chronic Gastritis

TYPE OF GASTRITIS	ETIOLOGY	SYNONYMS
NONATROPHIC	*Helicobacter pylori*	Superficial Diffuse antral gastritis Chronic antral gastritis Interstitial-follicular Hypersecretory Type B
ATROPHIC		
Autoimmune	Autoimmunity	Type A Diffuse corporal Pernicious anemia–associated
Multifocal atrophic	*H pylori* Environmental factors	Type B, Type AB Environmental Metaplastic Atrophic pangastritis Progressive intestinalizing 　pangastritis
SPECIAL FORMS		
Chemical	Chemical irritation Bile NSAIDs	Reactive Reflux
Radiation	Radiation injury	
Lymphocytic	Drugs Autoimmune mechanisms Idiopathic Gluten	Varioliform Celiac disease–associated
Noninfectious 　granulomatous	Crohn's disease Sarcoidosis Wegener granulomatosis Foreign substances	Isolated granulomatous
Eosinophilic	Food sensitivity	Allergic
Other infectious	Bacteria (other than *H pylori*) Viruses Parasites Fungi	Phlegmonous, syphilitic Cytomegalovirus Anisakiasis

ACUTE GASTRITIS

Etiology and Pathogenesis

Acute hemorrhagic or erosive gastritis may be caused by mucosal hypoxia associated with reduced gastric blood flow resulting from stress, trauma, burns, or sepsis. Alternatively, gastritis may be caused by bile reflux, exogenous substances such as

NSAIDs, or conditions such as central nervous system disorders (e.g., a Cushing ulcer, which is a peptic ulcer associated with lesions of the CNS). If mucosal defenses are breached, acid, proteases, and bile acids penetrate into the lamina propria, where they cause vascular injury, stimulate nerves, and activate the release of histamine and other mediators.

Clinical Features and Diagnosis

Acute hemorrhagic and erosive gastritis may present as acute upper gastrointestinal bleeding. Petechiae and small red or black erosions are visible in the endoscopic view. Stress-induced lesions generally involve the fundus and body of the stomach, whereas NSAID-induced hemorrhagic gastritis involves the entire stomach, including the antrum. Histological findings correlate poorly with endoscopically defined abnormalities and may show regenerating epithelium and sparse inflammation. Acute ulcers may occur in association with gastritis, especially with stress, and usually are multiple, large (0.5 to 2.0 cm in diameter), and located in the fundus and body.

The gastroenterologist who treats adults rarely diagnoses gastritis caused by acute *Helicobacter pylori* infection because most such infections occur in children. In research, however, acute *H pylori* gastritis has been shown to cause epigastric pain, nausea, and vomiting. Endoscopic evaluation shows striking antral abnormalities that mimic the appearance of lymphoma or carcinoma. Histologically, there are intense neutrophilic infiltration, edema, and hyperemia; these features clear with appropriate antibiotic therapy.

CHRONIC GASTRITIS

Helicobacter pylori Gastritis

Etiology and Pathogenesis

Although *H pylori* is present in many patients with nonulcer dyspepsia, it is doubtful that it has a major role in generating symptoms in most of these patients. The prevalence of dyspepsia is not different in infected and uninfected persons; in addition, among persons with nonulcer (functional) dyspepsia, the proportion of infected compared to uninfected persons is similar. In developing countries, the prevalence of *H pylori* infection in adults approaches 90%. In industrialized countries, the prevalence of infection parallels age as a result of a cohort effect, which means that the increased prevalence with age is not from acquiring infection over time. The prevalence of *H pylori* infection in the United States in persons age 50 is about 30%, whereas in Swedish and Danish schools in the year 2000 the rate was less than 1%.

Clinical Features and Diagnosis

Symptoms attributable to *H pylori* infection are reliably present only in peptic ulcer disease. Endoscopic findings in *H pylori* gastritis are variable and typically involve the entire stomach, although biopsies directed at the antrum alone may miss the diagnosis in up to 10% of cases. Techniques to detect *H pylori* include Giemsa and silver stains and the less reliable hematoxylin and eosin preparation. *H pylori* organisms are found in the mucus overlying the mucosa and adjacent to epithelial cells at the mucosal surface and in the pits. Gastric glands are rarely involved. *H pylori* gastritis is characterized by chronic superficial inflammation with lymphocytes, plasma cells, macrophages, and eosinophils, usually accompanied by acute inflammation consisting of neutrophilic infiltration of the surface and fove-olar epithelium and lamina propria. Lymphoid follicles, which are aggregates of lymphocytes with a central germinal center of pale mononuclear cells, are often seen and are virtually pathognomonic of *H pylori* gastritis. Acute inflammation is more common in antral than in proximal tissues. Other means of detecting *H pylori* infection with serologic tests, stool antigen tests, or functional tests of urease activity using breath tests or biopsies of gastric tissue are discussed in Chapter 31.

Chronic Chemical Gastritis

Etiology and Pathogenesis

NSAIDs and bile are the principal causes of chronic chemical gastritis, although iron and potassium supplements may also cause injury. Other terms denote similar conditions, including reactive gastritis or chemical gastropathy. Bile gastritis is a chronic condition in which bile-containing intestinal contents reflux into the stomach. Although most commonly diagnosed in patients who have undergone pyloroplasty or partial gastric resection, bile gastritis caused by duodenogastric reflux secondary to gastroduodenal motility disorders or cholecystectomy may occur in patients with intact stomachs. Bile acids and lysolecithin are known to induce acute gastric mucosal injury, which is enhanced by pancreatic enzymes. NSAIDs are also associated with the histopathological changes of chemical gastritis.

Clinical Features and Diagnosis

Patients with chronic chemical gastritis may present with symptoms of dyspepsia. On endoscopic examination, the stomach mucosa may appear congested and edematous with or without erosions. Biopsy specimens of affected areas may reveal minimal inflammation, but foveolar hyperplasia, edema, increased lamina propria smooth muscle fibers, and vascular dilation and congestion may be present. Fove-olae may have a tortuous corkscrew appearance, especially if biopsy specimens are taken near a gastroenterostomy. Foveolar hyperplasia secondary to bile reflux may regress if bile is diverted from a gastroenterostomy by a Roux-en-Y gastrojejunos-tomy. Although eosinophils may be prominent, only 30% of NSAID users exhibit neutrophils.

Atrophic Gastritis

Etiology and Pathogenesis

There are three subtypes of atrophic gastritis: autoimmune metaplastic, environmental metaplastic, and nonmetaplastic. Autoimmune metaplastic atrophic gastritis (AMAG) is an autosomal dominant disorder in which an immune response is directed against parietal cells and intrinsic factor in the proximal gastric mucosa, producing vitamin B_{12} deficiency and pernicious anemia. The mucosal changes of AMAG closely parallel elevations in serum antibodies to parietal cells and intrinsic factor. The loss of parietal cell mass produces profound hypochlorhydria. Affected patients may also exhibit other autoimmune diseases, including Hashimoto thyroiditis, Grave disease, myxedema, idiopathic adrenocortical insufficiency, hypoparathyroidism, and vitiligo. In AMAG, antral G cells release large amounts of gastrin, which causes an increase in the number of endocrine cells and may produce hyperplastic endocrine cell nodules in and around the gastric glands. This hyperplasia centers on the enterochromaffin-like (ECL) cell, which is the endocrine cell responsible for histamine secretion. In some patients, ECL hyperplasia progresses to carcinoid tumor. The malignant potential of these tumors is low, and only 9% metastasize. The risk of carcinoma in pernicious anemia, which usually is associated with AMAG, is 3- to 18-fold higher than in the general population, whereas the risk for AMAG alone is probably somewhat less. AMAG is not associated with *H pylori* infection.

Environmental metaplastic atrophic gastritis (EMAG) is most prevalent in Japan, South America, and China and is causally associated with *H pylori* infection, gastric bacterial overgrowth, coal dust exposure, tobacco smoking, and dietary salt and nitrate consumption. Nitroso compounds generated by the gastric bacterial metabolism of nitrates are thought to induce EMAG, metaplasia, and finally gastric cancer. Similarly, chronic *H pylori* infection is correlated with intestinal metaplasia and may be a risk factor in developing gastric carcinoma, although it is likely that other cofactors are also required for carcinogenesis.

Nonmetaplastic atrophic gastritis is associated with antral resection, in which the loss of oxyntic cells in the proximal gastric remnant results in vitamin B_{12} deficiency from insufficient intrinsic factor secretion. These patients have reduced circulating gastrin levels, which in turn fail to maintain the trophic effect on the oxyntic glands.

Clinical Features and Diagnosis

In general, atrophic gastritis is asymptomatic unless a complication develops. Hypochlorhydria may be present despite preservation of parietal cells, which suggests that antibodies to the proton pumps or inhibitory lymphokines released by inflammatory cells inhibit acid secretion. Achlorhydria typically occurs in the most advanced stages of disease. A low serum pepsinogen I level (<20 ng/mL) indicates corpus atrophy. Patients with autoimmune gastritis may present with iron deficiency or pernicious anemia. Achlorhydria appears to mediate the former (gastric acid is important in the absorption of nonheme iron), whereas the latter is a direct result of parietal cell damage. Manifestations of vitamin B_{12} deficiency include a sore tongue (smooth and beefy red), anorexia, and neurological complications (numbness, paresthesia, weakness, and ataxia). Autoimmune gastritis is a risk factor for gastric cancer.

Gastric biopsy specimens from patients with atrophic gastritis show a variety of patterns. Two types of metaplasia are seen with AMAG and EMAG. Pseudopyloric metaplasia is gastric metaplasia in which the parietal and chief cells are replaced with mucus-secreting and endocrine (gastrin) cells similar to those in prepyloric antral mucosa. Intestinal metaplasia is characterized by the replacement of the surface, foveolar, and glandular epithelium in the oxyntic or antral mucosa by intestinal epithelium. Type I intestinal metaplasia involves complete replacement of gastric mucosa by intestinal epithelium, whereas in type II and III metaplasia, the replacement is incomplete, with persistent gastric-type mucin cells. Goblet cells in type II metaplasia contain acidic sialomucins, whereas in type III metaplasia, goblet cells contain acidic sulfomucin. Incomplete intestinal metaplasia (especially type III) is associated with the highest risk of gastric adenocarcinoma. In AMAG, the metaplasia, glandular atrophy, and inflammation are limited to the gastric body and fundus. On upper gastrointestinal endoscopic examination, the rugae are inconspicuous and the submucosal vessels are clearly visible under the thinned mucosa. In the early stage of AMAG, termed *active autoimmune gastritis*, involvement is patchy, and multiple retained islands of normal mucosa that resemble pseudopolyps are visible. Pseudohypertrophy of parietal cells may be present and findings of chemical gastritis may be seen on antral biopsy specimens. In end-stage AMAG, replacement with metaplastic tissue is complete and the histological appearance is identical to that of the small intestine. Serum tests, which are useful to confirm AMAG, include elevations in the levels of antibodies to parietal cells and intrinsic factor and a reduction in the ratio of pepsinogen I to pepsinogen II.

EMAG is characterized by multiple localized areas of atrophy, metaplasia, and inflammation, which are most prominent in the antrum and to a lesser degree, in the gastric body. At least 20% of the available antral mucosa must be replaced by metaplasia or atrophy to diagnose EMAG. There often is a proximal migration of the transitional zone from normal mucosa to metaplastic tissue. Thinning of body and fundus mucosa may occur secondary to reduced gastrin levels. Gastric ulcers may form in regions of intestinal metaplasia. Pepsinogen ratios are abnormal in some but not all patients with EMAG, and some patients will have *H pylori* infection.

In nonmetaplastic atrophic gastritis, or postantrectomic mucosal atrophy, there is overall mucosal thinning associated with shortening of the oxyntic glands. Intestinal metaplasia may be prominent around the anastomosis, but it is not excessive in the more proximal gastric remnant.

Miscellaneous Forms of Chronic Gastritis

Eosinophilic Gastritis

Eosinophilic gastritis is characterized by eosinophilic infiltration of any or all layers of the stomach, often in association with peripheral eosinophilia and allergic conditions. Gastric mucosal involvement is most prevalent in the antrum, especially in children. Other biopsy findings include epithelial necrosis and regeneration.

Infectious Gastritis

Except for those infected with *H pylori*, healthy individuals rarely develop chronic infectious gastritis. Some dyspeptic patients are infected with a urease-positive, spirochete-like organism, *Helicobacter heilmannii*, which is similar to organisms found in the stomachs of cats, dogs, monkeys, and other animals. Alterations of gastric mucosal defenses that occur in atrophic gastritis or in acquired immunodeficiency syndrome (AIDS) may predispose patients with these conditions to bacterial, viral, parasitic, or fungal gastric infection. Phlegmonous gastritis is an overwhelming bacterial gastritis that produces acute epigastric pain, fever, and peritonitis in alcoholics, the elderly, and AIDS patients. The gastric wall and mucosa are grossly thickened from intense diffuse and suppurative inflammation. Streptococci, *Escherichia coli*, staphylococci, *Haemophilus* species, and gas-forming bacteria have been implicated in pathogenesis. Iatrogenic causes include gastric polypectomy and India-ink injection. The diagnosis usually is made at laparotomy, and treatment involves gastric resection and antibiotics. Gastric tuberculosis typically manifests with symptoms related to gastric obstruction and ulceration because of antropyloric involvement, although it may involve atypical sites in patients with AIDS. Cultures or polymerase chain reaction (PCR) examination of endoscopic biopsy specimens are required because acid-fast bacilli are rarely seen. The stomach may also be involved in infection with *Mycobacterium avium* complex in patients with AIDS. Syphilitic gastritis (secondary syphilis) can be associated with symptoms of anorexia, epigastric pain, and vomiting. Endoscopic examination reveals erosive antral gastritis, ulcers, or thickened rugae. Biopsy specimens show prominent spirochetes, acute and chronic inflammation with mucosal destruction, and mononuclear vasculitis in the submucosa and muscularis. Positive results of serologic tests for syphilis confirm the diagnosis. Rarely, gummas and fibrosis in tertiary syphilis may produce obstruction and the appearance of an infiltrating mass. Cytomegalovirus (CMV) is the most common viral cause of infectious gastritis and is a frequent finding in patients with AIDS. Symptoms include acute epigastric pain, nausea, and vomiting. On endoscopic examination, CMV infection appears as nonulcerative nodules of the body, fundus of the stomach, and ulceroerosive disease that mimics neoplasia. Biopsy specimens show atypical lymphocytosis and enlarged nuclei with intranuclear inclusions in glandular cells, macrophages, and endothelial cells. In children, CMV infection produces gastric fold enlargement with protein-losing enteropathy (i.e., childhood Ménétrier disease) and is characterized by intense eosinophilic infiltration of the lamina propria.

Parasitic infections that cause gastritis include cryptosporidiosis, anisakiasis, ascariasis, strongyloidiasis, and hookworm. Gastric cryptosporidiosis produces antral narrowing, erythema, edema, and inflammation and is a common infection in AIDS patients. Anisakiasis, the most common helminthiasis that affects the stomach, is associated with ingesting raw fish and is reported most frequently in Japan and the Netherlands. The *Anisakis* worm burrows into the mucosa. Infected patients present with severe pain, nausea, and vomiting. The histological findings include eosinophilic infiltration, necrosis, and multinucleated giant cells.

The stomach can be affected with disseminated histoplasmosis and can exhibit ulceration, rugal thickening, and organism-laden macrophages. *Cryptococcus* species may infect the stomach in AIDS. *Candida* commonly colonizes gastric ulcers, but invasive gastric candidiasis is rare in immunocompromised patients.

Crohn's Disease

One percent to 5% of patients with Crohn's disease have severe upper gastrointestinal involvement that is visually described as erythema, edema, nodularity, cobblestoning, erosions, ulcers, strictures, and obstruction. The antrum is most frequently involved and exhibits linear ulcerations and aphthous erosions. Biopsy specimens show focal, nonspecific, neutrophilic, and mononuclear infiltration. Histological proof of Crohn's gastritis is provided only by the demonstration of granulomas, which are found in only 7% to 34% of patients.

Granulomatous Gastritis

A variety of diseases may be associated with granulomatous gastritis. *Mycobacterium tuberculosis*, histoplasmosis, *H pylori*, and anisakiasis are infectious causes of gastric granulomata. Noninfectious associations include sarcoidosis, Crohn's disease, foreign bodies, adenocarcinomas (especially mucin-secreting tumors), immune-mediated vasculitic syndromes, and Wegener granulomatosis. Isolated granulomatous gastritis may affect the distal stomach and produce obstruction from wall thickening, lumenal narrowing, and transmural noncaseating granulomas. The cause of the disease is unknown. It may respond to treatment with corticosteroids, or surgery may be required.

Lymphocytic Gastritis

Lymphocytic gastritis, characterized by T-lymphocyte infiltration of the surface and foveolar epithelium, may be isolated, or it may occur in association with celiac sprue, lymphocytic and collagenous colitis, *H pylori* gastritis, or after using the antithrombotic agent ticlopidine. Hypertrophic lymphocytic gastritis produces large rugal folds, but it is distinct from Ménétrier disease. Varioliform gastritis generally occurs in the gastric body and is characterized by erosions overlying elevated lesions that resemble octopus suckers. Symptoms are common and include weight loss, anorexia, and epigastric pain. Hypoalbuminemia and protein-losing enteropathy may be present, associated with peripheral edema. Therapy generally is tailored to the inciting process and may entail steroids, sodium cromolyn, acid suppression, or dietary limitations.

Hypertrophic Gastropathies

Hypertrophic gastropathies (giant-fold gastropathies) include those conditions with enlarged rugae of the gastric body and fundus that exhibit increased numbers of mucosal epithelial cells, including Ménétrier disease (i.e., epithelial hyperplasia of the surface and foveolar mucous cells with atrophic or normal oxyntic glands); Zollinger-Ellison syndrome (i.e., increased numbers of parietal cells with normal numbers of mucous cells); and mixed hyperplastic gastropathy (i.e., increased numbers of mucous and oxyntic glandular cells) (Table 34-2). Patients with Ménétrier disease present with epigastric pain, weight loss, nausea, vomiting, gastrointestinal hemorrhage, and diarrhea, and are diagnosed by biopsy findings of extreme foveolar hyperplasia. Hypoalbuminemia from protein-losing enteropathy is found in 20% to 100% of patients with Ménétrier disease. Basal and stimulated acid secretion is low or normal, and gastrin levels may be slightly elevated. The risk of progression to gastric carcinoma is controversial; sepsis and vascular and thromboembolic complications are probably a greater threat to affected patients. No medications consistently improve Ménétrier disease, although anticholinergics reportedly increase albumin levels. Subtotal or total gastric resection may relieve pain and correct hypoalbuminemia. Transforming growth factor alpha (TGF-α) is markedly increased in gastric mucous cells in Ménétrier disease and may play a pathogenic role; successful treatment with a monoclonal antibody directed against the TGF-α receptor has been reported. Acute and chronic *H pylori* gastritis may cause rugal thickening so striking as to suggest Ménétrier disease and may produce glandular hyperplasia, gastric hypersecretion with or without hypoalbuminemia, and edema. Enlarged gastric folds may be caused by malignant neoplasms (e.g., lymphoma, adenocarcinoma), carcinoid tumors, or Cronkhite-Canada syndrome.

TABLE 34-2
Differential Diagnosis of Large Gastric Folds

Hypertrophic Gastropathies
  Ménétrier disease
  Zollinger-Ellison syndrome

Infections
  Helicobacter pylori
  Cytomegalovirus
  Syphilis
  Histoplasmosis

Neoplasia
  Carcinoma
  Lymphoma
  Carcinoid

Miscellaneous
  Lymphocytic gastritis
  Sarcoidosis
  Eosinophilic gastroenteritis
  Cronkhite-Canada syndrome

CHRONIC DUODENITIS

Peptic Duodenitis

Etiology and Pathogenesis

Peptic duodenitis is caused by chronic exposure to gastric acid. Acute or chronic inflammation may be present, especially with *H pylori* infection. Gastric mucous cell metaplasia (GMCM) is characterized by the replacement of duodenal mucosa with gastric-type mucus-secreting cells. It is an adaptive response to acid exposure and is most common in patients with duodenal ulcer, in men, and in tobacco smokers. In Zollinger-Ellison syndrome, GMCM may extend into the distal duodenum and jejunum. The association of *H pylori* with GMCM is very strong in active duodenitis and may represent a precursor to duodenal ulcer development. Brunner gland hyperplasia also occurs in the duodenal bulb in response to acid exposure and is an adaptive response that leads to increased bicarbonate secretion.

Clinical Features and Diagnosis

Patients with peptic duodenitis may be asymptomatic, or they may present with dyspeptic symptoms identical to those of peptic ulcer disease. Endoscopic evaluation may reveal erythema, edema, and erosions. Brunner gland hyperplasia gives a nodular appearance to the mucosa of the duodenal bulb. Duodenal biopsy specimens show neutrophilic and mononuclear infiltration. GMCM is characterized by gastric mucous cells as well as by metaplastic chief cells and parietal cells. *H pylori* colonization of metaplastic but not normal duodenal mucosa may be observed. Brunner gland acini are visible with hyperplasia but are rarely seen in normal histological resection specimens.

Miscellaneous Forms of Chronic Duodenitis

Crohn's Disease

Duodenal Crohn's disease may produce erosions, aphthous ulcers, linear ulcers, cobblestoning, nodules, fold thickening, and stenosis. Histological findings may be indistinguishable from those of peptic ulcer disease.

Celiac Sprue

Blunting of the villi and chronic inflammation occur with peptic duodenitis as well as with celiac sprue; therefore, if sprue is a diagnostic consideration, biopsy specimens should be obtained from the distal duodenum or jejunum.

Infectious Duodenitis

Infectious duodenitis caused by *M avium* complex or *Enterocytozoon bieneusi* may be seen in AIDS and in other forms of immunodeficiency.

CHAPTER 35

Tumors of the Stomach

ADENOCARCINOMA

Incidence and Epidemiology

Gastric cancer is the second most common cause of cancer mortality worldwide, with more than 600,000 deaths annually. Adenocarcinomas comprise by far the largest proportion of cancers of the stomach. In the United States, 21,500 cases of gastric cancer including 13,000 deaths were reported in the year 2000. Considerable geographic variation exists in age-adjusted annual incidence; for example, less than 5 cases per 100,000 of population in the United States compared to 35 per 100,000 in Japan or China. Even within countries, there is substantial ethnic variation. African Americans and Native Americans are 1.5 to 2.5 times more likely to get gastric cancer than whites, and in Singapore, Chinese have a higher incidence of cancer. Adenocarcinoma of the stomach occurs more commonly in men than in women, usually during the sixth and seventh decades.

Etiology and Pathogenesis

Risk Factors

The etiology of gastric cancer has been evaluated through multiple genetic and environmental factors, including diet, infections, and other exogenous agents. Gastric adenocarcinoma has been linked to diets that are high in carbohydrates and salt-preserved foods but deficient in fresh fruits and vegetables. A high dietary intake of salt is associated with atrophic gastritis and gastric cancer. Diets high in nitrates, nitrites, and secondary amines, which are precursors of carcinogenic N-nitrosamines, have been associated with gastric adenocarcinoma.

Several large case-control studies have illustrated an association between Helicobacter pylori infection and gastric adenocarcinoma. Patients infected with H pylori are twice as likely as uninfected persons to develop gastric adenocarcinoma, and animal models have demonstrated the direct gastric carcinogenic effect of infection with H pylori. Evaluation of data by the International Agency for Research on Cancer provided sufficient evidence to classify infection with H pylori as a group 1 carcinogen. H pylori is not linked to adenocarcinoma of the proximal stomach or gastroesophageal junction, which indicates that other pathogenic mechanisms lead to the development of these tumors. Epstein-Barr virus infection is associated with a subset of gastric cancer—a nonadenocarcinoma called lymphoepithelioma-like gastric carcinoma, which occurs primarily in the proximal stomach.

Prior gastric resection has also been associated with gastric cancer. Fifteen to 20 years after a Billroth II gastrectomy, and to a lesser extent after a Billroth I, patients have an increased risk for gastric cancer that has been estimated at as much as 3% annually. Anaerobic bacteria, nitrites, and bile reflux have all been implicated in the pathogenesis. Tobacco and alcohol use have not shown significant

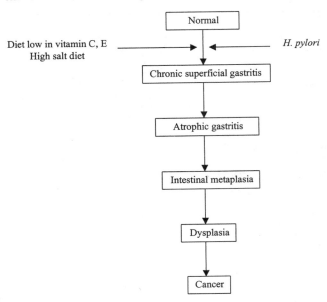

FIGURE 35-1. Sequences of gastric carcinogenesis.

correlation with the development of gastric cancer. Unlike colorectal cancer, there is no clearly defined mechanism for gastric carcinogenesis. However, there is evidence that mutations of tumor suppressor genes, *p53*, *APC*, or *ras* may be involved in carcinogenesis. Microsatellite instability is present in some gastric cancers, as is upregulation of cyclooxygenase (COX)–2 enzymes.

There is believed to be a stepwise progression from chronic gastritis, atrophy, and intestinal metaplasia to dysplasia and finally gastric cancer (Fig. 35-1). In regions where the risk for gastric adenocarcinoma is highest, atrophic gastritis is found in 80% to 90% of patients with gastric cancer, and intestinal metaplasia is present in the stomachs of 70% of patients with gastric adenocarcinoma. However, only 10% of patients with intestinal metaplasia and atrophic gastritis develop gastric cancer over a 15-year follow-up period. Chronic atrophic gastritis may result from type B antral gastritis associated with *H pylori* infection or from type A fundic gastritis associated with autoimmune disease. Patients with pernicious anemia and type A atrophic gastritis have an increased risk of gastric adenocarcinoma, but the magnitude and timing of this increased risk are poorly defined.

Tumors of the proximal stomach, particularly of the gastroesophageal junction, are associated with a separate group of risk factors. Adenocarcinoma of the gastroesophageal junction has increased in prevalence, unlike distal neoplasms, and presently accounts for 25% of gastric cancers. These proximal tumors often occur in Barrett metaplasia of the esophagus and may represent a variant of esophageal adenocarcinoma. Proximal stomach tumors are more likely to be associated with tobacco use; *H pylori* infection is not a risk factor. Based on these differences, adenocarcinoma of the gastroesophageal junction is often considered separately from tumors of the fundus, body, and antrum.

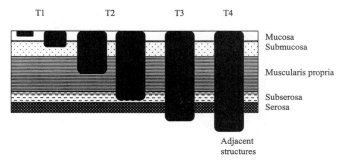

T1 T2 T3 T4

Mucosa
Submucosa

Muscularis propria

Subserosa
Serosa

Adjacent
structures

FIGURE 35-2. T classification of gastric carcinomas (TNM staging system).

Histopathology

The Borrmann classification of gastric adenocarcinoma contains four distinct morphologic subgroups, including polypoid, fungating, ulcerated, and diffusely infiltrating or linitis plastica. *Early gastric cancer* is a term that applies to tumors limited to the mucosa and submucosa. It is most commonly diagnosed during screening of asymptomatic high-risk populations and carries a favorable prognosis. The two best predictors of survival are depth of invasion (T stage) and metastases to lymph nodes (N stage) or distant sites (M stage) (Fig. 35-2). A TNM staging system categorizes gastric tumors into four stages that correlate with long-term survival (Table 35-1). Young patients, patients with linitis plastica, and patients with proximal tumors have poor prognoses.

Histologically, gastric cancer can be divided into an intestinal type, characterized by epithelial cells that form glandular structures, and a diffuse type, in which undifferentiated cells proliferate in sheets. The intestinal type is more common in countries where gastric cancer is endemic, whereas the diffuse type is more common in

TABLE 35-1
TNM Staging of Gastric Carcinomas

STAGE	T STAGE	N STAGE	M STAGE	5-YEAR SURVIVAL (%)
IA	T1	N0	M0	91
IB	T1	N1	M0	82
	T2	N0	M0	
II	T1	N2	M0	65
	T2	N1	M0	
	T3	N0	M0	
IIIA	T2	N2	M0	49
	T3	N1	M0	
	T4	N0	M0	
IIIB	T3	N2	M0	28
	T4	N1	M0	
IV	T4	N2	M0	5
	Any T	Any N	M1	

low-risk populations, such as that in the United States. The intestinal type is more likely to be associated with intestinal metaplasia and atrophic gastritis and has a more favorable prognosis than the diffuse type. Gastric malignancies rarely exhibit adenomatous and squamous features. The adenosquamous variant has a poor prognosis.

Clinical Features

Patients with early gastric cancer generally are asymptomatic. Rather, most individuals present at an advanced stage, usually with nonspecific symptoms such as epigastric pain, early satiety, bloating, nausea, vomiting, and weight loss. Gastrointestinal hemorrhage and gastric outlet obstruction are rarely the initial manifestations of a gastric tumor. The results of the physical examination may be normal, or evaluation may reveal occult or gross gastrointestinal blood loss, lymphadenopathy, or hepatomegaly with disease dissemination. A Virchow node indicates metastasis to the left supraclavicular lymph node, whereas a periumbilical nodule (Sister Mary Joseph node) may indicate tumor spread along peritoneal surfaces. An ovarian mass (Krukenberg tumor) or a mass in the cul-de-sac (Blumer shelf) may also be present. Paraneoplastic syndromes, such as acanthosis nigricans, membranous glomerulonephritis, microangiopathic hemolytic anemia, arterial and venous thrombi (Trousseau syndrome), seborrheic dermatitis (Leser-Trélat sign), or dermatomyositis, may also be present.

Findings on Diagnostic Testing

Upper Gastrointestinal Endoscopy

Suggestive symptoms or findings on physical examination require further evaluation by upper gastrointestinal endoscopy or double-contrast upper gastrointestinal barium radiography. Upper gastrointestinal endoscopy may provide evidence that strongly suggests a neoplasm, but endoscopic biopsy is necessary to confirm the diagnosis. The overall sensitivity and specificity of upper gastrointestinal endoscopy with biopsy are 95% and 99%, respectively. Multiple biopsies are necessary to achieve this accuracy. Further, the combined application of brush cytology then forceps biopsy may improve sensitivity. Biopsy specimens of ulcers are best obtained from the base and the four quadrants of the edge of the ulcer. Because of sampling error, any suggestion of malignancy in the appearance of a gastric ulcer warrants reevaluation by upper gastrointestinal endoscopy after therapy to confirm healing, and biopsy specimens should be taken of any persistent mucosal defect. Tumors that appear as thickened gastric folds with normal overlying mucosa are caused by infiltration of the tumor into the submucosa. These cancers can be diagnosed with cautious use of a snare to obtain a biopsy specimen from the submucosa. Light-induced fluorescence endoscopy is an emerging diagnostic technique that relies on the naturally occurring fluorescence (autofluorescence) of tissue after irradiation with blue or violet light to distinguish neoplastic from normal tissue.

Radiographic Studies

When performed by an experienced radiologist, upper gastrointestinal radiography detects more than 90% of gastric adenocarcinomas. Characteristic radiographic findings include an asymmetric ulcer crater, distorted or nodular folds radiating from an ulcer, a lack of distensibility of the stomach, or a polypoid mass. However, radiography does not have the capability of obtaining histological samples and has been largely replaced by endoscopy for diagnosing gastric malignancy.

Staging Evaluation

Endoscopic ultrasound (EUS) is ideally suited to the TNM classification for staging gastric cancer because it can accurately assess the depth of tumor penetration. Note, however, that EUS has limited ability to differentiate inflammatory from malignant adenopathy. And because EUS cannot detect the majority of distant metastases, computed tomographic (CT) scanning is required to evaluate the M stage. Magnetic resonance imaging (MRI) shows promise as a tool for excluding metastases, but it is not yet superior to CT for staging. Positron emission tomography (PET) appears to be sensitive in detecting gastric neoplasia; however, poor differentiation between primary and metastatic lesions precludes its use in staging.

Management and Course

Surgical Therapy

Complete surgical resection is the only therapy that offers a potential cure of gastric adenocarcinoma; however, the advanced stage at which more than half of patients present precludes curative surgery. The importance of surgical resection is reflected in the 5-year survival rate of 35% to 45% of patients with resectable tumors, compared with the 5-year survival rate of less than 5% of patients who undergo palliative resection.

Although surgery is recognized as the best treatment option for gastric cancer, there is little consensus on the optimal curative surgical procedure for gastric adenocarcinoma, especially concerning the extent of lymph node dissection. Adenocarcinomas of the proximal fundus are treated by proximal gastric resection. Tumors of the gastroesophageal junction require en bloc resection of the distal esophagus and proximal stomach, often by a combined thoracic and abdominal approach. Splenectomy usually is performed if tumors are located along the greater curvature. The role of resection of isolated hepatic metastases at the time of gastrectomy has not been determined in controlled clinical trials. Palliative surgery may be indicated for obstruction, perforation, or bleeding. Bypass procedures provide significantly shorter periods of palliation compared to resection.

Endoscopic Procedures

Endoscopic mucosal resection (EMR) has been shown to cure early gastric cancer in Japanese populations. A submucosal saline injection lifts the lesion away from the muscle layer. The targeted tissue is suctioned into a special cap on the end of the endoscope. Malignant tissue is then snared with electrocautery and removed. Palliative endoscopic therapy may consist of stent placement or Nd:YAG laser tumor ablation, both of which may be used to treat obstruction. Gastrointestinal hemorrhage may be controlled by Nd:YAG laser coagulation necrosis.

Medical Therapy

The role of chemotherapy and radiation therapy in treating gastric adenocarcinoma is evolving. Agents shown to decrease tumor mass include 5-fluorouracil, mitomycin C, doxorubicin, cisplatin, and hydroxyurea; however, there is no evidence of improved survival. Postoperative radiotherapy has likewise not been shown to increase survival.

Screening of High-Risk Populations

In Japan, screening asymptomatic adults every 1 to 2 years with upper gastrointestinal barium radiography or upper gastrointestinal endoscopy has resulted in earlier detection and decreased mortality from gastric cancer. In the United States, patients with pernicious anemia, persons who had gastric surgery more than

20 years previously, and persons with gastric adenomatous polyps represent high-risk populations. There is no evidence, however, that surveillance improves survival in patients with gastric cancer in the United States.

GASTRIC LYMPHOMA

Incidence and Epidemiology

Non-Hodgkin lymphoma is the second most common malignancy of the stomach; it constitutes 5% of gastric cancers. Seventy percent of gastrointestinal lymphomas occur in the stomach, and one third has no associated lymph node involvement.

Etiology and Pathogenesis

Similar to adenocarcinoma of the stomach, gastric lymphomas often occur in chronic atrophic gastritis and intestinal metaplasia. The tumors most commonly infiltrate the submucosal layers, producing thickened rugal folds or submucosal masses with overlying ulceration. There is evidence that more than 90% of low-grade gastric B-cell tumors, termed mucosa-associated lymphoid tissue (MALT) lymphomas, are associated with *H pylori* infection. The critical role of *H pylori* in the genesis of these tumors is supported by reports of complete regression of early stage tumors with antibiotic therapy.

Clinical Features

The presentation of gastric lymphoma is similar to that of gastric adenocarcinoma. Nonspecific symptoms include epigastric pain, weight loss, nausea, vomiting, early satiety, and anorexia. Gastrointestinal hemorrhage and perforation from extensive ulceration are less common manifestations. Physical examination may reveal an abdominal mass or peripheral adenopathy.

Findings on Diagnostic Testing

Upper gastrointestinal endoscopy and upper gastrointestinal barium radiography are the primary means for detecting gastric lymphoma; however, the ability to obtain biopsy specimens makes upper gastrointestinal endoscopy the procedure of choice. CT scans are required to determine extragastric involvement. Occasionally, lymphoma appears as a thickened fold on endoscopy and biopsy reveals a submucosal mass with normal overlying mucosa. In this setting, EUS can delineate which layers of the gastric wall are involved, and cytology or biopsy may confirm the diagnosis. Laparotomy may be necessary to define the extent of disease.

Management and Course

Gastric lymphoma has a favorable prognosis compared with gastric adenocarcinoma. The 5-year survival rate is 50%. The Ann Arbor staging system for gastric lymphoma is based on the extent of disease, which, once established, determines the appropriate course of management (Table 35-2). Patients with stage I tumors limited to the stomach have cure rates higher than 80% and should undergo total gastrectomy or limited gastrectomy with adequate margins. Postoperative chemotherapy and radiation therapy may improve survival of patients with this early stage disease. Patients with stage II to stage IV disease are best treated with

TABLE 35-2
Ann Arbor Staging System for Gastric Lymphoma

STAGE	EXTENT OF DISEASE	RELATIVE INCIDENCE (%)
I	Limited to stomach	26–38
II	Involvement of abdominal lymph nodes	43–49
III	Involvement of lymph nodes above the diaphragm	13–31
IV	Disseminated disease	

combination chemotherapy, but if bulky transmural stomach tumors are present, prophylactic gastrectomy is often performed to prevent treatment-related perforation. Patients with disseminated non-Hodgkin lymphoma rarely survive for 2 years. Most MALT lymphomas are stage I. Early mucosal tumors may respond to antibiotic therapy to eradicate *H pylori*, whereas more advanced MALT lymphomas require systemic chemotherapy. MALT lymphomas, in particular, have relatively favorable outcomes.

GASTROINTESTINAL STROMAL CELL TUMORS

Gastrointestinal stromal cell tumors (GISTs) are mesenchymal neoplasms that are thought to originate from the interstitial cells of Cajal, which is an innervated network of intestinal pacemaker cells. GISTs are composed of a heterogeneous group of neoplasms with predominantly myogenic, neural, or mixed features. Seventy percent of these uncommon tumors are located in the stomach. The peak incidence occurs in the fifth and sixth decades with equal gender distribution. Symptoms are similar to those of other gastric cancers, although bleeding is more common. Surgical resection is the treatment of choice for 50% to 80% of patients. No effective therapy exists for advanced metastatic disease. The 5-year survival rate is 28% to 65%.

METASTATIC TUMORS

Malignant neoplasms from distant sites may metastasize to the stomach. Common sources include melanoma, ovarian, colon, lung, and breast cancer. Tumors may be mucosal or submucosal with associated ulceration. Patients may experience epigastric pain, vomiting, and gastrointestinal hemorrhage.

MISCELLANEOUS BENIGN AND MALIGNANT GASTRIC TUMORS

Gastric Polyps

Most gastric polyps are hyperplastic with no malignant potential. They usually are less than 1 cm in diameter and rarely produce symptoms. Some patients with

Ménétrier disease (i.e., hypertrophic gastropathy) may have large numbers of fundic hyperplastic polyps. Adenomatous polyps account for 10% of gastric polyps. Their malignant potential dictates removal, followed by a program of endoscopic surveillance to detect recurrence. Patients with familial adenomatous polyposis (FAP) may have fundic gland polyposis. These polyps usually are hamartomatous, although some are adenomatous. Gastric adenomas in patients with FAP have the potential for malignant degeneration, necessitating excision and endoscopic surveillance.

Gastric Carcinoids

Only 3% of all carcinoid tumors are located in the stomach. There are three types of gastric carcinoids. The most common is type 1, which is characterized by generally small multiple tumors localized to the fundus and body. Type 1 gastric carcinoids have the lowest metastatic rate of the three types (9% to 23%). Associated findings include chronic atrophic gastritis, achlorhydria, and pernicious anemia. Type 2 is associated with multiple endocrine neoplasia type I (MEN I) and has an intermediate risk of metastasis. Type 3 is the least common but the most aggressive and most prone to metastasis. Type 3 gastric carcinoids are not associated with a hypergastrinemic state. The tumors are sporadic and generally solitary and large.

Gastric carcinoids are endocrine tumors that produce multiple bioactive substances, including serotonin, histamines, somatostatin, and kinins, but they rarely produce the carcinoid syndrome, which is characterized by flushing, diarrhea, and cardiopulmonary symptoms. Carcinoids usually are submucosal lesions, although they can cause ulceration of the overlying mucosa. Metastatic tumors may require systemic chemotherapy to control tumor bulk. The somatostatin analog octreotide improves symptoms in many patients with the carcinoid syndrome.

Leiomyoma and Leiomyosarcoma

Leiomyomas are the most common gastric submucosal masses. They usually cause no symptoms and are often detected incidentally during upper gastrointestinal endoscopy. Leiomyomas rarely undergo malignant transformation to leiomyosarcomas, which account for less than 1% of gastric malignancies. A leiomyosarcoma is a highly vascular tumor that often manifests with massive gastrointestinal hemorrhage. The differentiation of a leiomyoma from a leiomyosarcoma is often problematic and is based on the number of mitotic figures and invasiveness seen on histological examination. The 5-year survival rate of patients is about 50% after resection of a leiomyosarcoma.

CHAPTER 36

Structural Anomalies and Miscellaneous Diseases of the Small Intestine

EMBRYOLOGY AND ANATOMY

The small intestine is about 600 cm long and is divided into three segments: the duodenum, the jejunum, and the ileum. The ligament of Treitz separates the retroperitoneal duodenum from the jejunum and marks the reentrance of the small bowel into the peritoneum (the duodenal bulb possesses a mesentery and is also considered intraperitoneal). There is no similar landmark to differentiate the remaining two segments; however, the proximal two fifths of intraperitoneal small intestine is considered jejunum, and the remaining three fifths is ileum. The jejunum is thicker than the ileum and has more prominent plicae circulares, which are mucosal and submucosal invaginations.

The esophagus, stomach, duodenum (up to the ampulla of Vater), pharynx, respiratory tract, liver, pancreas, and biliary system begin to develop from the embryonic foregut in the fourth week of gestation. The midgut forms the distal duodenum, jejunum, ileum, cecum, appendix, ascending colon, and the proximal half of the transverse colon. The midgut initially communicates with the yolk sac and then narrows for connection to the omphalomesenteric or vitelline duct. The gut forms a U-shaped loop that herniates into the umbilical cord in the sixth week of gestation. The proximal limb of the loop rotates around the superior mesenteric artery axis and at 10 weeks, returns to the abdominal cavity with an additional counterclockwise rotation. The small intestine is attached to the posterior abdominal wall by a broad-based mesentery from the duodenojejunal junction to the ileocecal region.

The vascular and lymphatic systems of the small intestine travel through the mesentery. The hepatic artery originates from the celiac trunk and gives rise to the gastroduodenal artery, which divides into the anterior and posterior superior pancreaticoduodenal arteries. These arteries communicate with the anterior and posterior inferior pancreaticoduodenal arteries, which are branches of the superior mesenteric artery that supply the duodenum. The jejunum and ileum also receive arterial blood from branches of the superior mesenteric artery. The veins that drain the small intestine usually follow the arterial supply. Small lymph channels (i.e., lacteals) drain into mesenteric lymph nodes, which subsequently drain into the cisterna chyli and thoracic duct.

The small intestine has an extensive intrinsic neural system supplied by the myenteric (Auerbach) plexus, which lies between the longitudinal and circular muscle layers, and the submucosal (Meissner) plexus. The extrinsic autonomic innervation arises from the superior mesenteric ganglion (sympathetic) and the vagus nerve (parasympathetic). A rich sensory innervation comprises different nerves from the dorsal root and nodose ganglia.

Structurally, the small intestine is composed of four concentric layers: the mucosa, the submucosa, the muscularis propria, and the serosa. The mucosa is further divided into an epithelial layer, the lamina propria, and the muscularis mucosae. The epithelium is a continuous sheet of columnar cells that overlie the villi and form the crypts. Through the action of the columnar cells, the products of digestion are distributed via the vascular and lymphatic system to other areas of the body. Tight junctions between adjacent epithelial cells restrict hydrostatic and ionic flow. In a process of cellular renewal that lasts 3 to 5 days, undifferentiated stem cells in the crypts give rise to four major differentiated cell types: enterocytes, goblet cells, Paneth cells, and enteroendocrine cells. M cells and undifferentiated crypt cells are also present but in smaller numbers. Enterocytes are absorptive cells that exhibit prominent microvilli and possess numerous brush-border enzymes for digestion (e.g., disaccharidases, peptidases), lipid absorption proteins (e.g., apolipoproteins, fatty acid–binding proteins), as well as receptors, carriers, and transporters. Enterocytes possess cytoskeletal filaments that contribute to the structural rigidity of the brush border. Some of these filaments protrude from the cell membrane to form a surface coat called the glycocalyx. Goblet cells are present throughout the entire gastrointestinal tract, but they are most numerous in the ileum, where they produce the mucus that serves as a lubricant and a cytoprotective agent. Paneth cells are believed to be involved in host defense and mucosal barrier function because of their abundant expression of lysozyme and defensins and their ability to degranulate in response to bacteria. Enteroendocrine cells produce hormones and include D cells (somatostatin); L cells (glucagon-like immunoreactivity); enterochromaffin cells (serotonin); and cholecystokinin-secreting, substance P–secreting, and motilin-secreting cells. Other mucosal cell types include the "tuft" (caveolated) cells, intraepithelial lymphocytes, and M cells overlying Peyer patches. M cells engulf macromolecules, viruses, and bacteria by endocytosis and appear to regulate the immune response by presenting antigen to lymphocytes and macrophages.

The lamina propria contains immune cells (e.g., lymphocytes, macrophages, neutrophils, plasma cells, and mast cells). Plasma cells are responsible for immunoglobulin A (IgA) synthesis before complexing with secretory component from the enterocyte. Lymphoid follicles are collections of lymphocytes in the mucosa and submucosa. Peyer patches are organized follicular aggregates that contain M cells. Most numerous in the terminal ileum, Peyer patches play an important role in intestinal immunity. Other components of the lamina propria include fibroblasts, smooth muscle cells, arterioles, venules, and a central lacteal for delivering nutrients into the vascular system.

The submucosa contains connective tissue, blood vessels, the submucosal (Meissner) plexus, and, in the duodenum only, Brunner glands, which secrete mucus and bicarbonate. The muscularis propria consists of an outer longitudinal layer and an inner circular muscle layer, which generate peristalsis. The serosa is composed of mesothelial cells overlying loose connective tissue and is continuous with the mesentery.

DEVELOPMENTAL ABNORMALITIES

Meckel Diverticulum

Etiology and Pathogenesis

A Meckel diverticulum develops if the vitelline duct fails to resorb completely. Meckel diverticula, the most common gastrointestinal congenital anomaly, occur in 2% to 3% of the general population. The diverticula usually are 1 to 10 cm long and often are located within 100 cm of the ileocecal valve. One half contains heterotopic tissue, most commonly gastric, but pancreatic, colonic, or hepatobiliary tissue, or Brunner glands may also be present. *Helicobacter pylori* may colonize heterotopic gastric mucosa and produce inflammation.

Clinical Features, Diagnosis, and Management

Complications develop in 2% of cases, and include hemorrhage, intestinal obstruction, diverticulitis, perforation, and carcinoma. Gastrointestinal bleeding may occur as a result of ileal ulceration arising from acid production from heterotopic gastric mucosa. Diverticulitis is caused by enterolith impaction. Obstruction is caused by intussusception, volvulus, entrapment in hernias, or inflammation and scarring. Related malignancies include carcinoid, sarcoma, and adenocarcinoma. Children commonly present with gastrointestinal bleeding, whereas obstruction is by far the most frequent complication in adults. Meckel diverticulum may be diagnosed by radiolabeled technetium scanning, a highly sensitive and specific technique for children; however, for adults, it is fraught with high false-negative and false-positive rates (e.g., in Crohn's disease), even in bleeding patients. The sensitivity of the test may be improved by administering cimetidine, which inhibits release of the radiolabeled anion by the ectopic gastric mucosa, and pentagastrin, which enhances technetium uptake. Enteroclysis has better sensitivity than small bowel follow-through. Angiography may reveal active bleeding and thus document the persistent vitelline artery and its branches. Most asymptomatic Meckel diverticula do not require treatment. Surgical resection is indicated for hemorrhage, obstruction, or perforation and may need to include adjacent small intestine if it is ulcerated, inflamed, or obstructed. Resection of diverticula found incidentally during laparotomy has been advocated if the diverticula are large, if they have persistent fibrous bands, or if they have palpable masses.

Duplications

Etiology and Pathogenesis

Duplications may occur anywhere along the gastrointestinal tract. They contain all layers of the wall and may or may not communicate with the lumen. Most duplications of the small intestine occur in the ileum. Some tubular duplications may be lined with heterotopic mucosa of gastric, pancreatic, esophageal, thyroid, or bronchial origin.

Clinical Features, Diagnosis, and Management

Duplications vary greatly in presentation with symptoms of obstruction, pain, and hemorrhage. Obstructions result from a mass effect or from intussusception. Infrequently, they may penetrate into the head of the pancreas causing pancreatitis, or develop malignancies such as adenocarcinoma or carcinoid. Diagnosis may be made by barium radiography of the small intestine or by enteroclysis if the duplication communicates with the gut lumen. Computed tomographic (CT) or ultrasound studies may reveal a cystic mass. Radiolabeled technetium scans (i.e., Meckel scan) may show the duplication if gastric mucosa is present. The treatment of choice is complete surgical resection, if possible, or drainage into the adjacent intestinal lumen.

Atresia and Stenosis

Etiology and Pathogenesis

During embryological development, the lumen of the small intestine is initially occluded by epithelium. Failure of recanalization can result in stenosis, in which narrowing of the lumen leads to partial obstruction, or atresia, which is complete occlusion. Duodenal (and to a lesser extent, jejunal) stenosis and atresia may be associated with other congenital abnormalities, such as Down syndrome, malrotation, esophageal atresia, annular pancreas, imperforate anus, and growth retardation. Type I atresia is characterized by a membranous septum of mucosa and submucosa with intact bowel wall and mesentery. Type II atresia has two blind loops of small intestine connected by a fibrous cord. In type IIIa atresia, two blind loops are separated by a gap; in type IIIb, the distal superior mesenteric artery is absent. Type IV is characterized by the presence of multiple atresias. Although the pathogenesis of atresia is unknown, ischemia or a defect in recanalization of the gut lumen may be precipitating factors.

Clinical Features, Diagnosis, and Management

Polyhydramnios may occur in utero, and maternal ultrasound studies may detect proximal bowel dilation, fetal ascites, and extralumenal calcifications. Vomiting begins soon after birth, and if the obstruction is proximal to the ampulla of Vater, the vomitus is devoid of bile. Duodenal stenosis, which rarely occurs in adulthood, may produce a sensation of fullness, vomiting, and weight loss. Duodenal obstruction distal to the bulb gives a typical "double-bubble" signature in abdominal radiography. Upper gastrointestinal barium radiography can confirm the site of obstruction, but often it is not necessary for diagnosis. Barium enema radiography is recommended to exclude Hirschsprung disease and malrotation with volvulus. Treatment of infants begins with hydration, nasogastric suction, and correction of electrolyte abnormalities. Gastrojejunostomy is performed for proximal duodenal obstruction, and duodenojejunostomy for distal blockage. Type IIIb and type IV atresias may require extensive resection. All patients are given total parenteral nutrition postoperatively until normal intestinal function resumes.

Malrotation

Etiology and Pathogenesis

Malrotation is an anomalous rotation and fixation of the intestine during embryogenesis. The jejunum and ileum lie in the right side of the abdominal cavity and the colon in the left, with the cecum located in the left iliac fossa. The major clinical consequences of malrotation are volvulus and duodenal obstruction. The former is due to the presence of a narrow vascular pedicle instead of a broad mesentery anchoring the small intestine. Failure of the cecum to descend into the right lower quadrant causes a mobile cecum, also predisposing to volvulus. Duodenal obstruction can result from the presence of Ladd bands, peritoneal bands that pass from the cecum across the duodenum to the upper right quadrant. Reversed rotation produces a condition in which the mesentery of the small intestine passes in front of the transverse colon, producing colonic obstruction. One half of patients have other congenital anomalies, including duodenal atresia, annular pancreas, or Hirschsprung disease.

Clinical Features, Diagnosis, and Management

Most patients with midgut malrotation present primarily in infancy with bilious vomiting, distention, and visible peristalsis. Complications include intestinal or cecal volvulus or small bowel obstruction. Older children, adolescents, and adults may experience intermittent vomiting, failure to thrive, recurrent pain, or volvulus with acute abdominal pain, bloody stools, and distention. Abdominal radiography shows gastric and proximal intestinal dilation. Upper gastrointestinal barium radiography may show the site of obstruction and the characteristic "corkscrew" appearance of the twisted duodenum and proximal jejunum. CT scans may show reversed positioning of the superior mesenteric artery and vein. Treatment involves surgical division of the obstructing bands, resection of any infarcted segments, and fixation of the cecum to prevent volvulus. Most patients fare well postoperatively, but a subset of children experiences persistent nausea, vomiting, and pain because of dysmotility and damage to the small intestine from long-standing obstruction.

Superior Mesenteric Artery Syndrome

Etiology and Pathogenesis

Superior mesenteric artery syndrome is characterized by compression of the third portion of the duodenum against fixed retroperitoneal structures by the superior mesenteric artery, possibly because the artery is positioned at an acute angle to the aorta.

Clinical Features, Diagnosis, and Management

Symptoms may be acute or chronic and include epigastric distress and vomiting. Abdominal radiography may be normal or may reflect the "double-bubble" image indicative of duodenal obstruction, as discussed earlier. Upper gastrointestinal barium radiography reveals an abrupt cutoff of barium flow in the third duodenal portion. A narrowed angle of the superior mesenteric artery with respect to the aorta may be seen by angiography. Initial therapy involves small liquid feedings, and postprandially, the patient lies prone or on the left side. Duodenojejunostomy is reserved for refractory cases.

STRUCTURAL ABNORMALITIES

Volvulus

Etiology and Pathogenesis

Volvulus is an abnormal twisting of the intestine around its mesentery. Complications include strangulation and gangrene. In the United States, most cases of volvulus of the small intestine are associated with a predisposing condition such as an anomaly of rotation, postoperative adhesion, or congenital bands.

Clinical Features, Diagnosis, and Management

Patients with volvulus present with symptoms of small bowel obstruction or acute abdomen. Physical examination may reveal a distended abdomen, guarding and rigidity, and occasionally a palpable mass. Abdominal radiography may show distention with air-fluid levels, which indicates an obstruction. Upper gastrointestinal barium radiography may define anomalies of rotation. Angiography may show twisting of the superior mesenteric artery, confirming the diagnosis. Surgical treatment involves resection of the ischemic or gangrenous bowel, although occasionally derotation alone is sufficient.

Intussusception

Etiology and Pathogenesis

Intussusception occurs when a segment of bowel telescopes into adjacent distal bowel, resulting in obstruction and possibly ischemia. It is a common cause of small bowel obstruction in children and is usually idiopathic. However, a pathological lead point caused by a mass (e.g., leiomyoma or lymphoma), duplication, or intramural hematoma (as may occur with Henoch-Schönlein purpura), is present in 8% to 12% of pediatric cases. In contrast, a causative factor can be identified in 90% of adult patients in the form of an intestinal or extraintestinal mass (e.g., leiomyoma, neurofibroma, lipoma, lymphoma, polyp, metastatic tumor, Kaposi sarcoma), Meckel diverticulum, or after a Billroth II gastrojejunostomy.

Clinical Features, Diagnosis, and Management

Children with intussusception present with acute abdominal pain, vomiting, hematochezia, a palpable mass, diarrhea, and somnolence. The presentation in adults is more variable, with intermittent or chronic abdominal pain, nausea and vomiting, weight loss, or an abdominal mass. Abdominal radiography may show a crescent of gas capping the intussusception, a gas-free area corresponding to the intussusception itself, or a target sign comprising two concentric radiolucent circles outlining the intussusception. In children, barium enema radiography is useful because the ileocecal region often is involved and the enema may reduce the intussusception. If the lesion fails to recede or if perforation is present, surgery is required. Ultrasound may be advantageous, and CT scanning usually is not necessary. A definitive diagnosis in adults may require a combination of abdominal radiography, upper gastrointestinal and barium enema radiography, ultrasound, and CT studies. Adults should undergo surgical resection because most cases are associated with mass lesions.

Lymphangiectasia

Etiology and Pathogenesis

Intestinal lymphangiectasia is the dilation of lacteals caused by obstruction of lymph drainage from the small intestine. Consequences include malabsorption of chylomicrons and fat-soluble vitamins and development of protein-losing enteropathy. Lymphenteric fistulae may develop, resulting in loss of proteins, chylomicrons, and lymphocytes into the intestinal lumen. Lymphangiectasia may be a primary disorder (Milroy disease) or secondary to another disease that blocks intestinal lymph drainage, such as retroperitoneal carcinoma or lymphoma, retroperitoneal fibrosis, chronic pancreatitis, mesenteric tuberculosis or sarcoidosis, Crohn's disease, Whipple disease, scleroderma, celiac disease, or heart disease.

Clinical Features, Diagnosis, and Management

Patients exhibit malabsorption, steatorrhea, lymphocytopenia (mainly T lymphocytes), hypogammaglobulinemia, and hypoproteinemia. Milroy disease presents at any age with asymmetric lymphedema of an extremity. Less commonly, symptoms of abdominal pain, nausea and vomiting, gastrointestinal hemorrhage, or opportunistic infections (e.g., atypical mycobacteria, warts, or cellulitis) develop. Laboratory studies indicate increased amounts of fecal fat, prolonged prothrombin time, and reduced calcium or vitamin A levels. Fecal levels of α_1-antitrypsin usually are elevated, which is a diagnostic criterion for protein-losing enteropathy. If secondary lymphangiectasia is suspected, a CT scan may identify the etiology. Endoscopically dilated lacteals may cause the mucosa to develop opaque spots or white-tipped villi. The diagnosis of lymphangiectasia rests on biopsy specimens that show dilated lymphatic lacteals, villous atrophy, and mild inflammation. Managing secondary lymphangiectasia begins with identifying and treating the underlying cause. With primary disease, use of medium-chain triglycerides may reduce diarrhea, steatorrhea, and enteric protein loss. An octreotide regimen is reportedly efficacious, as is antiplasmin therapy for patients with elevated fibrinolytic activity. Peripheral edema is reduced by postural drainage and elastic stockings.

ULCERS OF THE SMALL INTESTINE

A variety of disorders are associated with ulcers of the small intestine (Table 36-1).

Medication-Induced Ulcers

Etiology and Pathogenesis

The most common causes of ulcers of the small intestine are nonsteroidal anti-inflammatory drugs (NSAIDs) and potassium supplements. Multiple small bowel ulcers (in 8.4% of patients), mucosal diaphragms, strictures, and perforations are associated with NSAID use. NSAID-induced ulcers of the small intestine typically involve the distal intestine. The risk of ulcer formation is increased by delayed intestinal transit, advanced age, and concurrent systemic illness. Other drugs that cause small bowel ulcers include corticosteroids, cytarabine, digoxin, and ferrous sulfate preparations.

Clinical Features, Diagnosis, and Management

Patients with medication-induced ulcers of the small intestine present with acute or chronic blood loss, obstruction, perforation, weight loss, hypoalbuminemia, and vague abdominal pain. Small intestine barium radiography, enteroclysis, endoscopy, enteroscopy, and capsule endoscopy are commonly used for diagnosis. If possible, the offending medication should be discontinued. Surgical intervention is necessary to treat complications such as hemorrhage, stricture, or perforation.

TABLE 36-1
Causes of Ulceration of the Small Intestine

Infection	***Vascular Causes***
Tuberculosis	Mesenteric insufficiency
Typhoid	Giant cell arteritis
Cytomegalovirus	Vasculitis
Syphilis	Vascular abnormality
Parasitic diseases	Amyloidosis
Strongyloidiasis	
Campylobacteriosis	***Hyperacidity***
Yersiniosis	Zollinger-Ellison syndrome
	Meckel diverticulum
Inflammatory Causes	Stomal ulceration
Crohn's disease	
Systemic lupus erythematosus	***Metabolic Causes***
Diverticulitis	Uremia
Mucosal Lesions	***Medications***
Ulcerative jejunoileitis	Potassium chloride
	NSAIDs
Tumors	Antimetabolites
Malignant histiocytosis	
Lymphoma	***Radiation Therapy***
Adenocarcinoma	
Melanoma	***Idiopathic Ulcers***
Kaposi sarcoma	Primary ulcer
	Behçet syndrome

Ulcers Associated with Systemic Disease

Etiology and Pathogenesis

Behçet syndrome affects the skin, joints, vascular system, central nervous system, and, in less than 1% of persons, the intestinal tract. Deep ulcers in the ileocecal region surrounded by a minimally inflamed mucosa are the characteristic intestinal manifestation. Patients with systemic lupus erythematosus may present with ulcers of the small intestine as a result of microthrombosis and vasculitis.

Clinical Features, Diagnosis, and Management

The optimal treatment of Behçet syndrome is not established, although intestinal resection may be necessary. No medical treatment consistently alters its course, and postoperative ulcer recurrence is common.

Ulcerative Jejunoileitis

Etiology and Pathogenesis

Chronic ulcerative jejunoileitis may be a complication stemming from long-standing celiac sprue. It is characterized by multiple ulcers in the small intestine in the setting of villous atrophy, mucosal inflammation, and crypt hyperplasia. Rarely, chronic ulcerative jejunoileitis occurs in patients who have no history of celiac sprue. This condition often is difficult to distinguish from lymphoma of the small intestine, which is associated with celiac sprue and chronic ulcerative jejunoileitis. Therefore, determination of lymphocyte cell surface markers is essential for proper diagnosis and treatment.

Clinical Features, Diagnosis, and Management

Patients present with chronic symptoms of malabsorption, including abdominal pain, fever, weight loss, diarrhea, and steatorrhea. Complications such as obstruction, melena, or perforation affect 20% to 30% of cases. The diagnosis is considered in patients with celiac sprue who have worsening malabsorption despite adherence to a gluten-free diet. Barium radiography of the small intestine may show strictures and intestinal fold thickening. CT scans may show mesenteric lymphadenopathy or splenic atrophy. Upper gastrointestinal endoscopy with biopsy has diagnostic value, but sufficient tissue must be obtained to exclude the diagnosis of lymphoma. Therapeutic options are limited, and most patients survive less than 2 years. Prednisone should be considered for patients without lymphoma. Surgical resection may be necessary to treat complications or lymphomatous involvement. Disseminated T-cell lymphoma is treated with aggressive chemotherapy.

DRUG-INDUCED DISEASE OF THE SMALL INTESTINE

Drugs That Cause Ischemia

Etiology and Pathogenesis

Drug-induced intestinal ischemia can result from arterial vasoconstriction, systemic or splanchnic hypotension, or mesenteric thrombosis. Antihypertensives (including diuretics) promote hypotension and hypovolemia, whereas catecholamines (e.g., dopamine, vasopressin, and norepinephrine) produce vasoconstriction. Digoxin reduces splanchnic blood flow. Cocaine-evoked peripheral vasoconstriction causes ischemia that is exacerbated by rebound vasodilation and reperfusion. Ergot alkaloids for treating migraines may cause splanchnic vasospasm with bowel infarction. Oral contraceptive use predisposes to mesenteric arterial or venous thrombosis. The risk of thromboembolism normalizes within 1 month after discontinuing oral contraceptives.

Clinical Features, Diagnosis, and Management

Drug-induced ischemia has a 70% to 90% mortality rate because of delays in presentation and comorbid disease. Patients present with incompletely localized pain, fever, hematochezia, distention, and ileus. Abdominal radiography may reveal perforation, obstruction, or ileus. CT studies may assist in diagnosing mesenteric infarction. Angiographic studies may appear normal with nonocclusive ischemia but may also show thrombosis or spasm secondary to digoxin or ergot alkaloids. Management should be conservative and should include fluids, electrolytes, and correction of acid-base disturbances. Nitroprusside may be used for vasoconstriction secondary to digoxin or ergot alkaloids. Surgical resection of infarcted segments is often required.

TABLE 36-2
Classification of Protein-Losing Enteropathy

Ulcerative diseases
    Erosive gastroenteritis
    Neoplasia
    Crohn's disease
    Pseudomembranous enterocolitis
    Acute graft-versus-host disease

Nonulcerative diseases
    Ménétrier disease
    Viral gastroenteritides
    Bacterial overgrowth
    Parasitic diseases
    Whipple disease
    Eosinophilic gastroenteritis
    Celiac sprue
    Tropical sprue
    Systemic lupus erythematosus

Disorders affecting the lymphatic system
    Congenital intestinal lymphangiectasia
    Mesenteric lymphatic obstruction
        Tuberculosis
        Sarcoidosis
        Lymphoma
        Retroperitoneal fibrosis
    Increased right heart pressure
        Constrictive pericarditis
        Congestive heart failure
    Whipple disease
    Crohn's disease

Protein-Losing Enteropathy

Etiology and Pathogenesis

Protein-losing enteropathy is abnormal loss of plasma protein from the gastrointestinal tract. Intestinal loss of serum proteins usually accounts for less than 10% of daily protein catabolism. Protein loss may increase fivefold in patients with protein-losing enteropathy, leading to hypoproteinemia. Causes of protein-losing enteropathy can be categorized into disorders causing small intestinal ulceration, nonulcerating diseases, and diseases that interfere with lymphatic drainage (Table 36-2). Nonulcerating diseases associated with protein-losing enteropathy include Ménétrier disease, atrophic gastritis, tropical sprue, celiac sprue, eosinophilic gastroenteritis, collagenous colitis, and colonic polyposis syndromes. Acute and chronic intestinal infections and bacterial overgrowth may produce protein-losing enteropathy. Rheumatologic disorders such as systemic lupus erythematosus and mixed connective tissue disease can be complicated by protein-losing enteropathy.

Clinical Features, Diagnosis, and Management

Protein-losing enteropathy may manifest with edema, steatorrhea, and lymphopenia. It is diagnosed by identifying elevated fecal α_1-antitrypsin clearance, which is calculated by dividing the product of daily stool volume and stool α_1-antitrypsin concentration by the serum α_1-antitrypsin concentration. Therapy consists of replacing long-chain triglycerides by medium-chain triglycerides. Mechanical therapy is used for dependent edema. Rarely, surgical lymphovenous anastomosis is effective.

CHAPTER 37

Dysmotility and Bacterial Overgrowth of the Small Intestine

DYSMOTILITY OF THE SMALL INTESTINE

Incidence and Epidemiology

Clinically recognized dysmotility syndromes that involve the small intestine are less prevalent than motor disorders that involve the esophagus, stomach, and colon. However, this may in part stem from nonspecific symptom presentations of small bowel motility abnormalities, as well as a paucity of reliable and available tests for their diagnoses.

Etiology and Pathogenesis

Small intestinal dysmotility may result from primary diseases of smooth muscle or enteric nerve tissue. Alternatively, motor dysfunction may be secondary to systemic neuromuscular diseases, endocrine disorders, or medications (Table 37-1).

TABLE 37-1
Causes of Dysmotility in the Small Intestine

Primary causes
  Familial types
    Familial visceral myopathies (types I, II, III)
    Familial visceral neuropathies (types I, II)
    Childhood visceral myopathies (types I, II)
  Nonfamilial or sporadic types
    Visceral myopathies
    Visceral neuropathies

Secondary causes
  Smooth muscle diseases
    Rheumatologic disease (e.g., scleroderma, polymyositis and dermatomyositis, systemic lupus erythematosus, mixed connective tissue disease)
    Muscular dystrophies (e.g., myotonic dystrophy, Duchenne muscular dystrophy)
    Amyloidosis
  Neurological diseases
    Chagas disease
    Intestinal ganglioneuromatosis
    Paraneoplastic pseudoobstruction
    Parkinson disease
    Spinal cord injury
  Endocrine disorders
    Diabetes mellitus
    Thyroid disease
    Hypoparathyroidism
  Medications
    Phenothiazines
    Tricyclic antidepressants
    Antiparkinsonian drugs
    Ganglionic blockers
    Clonidine
    Opiates
  Miscellaneous
    Celiac sprue
    Small intestinal diverticulosis
    Radiation enteritis
    Jejunoileal bypass
    Diffuse lymphoid infiltration of the small intestine
    Postgastrointestinal viral infection
    Anorexia nervosa and bulimia nervosa

Primary Causes

Familial Visceral Myopathies. Familial visceral myopathies (FVMs) are genetic diseases that produce degeneration and fibrosis of smooth muscle cells. They can involve the entire muscularis propria but may be confined to the longitudinal layer. Type I FVM is an autosomal dominant disorder characterized by esophageal dilation, megaduodenum, redundant colon, and megacystis. Megaduodenum manifests in adolescence; 10% percent develop intestinal pseudoobstruction. Twenty percent report dysphagia, whereas constipation occurs in one half. Volvulus has been reported. Megacystis rarely leads to urinary infection. Type II FVM (also known as mitochondrial neurogastrointestinal encephalomyopathy) is an autosomal recessive disorder. In adolescence to middle age, patients present with gastroparesis, small intestinal dilation and diverticula, striated muscle degeneration, peripheral neuropathy, deafness, ptosis, and ophthalmoplegia. Symptomatic intestinal pseudoobstruction often necessitates long-term parenteral nutrition. Screening tests for type II FVM include serum lactic acid, muscle enzymes, and leukocyte thymidine phophorylase. Skeletal muscle biopsies show characteristic mitochondrial ragged red fibers on modified Gomori stain. Type III FVM is an autosomal recessive condition characterized by diffuse intestinal dilation from the esophagus to the rectum that presents in middle age. All patients have chronic intestinal pseudoobstruction and require parenteral nutrition.

Familial Visceral Neuropathies. Familial visceral neuropathies (FVNs) are genetic diseases of myenteric plexus degeneration. Type I FVN is an autosomal dominant disease characterized by dilation of the distal small intestine and colon. Patients present with postprandial abdominal pain, distention, and diarrhea or constipation. One fourth of patients have gastroparesis. Histological study reveals marked reductions in argyrophilic myenteric neurons and nerve fibers. Most patients have mild malnutrition but require parenteral nutrition. Type II FVN is an autosomal recessive disease with hypertrophic pyloric stenosis, dilation, small intestinal malrotation, associated central nervous system malformations, and patent ductus arteriosus. In infancy, all patients present with fatal intestinal pseudoobstruction. Additional congenital neuropathic motility disorders may result from failed colonization of neural crest cells of the distal gut (as in Hirschsprung disease), disorders of enteric neuronal differentiation (as in intestinal ganglioneuromatosis), or impaired enteric nerve survival or maintenance (as in hypoganglionosis and congenital achalasia). Hirschsprung disease affects 1 in 5,000 births and is often associated with gene mutations in GDNF, RET, EDN-3, or EDNRB. Multiple endocrine neoplasia type IIB is a congenital neuropathic condition that presents with constipation or megacolon, mucosal neuromas, marfanoid habitus, medullated corneal nerve fibers, and endocrine neoplasms (medullary thyroid cancer, pheochromocytoma, parathyroid tumors). Pathological examination in this condition shows transmural intestinal ganglioneuromatosis with massive proliferation of neural tissue that appears like thickened nerve trunks. Other FVNs exhibit associated neurological symptoms, ptosis, ophthalmoplegia, mental retardation, and intestinal diverticula.

Childhood Visceral Myopathies. Childhood visceral myopathies (CVMs) are diseases distinct from FVMs. Patients with type I CVM present before 5 years of age with symptomatic dilation from the stomach to the rectum. The disease usually is fatal, but long-term parenteral nutrition may prolong life. Type II CVM is a more common autosomal recessive condition with intestinal pseudoobstruction, microcolon with malrotation and malfixation in the left abdomen, intestinal and colonic shortening, and megacystis with recurrent urinary infection. The disease occurs predominantly in female infants. Most patients die in infancy, although parenteral nutrition may prolong life.

Nonfamilial Visceral Myopathies and Neuropathies.   Rare cases of primary visceral myopathy appear to have no genetic predisposition. Histologically, there are no differences between the familial and nonfamilial types. Non-FVNs are more common than non-FVMs and may result from myenteric damage from chemicals, drugs, or viral infection. Patients with nonfamilial neuropathies exhibit active but nonperistaltic intestinal motor activity. Clinical manifestations are consistent with intestinal pseudoobstruction. Histological studies show reduced numbers of myenteric neurons, and those that remain are abnormal.

Secondary Causes

Scleroderma.   The small intestine is the second most frequently involved gastrointestinal organ in scleroderma, after the esophagus. Forty percent of patients exhibit gastric or intestinal stasis. Wide-mouth diverticula may be present, as may pneumatosis cystoides intestinalis, a finding that signifies a poor prognosis. Smooth muscle degeneration and collagen replacement, most prominently of the circular muscle layer, characterize the disorder. Manometric evaluation reveals a hypomotility pattern. Conventional stains do not detect myenteric plexus damage, but some patients exhibit a manometric pattern of uncoordinated intense contractions of the small intestine that suggests neuropathy in the early stages of disease.

Other Rheumatologic Disorders.   The gastrointestinal tract is involved in 50% of cases of dermatomyositis and polymyositis. A common presentation is dysphagia. Megaduodenum and delayed intestinal transit may be prominent; intestinal pseudoobstruction is rare. Smooth muscle dysfunction in systemic lupus erythematosus results in dilation of the small intestine and ileus, which is postulated to be secondary to vasculitis-related ischemia. Gastrointestinal involvement in mixed connective tissue disease, which is detected by high titers of antinuclear antibody against ribonucleoprotein, resembles that of scleroderma.

Myotonic Dystrophy.   Myotonic dystrophy is characterized by difficulty in muscle relaxation, a nasal voice, cataracts, and cardiac conduction defects. Dysphagia is the most common motor symptom, although diarrhea, constipation, and intestinal pseudoobstruction may occur. Radiographic findings include small intestinal dilation, hypomotility, and delayed transit, whereas manometry shows low-amplitude contractions, retrograde fasting motility, and increased tonic contractions. Histological evaluation shows swollen, degenerated, smooth muscle cells with fatty replacement, as well as rare degenerative changes in the colonic myenteric plexus.

Duchenne Muscular Dystrophy.   Duchenne muscular dystrophy is an X-linked recessive disorder that causes gastrointestinal smooth muscle degeneration, atrophy, and separation by connective tissue. Symptoms are usually related to esophageal or gastric dysmotility, although intestinal pseudoobstruction can occur.

Amyloidosis.   Amyloid protein is deposited in the small intestine in primary, secondary, myeloma-associated, or hereditary (familial Mediterranean fever) amyloidosis. In primary and myeloma-associated amyloidosis, muscle involvement produces dysmotility, whereas mucosal deposition in secondary and hereditary amyloidosis causes malabsorption. Amyloid rarely produces a visceral neuropathic pattern.

Other Neuromuscular Diseases.   Chagas disease is characterized by myenteric plexus destruction secondary to infection with *Trypanosoma cruzi*. Common manifestations are megaesophagus and megacolon, although megaduodenum and megajejunum may occur. Symptoms include constipation, diarrhea, and intestinal pseudoobstruction. Chronic intestinal pseudoobstruction may be a paraneoplastic consequence of small cell lung carcinoma, epidermoid lip carcinoma, or other malignancies. It is characterized by widespread myenteric and submucosal neuronal and axonal degeneration with mononuclear infiltration. Pheochromocytoma may produce intestinal pseudoobstruction from excess catecholamine production. Small bowel dysmotility with dilation and hypomotility occur with Parkinson disease. Medications used to treat the disease may exacerbate these symptoms. Histological studies show cytoplasmic hyaline inclusions (e.g., Lewy bodies) in the myenteric neurons of the esophagus and colon. Gastrointestinal neurofibromas occur in 10% of patients with neurofibromatosis and have very rarely been associated with intestinal pseudoobstruction. Spinal cord injury produces minimal chronic effects on small intestine motor activity, although constipation and postprandial distention are prevalent secondary to constipation. Ileus and distention are common immediately after spinal damage.

Endocrine Disorders.   The small intestine tends to be involved less frequently and later in the course of diabetes mellitus. There are no morphologic abnormalities of the myenteric or submucosal plexuses. Although smooth muscle thickening with eosinophilic hyaline body deposition has been observed, myopathy does not occur in most diabetics. Many individuals with long-standing diabetes develop small intestinal bacterial overgrowth, which may be a consequence of dysmotility. Hyperthyroidism stimulates intestinal transit, causing diarrhea and malabsorption, whereas hypothyroidism retards propulsion, producing constipation, ileus, and pseudoobstruction. Hypoparathyroidism may lead to intestinal pseudoobstruction as a consequence of hypocalcemia.

Medication-Induced Dysmotility.   Although medications more often affect colonic motor activity, small bowel contractile function is inhibited by phenothiazines, antiparkinsonian agents, tricyclic antidepressants, anticholinergics, opiates (including loperamide), and calcium channel antagonists. Conversely, tegaserod, erythromycin, cholinergic agonists, and octreotide can stimulate small bowel contractile activity.

Miscellaneous Causes of Dysmotility of the Small Intestine.   Intestinal pseudoobstruction has been reported with celiac sprue. Jejunal diverticulosis results from altered small bowel motility and is a complication of celiac sprue, Fabry non possessive disease, type II FVM, and Cronkhite-Canada syndrome. Abdominal irradiation can produce acute small bowel dysmotility as well as chronic motor disruption with development of bacterial overgrowth, diarrhea, malabsorption, and intestinal pseudoobstruction. Diffuse lymphoid infiltration of the small intestinal lamina propria, muscularis propria, and myenteric plexus reportedly causes intestinal pseudoobstruction. Recurrent episodes of pseudoobstruction occur after jejunoileal bypass for morbid obesity; bacterial overgrowth in the bypassed segment is believed to be the cause. Anorexia nervosa and bulimia nervosa are associated with delayed intestinal transit, but the significance of this finding is uncertain.

Clinical Features

Most patients with small intestinal dysmotility have similar clinical manifestations, regardless of the underlying disease. Individuals with mild disease are asymptomatic. Severely affected patients suffer from chronic intestinal pseudoobstruction, which is defined as the presence of symptoms and signs of obstruction without mechanical blockage. Most cases present with an intermediate pattern of postprandial, crampy abdominal pain, bloating, nausea, and vomiting. Diarrhea and malabsorption may result from bacterial overgrowth. On examination, patients may be cachectic and malnourished. The abdomen may be silent with smooth muscle dysfunction or exhibit hyperactive, high-pitched bowel sounds with neuropathic disease. Extraintestinal manifestations that involve the urinary tract and peripheral or central nervous structures may be evident with primary intestinal dysmotility; specific organ systems may be involved in secondary disease (e.g., sclerodactyly with scleroderma).

Findings on Diagnostic Testing

Laboratory Studies

Blood tests provide evidence of malnutrition or malabsorption, including anemia (iron, folate, or vitamin B_{12} deficiency), low cholesterol, hypocalcemia, and hypoalbuminemia. Blood tests detect secondary causes of intestinal dysmotility: hyperglycemia with diabetes, abnormal thyroid chemistry levels with hyper- or hypothyroidism, hypocalcemia with hypoparathyroidism, positive serologic findings with rheumatologic disease, elevated creatine phosphokinase levels with muscular dystrophy, positive leukocyte thymidine phosphorylase with type II FVM, the presence of antimyenteric neuronal antibodies with paraneoplastic intestinal dysmotility, and positive findings on hemagglutination and complement fixation studies in Chagas disease.

Radiographic Studies

Abdominal radiographs may show diffuse or localized intestinal dilation with or without air-fluid levels. Barium radiography of the small intestine may confirm dilation with delayed transit and altered motor patterns on fluoroscopy. Enteroclysis may be necessary to exclude mechanical obstruction confidently in some cases. Barium enema radiography and intravenous pyelography may detect colonic or urinary motor dysfunction. Radiopaque marker tests or scintigraphy can quantify colonic transit in cases of diffuse gastrointestinal dysmotility. Chest radiography and chest and abdominal computed tomography (CT) scans may confirm a diagnosis of paraneoplastic intestinal dysmotility.

Small Intestinal and Colonic Manometry

Small intestinal manometry characterizes abnormal motor patterns during fasting and after a meal. The migrating motor complex is a stereotypical pattern consisting of three phases that recur every 90 to 120 minutes during fasting. The fed motor pattern is characterized by irregular phasic contractions in the small intestine that begin soon after ingesting a meal and persist for more than 2 hours until the digested nutrients pass the intestine. Myopathic disease produces diffuse reductions in contractile amplitude, but the migrating motor complex and fed patterns usually are preserved. Visceral neuropathies produce abnormal or absent migrating motor complex activity, abnormal migration of contractions, or loss of the normal fed pattern. The amplitude and frequency of contractions may be increased with neuropathic disease. A manometric pattern of clustered contractions separated by periods of motor quiescence lasting longer than 1 minute has been described in association with mechanical obstruction. Manometry of the colon typically detects irregular contractions of varying frequency and amplitude. The gastrocolonic response, an increase in colon contractions, persists for more than 1 hour after healthy individuals eat a caloric meal. Patients with diffuse dysmotility or dysmotility restricted to the colon often exhibit absent phasic colon contractions and loss of the gastrocolonic response.

The Role of Surgery in Diagnosis

Visceral myopathy and neuropathy are definitively diagnosed in selected cases by surgical full-thickness intestinal biopsy with trichrome staining of the specimen, which detects smooth muscle fibrosis, and by silver staining, which assesses the myenteric plexus. In many instances, this procedure can be performed with a laparoscope to reduce morbidity. Surgery is also necessary in rare cases in which small intestinal obstruction is still a consideration after negative findings from barium radiography of the small intestine. Biopsy specimens of striated muscle may diagnose muscular dystrophy.

Management and Course

Dietary Therapy

Postprandial symptoms may respond to dietary supplements that provide 1500 to 1800 kcal per day in three to four equally sized feedings. Liquid nutrient supplements empty faster from the stomach and progress through the small intestine more easily than solid food. Elemental formulations that are low in fat and lactose-free are well absorbed. Carbonated beverages produce gaseous distention and should be avoided. For severe pseudoobstruction, feedings should be withheld, and intravenous hydration and nasogastric suction should be instituted. If symptoms are prolonged, permanent, home total parenteral nutrition may be necessary.

Medication Therapy

Prokinetic medications are often prescribed for intestinal dysmotility, but they often are less effective than in gastroparesis. Octreotide may reduce nausea, vomiting, bloating, and pain for the short term in patients with bacterial overgrowth secondary to intestinal pseudoobstruction with scleroderma. Long-term use of octreotide plus erythromycin may produce benefits in some patients with chronic intestinal pseudoobstruction. The utility of other drugs that stimulate intestinal contractions (tegaserod, metoclopramide, bethanechol, neostigmine) in small intestinal dysmotility syndromes is not proven. Pain control with narcotics is discouraged because they inhibit gut motor activity and have a potential for drug dependence. Constipation may respond to osmotic laxatives (e.g., milk of magnesia), isotonic laxatives that contain polyethylene glycol, or tap water enemas. Bulk laxatives may exacerbate symptoms and are not advocated.

Surgical Therapy

In patients with megaduodenum, the duodenum may be drained with side-to-side duodenojejunostomy, or it may be partially resected. Surgery should be avoided if the dysfunctional segments are longer because adhesions may develop that could exacerbate obstructive symptoms. Small intestinal venting may reduce some symptoms secondary to gaseous distention. Small bowel transplantation is rarely considered because of high complication rates and the low likelihood of long-term postoperative survival.

SMALL INTESTINAL BACTERIAL OVERGROWTH

Incidence and Epidemiology

Small intestinal bacterial overgrowth is characterized by nutrient malabsorption caused by excessive numbers of bacteria in the small bowel lumen. Various structural and functional disorders of the gastrointestinal tract predispose to the development of bacterial overgrowth. Recent reports suggest the condition may be more common than previously thought and may contribute to diarrhea in the elderly and bowel symptoms in persons with irritable bowel syndrome.

Etiology and Pathogenesis

Causes of Bacterial Overgrowth

Conditions favoring bacterial overgrowth include intestinal stasis, abnormal proximal connections to the colon, reduced acid secretion, immunodeficiency, and advanced age (Table 37-2). Chronic strictures from Crohn's disease, lymphoma, and radiation injury cause stasis, as do intestinal diverticula and blind loops resulting from Billroth II anastomoses, Roux-en-Y gastrojejunostomy, jejunoileal bypass for morbid obesity, and Kock continent ileostomy. Primary and secondary causes of intestinal hypomotility and pseudoobstruction predispose to bacterial overgrowth. Abnormal connections that cause bacterial overgrowth include gastrocolic and gastrojejunocolic fistulae and resection of the ileocecal junction. Gastric acid decreases the bacterial inoculum reaching the proximal small intestine. Thus, hypochlorhydria from atrophic gastritis, ulcer surgery, and possibly acid-suppressive medications predisposes to bacterial overgrowth, especially if conditions promoting stasis

---

TABLE 37-2
Conditions Favoring Development of Bacterial Overgrowth

Intestinal stasis
  Anatomic
    Strictures
    Diverticulosis of the small intestine
    Surgery (e.g., enteroenteric anastomosis, Billroth II gastrojejunostomy, jejunoileal
      bypass, Kock continent ileostomy)
  Dysmotility of the small intestine
    Scleroderma
    Idiopathic intestinal pseudoobstruction
    Diabetic autonomic neuropathy

Abnormal connection between proximal and distal intestine
  Fistulae
    Gastrocolic
    Gastrojejunocolic
  Resection of the ileocecal junction

Hypochlorhydria
    Atrophic gastritis
    Hypochlorhydric medications
    Surgery for peptic ulcer disease

Immunodeficiency
    Primary immunodeficiency
    Acquired immunodeficiency syndrome
    Malnutrition

Age

?Irritable bowel syndrome

are also present. Bacterial colonization of the small intestine occurs with common variable immunodeficiency and acquired immunodeficiency syndrome. The prevalence of bacterial overgrowth increases with advancing age, and is secondary to hypochlorhydria, intestinal stasis, or both. Recently, bacterial overgrowth was proposed as a contributor to symptoms in subsets of patients with irritable bowel syndrome. However, this association requires confirmation.

Consequences of Bacterial Overgrowth
Bacterial overgrowth results in malabsorption of fats, carbohydrates, and protein in the absence of intestinal invasion. Bacterial deconjugation of bile acids, particularly by anaerobic organisms, is the primary mechanism for malabsorption of fats and fat-soluble vitamins (vitamins A, D, and E). Vitamin K synthesis by lumenal bacteria accounts for the absence of coagulopathy. Bacterial metabolites (e.g., hydroxylated fatty acids, unconjugated bile acids) may have a toxic effect on the intestinal mucosa. Reduction of brush border disaccharidases by bacterial proteases and decreased monosaccharide uptake may produce carbohydrate malabsorption. Diarrhea results from the generation of osmotically active carbohydrate fragments. Bacterial formation of hydrogen and carbon dioxide can produce abdominal gas and pain. Hypoproteinemia is a consequence of bacterial competition for ingested proteins, decreased amino acid and peptide uptake, decreased levels of pancreatic enterokinase, and protein-losing enteropathy. Anaerobic bacteria compete with the host for vitamin B_{12}, which leads to macrocytic anemia in some patients. In contrast, lumenal bacteria synthesize folate that leads to normal or increased levels of serum folate. Bacterial overgrowth can also produce thiamine and nicotinamide deficiency.

Bacteria-Induced Intestinal Mucosal Injury
Histological evidence of mucosal damage is observed in some cases of small intestinal bacterial overgrowth, with subtotal villous atrophy and increased inflammatory cells in the lamina propria. Focal ulcerations and erosions have been seen, especially in cases of pouchitis secondary to ileal pouch–anal canal anastomosis or Kock continent ileostomy.

Clinical Features

Diarrhea and weight loss are prominent symptoms of bacterial overgrowth as a result of malabsorption, maldigestion, and reduced oral intake. Vitamin B_{12} deficiency may produce macrocytic anemia or neurological changes. Other manifestations of vitamin deficiencies include night blindness, osteomalacia, tetany, peripheral neuropathy, and edema. Extraintestinal consequences of bacterial overgrowth include dermatitis, hepatic injury, nephrotoxicity, and arthritis.

Findings on Diagnostic Testing
Microbiologic Studies
Microbiologic cultures of small intestinal aspirates are the standard for diagnosing bacterial overgrowth. Fluid samples are aspirated using fluoroscopically placed catheters or capsules or endoscopic suction and are transferred immediately to an anaerobic transport vial and plated for aerobic and anaerobic organisms. Symptomatic bacterial overgrowth is usually associated with detection of anaerobes. The presence of more than 10^5 colony-forming units per milliliter in the duodenum is diagnostic of bacterial overgrowth.

Breath Tests

Breath tests measure excretion of hydrogen or carbon dioxide produced by intralumenal bacterial metabolism of an administered substrate. These tests are less invasive alternatives to small bowel intubation. The hydrogen breath test after ingesting a carbohydrate substrate (e.g., glucose, lactulose) is advantageous because no radiolabeled compounds are ingested. However, false-negative results are common because 15% to 20% of healthy individuals harbor flora that do not produce hydrogen. In some patients, elevations in fasting breath hydrogen levels suggest bacterial overgrowth. Hydrogen breath testing provides 62% to 68% sensitivity and 44% to 83% specificity for diagnosis compared with intestinal fluid culture. ^{14}C-D-xylose is a good substrate for breath testing because of its minimal metabolism by the host. ^{14}C-D-xylose breath testing exhibits 30% to 100% sensitivity and 89% to 100% specificity in diagnosing bacterial overgrowth. Radiolabeled bile acid breath tests are no longer used because of poor sensitivity and specificity.

Other Tests

Other diagnostic studies that suggest bacterial overgrowth include vitamin B_{12} levels and the Schilling test. If not already known, the underlying cause of bacterial overgrowth may be diagnosed by specific endoscopic, radiographic, and manometric techniques.

Management and Course

Initial management of bacterial overgrowth consists of fluid and nutritional support, including vitamin replacement. Antibiotics with efficacy in treating bacterial overgrowth include tetracycline, ampicillin, erythromycin, clindamycin, metronidazole, oral aminoglycosides, and quinolones. Most patients respond to a single 7- to 10-day course, but some require intermittent antibiotic therapy or a continuous course of alternating antibiotics to minimize the development of resistant organisms. Most prokinetic agents have limited efficacy in treating bacterial overgrowth secondary to intestinal dysmotility, although octreotide may produce benefits in selected individuals. Probiotic treatments with *Lactobacillus* organisms may prolong remission after antibiotic therapy. Surgical correction of anatomic causes of intestinal stasis can be considered.

CHAPTER 38

Infections of the Small Intestine with Bacterial and Viral Pathogens

INCIDENCE AND EPIDEMIOLOGY

Bacterial and viral infections of the small intestine cause disease mediated by toxins or by direct destruction of intestinal epithelial cells. Ingesting food or water contaminated with pathogens accounts for most cases (Table 38-1). An estimated 76 million cases of foodborne disease occur per year in the United States, accounting for 325,000 hospitalizations and 5000 deaths. The annual economic impact has been assessed at $5 billion or more annually. Bacterial pathogens, including *Escherichia coli*, *Salmonella*, *Shigella*, and *Campylobacter*, are typically the cause of foodborne illness. The latter two genera usually are colonic pathogens and are discussed in Chapter 45.

ILLNESS FROM BACTERIAL TOXINS

Staphylococcus aureus

Etiology and Pathogenesis

Staphylococcus aureus is a gram-positive coccus that accounts for 1% to 2% of recognized foodborne illness in the United States. Epidemics often occur during warm weather, reflecting the association of *S aureus* outbreaks with large gatherings (e.g., picnics). The high sugar or salt content of certain foods (e.g., salads, pastries, and meats) allows selective growth of the organism. The organism produces at least seven enterotoxins and a delta-toxin that can evoke fluid secretion in the intestine.

Clinical Features, Diagnosis, and Management

The clinical features of food poisoning with *S aureus* include nausea, vomiting, and diarrhea. These symptoms occur with an attack rate of 80% to 100% within 8 hours after ingesting preformed enterotoxin. Full recovery usually occurs within 48 hours. The diagnosis is clinical but may be confirmed by culturing the organism from the food or food handler.

Bacillus cereus

Etiology and Pathogenesis

Bacillus cereus is an aerobic, motile, spore-forming gram-positive rod. It accounts for less than 1% of foodborne disease in the United States. The organism produces two types of toxins, depending on the media upon which it grows.

TABLE 38-1
Clinical and Epidemiologic Features of Agent-Specific Foodborne Diseases

ORGANISM OR AGENT	PATHOGENESIS: TOXIN (T)/INVASION (I)	FOODS MOST COMMONLY IMPLICATED
Staphylococcus aureus	T	Salads, cream-filled pastries, meats (pork, beef, poultry)
Bacillus cereus		
Emetic illness	T	Fried rice
Diarrheal illness	T	Meats, vanilla sauce, cream, baked goods, salads, chicken soup
Clostridium botulinum	T	Raw honey (infants), improperly canned products
Clostridium perfringens	T	Improperly stored beef, fish, or poultry dishes (after preparation), pasta, salads, dairy products, Mexican foods
Puffer fish	T	Fugu (especially prepared Japanese puffer fish)
Paralytic shellfish	T (saxitoxin)	Most bivalved mollusks (shellfish), especially from infectious waters with red tide blooms
Ciguatera	T (ciguatoxin)	Barracuda, groupers, snappers, jacks, reef sharks
Scromboid	—	"Blood fish" (tuna, albacore, mackerel)
Salmonella species	T/I (little mucosal damage)	Eggs, poultry, beef, dairy products
Shigella species	T/I	Salads (egg, tuna, poultry), milk
Yersinia species	T/I	Milk (raw or chocolate)
Vibrio parahaemolyticus	T	Oysters, crabs, shellfish, seawater, contaminated food
Vibrio cholerae (non-O1)	T (a few produce cholera toxin)	Seafood, grated eggs
Vibrio cholerae (O1)	T	Seafood, fecally contaminated water
Campylobacter species	T/I	Raw milk, poultry, beef, clams, pet animals
Escherichia coli		
Enterotoxigenic	T	Salads, peeled fruits, meats dishes, pastries
Enteroinvasive	I	Salads, cheese
Rotavirus	T (proposed), superficial mucosal damage	Fresh water, seafood
Norwalk virus	— (superficial mucosal damage)	Shellfish, drinking water

Clinical Features, Diagnosis, and Management

Two distinct clinical syndromes are associated with foodborne illness caused by *B cereus*. Patients with the emetic illness present with vomiting and cramping. Symptoms appear 1 to 6 hours after ingestion and persist for 2 to 10 hours. Patients with the diarrheal illness have profuse watery diarrhea, abdominal cramping, and occasional vomiting. The illness has an incubation period of 6 to 24 hours and lasts for 16 to 48 hours. The diagnosis is based primarily on clinical information. Both syndromes are self-limited. Prevention of *B cereus* infection requires proper food handling and storage.

Clostridium botulinum

Etiology and Pathogenesis

Clostridium botulinum is a ubiquitous, anaerobic, spore-forming, gram-positive bacterium that produces a neurotoxin capable of blocking acetylcholine release at the neuromuscular junction. Improperly canned food is the usual source of infection.

Clinical Features, Diagnosis, and Management

Mild nausea, vomiting, abdominal pain, and diarrhea occur within 12 to 36 hours after ingestion. Associated neurological symptoms may also be present, including diplopia, ophthalmoplegia, dysarthria, dysphagia, dysphonia, descending weakness, paralysis, postural hypotension, and respiratory muscle paralysis. The latter is the major cause of mortality and occurs in 15% of patients; otherwise, full recovery may take months. The diagnosis is confirmed by detecting botulinum toxin in the stool and vomitus of infected patients or in the contaminated food. Electromyography can be used to differentiate this illness from Guillain-Barré syndrome. Treatment is supportive in addition to administering the antitoxin early in the course of disease.

Clostridium perfringens

Etiology and Pathogenesis

Clostridium perfringens is a nonmotile, obligate anaerobe that is responsible for approximately 2% of all foodborne cases reported to the Centers for Disease Control and Prevention (CDC). Spores are heat-resistant and grow in temperatures that vary from 15° to 50°C. The organism produces a heat-labile enterotoxin that binds to mucosal cell surfaces, causing structural damage and leading to loss of electrolytes, fluids, and proteins. Most outbreaks occur in the autumn and winter and result from ingesting improperly stored beef, fish, poultry, pasta salads, and dairy products.

Clinical Features, Diagnosis, and Management

C perfringens causes watery diarrhea and cramping abdominal pain 8 to 24 hours after ingestion of contaminated food. The disease is self-limited, and full recovery is expected within 24 hours, although dehydration may cause death of elderly patients. *C perfringens* has also been implicated in antibiotic-associated diarrhea. Other toxins (e.g., alpha-toxin and beta-toxin) can produce necrotizing enterocolitis, ileus, and pneumatosis intestinalis. Definitive diagnosis is made by demonstrating more than 10^5 organisms per gram in contaminated food or more than 10^6 spores per gram in stools of affected individuals, or by detecting *C perfringens* enterotoxin in assays. Therapy for infection with *C perfringens* is supportive, although oral metronidazole (400 mg, three times per day for 7 to 10 days) may facilitate eradication of the infection.

Listeria monocytogenes

Etiology and Pathogenesis

Listeria monocytogenes is a non–spore-forming, gram-positive bacillus that is notorious for causing gastrointestinal illness from ingesting unpasteurized milk products, although an association with ingesting contaminated meats, fruits, vegetables, and seafood is also known. It is uncommon and is reported to the CDC in only 0.1% of foodborne outbreaks. Populations at risk include pregnant women, infants, immunosuppressed individuals, the elderly, veterinarians, and laboratory workers.

Clinical Features, Diagnosis, and Management

The varied clinical presentation of *Listeria* ranges from mild febrile illness to an overt episode of bacteremia, meningitis, and sepsis. Complications include perinatal listeric septicemia (granulomas and abscesses in multiple organs), cervical adenitis, endocarditis, arthritis, osteomyelitis, brain abscess, peritonitis, and cholecystitis. It is diagnosed by isolating the organism with "tumbling motility." Early treatment with ampicillin and an aminoglycoside is indicated because of the seriousness of the illness. Trimethoprim-sulfamethoxazole, macrolides, and tetracycline have also been advocated; cephalosporins are not effective. The duration of therapy has not been well studied, but at least 2 weeks, and up to 6 weeks, is recommended.

Vibrio cholerae

Etiology and Pathogenesis

Cholera causes an estimated 100,000 deaths worldwide each year out of 5.5 million total cases annually. Cholera is caused by *Vibrio cholerae*, a motile, monoflagellated, gram-negative, curved rod that classically causes voluminous watery diarrhea by elaborating an enterotoxin. The disease is endemic in southern Asia, Africa, and Latin America. Cholera is transmitted mainly via seafood or fecally contaminated water, and the disease primarily affects children (age 2 to 9) and women of childbearing age who live in crowded conditions with poor water and waste sanitation. Other persons at increased risk of infection include those with hypochlorhydria or impaired immune function. Person-to-person transmission is not considered important. There are seven *Vibrio* species that are known to cause gastroenteritis. Although the risk of cholera in the United States is small, cases involving serogroups O1 and O139 have been reported. Cholera toxin consists of an "A" subunit, which is internalized and irreversibly activates mucosal adenylate cyclase, thus producing massive electrolyte and fluid secretion, and a "B" subunit, which binds to specific surface receptors and enables the A subunit to enter into the cell. The inoculum required to produce illness is larger than 10^6 organisms.

Clinical Features, Diagnosis, and Management

The clinical presentation of cholera is highly variable, ranging from subclinical gastroenteritis to severe cholera (cholera gravis) that may lead to hypovolemic shock within 1 hour. After an incubation period of a few hours to 7 days, cholera manifests with diarrhea, which is described as having the consistency of rice water. Associated symptoms include vomiting, metabolic acidosis, hyponatremia, hypokalemia, hypoglycemia, lethargy, altered sensorium, and seizures. Paralytic ileus, muscle cramps, weakness, and cardiac arrhythmias may result secondary to electrolyte abnormalities. The diagnosis is based on the characteristic clinical presentation, direct stool examination identifying the "shooting star" motility under dark-field or phase microscopy or stool culturing of *V cholerae* O1 or *V cholerae* O139 Bengal. The mainstay of therapy is prompt initiation of oral rehydration with glucose and electrolyte solutions endorsed by the World Health Organization. Intravenous lactated Ringer solution may be required to treat severe dehydration or concomitant vomiting. Antibiotics reduce the volume and duration of diarrhea and shorten the period of excretion of *V cholerae*. Tetracycline (250 to 500 mg, four times daily for 3 days) and doxycycline are effective, as are streptomycin, chloramphenicol, trimethoprim-sulfamethoxazole, nalidixic acid, ampicillin, and furazolidone. Eradication with a single 1-g dose of ciprofloxacin has been effective. Primary infection with *V cholerae* confers immunity to subsequent infection for at least 3 years. Parenteral and oral vaccines have been formulated, but they confer only about 50% protection.

Other Vibrio Species
Etiology and Pathogenesis
Vibrio parahaemolyticus is found in salt water or in its inhabitants and frequently causes foodborne illness in the United States. Reported cases generally involve ingestion of raw or improperly stored seafood or contamination of food with seawater. It elaborates an enterotoxin and produces inflammation in the small intestine. In addition to *V parahaemolyticus*, a group of vibrios termed non-O1 cholera vibrios (they do not agglutinate in antiserum against O-group 1 antigen) can cause gastroenteritis. Infection may result from ingesting oysters, eggs, and potatoes or from exposure to dogs. Other vibrios (e.g., *Vibrio fluvialis*, *Vibrio furnissii*, *Vibrio hollisae*, and *Vibrio mimicus*) may also cause diarrheal illness.

Clinical Features, Diagnosis, and Management
V parahaemolyticus produces a range of illness from mild diarrhea to dysentery after an incubation of longer than 24 hours, with associated nausea, vomiting, headache, and fever. Non-O1 cholera vibrio illness presents with diarrhea, which lasts 1 to 6 days, and is associated with abdominal cramping, fever, nausea, and vomiting. Most cases of gastroenteritis caused by *V parahaemolyticus* and non-O1 cholera vibrios are self-limited, and antibiotics do not shorten the duration of symptoms. Severe illness, however, may be effectively treated with tetracycline.

Escherichia coli Enteropathogens

Most strains of *E coli* do not produce disease. However, four clinically and epidemiologically distinct syndromes are associated with *E coli*: enterotoxigenic, enteropathogenic, enteroinvasive, and enterohemorrhagic infections. Enterotoxigenic and enteropathogenic *E coli* infections affect the small intestine and are discussed here. Enteroinvasive and enterohemorrhagic *E coli* infections primarily affect the colon and are discussed in Chapter 45.

Enterotoxigenic Escherichia coli
Etiology and Pathogenesis
Enterotoxigenic *E coli* (ETEC) causes disease by producing a heat-labile toxin and two heat-stable toxins. The heat-labile toxin increases cAMP levels, leading to chloride secretion and secretory diarrhea. One of the heat-stable toxins activates guanylate cyclase. Disease occurs in the absence of invasion or damage to intestinal epithelial cells. ETEC is a major cause of diarrhea in children in developing countries and accounts for most cases of traveler's diarrhea resulting from ingesting food contaminated by human waste.

Clinical Features, Diagnosis, and Management

Patients with ETEC present with watery diarrhea, abdominal cramping or pain, headache, arthralgias, myalgias, vomiting, and low-grade fever. The period of illness is generally 2 to 5 days. Less than 10% of patients complain of symptoms for more than 1 week. Dehydration is severe only in the very young or very old. Fluid and electrolyte replacement are emphasized. Therapy includes trimethoprim-sulfamethoxazole (DS twice daily for 3 days), fluoroquinolone twice daily for 3 days (ciprofloxacin 500 mg, norfloxacin 400 mg, ofloxacin 300 mg), or ciprofloxacin (one 750-mg dose). Prophylaxis with bismuth subsalicylate, two 262-mg tablets, four times daily, is more than 60% effective in preventing illness. Probiotic prophylaxis using *Lactobacillus* species also may be efficacious. Vaccine trials have met with variable success.

Enteropathogenic Escherichia coli

Etiology and Pathogenesis

Enteropathogenic *E coli* (EPEC) produces disease as a result of its ability to adhere to the epithelial cell and destroy microvilli. It is an endemic pathogen with fecal-oral transmission and affects primarily infants and children younger than 2 years. Older children and adults may serve as reservoirs for this illness.

Clinical Features, Diagnosis, and Management

Patients with EPEC present with profuse watery diarrhea and associated symptoms of vomiting, fever, failure to thrive, metabolic acidosis, and possibly life-threatening dehydration. The diagnosis is by stool culture with serotyping, documentation of tissue culture adherence, or detecting the adherence factor by DNA probe techniques. Therapy relies on fluid and electrolyte replacement, as the illness is usually self-limited.

Nontyphoidal Salmonella Species

Etiology and Pathogenesis

Although all *Salmonella* are grouped into a single species, *Salmonella choleraesuis*, there are seven species subgroups, of which subgroup I contains almost all the serotypes that cause human disease. Nontyphoidal *Salmonella* species account for 1.5 million cases of foodborne enteric illness in the United States annually. *Salmonella* may be acquired from infected eggs, poultry, beef, dairy products, pet turtles, carmine red dye, aerosols, marijuana, thermometers, endoscopes, and platelet transfusions. Outbreaks of infection tend to be during the summer and autumn, likely from picnics and barbecues during which food is not cooked at temperatures necessary to kill the organism (>150°F for 12 minutes). Person-to-person transfer is important only in institutional settings where fecal contamination is prevalent. Other persons at risk include patients with malignancy, immunosuppression, alcoholism, hypochlorhydria, sickle cell anemia, cardiovascular disease, hemolytic anemia, or schistosomiasis, and those who have recently undergone surgery.

The development of symptomatic infection depends on the volume of organisms ingested and various host factors. Diarrhea develops only if the mucosa of the small intestine is invaded. The pathogenicity is poorly understood but is thought to involve regulatory proteins that control the synthesis of proteins at the level of transcription. Unlike *Shigella* infection, *Salmonella* only rarely causes ulceration, hemorrhage, and microabscesses. Invasion of the bloodstream by nontyphoidal *Salmonella* species is infrequently beyond the mesenteric lymph nodes, and blood cultures are positive in less than 10% of cases.

Clinical Features, Diagnosis, and Management

Nontyphoidal *Salmonella* species are associated with a spectrum of disease severity ranging from infrequent loose stools to a cholera-like diarrhea with dehydration. Associated symptoms include fever, abdominal pain, nausea, and vomiting. Symptoms manifest within 48 hours of exposure and persist for 3 to 7 days. Complications include osteomyelitis, focal abscesses, bacteremia, sepsis, and infection of aortic or iliac aneurysms. Diagnosis is by stool culture and the mainstay of treatment is supportive care. Antimicrobials are not recommended for mild to moderate disease because they may prolong intestinal carriage of the organism and increase the risk of relapse. Antimicrobials do not shorten symptom duration. Indications for antibiotics include extremes of age, immunodeficiency, sepsis, abscess, osteomyelitis, and chronic typhoid carrier states. Multidrug resistance is emerging in the United States, mediated by large complex plasmids. In seriously ill patients, administration of two antimicrobial agents of different classes for 10 to 14 days orally or parenterally is indicated. Antibiotics with proven efficacy include ampicillin, amoxicillin, trimethoprim-sulfamethoxazole, chloramphenicol, cefotaxime, ceftriaxone, and quinolones. To eradicate the chronic carrier state, 6-week regimens of amoxicillin and trimethoprim-sulfamethoxazole and norfloxacin or ciprofloxacin for 3 weeks have known efficacy.

Salmonella typhi

Etiology and Pathogenesis

The pathogenesis of *Salmonella typhi* resides with the Vi antigen, which prevents antibody binding and subsequent phagocytosis by the host. The organism is transmitted by the fecal-oral route, and humans are the only known reservoir. Initially, transient bacteremia results from organism release from dying macrophages in Peyer patches. Persistence of *Salmonella typhi* in the circulating macrophages leads to seeding of distant sites and a second phase of bacteremia that coincides with enteric fever.

Clinical Features, Diagnosis, and Management

After an incubation period of about 1 week (range 3 to 60 days), enteric fever (temperature of 39° to 40°C) develops and persists for 2 to 3 weeks. Associated symptoms include headache, malaise, mental confusion, anorexia, abdominal discomfort, bloating, and upper respiratory symptoms. Initially, diarrhea may be short-lived and resolves prior to the onset of fever, only to recur in the late phase of illness. The liver and spleen may be enlarged, and abdominal tenderness may mimic appendicitis. Rose spots—a faint salmon-colored maculopapular rash on the anterior trunk—develop in 30% of patients but last only 3 to 4 days. Relative bradycardia (pulse slow for degree of fever) may be seen. Hematologic abnormalities include leukopenia and anemia. Complications include hemorrhage, intestinal perforation, pericarditis, orchitis, and splenic or liver abscess.

A combination of cultures from blood, bone marrow, and intestinal secretions will provide the diagnosis in more than 90% of patients, although the sensitivity of blood culture alone is 50% to 70%. Third-generation cephalosporins and fluoroquinolones are effective in treating typhoid fever and have replaced chloramphenicol as the treatment of choice. Symptom relapse occurs in 3% to 13% of cases. Oral (live attenuated virus) and parenteral (whole-cell and purified capsular polysaccharide) vaccines are effective in preventing illness.

Yersinia Organisms

Etiology and Pathogenesis

Yersinia species are gram-negative, non–lactose-fermenting coccobacilli that cause gastrointestinal illness primarily in children. *Yersinia enterocolitica* causes 0.1% of reported foodborne illness in the United States. The organism is transmitted by the fecal-oral route; by animals (e.g., dogs); and by contaminated milk, ice cream, tofu, and water.

Clinical Features, Diagnosis, and Management

Yersinia enterocolitica manifests clinically as a self-limited, febrile, diarrheal illness. Abdominal pain often occurs in the right lower quadrant and may mimic appendicitis. Other symptoms include vomiting, dysentery, arthritis, and pharyngitis. Most cases resolve over 2 to 3 days, although diarrhea can persist for months, especially in children. Rare complications of appendicitis, intestinal perforation, ileocolic intussusception, peritonitis, toxic megacolon, or cholangitis have been reported. Sepsis is uncommon but is associated with iron overload states (e.g., hemochromatosis, cirrhosis, and hemolysis). Focal *Yersinia* infections may involve the meninges, joints, bone, sinuses, and pleural spaces. Thyroiditis or glomerulopathy have developed in the postinfectious state. Moreover, patients who are HLA-B27–positive are susceptible to postinfectious Reiter syndrome, carditis, arthritis, rashes, erythema nodosum, ankylosing spondylitis, and inflammatory bowel disease.

Yersinia is diagnosed by stool examination that shows leukocytes and erythrocytes and by stool cultures using special techniques specific for *Yersinia* species. There is no evidence supporting the general use of antimicrobial therapy because the disease is usually self-limited and antibiotics do not decrease the risk of postinfectious complications. If septicemia occurs, however, therapy may consist of aminoglycosides, tetracycline, chloramphenicol, trimethoprim-sulfamethoxazole, piperacillin, or third-generation cephalosporins.

Aeromonas, Plesiomonas, and Edwardsiella
Etiology and Pathogenesis

Aeromonas species, *Plesiomonas shigelloides*, and *Edwardsiella tarda* are pathogens responsible for gastroenteritis (including traveler's diarrhea), wound infection, and meningitis. All are waterborne: *Aeromonas* species are commonly identified and isolated from freshwater fish and shrimp, *P shigelloides* is present in contaminated oysters and seafood, and *E tarda* is found primarily in water and aquatic animals. All produce illness by elaborating an enterotoxin and by cytotoxic activity.

Clinical Features, Diagnosis, and Management

Symptoms of infection with *Aeromonas hydrophila* include watery diarrhea with blood and mucus and fever. Symptoms usually last less than 1 week but in rare cases may persist for more than 1 year. The organism is sensitive to quinolones, aminoglycosides, trimethoprim-sulfamethoxazole, tetracycline, third-generation cephalosporins, and fluoroquinolones, but resistant to ampicillin. Infections with *P shigelloides* most commonly produce vomiting, dehydration, fever, and bloody diarrhea for 2 to 14 days. *P shigelloides* is susceptible to chloramphenicol, aminoglycosides, trimethoprim-sulfamethoxazole, tetracycline, third-generation cephalosporins, and quinolones. *E tarda* can cause either a secretory diarrhea or a more invasive dysentery-like illness. Data on treatment are limited, but the organism appears to be sensitive to ampicillin, trimethoprim-sulfamethoxazole, and ciprofloxacin.

VIRAL GASTROENTERITIS

Five distinct families of viruses produce human illness: rotavirus, Norwalk and Norwalk-like viruses, adenovirus, calicivirus, and astrovirus.

Rotavirus

Epidemiology and Pathogenesis

Rotavirus is a nonenveloped, spherical, segmented, double-stranded, RNA virus that is the single most important cause of severe diarrhea in young children worldwide. It is estimated that rotavirus infects 1 million people annually in the United States, mainly children from age 3 months to 36 months, although it also causes symptomatic infection in elderly or immunocompromised adults. In the United States, rotavirus infections usually occur in the fall, although infection occurs year-round in tropical regions. Transmission is by fecal-oral transfer, most likely person-to-person, and children and asymptomatic adults are the major reservoirs. Recurrent infections with differing serotypes are not uncommon. Infection with rotavirus causes loss of mature villus absorptive cells and loss of brush border hydrolases, causing fluid loss and osmotic diarrhea. In addition, a nonstructural protein of the virus appears to have enterotoxin-like activity and may augment diarrhea.

Clinical Features, Diagnosis, and Management

Most rotavirus infections are not associated with symptomatic disease. Clinical cases present after an incubation period of 1 to 3 days with a rapid onset of fever, malaise, vomiting, and watery diarrhea. The illness typically lasts 3 to 8 days. A mild elevation of blood urea nitrogen and metabolic acidosis are common. Stools are watery but devoid of red or white blood cells. A number of diagnostic assays have been developed to detect rotavirus infection. Solid-phase immunoassays have sensitivities and specificities higher than 90%. Nucleic acid hybridization assays are also available, as are reverse transcriptase–polymerase chain reaction (PCR) assays; however, both are generally more expensive than solid-phase immunoassays. Electrophoretic analysis of stool RNA is both sensitive and inexpensive. Culture of the virus from fecal specimens is also feasible. Therapy for rotaviral diarrhea is supportive. Oral rehydration therapy is the cornerstone of treatment; no effective antiviral medication is available. Several live, attenuated, rotavirus vaccines are being tested.

Norwalk and Norwalk-like Caliciviruses

Epidemiology and Pathogenesis

Norwalk virus is a nonenveloped, round, viral particle that causes epidemic diarrhea in both developed and underdeveloped countries. The virus, named after the 1968 outbreak of gastroenteritis that affected half of the teachers and students of an elementary school in Norwalk, Ohio, was the first evidence of a viral etiology for diarrhea. The settings of Norwalk virus outbreaks include homes, schools, cruise ships, swimming pools, and military facilities. Transmission is primarily through the fecal-oral route, although person-to-person, airborne, and fomite transmissions have also been implicated. Primary and secondary attack rates higher than 50% and higher than 30%, respectively, have been reported. Biopsy specimens of the small intestine show broad and blunted villi, crypt cell hyperplasia, cytoplasmic vacuoles, and infiltration of the lamina propria with polymorphonuclear and mononuclear cells. Brush border enzymes are reduced and gastric emptying may be delayed.

Clinical Features, Diagnosis, and Management

The incubation period is 10 to 50 hours. The most frequently reported symptoms are nausea, abdominal cramps, headache, diarrhea and fever, which last 12 to 72 hours. There are no commercially available diagnostic tests for Norwalk virus infection. Research centers have diagnosed infection through detection of viral antigen by enzyme-linked immunosorbent assay (ELISA), the presence of viral RNA by reverse transcriptase–PCR, or the serologic response to infection. Therapy centers on fluid and electrolyte replacement and symptomatic treatment of diarrhea. Prevention should be directed toward hand washing and hygienic food preparation.

"Classic" Human Calicivirus

Epidemiology and Pathogenesis

Typical caliciviruses, or Sapporo-like viruses, resemble animal caliciviruses more than Norwalk-like viruses. Although first described in children, infection can also occur in adults. Fecal-oral transmission is suspected; oysters and cold foods have been identified as potential sources of foodborne illness.

Clinical Features, Diagnosis and Management

Symptoms include vomiting and diarrhea, which may be associated with abdominal pain, fever, and respiratory symptoms. The incubation period is 1 to 3 days, followed by a symptomatic course lasting 1 to 2 days. Direct electron microscopy may detect the virus, in addition to an ELISA test. Treatment is supportive and focuses on rehydration.

Astrovirus

Epidemiology and Pathogenesis

Astrovirus infection mainly affects children, but it also occurs in institutionalized elderly patients. Other groups at risk of infection are bone marrow transplant recipients and patients infected with human immunodeficiency virus. Viral aggregates are seen in enterocytes, which appear to cause villus atrophy and crypt cell hyperplasia.

Clinical Features, Diagnosis and Management

After an incubation period of 1 to 4 days, symptoms that consist of watery diarrhea with vomiting, fever, and abdominal pain ensue for about 2 to 3 days. An ELISA based on monoclonal antibodies to all 8 types of human astroviruses is commercially available. Supportive therapy is advocated. Immunoglobulin administered intravenously, orally, or by a combination of routes has been reportedly efficacious, although not yet studied in controlled clinical trials.

Enteric Adenoviruses

Epidemiology and Pathogenesis

Adenoviruses are DNA viruses, of which serotypes 40 and 41 in particular are known to cause gastroenteritis. The infection affects mainly children younger than age 2. Viral infection appears to vary geographically but does not exhibit seasonal variation. Infection is transmitted from person to person.

Clinical Features, Diagnosis and Management

The presentation of adenovirus is similar to that of other viral agents. The incubation period is about 7 days. Symptoms include watery diarrhea and vomiting, in addition to respiratory complaints and fever. An ELISA kit is available for diagnosis. Viral particles can be evaluated directly by electron microscopy and by PCR. The goal of therapy is rehydration and adequate nutritional intake.

Toxins Associated with Seafood Consumption

Etiology and Pathogenesis

Toxins associated with consumption of seafood include tetrodotoxin (puffer fish), saxitoxin (shellfish), and ciguatoxin (ciguatera; contaminated fish include barracuda, groupers, snappers, jacks, and reef sharks). Saxitoxin and ciguatoxin are produced by unicellular organisms called dinoflagellates. Scombroid fish poisoning results from ingesting saurine generated by *Proteus* species or *Klebsiella* species that are present in spoiled tuna, albacore, mackerel, and skip jacks.

Clinical Features, Diagnosis, and Management

Paresthesias, ataxia, hypotension, seizures, cardiac arrhythmias, respiratory and skeletal muscle paralysis are caused by tetrodotoxin, saxitoxin, and ciguatoxin. Death results in 5% to 18% of saxitoxin ingestions and 30% to 60% of tetrodotoxin ingestions. Ciguatoxin can be detected by an ELISA. Therapy for these syndromes is generally supportive, although intravenous mannitol relieves symptoms produced by ciguatoxin, a sodium channel agonist. Patients with scombroid fish poisoning exhibit flushing, erythema, vertigo, and a generalized burning sensation caused by the histamine-like properties of saurine. Scombroid poisoning may be effectively treated with antihistamines.

CHAPTER 39

Celiac Disease

INCIDENCE AND EPIDEMIOLOGY

Celiac disease, also known as celiac sprue and gluten-sensitive enteropathy, is characterized by intestinal mucosal damage and malabsorption from dietary intake of wheat, rye, barley, or oats. Symptoms may appear with the introduction of cereal into the diet in the first 3 years of life. A second peak in symptomatic disease occurs in adults during the third or fourth decade, although disease onset as late as the eighth decade has been reported. Serologic testing of blood donors indicates that the prevalence of celiac disease is approximately 1 in 250 adults. In Ireland, the prevalence may be as high as 1 in 120. The disorder occurs in Arabs, Hispanics, and Israeli Jews, but is rare in individuals with a pure Afro-Caribbean or Chinese background.

ETIOLOGY AND PATHOGENESIS

Celiac disease results from an interplay of environmental factors, genetic predisposition, and immunologic interactions (Table 39-1).

TABLE 39-1
Factors and Diseases Associated with Celiac Disease

FACTOR/DISEASE	INCIDENCE
First-degree relative of celiac patient	10%
HLA-DQ2 or HLA-DQ8	99%
IgA deficiency	2.5%
Hyposplenism	100%
Aphthous ulceration	5%
Thyroid disease	6%
Diabetes mellitus	6%
Small intestinal T-cell lymphoma	10%
Dermatitis herpetiformis	Unknown
Other immune diseases	Unknown
Down syndrome	Unknown

Cereal Chemistry

The alcohol-soluble gliadin fraction of wheat gluten and similar alcohol-soluble proteins (prolamins) in rye, barley, and oats contain the disease-promoting moieties in these grains. A single variety of wheat may contain 40 or more different, closely related gliadins. Gliadins are subdivided according to their electrophoretic mobility patterns and by their N-terminal amino acid sequences. The α, β, γ, and ω subfractions of gliadin are toxic to celiac small intestinal mucosa and exacerbate clinical disease. There is a shared amino acid sequence between A-gliadin and the 54-kd E1b coat protein of adenovirus 12, raising the possibility that an encounter with this virus may play a pathogenic role in inducing celiac disease.

Immune Factors

Jejunal biopsies from celiac disease patients show dense lamina propria lymphocyte and plasma cell infiltrates as well as increased intraepithelial lymphocytes. Patients with untreated celiac disease have high circulating antibody titers to gliadin, reticulin, and endomysium. The antigen for antiendomysial antibody is tissue transglutaminase (tTG). The action of tTG on gliadin peptides is crucial for T-lymphocyte activation. tTG may generate additional antigenic T-cell neoepitopes by cross-linking extracellular matrix proteins with gliadin. Celiac disease is associated with increased cells that express proinflammatory cytokines, including interferon-γ and tumor necrosis factor–α. It has been suggested that gliadin reaches the dendritic cells of the lamina propria, which present it to sensitized T cells. These sensitized lymphocytes generate immune products that damage the enterocytes. Interferon-γ induces HLA class II gene product expression in the enterocytes, which then present further antigen to the sensitized T cells. Cloned T cells from celiac disease patients respond to peptides from different gliadin subfractions.

Genetic Factors

Symptomatic or asymptomatic celiac disease can occur in 10% of first-degree relatives of patients with defined celiac sprue. Three fourths of identical twins are concordant for the disorder. Celiac sprue is strongly associated with HLA class II

D region genes, which may be important determinants of disease susceptibility. Associations of the HLA-DP region with tumor necrosis factor–α genes have been reported. It is estimated that HLA associations account for 30% of the genetic susceptibility to celiac disease.

CLINICAL FEATURES

Adult patients with celiac disease often, but not always, have gastrointestinal symptoms, fatigue, weight loss, or pallor when diagnosed. Typically, affected individuals pass 3 to 4 loose stools daily, which are frothy or difficult to flush, in association with flatulence, loud borborygmi, as well as rare nausea, vomiting, or abdominal pain. Some patients report anorexia, whereas others experience voracious appetites. The magnitude of weight loss depends on the extent (lesions begin proximally in the duodenum), the severity of the intestinal lesion, and the degree to which the patient increases dietary intake. Rare cases of celiac disease present with intestinal pseudoobstruction. Conversely, some patients are asymptomatic and the diagnosis is considered after detecting unexplained iron deficiency anemia. In children, celiac disease produces failure to thrive, pallor, developmental delay, and short stature, in addition to variable abdominal symptoms. Children with celiac sprue typically present in the first to third years of life. Symptoms often disappear during adolescence but may recur during early adulthood.

Other regions of the gastrointestinal tract may exhibit inflammatory changes in patients with celiac disease. Ten percent of patients also have lymphocytic gastritis. Microscopic colits represents a cause of unexplained watery diarrhea and is diagnosed on colonic biopsy. When this is diagnosed, coexistent celiac disease should be entertained. Depending on whether a thickened subepithelial collagen band is demonstrated, microscopic colitis may be subclassified as collagenous or lymphocytic colitis.

Patients with celiac disease can present with extraintestinal manifestations (Table 39-1). Anemia may be secondary to iron or folate malabsorption or, in the case of severe ileal disease, vitamin B_{12} deficiency. Osteopenic bone disease results from calcium and vitamin D malabsorption. Hypocalcemia (and hypomagnesemia) may be associated with tetany and may lead to secondary hyperparathyroidism. Cutaneous bleeding, epistaxis, hematuria, and gastrointestinal hemorrhage may result from vitamin K malabsorption. Neurological manifestations include peripheral sensory neuropathy, patchy demyelination of the spinal cord, and cerebellar atrophy with ataxia. Psychiatric findings include mood changes, irritability, and depression. The cause of the neurological and psychiatric manifestations is unknown; furthermore, these symptoms may not resolve by excluding gluten from the diet. Muscle weakness may result from a proximal myopathy. Vitamin A deficiency may lead to night blindness. Women may experience amenorrhea, delayed menarche, and disturbed fertility. Men may report impotence and infertility. Some patients exhibit hyposplenism, which may increase the risk of bacterial infection. These persons should be given prophylactic antibiotics before invasive procedures or dental work.

A number of immunologic conditions are associated with celiac disease (Table 39-1). The main cutaneous complication is dermatitis herpetiformis, a skin disease with intensely pruritic papulovesicular lesions on the elbows, knees, buttocks, sacrum, face, scalp, neck, and trunk. Approximately 5% of patients with celiac disease report symptomatic dermatitis herpetiformis. Most patients who present initially with dermatitis herpetiformis exhibit celiac sprue–like findings on intestinal biopsy specimens and may respond slowly to a gluten-free diet, although this is not universal. In most patients, a granular or speckled pattern of IgA deposits is noted at the epidermal-dermal junction of uninvolved skin; a linear pattern is less common. Celiac disease exhibits clinical associations with other immune-mediated diseases such as insulin-dependent diabetes mellitus, thyroid disease, IgA deficiency, Sjögren syndrome, systemic lupus erythematosus, mixed cryoglobulinemia, vasculitis, pulmonary disease, pericarditis, mesenteric lymph node cavitation, inflammatory bowel disease, neurological disorders, ocular abnormalities, IgA mesangial nephropathy, primary sclerosing cholangitis, and primary biliary cirrhosis. Other skin diseases found in patients with celiac sprue include psoriasis, eczema, pustular dermatitis, cutaneous amyloid, cutaneous vasculitis, nodular prurigo, and mycosis fungoides.

Physical findings depend on disease severity. Patients with mild disease exhibit no abnormal physical symptoms. In more severe disease, emaciation, clubbed nails, dependent edema, ascites, ecchymoses, pallor, cheilosis, glossitis, decreased peripheral sensation, and a positive Chvostek or Trousseau sign may be detected. Hyperkeratosis follicularis may result from vitamin A deficiency. The abdomen may be distended and tympanitic and have a doughy consistency.

FINDINGS ON DIAGNOSTIC TESTING

Laboratory Studies

Screening blood tests for celiac disease may detect anemia (microcytic resulting from iron deficiency or macrocytic resulting from folate or vitamin B_{12} deficiency), hypocalcemia, hypophosphatemia, hypomagnesemia, metabolic acidosis, hypoalbuminemia, hypoglobulinemia, low serum vitamin A levels, prolonged prothrombin time, and an elevated serum alkaline phosphatase level. Fecal fat levels may be increased on qualitative (i.e., Sudan stain) or quantitative assessment. Patients with celiac disease may have flat, glucose tolerance test results.

Antibody Testing

If celiac disease is a diagnostic consideration in a patient with unexplained gastrointestinal symptoms, serologic antibody tests are informative but do not replace the need for small intestinal biopsy. The sensitivity and specificity of IgA antigliadin antibodies are 83% and 82%, respectively. More recently developed antibody tests provide more reliable screens for celiac disease. Antiendomysial antibodies have a sensitivity and specificity for disease detection of 90% and 99%, whereas tTG serologic testing is 93% sensitive and 95% specific. Of patients with celiac disease, 2% to 3% have selective IgA deficiency, which may produce false-negative tests in antigliadin, antiendomysial, and anti-tTG antibody testing. Some clinicians obtain IgG titers of the same antibodies or measure serum IgA levels to exclude this possibility.

Histology of the Small Intestine

To confirm the diagnosis of celiac disease, biopsy of the small intestinal mucosa is mandatory. With active disease, the endoscopic appearance of the duodenal mucosa is a loss of normal folds with scalloping. Different grades of enteropathy can be graded on microscopic examination. Grade 0, or preinfiltrative, histology appears normal but can produce antibody to gluten and endomysium, is found in some cases of dermatitis herpetiformis, and characterizes latent disease. Grade 1 is an infiltrative lesion with increased epithelial lymphocytes but no villous atrophy, it usually does not produce gastrointestinal symptoms. Grade 2 is similar to grade 1, but the crypts are hypertrophic. The destructive grade 3 lesion is characterized by the typical flat mucosa of untreated celiac disease. With this finding, the total thickness of the mucosa is increased by crypt hyperplasia and lamina propria infiltration by plasma cells and lymphocytes. Epithelial cells lose their columnar appearance and become pseudostratified. Subtotal villous atrophy may be observed in milder disease or in disease that has been treated with a gluten-restricted diet. The grade 4 lesion is a hypoplastic histology that is not responsive to a gluten-free diet and is associated with nonneoplastic and neoplastic complications of celiac disease (see Complications). Other infectious or inflammatory diseases produce histological findings similar to celiac disease. Thus, a presumptive diagnosis of celiac disease should be supported by the response to a gluten-free diet.

Findings of Imaging Studies

In 85% of celiac disease patients, barium radiography of the small intestine exhibits the loss of the fine, feathery mucosal pattern with thin mucosal folds. Additional findings in some individuals include straightening of the valvulae conniventes, thickened mucosal folds, lumenal dilation, and flocculation of contrast. Such radiographic exams are most important in excluding ulcerative and neoplastic complications of celiac disease. Abdominal computed tomography and magnetic resonance imaging may detect hyposplenism and abdominal lymphadenopathy in some patients. The bone density of patients with celiac disease is measured to exclude osteopenia.

MANAGEMENT AND COURSE

The mainstay for treating celiac sprue is the initiation of a gluten-free diet. Commitment to this diet is lifelong. It requires completely eliminating wheat (including triticale, spelt, and semolina), rye, barley, and oat products from the diet. Corn, rice, sorghum, buckwheat, and millet do not activate the disease. Gluten is not present in distilled liquor; therefore, whisky and other spirits are well tolerated. However, barley-containing beer and ale should be avoided. Because of the loss of brush border lactase activity, dairy products should initially be avoided, but these substances can be reintroduced after symptoms improve on a gluten-restricted diet. Symptomatic improvement with these dietary recommendations may be reported as soon as 48 hours after they are initiated. Recovery of normal intestinal histological features often takes much longer (i.e., months), and abnormalities persist in 50% of patients, despite strict adherence to the diet. The distal intestinal mucosa heals more rapidly than the proximal mucosa. Supplemental iron or folate (and rarely vitamin B_{12}) may be needed to treat anemia early in therapy. Vitamin K may be required to treat a coagulation deficit. Osteopenic bone disease is treated with calcium and vitamin D replacement or bisphosphonate therapy. Corticosteroid therapy should be reserved for patients unresponsive to dietary gluten restriction or for patients with complications. Azathioprine or 6-mercaptopurine can be used as steroid-sparing agents, if needed. The benefits of cyclosporine are unproven. Dermatitis herpetiformis is treated with dapsone, in addition to initiating a gluten-free diet.

Complications

Enteropathy-associated T-cell lymphoma of the small intestine may complicate long-standing celiac disease and is often multifocal and diffuse. Diagnosing lymphoma may be difficult because of the insidious onset of symptoms in many patients. Carcinoma of the small intestine as well as of the mouth, pharynx, and esophagus are more common in patients with celiac disease than in the normal population. Evidence strongly suggests that adherence to a gluten-free diet reduces the subsequent incidence of malignancy. Chronic ulcerative jejunoileitis is characterized by multiple ulcers and strictures of the small intestine and presents with anemia, hemorrhage, perforation, or stricture. Patients with celiac disease who have this complication often are refractory to gluten restriction and are further predisposed to developing lymphoma. Other causes of refractoriness to dietary therapy include refractory sprue and collagenous sprue in which a thick band of collagen-like material is deposited under the intestinal epithelial cells. Some patients with refractory sprue have circulating antienterocyte antibodies. Although many refractory patients respond to corticosteroids or other immunosuppressive drugs, some individuals require permanent parenteral hyperalimentation to maintain adequate nutrition and hydration.

CHAPTER **40**

Disorders of Epithelial Transport in the Small Intestine

DISORDERS OF CARBOHYDRATE ABSORPTION

Starch, sucrose, lactose, and fructose are the major dietary carbohydrates. Assimilating them requires hydrolysis to and subsequent small intestine mucosal uptake of monosaccharide components. Maldigested or malabsorbed intralumenal carbohydrates draw fluid into the small intestine by osmosis. On delivery to the colon, the sugars become substrates for bacterial fermentation and are converted from oligosaccharides or disaccharides to monosaccharides, further increasing the osmotic load. Bacterial conversion of carbohydrates to short-chain fatty acids that are absorbed across the colon wall partially compensates for this increased load.

Lactase Deficiency
Etiology and Pathogenesis
Adult lactase deficiency, the most prevalent genetic deficiency syndrome worldwide, affects more than 50% of the population. In most populations, lactase activity decreases after age 5 to levels approximately 5% to 10% of those at birth. Clinically relevant lactose intolerance primarily affects African American, Asian,

Mediterranean, Native American, and Mexican American populations and spares all but 5% to 15% of people of Northern European descent (Table 40-1). Congenital lactase deficiency, a second disorder, is a rare autosomal recessive condition that is characterized by watery diarrhea in infancy. Lactose intolerance also develops secondary to other injury to the intestine, such as infections or inflammatory conditions (e.g., celiac disease, rotavirus, giardiasis, radiation enteritis, Crohn's disease) that result in reduced absorptive surface area, insufficient contact time, and reduced mucosal enzyme levels. In many of these conditions, recovery of normal lactase activity is prolonged after adequate treatment of the primary disorder. Milk intolerance also may be a consequence of sensitization to a protein component of cow's milk, rather than reduced lactase levels. This sensitivity can follow an infection (e.g., with rotavirus in infants).

Clinical Features, Diagnosis, and Management

Lactase-deficient adults report distention, bloating, abdominal pain, flatulence, and diarrhea after ingesting dairy products. In severe cases in infants, acidosis and dehydration may develop. Adult-onset lactase decline has been associated with osteoporosis, presumably due to milk avoidance. Confirmation of lactase deficiency depends on reproducing symptoms with lactose ingestion. Lactose absorption tests have been used with sensitivities of 75% and specificities of 96%; however, these tests are time-consuming and are infrequently performed. Breath hydrogen testing is an alternative diagnostic method that involves gas chromatographic analysis of expired breath to detect hydrogen after ingesting lactose. Lactase deficiency is diagnosed if the rise in breath hydrogen is higher than 20 ppm. The magnitude of the increase above 20 ppm correlates semiquantitatively with the degree of malabsorption. False-positive tests occur with bacterial overgrowth. False-negative results are caused when patients have recently taken antibiotics or are not hydrogen producers. The definitive test for for diagnosing lactase deficiency is assaying disaccharidase activity on intestinal biopsy specimens, but this test is rarely necessary.

Managing lactase deficiency relies on reducing dietary lactose, substituting alternate nutrient sources, regulating calcium intake, and using commercial lactase preparations. Complete elimination of lactose from the diet is mandated in only a minority of patients. Calcium may be given in the form of calcium carbonate or calcium gluconate. Commercial lactase products contain bacterial or yeast β-galactosidases. Similarly, live yogurt culture contains β-galactosidase that may provide an alternate source of calcium for many lactose-intolerant patients.

TABLE 40-1
Ethnic Distribution of Lactase Deficiency

POPULATION	PREVALENCE OF LACTASE DEFICIENCY (%)
Swedish	1
Austrian	20
US White	7–22
French	32–44
Italian	50–72
African American	65
Native American	95
Vietnamese	100

Sucrase-Isomaltase Deficiency

Etiology and Pathogenesis

Sucrase-isomaltase deficiency is an autosomal recessive disorder characterized by undetectable intestinal sucrase activity and reduced isomaltase activity. The diagnosis is made in patients ranging in age from infants to young adults. At least 6 gene defects have been identified, which include impairments of enzyme processing, inappropriate transport to sites other than the brush border, and altered intracellular degradation.

Clinical Features, Diagnosis, and Management

In infants, diarrhea, secondary malabsorption, and failure to thrive develop with the introduction of sucrose-containing formulas. In adults, diarrhea, cramps, and flatulence may develop after an attack of gastroenteritis. Diagnosis is most easily made by sucrose hydrogen breath testing; however, false-positive tests occur in 20% to 30% of patients. In some cases, intestinal biopsy with disaccharidase determination may be needed. Instituting a sucrose-free diet results in cessation of diarrhea and weight gain. Oral sacrosidase supplements (from *Saccharomyces cerevisiae*) show promise for reducing the symptoms of this condition.

Trehalase Deficiency

Etiology and Pathogenesis

Trehalose intolerance is a rare condition of carbohydrate malabsorption, probably because young mushrooms are the only major dietary source of this sugar. Relative trehalose deficiencies are common in Greenland.

Clinical Features, Diagnosis, and Management

Affected individuals develop abdominal pain, bloating, and diarrhea after ingesting the mushrooms. Diagnosis is made by oral tolerance tests. Treatment is avoidance of young mushrooms.

Glucose-Galactose Malabsorption

Etiology and Pathogenesis

Congenital glucose-galactose malabsorption is a rare autosomal recessive condition characterized by impaired sodium-coupled glucose-galactose transport caused by 1 of 20 or more mutations in the transporter protein. Transient glucose malabsorption may develop in infants after gastrointestinal surgery or gastroenteritis (caused by rotavirus). It usually resolves rapidly.

Clinical Features, Diagnosis, and Management

Infants present with profuse watery diarrhea, dehydration, distention, vomiting, and failure to thrive in the first week of life. Fecal analysis reveals a low pH and the presence of reducing substances. The most reliable diagnostic test is hydrogen breath testing. Replacement of dietary glucose and galactose with fructose improves symptoms immediately.

Intolerance to Other Carbohydrates

Etiology and Pathogenesis

Fructose and sorbitol are poorly absorbed dietary carbohydrates. Malabsorption of these two sugars produces symptoms in the absence of any heritable enzyme deficiency. Fructose is prevalent in fruits, sucrose, and soft drinks, whereas sorbitol is present in fruits, dietetic candies, and chewing gum. Malabsorption of starch from wheat, corn, oat, potato, and bean sources is observed in susceptible populations. Rice generally does not provoke symptoms. Starch from refined or gluten-free flour is better absorbed, suggesting that fiber or protein components rather than the starch itself may be responsible for the symptoms.

Clinical Features, Diagnosis, and Management

Susceptible patients present with bloating, flatulence, pain, or diarrhea after ingesting relatively small amounts of these carbohydrates (e.g., two soft drink cans or four sticks of gum). Hydrogen breath testing after ingestion of fructose, sorbitol, or starch can be performed, but the clinical utility of these tests is undefined. When suspected or documented, reducing dietary consumption of the offending carbohydrate is recommended. Administration of supplemental β-galactosidase supplements to hydrolyze dietary oligosaccharides has met with limited success in alleviating symptoms.

DISORDERS OF PROTEIN AND AMINO ACID ABSORPTION

Enterokinase Deficiency
Etiology and Pathogenesis

Congenital enterokinase deficiency produces low proteolytic activity in the duodenal juice, despite normal levels of amylase and lipase. The addition of exogenous enterokinase converts trypsinogen to trypsin, resulting in activation of other proteolytic enzymes.

Clinical Features, Diagnosis, and Management

Infants with enterokinase deficiency present with diarrhea, retarded growth, and hypoproteinemia with edema. Steatorrhea may result from secondary mucosal changes and pancreatic insufficiency. The diagnosis is confirmed by enzyme assay of a mucosal biopsy specimen or by activation of proteolytic activity in the duodenal fluid by adding enterokinase. Patients are treated with pancreatic enzyme supplements.

DISORDERS OF AMINO ACID TRANSPORT

Etiology and Pathogenesis

A number of defects in amino acid transport have been described. Clinical protein malnutrition and essential amino acid deficiency are rare in most cases. Hartnup disease is an autosomal recessive condition characterized by a defect in the transport of neutral amino acids. Cystinuria is an autosomal recessive defect of cystine and dibasic amino acid transport. Other disorders of amino acid transport include lysinuric protein intolerance (dibasic amino acids), blue diaper syndrome (tryptophan), oasthouse urine disease (methionine), Lowe syndrome (lysine, arginine), and Joseph syndrome (glycine, proline, hydroxyproline).

Clinical Features

Disorders of intestinal amino acid transport generally present with extraintestinal manifestations: pellagra-like rash and neuropsychiatric symptoms in Hartnup disease; renal calculi and chronic pancreatitis in cystinuria; growth retardation and hepatosplenomegaly in lysinuric protein intolerance; hypercalcemia and nephrocalcinosis in blue diaper syndrome; mental retardation and seizures in oasthouse urine disease; aminoaciduria in Joseph syndrome; and mental retardation, cataracts, and renal failure in Lowe syndrome. Management relies on controlling the sequelae of these disorders. Nicotinamide relieves skin lesions associated with Hartnup disease. Consumption of sodium bicarbonate reduces nephrolithiasis in cystinuria. Lysinuric protein intolerance is managed with a low protein diet coupled with citrulline supplementation.

DISORDERS OF FAT ABSORPTION

Abetalipoproteinemia

Etiology and Pathogenesis

Abetalipoproteinemia is an autosomal recessive disorder in which plasma apolipoprotein B–containing lipoproteins (B100 and B48) are absent, producing very low plasma cholesterol and triglyceride levels. The disorder results from a defect in the intestinal microsomal transfer protein responsible for triglyceride, cholesteryl ester, and phosphatidylcholine transfer. Variants of abetalipoproteinemia include chylomicron retention disease (or Anderson disease, serum B48 is absent) and the autosomal codominant disorder, familial hypobetalipoproteinemia.

Clinical Features, Diagnosis, and Management

The initial clinical manifestations of abetalipoproteinemia are fat malabsorption, failure to thrive, and hemolysis with erythrocyte acanthosis at birth. Low cholesterol, triglyceride, chylomicron, low and very low density lipoprotein, apoprotein B, and vitamin A and E blood levels are found. Long-term sequelae in adolesence and young adulthood include fat-soluble vitamin deficiency and development of retinopathy and fatal spinocerebellar degeneration. Small intestinal biopsies show that the mucosa is engorged with fat droplets, reflecting the inability to synthesize and secrete chylomicrons. Anderson disease is not associated with acanthosis or low triglyceride levels. Clinical manifestations occur later in familial hypobetalipoproteinemia. Management of these conditions includes dietary fat restriction and vitamin A, E, and K supplementation.

DISORDERS OF ELECTROLYTE AND MINERAL TRANSPORT

Etiology and Pathogenesis

Congenital chloride diarrhea is inherited in autosomal recessive fashion and results from a defect of Cl^-/HCO_3^- exchange in the small intestine and colon that results in the loss of chloride absorption, intestinal acidification, and secondary impairment of sodium absorption. Isolated cases of congenital sodium diarrhea have been ascribed to defects in intestinal sodium absorption. Familial hypomagnesemia is characterized by impaired intestinal magnesium absorption in the intestine. Acrodermatitis enteropathica is an autosomal recessive disorder of altered zinc uptake. Menkes (steely hair) syndrome is a generalized X-linked recessive disorder of cellular copper transport.

Clinical Features, Diagnosis, and Management

A pathognomonic feature of congenital chloride diarrhea is fetal onset of diarrhea with polyhydramnios. At birth, infants develop severe watery diarrhea, hyponatremia, hypochloremia, dehydration, metabolic alkalosis, and hypokalemia. The diagnosis is confirmed by documenting elevated levels of fecal chloride (>90 mEq/L) with a negative anion gap and a low fecal pH. Patients are treated with oral sodium chloride and potassium chloride solutions. Patients with congenital sodium diarrhea also present with dehydration, metabolic acidosis, and profound fecal sodium losses. Therapy consists of fluid and sodium citrate supplements. Patients with familial hypomagnesemia present with tetany and seizures in infancy and are treated with oral magnesium therapy. Acrodermatitis enteropathica, an illness characterized by diarrhea, alopecia, failure to thrive, and a rash of the perioral and perianal regions and extremities, is treated with oral zinc. Menke syndrome is characterized by retarded growth, abnormal hair, hypopigmentation, bone changes, and cerebral degeneration with seizures and usually is fatal by the age of 3 years. Parenteral copper histidine supplements are given but do not arrest cerebral degeneration.

MICROVILLOUS INCLUSION DISEASE

Etiology and Pathogenesis

Microvillous inclusion disease results from defective brush border assembly and differentiation caused by an error of intracellular assembly. The enterocytes lack microvilli, or they have disordered microvilli as well as vesicular bodies and intracytoplasmic vacuoles.

Clinical Features, Diagnosis, and Management

Infants present with severe diarrhea after birth. The diagnosis is made by electron microscopic demonstration of microvillous inclusions in biopsy specimens from the rectal mucosa. Lifelong total parenteral nutrition is required in most cases, although octreotide, clonidine, and epidermal growth factor have had limited success. Enterectomy may be needed to reduce fluid losses. Intestinal transplantation may become standard therapy for this disease.

DISORDERS OF COBALAMIN (VITAMIN B$_{12}$) ABSORPTION

Etiology and Pathogenesis

Congenital pernicious anemia results from the absence of functional intrinsic factor either due to reduced synthesis or synthesis of a nonfunctional form. Ileal defect syndrome (Imerslund-Grasbeck syndrome) is caused by defective transport of the intrinsic factor–cobolamin complex at the level of the ileal enterocyte. Three forms of transcobalamin II (TCII) deficiency have been described, including absent TCII, defective TCII unable to bind cobalamin, and defective TCII unable to promote cobalamin uptake into cells. Other reported defects include transcobalamin I (R binder) deficiency and Addisonian pernicious anemia.

Clinical Features, Diagnosis, and Management

Congenital pernicious anemia presents with megaloblastic anemia and developmental delay, usually between the ages of 1 and 5 years. Vitamin B_{12} malabsorption is characterized by megaloblastic anemia and neurological disease with low serum vitamin B_{12} levels in childhood. The Schilling test shows impaired absorption of vitamin B_{12}, which corrects with exogenous intrinsic factor. Therapy involves monthly injections of vitamin B_{12}. Ileal defect syndrome is suggested by abnormal Schilling tests that do not correct with exogenous intrinsic factor. Infants with TC II deficiency present with megaloblastic anemia in infancy and normal levels of vitamin B_{12} with vomiting, diarrhea, and hypotonia. This disorder is treated with massive doses of vitamin B_{12} to ensure that the vitamin will enter tissues by passive diffusion.

PRIMARY BILE SALT MALABSORPTION

Etiology and Pathogenesis

Primary bile salt malabsorption is classified into three types: type I is secondary to ileopathy or ileal resection; type II is an idiopathic disorder with normal intestinal histology; and type III occurs in other disorders, including chronic pancreatitis, diabetes, after peptic ulcer surgery, and after cholecystectomy. Symptoms result from stimulation of colonic secretion secondary to impaired absorption of dihydroxy bile acids. In children, bile salt malabsorption may be secondary to a defect in the ileal sodium/bile acid cotransporter.

Clinical Features, Diagnosis, and Management

Patients present with chronic diarrhea with exaggerated fecal losses of bile salts. Bile acid malabsorption can be documented using ^{75}SeHCAT (23-seleno-25-homotaurocholic acid) to measure fecal radioactivity or retained abdominal radioactivity. However, in most clinical settings, the diagnosis of primary bile salt malabsorption is one of exclusion. Therapy involves long-term administration of bile acid–binding agents such as cholestyramine.

CHAPTER 41

Short Bowel Syndrome

INCIDENCE AND EPIDEMIOLOGY

Short bowel syndrome refers to the symptoms and pathological disorders associated with a malabsorptive state that results from removing a large portion of the small intestine or colon. The consequences of small bowel resection are variable, but in general relate to the extent of resection, the site of resection, and subsequent adaptive processes.

ETIOLOGY AND PATHOGENESIS

Causes of Short Bowel Syndrome

The most common disorders in adults that lead to massive resection of the small intestine are vascular insults and Crohn's disease (Table 41-1). Risk factors for vascular disease include advanced age, congestive heart failure, atherosclerotic and valvular heart disease, chronic diuretic use, hypercoagulable states, and oral contraceptive use. Less common adult causes include jejunoileal bypass, abdominal trauma, neoplasm, radiation enteropathy, and gastrocolic fistulae. Pediatric causes of short bowel syndrome are intestinal atresia, midgut or segmental volvulus, abdominal wall defects, necrotizing enterocolitis, Hirschsprung disease, hypercoagulable states, cardiac valvular vegetations, Crohn's disease, and abdominal trauma.

Factors That Influence Absorption after Intestinal Resection

The amount of small intestine that remains after resection determines the transit time as well as the surface area available for nutrient, fluid, and electrolyte absorption. Approximately 50% of the small intestine can be resected without significant nutritional sequelae, but resections of 75% or more almost invariably produce severe malabsorption that requires enteral or parenteral replacement therapy. Long-term survival has been reported with only 15 to 48 cm of residual jejunum in addition to the duodenum.

Resection of different small intestinal regions produces distinct consequences. Removal of the jejunum causes only limited defects in macronutrient, electrolyte, and water absorption. Jejunal resection reduces secretion of mucosal hormones that leads to gastric hypersecretion and pancreatic insufficiency. Removal of more than 100 cm of ileum usually precludes bile acid absorption and leads to bile salt induced secretory diarrhea. The body compensates for this loss by increasing bile acid synthesis up to eightfold. Steatorrhea also results from loss of long ileal segments. The ileum is the primary site for vitamin B_{12} absorption. Malabsorption of vitamin B_{12} occurs with resection of as little as 60 cm. Because ileal nutrients regulate gastric emptying and small bowel transit, ileal resection may shorten intestinal transit

---

TABLE 41-1
Causes of Short Bowel Syndrome

Adult Causes

Intestinal vascular insults
Superior mesenteric artery embolus or thrombosis
Superior mesenteric vein thrombosis
Volvulus of the small intestine
Strangulated hernia

Postsurgical causes
Jejunoileal bypass
Abdominal trauma with resultant resection
Inadvertent gastroileal anastomosis for peptic ulcer disease

Miscellaneous
Crohn's disease
Radiation enteritis
Neoplasms

Pediatric Causes

Prenatal causes
Vascular accidents
Intestinal atresia
Midgut or segmental volvulus
Abdominal wall defect

Postnatal causes
Necrotizing enterocolitis
Trauma
Inflammatory bowel disease
Midgut segmental volvulus
Hirschsprung disease
Radiation enteritis
Venous thrombosis
Arterial embolus or thrombosis

---

times, magnifying the absorptive defect. A combined resection of the small intestine and colon usually increases dehydration and sodium and potassium depletion compared with a resection of the small intestine alone. Preservation of at least 50% of the colon reduces morbidity and mortality after massive small intestinal resection. Removal of the ileocecal junction accelerates small intestinal transit and increases bacterial colonization of the residual intestine, producing bile salt deconjugation, fat and fat-soluble vitamin malabsorption, vitamin B_{12} malabsorption, and bile salt diarrhea.

Animal models suggest that intestinal villi lengthen and become thicker after small bowel resection. In human biopsy specimens, mucosal hyperplasia has been demonstrated. Increased ileal absorption of glucose, maltose, sucrose, bile acids, vitamin B_{12}, and calcium after proximal resection has been documented in animals, as has increased activity of the enzymes involved in DNA and pyrimidine synthesis. In humans, there is a gradual improvement in the absorption of fat, nitrogen, and carbohydrate after extensive resection of the small intestine, which may take 1 or more years. The colon also undergoes adaptive dilation, lengthening, and mucosal proliferation and acquires the ability to absorb glucose and amino acids to a limited degree. Enteral nutrients elicit intestinal adaptation by direct effects on epithelial cells and by stimulating trophic gastrointestinal and pancreaticobiliary hormone secretion. Disaccharides are more potent stimulants of adaptation than monosaccharides, whereas highly saturated fats are more effective than those that are less saturated. Hormones that may have relevant trophic effects include gastrin, cholecystokinin, enteroglucagon, and neurotensin. Growth factors such as epithelial growth factor and insulin-like growth factor I, prostaglandins, glutamine, arginine, short-chain fatty acids, and polyamines such as putrescine, spermidine, and spermine also may participate in the adaptation process. Conversely, intestinal hypoplasia may result from complete reliance on parenteral nutrition.

CLINICAL FEATURES

The clinical presentation of short bowel syndrome is divided into three phases: early (1 to 2 weeks after surgery), intermediate, and late. In the immediate postoperative period after 75% or more of the small bowel has been resected, gastric hypersecretion, diarrhea, dehydration, and electrolyte deficiencies (hyponatremia, hypokalemia, hypocalcemia, and hypomagnesemia) supervene. During this phase, parenteral supplements are given. An intermediate phase follows during which intestinal adaptation occurs and oral feedings may be started. Because of ongoing malabsorption, weight loss, and malnutrition, enteral or parenteral supplements may still be needed. During the late phase with complete adaptation, weight often stabilizes and normal oral intake may be possible. Some patients never reach a stage where they can supply all needs orally, and home parenteral nutrition may be needed.

Diarrhea results from decreased transit time, increased osmolarity of the lumenal contents (as a result of carbohydrate malabsorption), bacterial overgrowth, gastric hypersecretion, and increased water and electrolyte secretion. After surgery, fluid losses may exceed 5 L per day, especially with concomitant colectomy. Gastric hypersecretion evokes intestinal mucosal damage, impaired micelle formation, and inhibition of pancreatic enzyme function. Nutritional deficiencies produce weight loss, weakness, fatigue, and growth retardation (in children). Consequences of fatty acid malabsorption include tetany, osteomalacia, and osteoporosis secondary to hypocalcemia and hypomagnesemia. Depletion of the bile salt pool with ileal resection contributes to steatorrhea. Undigested and unabsorbed carbohydrates may be metabolized by colonic bacteria to short-chain fatty acids that cause diarrhea by osmotic and secretory effects. Proteins also are metabolized by colonic flora and contribute to osmotic diarrhea to a lesser degree. Fat-soluble vitamin deficiency is common, as is vitamin B_{12} deficiency, but other water-soluble vitamins and trace metals are generally well absorbed even if the resection is extensive. However, zinc deficiency, which may impair intestinal adaptation, occurs rapidly.

Short bowel syndrome has significant systemic sequelae. Calcium oxalate renal calculi develop because of increased colonic absorption of dietary oxalate, decreased urinary concentrations of phosphate and citrate, and reduced urinary volume. The incidence of gallstones is increased twofold to threefold by ileal resection This phenomenon has been attributed to bile salt malabsorption, which secondarily causes cholesterol supersaturation of gallbladder bile. However, calcium-containing cholesterol stones and pigment stones are also prevalent after small bowel resection, indicating that other mechanisms are involved. Intrahepatic steatosis and hepatic dysfunction occur secondary to parenteral nutrition and sepsis and may lead to liver failure especially in children.

FINDINGS ON DIAGNOSTIC TESTING

Laboratory Testing

Laboratory abnormalities relate to the severity of nutrient, vitamin, and mineral deficiencies. Electrolyte determinations may reveal hyponatremia, hypokalemia, hypocalcemia, and hypomagnesemia, whereas a complete blood count may show anemia caused by vitamin B_{12} deficiency or, less commonly, folate and iron deficiencies. Fat-soluble vitamin deficiencies (i.e., A, D, E, and rarely K) may be evident. Urine oxalate levels may be elevated in patients predisposed to oxalate calculi. Fecal analysis reveals elevated fat levels. Bacterial overgrowth is diagnosed by quantitative culture of intestinal fluid obtained endoscopically or from a fluoroscopically placed aspiration catheter. Hydrogen breath testing is less reliable because of rapid transit of the substrate into the colon.

Radiographic Studies

Small intestinal barium radiography can be performed if the length of residual bowel is uncertain. Bone radiography and bone densitometry can be used to assess for osteomalacia and osteoporosis in a patient with calcium and vitamin D malabsorption. Ultrasound may be of value in detecting gallstones. Computed tomography, intravenous pyelography, or renal ultrasound may detect renal calculi.

MANAGEMENT AND COURSE

Medical Therapy

Controlling diarrhea and malnutrition is a major goal of treating a patient with short bowel syndrome Opiate agents, the most effective antidiarrheal agents for this condition, act by delaying transit in the small intestine and increasing intestinal capacity. Loperamide may be effective in some cases, but many patients require more potent opiates such as codeine or tincture of opium to control symptoms. In patients with limited ileal resection, cholestyramine may be effective for treating bile salt diarrhea. Subcutaneous octreotide reduces fluid and electrolyte losses in some patients with short bowel syndrome as a result of retarded propulsion, decreased digestive juice secretion, and altered mucosal fluid and electrolyte transport. Proton pump inhibitors may reduce gastric hypersecretion, minimizing ulcer complications and inhibiting the gastric secretory contribution to diarrhea. Oral broad-spectrum antibiotics are warranted if intestinal bacterial overgrowth is suspected. Pancreatic enzyme supplements are given to patients with proximal intestinal resections because of the loss of cholecystokinin and secretin release and to those with severe protein-calorie malnutrition.

Nutritional Therapy

During the initial postoperative phase, total parenteral nutrition is required to prevent diarrhea, dehydration, and fluid and electrolyte losses. Over time, many patients can be slowly weaned from intravenous feedings. If more than 25% of the intestine remains, it should be possible to stop parenteral nutrition eventually. The length of remaining small intestine, preservation of the colon, and ileo-colonic anastomosis predict the ability to wean from intravenous hyperalimentation.

Patients who receive long-term parenteral nutrition at home require a permanent intravenous catheter that must be placed surgically.

Limited oral intake to stimulate intestinal adaptation should be resumed when stool output is less than 2 L per day. A liquid solution that contains an isotonic sodium and glucose mixture takes advantage of the small intestinal sodium/glucose cotransport carrier to enhance fluid absorption. For patients with more than 60 to 80 cm of remaining small intestine, consumption of dry solids can be started slowly. Foods low in lactose content may be needed to limit diarrhea. If oxalate stones are a concern, administering oral calcium or cholestyramine may reduce dietary oxalate absorption. Fat content may need to be limited in a patient with an intact colon because colonic bacterial fat metabolites such as hydroxyl fatty acids promote secretory diarrhea. Medium-chain triglycerides can be used as nutritional supplements because they are absorbed directly from the proximal intestine into the portal circulation in the absence of bile salts. However, medium-chain triglycerides are unpalatable, may induce diarrhea, and do not provide essential fatty acids. The role of fiber supplements is controversial. In some patients, oral conjugated bile acids may improve fat absorption.

Patients who cannot tolerate oral feedings and those with less than 60 to 80 cm of remaining small intestine may benefit from enteral feedings. Elemental or semielemental formulas are recommended initially because they require minimal absorptive surface area. These formulas contain sucrose or glucose polymers, easily digested proteins, or free amino acids or short peptides, vitamins and minerals, and minimal amounts of fat. Because of their poor taste and their propensity to induce osmotic diarrhea, these formulas are often administered by slow infusion through a nasogastric or nasoenteric tube. Polymeric formulations provide 30% of calories as fat and contain intact protein sources. These solutions are more palatable and can be introduced when adaptation has progressed.

In general, vitamin and mineral supplements are included in oral feedings and enteral and parenteral solutions. Liquid solutions should be given because the hard matrix of solid pills may not dissolve during rapid transit through the shortened small intestine. Multivitamin preparations that contain two to five times the recommended dietary allowances are advocated. Patients with ileal resections of more than 90 cm should receive intramuscular vitamin B_{12}. Serum retinol, calcium 25-hydroxyvitamin D, and urinary calcium are monitored to assess the adequacy of vitamin A and D supplementation. Calcium intake of 1000 to 1500 mg per day is encouraged. Symptomatic hypomagnesemia may mandate intravenous magnesium replacement because oral magnesium supplements worsen diarrhea. Iron and zinc deficiency can develop, requiring specific supplementation. Deficiencies of other minerals usually are averted by multivitamins.

Surgical Therapy

A variety of surgical procedures may benefit selected patients with short bowel syndrome. Antiperistaltic segments that retard intestinal transit can increase water, fat, and nitrogen absorption in 70% of patients. Interposition of colonic segment into the shortened small intestine also has been tried to slow propulsion. Tapering enteroplasty may improve intestinal function in patients with short bowel syndrome who have had a dilated small intestine. In children, a technique of lengthening the small intestine by using redundant small intestine from a tapering procedure has been tried.

Small intestinal transplantation has become a life-saving treatment for patients with irreversible intestinal failure who cannot be maintained on parenteral nutrition because of liver disease, recurrent sepsis, or loss of venous access. Contraindications to intestinal transplant include profound neurological difficulty, life-threatening illness, and multiple system immune disease. Transplantation should be considered prior to development of parenteral nutrition–associated cirrhosis because combined liver-intestine transplants have higher mortality rates than that of intestinal transplantation alone. One-year survival rates after intestinal transplantation range from 66% to 75%, depending on the need for other grafts or transplanted organs. Causes of death after intestinal transplant include sepsis, lymphoproliferative disease, nontransplant organ failure, thrombosis, ischemia, bleeding, and graft rejection.

CHAPTER 42

Tumors and Other Neoplastic Diseases of the Small Intestine

Tumors of the small intestine account for less than 2% of all gastrointestinal malignancies. Primary cancers of the small intestine include adenocarcinomas, carcinoids, lymphomas, sarcomas, and leiomyosarcomas; however, benign neoplasms such as adenomas, leiomyomas, lipomas, and hamartomas are more common (Table 42-1).

ADENOCARCINOMA

Incidence and Epidemiology

Although adenocarcinoma is the most common primary cancer of the small intestine, the annual incidence is 4 cases per 1 million people. Most adenocarcinomas develop in the duodenum and jejunum. They occur more frequently in patients with familial adenomatous polyposis (FAP), which carries an increased relative risk of adenocarcinoma of the duodenum and periampullary region. Other conditions associated with an increased frequency of adenocarcinoma include long-standing Crohn's disease, celiac sprue, and urologic ileal conduits. The overall 5-year survival is 30%; median life expectancy after diagnosis is less than 20 months.

Etiology and Pathogenesis

There appears to be an adenoma-to-carcinoma sequence leading to adenocarcinoma of the small intestine, similar to the well-recognized pathogenesis of colorectal cancer. The high incidence of duodenal adenomas and carcinomas in patients with FAP suggests that the genetic and molecular mechanisms of carcinogenesis in the small intestine are similar to those of colorectal cancer. Hereditary nonpolyposis colorectal cancer (HNPCC), hamartomatous polyposis (Peutz-Jeghers syndrome), Crohn's disease, gluten-sensitive enteropathy

TABLE 42-1
Classification of Tumors of the Small Intestine

Benign Epithelial Tumors
    Adenoma
    Hamartomas (Peutz-Jeghers syndrome, Cronkite-Canada syndrome, juvenile
       polyposis, Cowden disease, Bannayan-Riley-Ruvalcaba syndrome)

Malignant Epithelial Tumors
    Primary adenocarcinoma
    Metastatic carcinoma
    Carcinoid tumors

Lymphoproliferative Disorders
    B-cell
      Diffuse large cell lymphoma
      Small, noncleaved cell lymphoma
      Mucosa-associated lymphoid tissue (MALT) lymphoma
      Mantle cell lymphoma (multiple lymphomatous polyposis)
      Immunoproliferative small intestinal disease (IPSID)
    T-cell
      Enteropathy-associated T-cell lymphoma

Mesenchymal Tumors
    Gastrointestinal stromal cell tumors (GISTs)
    Fatty tumors (lipoma, liposarcoma)
    Neural tumors (schwannomas, neurofibromas, ganglioneuromas)
    Paragangliomas
    Smooth muscle tumors (leiomyoma, leiomyosarcoma)
    Vascular tumors (hemangioma, angiosarcoma, lymphangioma, Kaposi sarcoma)

(celiac sprue), and the diversion of bile are associated with an increased risk of small intestinal adenocarcinoma. The risk of carcinoma also increases for persons who smoke cigarettes and those who consume more than 80 g ethanol per day.

Clinical Features

Eighty-five percent of patients with small intestinal adenocarcinomas present after age 50. Symptoms may include abdominal pain, nausea, vomiting, and weight loss. Occult blood loss with anemia may be present. Ileal tumors may cause intussusception, and periampullary tumors (i.e., tumors of the ampulla of Vater) may cause gastric outlet obstruction, biliary obstruction with jaundice, or pancreatitis. Patients with celiac sprue may present with new-onset weight loss and abdominal pain after years of quiescent disease. Similarly, patients with Crohn's disease exhibit symptoms of obstruction that may mistakenly be attributed to a flare of their underlying disease.

The physical examination of patients with adenomas and adenocarcinomas of the small intestine is often normal. A minority of patients have abdominal distention, abdominal masses, gastric outlet obstructions, or evidence of fecal occult blood loss.

TABLE 42-2
Distribution of Malignant Tumors of the Small Intestine

TUMOR	DUODENUM (%)	JEJUNUM (%)	ILEUM (%)
Primary adenocarcinoma	40	38	22
Malignant carcinoid	18	4	78
Primary lymphoma	6	36	58
Leiomyosarcoma	3	53	44

Findings on Diagnostic Testing

Upper gastrointestinal endoscopy using both forward-viewing and side-viewing endoscopes may be necessary to diagnose small intestinal adenocarcinoma. Most adenomas in patients with FAP are located in the proximal duodenum and periampullary region, whereas up to one half of sporadic carcinomas occur in the jejunum and ileum (Table 42-2). Lesions in the proximal or middle jejunum can be identified and biopsies specimens obtained with push enteroscopy. Distal lesions may require barium radiography of the small intestine for diagnosis. Enteroclysis, which is more sensitive than routine barium radiography, may be necessary to detect diminutive mass lesions. Patients who exhibit gastrointestinal bleeding may benefit from angiography if no source can be identified by upper gastrointestinal endoscopy or colonoscopy. Adenocarcinomas appear as hypovascular masses with associated encasement of the surrounding vessels. Wireless capsule endoscopy of the small intestine may be useful for visualizing tumors that are too small to detect by radiographic techniques if clinical suspicion remains elevated despite normal radiographic studies. Computed tomographic (CT) scans are helpful in staging tumors of the small intestine by identifying lymph node and hepatic metastases.

Management and Course

Surgical resection is the treatment of choice for adenocarcinoma of the small intestine. Tumors in the jejunum and proximal ileum are treated with segmental resection. A right hemicolectomy is required to treat adenocarcinoma of the distal ileum. Lesions that involve the ampulla of Vater require pancreaticoduodenectomy (i.e., the Whipple procedure). The long-term survival for primary small bowel adenocarcinoma is 47.6% (local disease), 33% (regional disease), and 3.9% (distal disease). Neither chemotherapy nor radiation therapy is effective for small bowel adenocarcinoma.

CARCINOIDS

Incidence and Epidemiology

Seventy-four percent of carcinoid tumors develop in the gastrointestinal tract. After the appendix, the small intestine is the second most common gastrointestinal site for the development of carcinoid tumors; the majority of small bowel carcinoids occur in the ileum. Carcinoids account for 20% to 40% of all malignant small bowel tumors; the annual incidence is 1.2 to 6.5 per 1 million persons. The median age at diagnosis is 60, but there is a wide range (22 to 84 years). Carcinoids are more common in men and in African Americans.

Etiology and Pathogenesis

Carcinoid tumors are a type of endocrine neoplasm termed *amine precursor uptake and decarboxylation tumors* (APUDomas). Histologically, carcinoids resemble other neuroendocrine tumors and are characterized by clumps of uniform cells with hyperchromatic nuclei. Carcinoid tumors are malignant and are classified by their products of secretion. Serotonin is responsible for most symptoms in the carcinoid syndrome, but prostaglandins, gastrin, bradykinin, and other substances also produced by carcinoid tumors may affect the clinical presentation. Overall 5-year survival is 55%; breakdown by stage is 65% (local disease), 64% (regional), and 36% (metastatic). Seventy percent of carcinoids in the small intestine are detected incidentally during upper gastrointestinal endoscopy, surgery, or autopsy.

Clinical Features

The most common clinical presentation of a symptomatic carcinoid tumor of the small intestine is intermittent abdominal pain. Additional complications include intestinal ischemia, intussusception, and gastrointestinal hemorrhage.

  The carcinoid syndrome affects 10% to 18% of patients with small bowel carcinoids. Although localized foregut carcinoids may produce the carcinoid syndrome, carcinoids of the small intestine cause this syndrome only after hepatic metastasis. The characteristic symptoms of the carcinoid syndrome are flushing of the face and neck and intermittent watery diarrhea. Less common symptoms include bronchospasm and right-sided heart failure. Patients with carcinoid syndrome may experience a hypotensive crisis during the induction of general anesthesia.

Findings on Diagnostic Testing

Laboratory Testing

Measuring the urinary excretion of 5-hydroxyindoleacetic acid (5-HIAA), the major metabolite of serotonin, is a sensitive and specific test for the carcinoid syndrome, but it is less accurate for detecting localized carcinoids. Excretion of more than 30 mg of 5-HIAA in a 24-hour urine sample after provocative testing is diagnostic of the carcinoid syndrome. False-positive tests may be caused by celiac disease, Whipple disease, tropical sprue, and ingesting food rich in serotonin (e.g., walnuts, bananas, and avocados). Elevation of chromogranin A can also be used for diagnosing carcinoid tumors, as well as for monitoring treatment response or recurrence. The measurement of neuron-specific enolase levels has also been used, but it is a less accurate diagnostic test for carcinoid tumors than the measurement of chromogranin A.

Imaging Studies

Because most carcinoids occur in the ileum, upper gastrointestinal endoscopy and colonoscopy have limited roles in identifying these tumors. Most symptomatic lesions are visible in barium radiographs of the small intestine. The desmoplastic distortion of the mesentery may be evident as kinking and tethering of the intestine. A CT scan is also helpful in demonstrating these mesenteric changes; it is the procedure of choice for documenting hepatic metastases. Scintigraphy with iodine-123 (^{123}I) or ^{131}I-labeled metaiodobenzylguanidine (I-MIBG), indium-labeled pentetreotide, or octreotide may identify primary and metastatic carcinoids not detected by conventional imaging techniques. Positron-emission tomography (PET) can also be used to identify metastatic carcinoids.

Management and Course

Localized carcinoids of the small intestine should be completely resected, either endoscopically or surgically. Asymptomatic lesions smaller than 1 cm in diameter may be treated with local excision, but lesions larger than 1 cm require a wide surgical excision. Duodenal lesions require a Whipple procedure, whereas distal ileal lesions require ileocecectomy and lesions in the jejunum and proximal ileum require segmental resection with 10-cm margins. When localized disease is resected, the overall 5-year survival is 75%, compared with 20% for metastatic disease.

Tumors with regional spread require wide surgical resection. Five-year survival after resection and nodal dissection for regional disease is 65% to 71%, compared to 38% for patients who do not have surgery.

Patients with metastatic disease and the carcinoid syndrome may benefit from debulking surgery. The somatostatin analog octreotide inhibits serotonin release and reduces flushing in more than 70% and reduces diarrhea in more than 60% of patients with carcinoid syndrome. Initial doses range from 50 to 250 μg subcutaneously, two to three times daily, but as the disease progresses, larger doses may be necessary. Treatment with interferon is associated with substantially longer survival (median 80 months) compared to combination chemotherapy with streptozocin and 5-fluorouracil (8 months); the addition of hepatic chemoembolization to interferon may be associated with even longer survival.

MESENCHYMAL TUMORS

Incidence and Epidemiology

Gastrointestinal stromal cell tumors (GISTs) describe a heterogeneous collection of mesenchymal tumors previously thought to be of "smooth muscle" origin. The most common variant found in the small intestine is the mesenchymal spindle cell tumor. Twenty percent to 30% of GISTs occur in the small intestine (60% occur in the stomach). Malignant GISTs are sarcomas with an incidence of 1.2 to 1.5 cases per million population.

Etiology and Pathogenesis

GISTs of the small intestine are classified by phenotype: myoid, neural, or ganglionic. Almost all GISTs express CD117 antigen (protooncogene protein c-kit), and 70% express CD34 antigen, in contrast to true leiomyomas, leiomyosarcomas, and schwannomas. Because intestinal cells of Cajal express similar proteins, it has been postulated that GISTs have the same embryonic origin.

Clinical Features and Diagnosis

Most small GISTs are discovered incidentally and are asymptomatic. Larger tumors may be associated with symptoms of abdominal pain, nausea, vomiting, weight loss, or gastrointestinal hemorrhage. In some series, up to 40% of patients with ileal GISTs present with intussusception.

Small bowel radiography, CT scan, and angiography are useful in diagnosing GISTs. Because the lesions are submucosal, endoscopic diagnosis is often difficult unless ulceration is present. Endoscopic ultrasound has been shown to differentiate malignant from benign GISTs based on the following criteria: tumor size larger than 4 cm, irregular extralumenal margins, and the presence of cystic spaces. Biopsy specimens or resected tissue should be stained for CD117 to confirm the diagnosis of a GIST.

Treatment

The treatment of choice for small bowel GISTs is segmental intestinal resection. Despite complete resection with negative margins, recurrence rates approach 50% to 80%. Neither chemotherapy nor radiation therapy benefits patients with unresectable metastatic or recurrent disease.

LYMPHOMA

Incidence and Epidemiology

Primary lymphoma accounts for 7% to 25% of the malignancies of the small intestine; the annual incidence is 1 to 3 per million persons. The small intestine is second to the stomach as a site for development of primary gastrointestinal lymphoma. There are two major variants of lymphoma with distinct epidemiologic associations. Primary small bowel lymphomas (PSBLs) are characterized by the absence of peripheral or mediastinal lymphadenopathy, a normal leukocyte count and differential, and lack of liver or spleen involvement. They are more prevalent in Western countries; are of the non-Hodgkin variety; and are associated with celiac sprue, diffuse nodular lymphoid hyperplasia, and acquired or congenital immunodeficiency. Immunoproliferative small intestinal disease (IPSID) occurs almost exclusively in developing countries. Patients usually present in young adulthood with diffuse intestinal involvement.

Etiology and Pathogenesis

PSBLs occur more commonly in the distal small intestine and generally are localized to one section of the bowel, in contrast to the diffuse nature of IPSID. Most are B-cell lymphomas; the most common type is small, noncleaved cell lymphomas. Mucosa-associated lymphoid tissue (MALT) lymphomas can occur in the small intestine, as can mantle cell lymphomas (multiple lymphoid polyposis). The latter is an aggressive tumor that often presents with distant lymph node and bone marrow involvement. In contrast to sporadic lymphomas in the small intestine, those associated with celiac sprue usually are of T-cell origin.

Evidence suggests that an infectious agent may cause the IPSID variant of lymphoma of the small intestine. The disease occurs almost exclusively in geographic regions where parasitic and other enteric infections are endemic. Tetracycline given early in the course of the disease can induce complete remission. A lack of response to antibiotics in patients with later stage disease, however, suggests that other factors are also involved.

Clinical Features

A discrete mass lesion characterizes PSBL. Intermittent abdominal pain caused by obstruction is the most common complaint. Weight loss is often marked, and a small percentage of patients presents with perforations. Lymphoma should be suspected in patients with celiac sprue who complain of abdominal pain and weight loss after years or decades of quiescent disease. Misinterpreting these symptoms as a flare of celiac sprue may delay diagnosis.

Patients with IPSID present earlier than those with PSBL. Patients report profuse diarrhea and weight loss in addition to symptoms of obstruction. Many patients have associated clubbing of the digits. Unlike PSBL, a palpable abdominal mass is uncommon.

Findings on Diagnostic Testing

Barium radiography of the small intestine is the primary means of detecting small bowel lymphomas. Because most PSBLs occur in the ileum, upper gastrointestinal endoscopy may not visualize the lesion. Tumors within the distal 5 to 10 cm of the terminal ileum are accessible to colonoscopic biopsy. CT scans may be able to stage the tumor based on detecting malignant intra-abdominal and intrathoracic lymph nodes. Because of the diffuse nature of IPSID, a laparotomy may be required to establish the diagnosis. There are no specific laboratory features of PSBL, but serum protein electrophoresis demonstrates an α-heavy chain paraprotein in 20 to 70% of patients with IPSID.

Management and Course

Staging lymphomas of the small intestine is similar to that of gastric lymphomas. Patients with PSBL should be treated with surgical resection with lymph node sampling. Even if curative resection is not possible, palliative resection will prevent perforation resulting from chemotherapy-induced tumor necrosis. Combination chemotherapy is indicated for disease that is incompletely resected or unresectable, but the role of adjuvant therapy after curative resection is undefined. Patients with IPSID may respond to antibiotic therapy in the prelymphomatous stage (tetracycline or metronidazole for 6 to 12 months). Nonresponders or patients in the lymphomatous stage have responded to anthracycline-based chemotherapy. The 5-year survival rate after curative resection for PSBL is 44% to 65%, whereas the corresponding survival rate for unresectable disease is only 20%. A poor prognosis is associated with IPSID, enteropathy-associated T-cell lymphoma, and mantle cell lymphoma.

CHAPTER 43

Structural Anomalies and Diverticular Disease of the Colon

COLONIC EMBRYOLOGY AND ANATOMY

The colon begins to develop during the fourth gestational week, originating from the embryonic midgut (from which the appendix, cecum, ascending colon, and proximal transverse colon are derived) and hindgut (from which the distal transverse colon, descending colon, sigmoid colon, and rectum are derived). The anorectal septum, which initially divides the cloaca into the ventral urogenital sinus and the dorsal rectum, ruptures in the eighth week, creating the anal canal. Development of the colonic epithelium is similar to that of the small intestine and occurs with the formation of the lumen at 8 weeks of gestation. Epithelial ridges form at 10 to 11 weeks of gestation. Small lumens form at the base of these ridges and subsequently extend to the main lumen, resulting in the formation of broad primary villi. Between weeks 12 to 15, the formation of cyst-like spaces within these primary villi and the accompanying upgrowth of mesenchyme results in the division of primary villi into numerous secondary villi. Epithelial cells proliferate, leading to the formation of the colonic crypts. The colonic villi disappear between the twenty-ninth week and term, leaving only the colonic crypts. The fetal colonic epithelium contains several small intestinal cell types, including goblet cells, columnar epithelial cells with microvilli, and enteroendocrine cells, which appear to secrete trophic factors. Smooth muscle cells and muscular structures such as the taenia coli and haustra appear in the tenth week. The enteric nervous system develops within the first 12 weeks, and by the end of this period, the Auerbach and Meissner plexuses work in concert with the muscles to initiate colonic motility.

The adult colon is 3 to 5 feet long and extends from the ileocecal junction to the rectum. The lumenal diameter progressively decreases from the cecum (7.5 to 8.5 cm) to the sigmoid colon (2.5 cm). The ascending and descending colons, rectum, and posterior surfaces of the hepatic and splenic flexures are fixed retroperitoneal structures; whereas the cecum, transverse colon, and sigmoid colon are intraperitoneal. Circular muscle envelops the full circumference of the colon, whereas the outer longitudinal muscle layer is confined to three bands, the taenia coli, located 120 degrees apart around the circumference. The haustra are sacculations separated by the plicae semilunares. The rectum is a 12- to 15-cm-long structure extending from the sigmoid colon to the anus. It is composed of mucosal, submucosal, and circumferential inner circular and outer longitudinal muscle layers. In contrast to the colon, the rectum has no serosal layer. The anal canal is 4 cm long and is lined by squamous epithelium that lacks hair follicles, sebaceous glands, and sweat glands. The mucocutaneous junction (dentate line) is located 1.0 to 1.5 cm above the anal verge. The columns of Morgagni are mucosal folds above the dentate line. The anorectal ring is the palpable upper border of the anal sphincter, located 1.0 to 1.5 cm proximal to the dentate line.

The superior mesenteric artery branches into the ileocolic, right colic, and middle colic arteries that supply arterial blood to the cecum, ascending colon, and transverse colon. The inferior mesenteric artery supplies the descending colon, sigmoid colon, and upper rectum through its left colic, sigmoidal, and superior rectal branches. Collateral vessels interconnect these arterial sources, including the marginal artery of Drummond that runs along the mesenteric border of the colon and the arc of Riolan that connects the middle colic to the left colic artery. The middle and inferior rectal arteries that originate from the internal iliac and internal pudendal arteries, respectively, supply the distal rectum. Hemorrhoidal tissue also receives blood from the rectal arteries.

The venous drainage of the colon parallels the arterial supply except for the inferior mesenteric vein, which runs retroperitoneally before entering the splenic vein. The internal hemorrhoids drain into the superior rectal vein, and the external hemorrhoids drain into the pudendal veins. Lymphatic capillaries encircle the colon in the submucosa and muscularis mucosae. Lymph nodes are located on the bowel wall (epicolic), along the inner margin (paracolic), around the mesenteric arteries (intermediate), and at the origin of the superior mesenteric artery and the inferior mesenteric artery (main). Lymph from the lower rectum and anal canal above the dentate line enters the inferior mesenteric nodes and iliac nodes and subsequently drains to the periaortic nodes. Below the dentate line, lymph drains to the inguinal nodes and to the rectal lymph nodes.

The sympathetic and parasympathetic nerves to the colon follow the course of the blood vessels. The sympathetic nerves arise from the superior mesenteric plexus, which supplies the proximal colon, and from the inferior mesenteric plexus, which supplies the left colon and rectum. The parasympathetic innervation to the right colon comes from the vagus, and the distal colon from the pelvic nerve. Distal sympathetic and parasympathetic fibers also innervate the bladder, prostate, and sexual organs, all of which may be injured during dissection of the rectum. Afferent fibers from the pudendal nerve innervate the anal epithelium.

The mucosa of the colon is similar histologically to that of the small intestine. Both are lined by simple columnar epithelium; however, mature colonic mucosa lacks villi. The lamina propria contains plasma cells, macrophages, lymphocytes, and abundant lymphoid nodules that often extend into the submucosa. Subepithelial fibroblasts produce many of the components of the basal lamina. The epithelial cells undergo renewal every 6 days and are replaced by descendants of stem cells from the lower third of the crypts. There are three main epithelial cell types: colonocytes, goblet cells, and enteroendocrine cells. Colonocytes can absorb sodium, chloride, and water but not glucose or amino acids. These cells have a limited ability to absorb fatty acids and package them into chylomicrons. Goblet cells secrete mucus that lubricates and protects the epithelium from adherence of pathogens. Enteroendocrine cells secrete enteroglucagon, peptide YY, serotonin, substance P, pancreatic polypeptide, and somatostatin. These cells are more numerous in the rectum and appendix, which may explain the frequent occurrence of neuroendocrine tumors at these sites.

DEVELOPMENTAL ABNORMALITIES OF THE COLON

Hirschsprung Disease

Etiology and Pathogenesis

Hirschsprung disease results from the failure of the neural crest cells to complete their caudal migration to the anus during fetal development. The resulting aganglionic segment of colon does not relax and causes functional obstruction. The rectosigmoid is involved in 75% to 80% of cases, whereas the entire colon and parts of the small intestine are involved in 5% to 10% of cases.

Clinical Features, Diagnosis, and Management

Newborns with Hirschsprung disease may present with abdominal distention and delayed passage of meconium, whereas older children may present with chronic constipation, distention, volvulus, or perforation. Adults with a very short segment of involvement may report a history of constipation that dates back to childhood. Digital examination may show an empty rectal vault in Hirschsprung disease, differentiating this entity from idiopathic megacolon, in which voluminous stool is present in the vault. Abdominal radiography may show colonic dilation with a paucity of gas, and barium enema examination may reveal a short, narrow, transition zone. However, barium enema radiographs may appear normal in patients with total colonic aganglionosis, very short segment involvement, or neonatal Hirschsprung disease. Anorectal manometry typically demonstrates a loss of the rectoanal inhibitory reflex, characterized by an absence of the normal relaxation of the internal anal sphincter in response to rectal distention. Deep rectal biopsy specimens that include the mucosa and submucosa are necessary for diagnosing Hirschsprung disease, and in some patients, full-thickness operative biopsy specimens may be required. Biopsy specimens from affected persons exhibit hyperplastic or hypertrophic nerve fibers with an absence of ganglion cells. Special stains of the specimen reveal an increase in acetylcholinesterase content. A colostomy is often performed before definitive surgical repair to allow the bowel to stabilize and resume a normal caliber. Pull-through operations (Swenson, Duhamel, and Soave) can anastomose normally innervated bowel to the anus with or without resection of affected bowel. Rectal myotomy may cure patients with short segment involvement.

Colonic Duplications

Etiology and Pathogenesis

Intestinal duplications can occur anywhere along the gastrointestinal tract; the colon and rectum account for 5% to 10% of gastrointestinal duplications. Colonic duplications are thought to result from failure of the colon to recanalize in utero, from caudal twinning, or from incomplete separation of the notochord from the ectoderm. These duplications may communicate with the colonic lumen or they may be closed cysts.

Clinical Features, Diagnosis, and Management

Duplications can produce symptoms of obstruction, volvulus, and hemorrhage. Less common complications include infection and malignant degeneration. Abdominal radiography, barium enema radiography, or computed tomographic (CT) scanning may reveal masses with or without communication with the colon. Rectal duplications are resected, even if asymptomatic, because of the risk of malignancy. Cystic duplications may be excised, whereas tubular duplications in direct apposition with the colon wall can be treated by dividing the common wall. Mucosal excision may be required if heterotopic gastric mucosa is present.

Malrotation

Etiology and Pathogenesis

Malrotation occurs when the midgut fails to complete the 270-degree rotation before reentering the abdomen at 10 to 12 weeks of gestation. The cecum and right colon overlie the duodenum in the right upper quadrant and the duodenojejunal junction is positioned to the right of the spine. Malrotation is associated with intestinal atresia, intussusception, Hirschsprung disease, and abdominal wall defects in 30% to 60% of cases.

Clinical Features, Diagnosis, and Management

Infants usually present within the first month of birth with bilious vomiting, a flat abdomen, and bloody stools due to ischemia. There may also be evidence of proximal intestinal obstruction or volvulus. Abdominal radiography may show gastric or duodenal obstruction. Upper gastrointestinal barium radiography may reveal displacement of the ligament of Treitz on the right, whereas barium enema radiography may demonstrate the cecum in the right upper quadrant. Surgery for malrotation involves reducing any volvulus, severing the Ladd bands that overlie

he right colon and duodenum, removing the appendix, and fixing the duodenum
a the right upper quadrant and the cecum in the left upper quadrant.

mperforate Anus

tiology and Pathogenesis

n imperforate anus is classified according to the anatomic level of the defect. A
igh lesion (more common in males) involves termination of the bowel above the
evator ani muscles, whereas a low imperforate anus (more common in females)
nvolves termination of the rectum below the levator ani and may be accompanied
y fistulous connections to the perineum, vagina, or other organs. Imperforate
nus has an incidence of 1 in 20,000 live births and is associated with congenital
genitourinary, sacral, cardiac, or gastrointestinal anomalies (e.g., esophageal atresia)
n 50% of cases.

Clinical Features, Diagnosis, and Management

nfants present with a failure to pass meconium, unless a fistula is present. Char-
cterization of the defect relies on air invertograms (to identify the location of
he rectum), fistulograms, CT scans, or magnetic resonance imaging studies. The
rinary tract requires examination by intravenous pyelography and voiding cys-
ourethrograms. Low lesions can be treated by dilating fistulous tracts with or without anoplasty. High lesions are treated with an initial diverting colostomy followed
by a pull-through operation—for example, the Pena and deVries procedure—that
as a 70% to 80% success rate.

VOLVULUS

Etiology and Pathogenesis

Volvulus is the twisting of an air-filled segment of bowel about its mesentery.
A dilated, redundant colon is required for the development of volvulus, which
causes less than 10% of colonic obstructions in the United States. Sigmoid volvulus
(60% of cases) occurs in elderly and institutionalized persons and in patients with
neuropsychiatric disease, chronic constipation, or colonic atony after laxative abuse.
Cecal volvulus (<20% of cases) occurs in younger patients and is believed to be
caused by adhesions from prior surgery, pregnancy, left colon obstruction, or an
anomalous fixation of the right colon with a mobile cecum. Most patients with
cecal volvulus have full axial twisting of the associated mesentery and blood vessels,
but in some, the cecum is folded in an anterior cephalad direction (cecal bascule).
The resulting tension on the colonic wall may produce gangrene.

Clinical Features, Diagnosis, and Management

Abdominal pain, distention, and obstipation are the typical symptoms of sigmoid
volvulus. Gangrene is manifested by fever, signs of peritoneal irritation, or leukocytosis. Abdominal radiography demonstrates an inverted U-shaped loop with a
dense line running to the point of torsion. In uncomplicated cases, radiography
enhanced with water-soluble contrast (Gastrografin) or barium enema may define
the site of volvulus and lead to therapeutic reduction of the twisted loop. These
techniques are avoided in patients with possible peritonitis, however. In the absence
of peritonitis, sigmoidoscopy with placement of a rectal tube may result in dramatic
decompression. Elective resection of the involved colon should follow. Emergency

surgery is indicated if there is evidence of ischemia, gangrene, or unsuccessful detorsion.

Cecal volvulus is characterized by pain, nausea, vomiting, and obstipation. The symptoms are intermittent in many patients. Abdominal radiography may show a kidney-shaped, air-filled structure in the left upper quadrant and multiple air-fluid levels in the small intestine. Barium or Gastrografin enema radiography may show the site of torsion but is not indicated if plain radiography provides the diagnosis. Colonoscopy may reduce the volvulus, but success is limited. Right hemicolectomy with primary anastomosis or cecopexy and cecostomy are recommended if gangrene is not present. Resection, ileostomy, and construction of a mucous fistula are indicated for cases complicated by gangrene.

Volvulus of the transverse colon is rare due to the short mesentery of this segment of the colon. Patients present with symptoms of colonic obstruction, and barium enema radiography provides a diagnosis. Most patients require operative detorsion and resection of the involved colonic segment.

UNCOMPLICATED DIVERTICULOSIS

Etiology and Pathogenesis

Diverticulosis is an acquired condition characterized by the presence of diverticula, saclike protrusions of the colonic wall. Typical colonic diverticula herniate through defects in the muscle layer where arteries pass (vasa recta), on either side of the mesenteric tenia and on the mesenteric aspect of the antimesenteric teniae (Fig. 43-1). Because they do not possess muscular layers, they are false or pulsion diverticula. In industrialized nations, 33% to 50% of the population older than age 50 has colonic diverticula, which may relate to low levels of dietary fiber. Ninety-five percent of patients with diverticulosis have diverticula in the sigmoid colon. Twenty-four percent of patients have diverticula in other regions in addition to the sigmoid colon; 7% have pancolic involvement. Sigmoid diverticulosis is accompanied by thickening of the circular muscle, shortening of the taenia coli, and narrowing of the lumen. Most diverticula are 0.1 to 1.0 cm in diameter, whereas larger diverticula may be the consequence of prior diverticulitis. Rectal diverticula are rare because of the presence of the circumferential longitudinal muscle layer.

Development of diverticulosis depends on the strength of the colon wall and the pressure difference between the lumen of the colon and the peritoneal cavity. Muscle thickening in the sigmoid colon is likely to represent a prediverticular condition resulting from high intralumenal pressures in an area of small diameter, with no corresponding increase in wall strength. The elasticity and tensile strength of the colon decrease with age, an effect that is most marked in the sigmoid colon. Deterioration in colonic structural proteins in Ehlers-Danlos and Marfan syndromes may explain the premature development of diverticula in these conditions. The role of primary colonic motor disorders in the pathogenesis of diverticulosis is undefined, and the relation of diverticulosis and irritable bowel syndrome is controversial.

Clinical Features, Diagnosis, and Management

Eighty percent to 85% of persons with diverticulosis never develop significant symptoms. Some patients have mild, intermittent abdominal pain, bloating, flatulence, and altered defecation, although coexistence of irritable bowel syndrome is possible. Three fourths of the remaining patients develop diverticulitis and one fourth report hemorrhage. On barium enema radiography, diverticula appear as

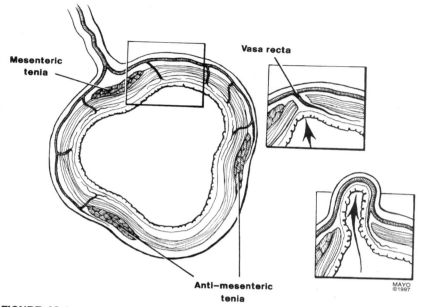

FIGURE 43-1. Cross section of the sigmoid colon. The main illustration indicates the points of penetration of the vasa recta around the bowel circumference. *Inset:* The development of a diverticulum at one such point of weakness. (From Young-Fadok TM, Pemberton JH. Colonic diverticular disease: epidemiology and pathophysiology. In: Rose BD, ed. *UpToDate in Medicine* [CD-ROM]. Wellesley, MA: UpToDate; 1997.)

contrast-filled colonic protrusions that may persist after evacuation. The presence of diverticula may reduce the accuracy of barium enema radiography to 50% in detecting coexisting colonic neoplasia. Colonoscopy may reveal diverticular orifices, sigmoid tortuosity, and thickened folds consistent with prior diverticulitis. Therapy for symptomatic but uncomplicated diverticular disease relies on increased intake of dietary fiber or the use of fiber supplements.

DIVERTICULITIS

Etiology and Pathogenesis

Diverticulitis is symptomatic inflammation of a diverticulum and begins as peridiverticulitis caused by a microperforation of the colon. The incidence of diverticulitis increases with age. Most cases of diverticulitis in westernized countries are left-sided, but inflammation of diverticula at other sites, including the rectum and appendix, may occur.

Clinical Features, Diagnosis, and Management

Early manifestations of diverticulitis include pain and tenderness over the site of inflammation (usually in the lower abdomen or pelvis), nausea and vomiting, ileus,

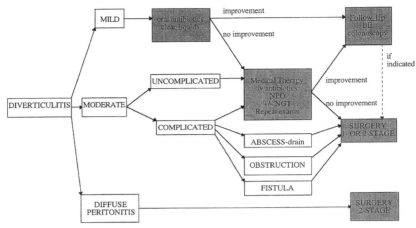

FIGURE 43-2. Algorithm for treating acute diverticulitis. (From Young-Fadok TM, Pemberton JH. Colonic diverticular disease: acute diverticulitis. In: Rose BD, ed. *UpToDate in Medicine* [CD-ROM]. Wellesley, MA: UpToDate; 1997.)

fever, a possible palpable mass, and tenderness or a mass effect on rectal examination. Complications of progressive inflammation include abscess, perforation, fistulization, and obstruction. CT scanning is indicated if the diagnosis is uncertain, complications are suspected, medical therapy has failed, or the patient is immunocompromised. CT scans may reveal thickening of the colon wall, pericolic inflammation, fistulae, sinuses, abscess cavities, and obstruction. Ultrasound is occasionally useful for detecting and draining pericolonic fluid collections. Barium enema radiography is not recommended during the acute attack, although water-soluble contrast enemas may be used to detect diverticula. Careful flexible sigmoidoscopy is used during an episode of suspected diverticulitis to differentiate a neoplasm from an inflammatory diverticular mass, but colonoscopy is contraindicated in cases of acute diverticulitis because of the risk of complications, including perforation.

The initial management of diverticulitis includes fluid replacement, nasogastric suction for ileus or obstruction, and broad-spectrum antibiotics to treat possible infection with anaerobes, gram-negative bacilli, and gram-positive coliform organisms (Fig. 43-2). Unstable patients should receive ampicillin, gentamicin, and metronidazole, whereas stable patients with local peritoneal signs may be given ampicillin/sulbactam, imipenem/cilastatin, or ticarcillin/clavulanate for 7 to 10 days. When necessary, clindamycin may be substituted for metronidazole, vancomycin for penicillin, and aztreonam for gentamicin. Oral quinolones, amoxicillin/clavulanate, or a cephalosporin may be given to outpatients who have no peritoneal signs. Indications for surgery include perforation, abscess, fistula, obstruction, recurrent diverticulitis, or the inability to exclude carcinoma. In the case of urgent surgery, primary anastomosis is not attempted because anastomotic breakdown is possible. However, a one-stage operation with anastomosis can be performed in the absence of advanced age, sepsis, hemodynamic instability, an unprepared colon, local contamination, friable tissues, malnutrition, steroid use, or poor blood supply. Percutaneous CT-guided abscess drainage may benefit patients who are stable and without signs of sepsis. Fistulae usually can be resected in a one-stage procedure.

whereas obstruction usually mandates a two-stage operative approach. Surgical resection can reduce the likelihood of recurrent diverticulitis from 30% to between 5% and 10%. In most cases, distal sigmoid resection must be complete to minimize recurrent diverticular inflammation.

DIVERTICULAR HEMORRHAGE

Etiology and Pathogenesis

Diverticular hemorrhage is the most common cause of acute massive colonic blood loss. Massive bleeding from colonic diverticula occurs in 5% of patients; minor bleeding occurs in up to 47%. The close proximity of diverticula and arteries accounts for the propensity of these lesions to bleed. Paradoxically, although most diverticula are sigmoid in location, half of diverticular hemorrhages emanate from a right colonic source.

Clinical Features, Diagnosis, and Management

Diverticular hemorrhage is characterized by the sudden, painless passage of large amounts of bright-red blood from the rectum and may be associated with hypotension, tachycardia, or syncope. Bleeding stops spontaneously in 80% of patients. Complications of diverticular hemorrhage are related to hypovolemia and involve the heart, brain, kidneys, and lungs. The initial management of diverticular hemorrhage, as for other types of gastrointestinal hemorrhage, requires aggressive fluid resuscitation and replacement of colloid including blood products. The patient's cardiovascular system must be stabilized, the airway protected, and ventilation support established. Because massive hemorrhage is statistically more likely to be from an upper rather than lower gastrointestinal source, upper gastrointestinal lavage or upper gastrointestinal endoscopy should be performed to exclude definitively a source proximal to the ligament of Treitz. Combinations of radionuclide imaging, mesenteric angiography, and colonoscopy may be required to determine the type and location of the bleeding lesion. Methods to increase the accuracy of colonoscopy include high-flux irrigation and intraoperative colonoscopy with antegrade colonic lavage through a cecostomy. Although endoscopic therapy to stop diverticular hemorrhage often fails, localization of the bleeding site may allow limited resection of the appropriate colonic segment. Scintigraphy with technetium-99m (^{99m}Tc) sulfur colloid or ^{99m}Tc-tagged erythrocytes in conjunction with angiography may confirm the presence of active bleeding and assists in localizing the approximate site of hemorrhage. The rate of bleeding must be 0.1 mL/min or more for this modality to reveal the source. Selective mesenteric angiography may show extravasation of the contrast agent if the bleeding rate is higher than 0.5 mL/min. In such cases, the angiocatheter may also be used to deliver intra-arterial vasopressin or synthetic emboli to stop bleeding in patients who are not surgical candidates.

Minor hemorrhage (<2 units transfused) with spontaneous cessation is managed conservatively. Persistent hemorrhage (2 to 4 units transfused) mandates the use of scintigraphy and angiography to localize the site of bleeding and to reduce the rate of blood loss so that the involved segment may be surgically resected on a semielective basis. More urgent surgery is necessary for major hemorrhage (>4 units transfused) that does not stop. If the site of bleeding cannot be determined, total abdominal colectomy may be needed.

CHAPTER 44

Irritable Bowel Syndrome and Motor Disorders of the Colon

IRRITABLE BOWEL SYNDROME

Incidence and Epidemiology

Irritable bowel syndrome (IBS) is a disorder characterized by abdominal pain or discomfort with altered bowel habits in the absence of organic disease. The most widely accepted definition is provided by the Rome II criteria—at least 12 weeks, during the previous 12 months, of abdominal pain or discomfort associated with two or more of the following three features related to bowel habit: (1) relief of discomfort by defecation, (2) association of discomfort with altered stool form, and (3) association of discomfort with altered stool passage (Table 44-1). Using symptom based criteria, approximately 14% of the United States population reports symptoms consistent with a diagnosis of IBS. Only one quarter of this number seeks medical attention because of symptom severity and other factors including psychosocial dysfunction. Most affected individuals report disease onset before age 45, although the condition is recognized in both adolescents and the elderly. IBS is two to four times more common in women.

Etiology and Pathogenesis

The pathogenesis of IBS involves contributions from altered gastrointestinal motor and sensory function, central nervous system dysfunction, and miscellaneous factors.

Gastrointestinal Motor Abnormalities

A variety of gastrointestinal motor abnormalities have been characterized in IBS. The gastrocolonic response, the increase in colon contractile activity after ingesting a meal, is more intense and prolonged in IBS. Increases in clustered contractions and intense propagating contractions in the small intestine also have been reported. Exaggerated colonic motor responses are observed in IBS patients after cholecystokinin injection, rectal balloon inflation, and colonic bile acid perfusion, whereas the small intestine exhibits increased contractile responses to cholecystokinin and neostigmine. Abnormalities in esophageal motility, gastric motor and myoelectric activity, and gallbladder contractile function have been reported in subsets of patients with IBS. The relevance of many of these contractile abnormalities is uncertain because they correlate incompletely with symptoms and with clinical responses to therapy.

Gastrointestinal Sensory Abnormalities

IBS patients also exhibit evidence of hypersensitive visceral nerve function. Abnormal perception of balloon distention of the rectum, colon, and other lumenal

TABLE 44-1
Rome II Criteria for Irritable Bowel Syndrome

At least 12 weeks during the previous 12 months of abdominal pain or discomfort associated with two or more of the following three features related to bowel habit:
1. Relief of discomfort by defecation
2. Association of discomfort with altered stool form
3. Association of discomfort with altered stool passage

sites has been observed in 60% to 94% of patients (especially those with diarrhea), including increased discomfort and abnormal referral patterns in which inflation in one region is perceived in a distant anatomic site. Conversely, IBS patients have normal sensitivity to noxious cutaneous stimulation, localizing the sensory defect to the visceral nervous system. Patients with IBS may perceive physiological motor activity in the small intestine that healthy controls do not sense. Those with gaseous complaints including bloating can sense lower intralumenal gas volumes than asymptomatic persons.

Central Nervous System Dysfunction

The central nervous system has potent effects on gastrointestinal function in both healthy persons and in patients with IBS. In healthy volunteers, painful somatic stimulation and experimental stress increase rectal contractions, alter physiological small intestinal motor patterns, and delay gastric emptying. Many IBS patients report increases in symptoms during stress and also have increased levels of lifetime stress. Abnormal psychiatric features, including major depression, somatization disorder, anxiety disorder, panic disorder, neuroticism, hostility, hypochondriasis, and phobias, are reported in up to 80% of individuals with IBS. Women with IBS report histories of physical or sexual abuse at rates two to eleven times that of the control population. Recent studies using functional imaging techniques such as positron emission tomography and functional magnetic resonance imaging show altered blood flow in regions of the brain that regulate the emotional components of pain, suggesting underlying pathogenic factors within the central nervous system.

Other Proposed Pathogenic Factors

Other factors play roles in subsets of patients with IBS. Approximately 25% of patients report symptom onset after an attack of bacterial gastroenteritis. These individuals exhibit increases in lymphocyte and enterochromaffin cell populations in the colonic mucosa, with associated elevations in mucosal cytokine production that suggest an inflammatory basis for some cases of IBS. Other studies suggest an increased prevalence of celiac disease in patients with IBS symptoms. Minor roles have been proposed for malabsorption of simple carbohydrates (lactose, fructose, sorbitol), food intolerance, bile salt–induced colonic secretion and dysmotility, and altered gastrointestinal hormone release.

Clinical Features

The intensity, location, and timing of abdominal discomfort or pain in patients with IBS are highly variable. The pain may be so intense as to interfere with daily activities. Pain is most often described as crampy or achy, but sharp, dull, and gaslike pains are also reported. Abdominal pain in IBS commonly is exacerbated by ingesting a meal or by stress and may be relieved by defecation or passage of flatus. Despite this, the pain rarely leads to significant weight loss or malnutrition and infrequently interrupts sleep. Abdominal discomfort may be associated with significant complaints of bloating, which may or may not produce visible distention.

Different bowel habit disturbances characterize distinct IBS subsets. Constipation-predominant IBS patients report stools that are hard or pellet-like, are difficult to pass, and are associated with a sensation of incomplete fecal evacuation. Diarrhea-predominant patients pass soft or loose stools of normal daily volume, which may occur after eating or during stress. Many individuals exhibit a pattern of diarrhea alternating with constipation and report characteristics of each subtype. Passage of fecal mucus is reported by 50% of patients. Rectal bleeding, nocturnal diarrhea, malabsorption, or weight loss warrants an aggressive search for organic disease.

IBS patients frequently report symptoms referable to other organs. Large subsets have associated heartburn, early satiety, nausea, vomiting, and dyspepsia. High incidences of genitourinary dysfunction (dysmenorrhea, dyspareunia, impotence, urinary frequency, and incomplete urinary evacuation), fibromyalgia, low back pain, headaches, fatigue, insomnia, and impaired concentration have been observed in individuals with IBS.

Physical examination of the person with IBS usually is unimpressive. The patient may appear anxious and have cold, clammy hands. Diffuse tenderness or a palpable bowel loop may be evident on abdominal examination. Organomegaly, adenopathy, or occult fecal blood is not consistent with a diagnosis of IBS and warrants a search for organic disease.

Findings on Diagnostic Testing

Diagnosing IBS confidently involves a directed evaluation to confirm that organic disease is not present. The extent of the diagnostic investigation depends on patient age and the predominant symptoms.

Laboratory Studies

Normal values of selected laboratory tests help to confirm a diagnosis of IBS. In contrast, anemia, leukocytosis, or leukopenia or elevations of the sedimentation rate suggest organic disease. Thyroid chemistries are performed in some cases of diarrhea-predominant or constipation-predominant disease to exclude hyperthyroidism or hypothyroidism, respectively. Celiac disease serologies, including endomysial and tissue transglutaminase antibodies, are obtained in individuals with possible celiac disease. Stool samples may be obtained to exclude giardiasis in some patients with diarrhea-predominant disease.

Structural Studies

Structural testing is recommended for many patients with suspected IBS. In patients older than age 45 to 50, colonoscopy is recommended to screen for colorectal cancer. Sigmoidoscopy or colonoscopy may be performed in younger individuals, especially if the diagnosis is uncertain. Biopsy of the colon during lower endoscopy is indicated in some patients with prominent diarrhea to rule out microscopic colitis as a cause of symptoms. Upper endoscopy may be performed for reflux or dyspeptic symptoms. Endoscopic small intestinal biopsy is indicated if serologic testing suggests celiac disease.

Other Testing

Other tests occasionally are indicated to evaluate for other diagnostic possibilities in patients with IBS symptoms. Hydrogen breath testing often is used to exclude lactase deficiency or small intestinal bacterial overgrowth. Patients with constipation refractory to medical management may undergo colonic transit testing using radiopaque markers, anorectal manometry, and defecography to test for slow transit constipation, pelvic floor abnormalities, and anal sphincter dysfunction. Individuals with severe diarrhea may be evaluated for secretory or malabsorptive processes. Screening for laxatives should be considered because laxative abuse is common in patients with unexplained diarrhea. Liver chemistry studies and ultrasound are performed for suspected biliary tract disease. Computed tomography is obtained if malignancy is a concern in a patient with prominent pain, whereas gastric scintigraphy or gastroduodenal manometry may be indicated for a patient with prominent nausea, vomiting, or early satiety. In very rare instances, screening for porphyria or heavy metal intoxication is performed.

Management and Course

After a confident diagnosis of IBS, the clinician should provide reassurance and education to the patient and impart awareness that IBS is a functional disorder without long-term health risks. In some individuals, education and dietary advice will be sufficient. However, most patients receive medications to reduce their symptoms. Some affected persons will be refractory to drug treatment and are considered for psychological therapies. IBS usually persists in a waxing and waning fashion for many years. Despite this, the quality of life for patients with IBS can be improved by appropriate physician involvement; patients can cope with their symptoms and experience an improved sense of well-being. Patients likely to report good outcomes include those who are male, have a brief history of symptoms, have acute symptom onset, exhibit predominant constipation, and have a good initial response to therapy.

Dietary Recommendations

Changes in diet can be recommended for selected patients with IBS. Reducing fat content may decrease abdominal discomfort evoked by lipid-stimulated motor activity. Increasing fiber content in the diet or consuming a fiber supplement (psyllium, polycarbophil, or methylcellulose) may improve bowel function in constipated IBS patients. Fiber supplements may take several weeks to produce satisfactory results and can produce gaseous symptoms if large quantities are ingested rapidly. Low-gas diets have been devised to reduce bloating and excess flatulence in patients with IBS (Table 44-2). Some patients with diarrhea and excess gas may respond to exclusion of dairy products or fruits and soft drinks that contain the poorly absorbed sugars fructose and sorbitol.

Medication Therapy

Medication regimens for patients with IBS should be customized to treat the predominant symptoms of each individual. Individuals with constipation who do not respond to fiber supplements may experience relief with osmotic laxatives such as milk of magnesia or a poorly absorbed sugar (e.g., lactulose, sorbitol). Isotonic solutions that contain polyethylene glycol are useful for constipation and may produce fewer side effects than hypertonic osmotic laxatives. The prokinetic drug tegaserod improves bowel function, decreases abdominal pain, and reduces bloating in patients with constipation-predominant IBS. Opiate agents (e.g., loperamide, diphenoxylate with atropine) are the most useful initial agents for treating diarrhea-predominant IBS. Other medications used for some individuals with diarrhea include the bile acid binder cholestyramine and disodium cromoglycate for rare cases of food hypersensitivity. The 5-HT_3 receptor antagonist alosetron is a potent treatment for refractory diarrhea-predominant IBS. Because this agent

TABLE 44-2
Foods and Flatus Production

Normoflatulogenic Foods
  Meat, poultry, and fish
  Vegetables (e.g., lettuce, cucumber, broccoli, pepper, avocado, cauliflower, tomato,
    asparagus, zucchini, okra, olives)
  Fruits (e.g., cantaloupe, grapes, berries)
  Carbohydrates (e.g., rice, corn chips, potato chips, popcorn, graham crackers)
  Nuts
  Miscellaneous (e.g., eggs, non–milk chocolate, gelatin, fruit ice)

Moderately Flatulogenic Foods
  Pastries
  Potatoes
  Eggplant
  Citrus
  Apple bread

Extremely Flatulogenic Foods
  Milk and milk products
  Vegetables (e.g., onions, beans, celery, carrots, brussels sprouts)
  Fruits (e.g., raisins, bananas, apricots, prune juice)
  Miscellaneous (e.g., pretzels, bagels, wheat germ)

Adapted from Van Ness MM, Cattou EL, Flatulence: pathophysiology and treatment. Am Fam Physician 1985; 31:198.

increases the risks of severe constipation and ischemic colitis, it is prescribed only through a restricted program. Antispasmodic anticholinergic agents are the initial therapy of choice to reduce pain in IBS. These drugs also blunt the gastrocolonic response and may also be useful in preventing postprandial diarrhea. Tricyclic antidepressants exhibit significant potency in patients with significant pain. Tricyclics may also reduce symptoms in those with prominent diarrhea. Conversely, this class of drugs can exacerbate constipation. The gonadotropin-releasing hormone analog leuprolide has been evaluated for patients with severe pain. However, this agent induces amenorrhea and osteoporosis and should be used with care.

Over-the-counter and alternative therapies are sometimes used for treating IBS. Antigas products, such as simethicone, activated charcoal, and bacterial α-galactosidase, have been proposed for patients with bloating, but controlled trials of these agents have not been performed. Selected herbal remedies reportedly provide benefits to some patients. Probiotic compounds reduce gaseous symptoms in some IBS trials. Oral antibiotics provide benefit to some individuals with IBS and associated bacterial overgrowth.

Psychological Therapies

The involvement of psychiatrists and psychologists is reserved for IBS patients who exhibit psychosocial dysfunctional behavior or who fail to respond to aggressive medication therapy. Some studies of psychotherapy report reductions in abdominal pain, diarrhea, and somatic symptoms as well as anxiety. Biofeedback and relaxation training may reduce symptoms. Hypnosis has been effective in selected patients with medically refractory symptoms. Consistent problems with most of these

investigations include poor definitions of symptom response or lack of appropriate control populations.

SLOW TRANSIT CONSTIPATION AND COLONIC PSEUDOOBSTRUCTION

Etiology and Pathogenesis

Patients consider that they are constipated when they experience infrequent defecation, straining on defecation, hard stools, or a sensation of incomplete fecal evacuation. Difficult evacuation of stools of normal consistency with associated straining and the need to apply pelvic pressure to effect defecation usually indicates pelvic floor or anal sphincter dysfunction. Infrequent passage of hard stools is more consistent with slow-transit constipation (also referred to as colonic inertia), in which motor activity is diffusely impaired throughout the colon. High-amplitude propagating pressure waves are reduced in slow transit constipation. Histological examination of resected colonic tissue from patients with severe slow transit constipation reveals loss of enteric neurons and interstitial cells of Cajal populations that are responsible for neuromuscular coordination in the gut.

Chronic colonic pseudoobstruction may result from neurological disease (Chagas disease, Parkinson disease, diabetic neuropathy, dysautonomias, Hirschsprung disease, paraneoplastic disease), myopathic conditions (scleroderma, amyloidosis, other collagen diseases), or metabolic disorders (hypothyroidism, porphyria, pheochromocytoma). Some patients exhibit megacolon. Other individuals with localized disease show evidence of megarectum. Chronic colonic pseudoobstruction also is a component of the more generalized dysmotility syndrome known as chronic intestinal pseudoobstruction, which can be due to hereditary disorders of gut smooth muscle or nerves or may be idiopathic. In addition to Hirschsprung disease, the differential diagnosis of colonic pseudoobstruction in children includes Kawasaki disease, Duchenne muscular dystrophy, and familial visceral myopathies and neuropathies.

Clinical Features, Diagnosis, and Management

Slow transit constipation and most cases of chronic colonic pseudoobstruction are characterized by infrequent defecation and stools that are desiccated and difficult to pass. In severe cases, patients may defecate less than once per week. The presence of extracolonic symptoms raises concern for a generalized dysmotility syndrome. Esophageal involvement is suggested by dysphagia, heartburn, and regurgitation. Gastric and small bowel involvement produces nausea, vomiting, bloating, distention, constipation, or diarrhea if there is concurrent bacterial overgrowth in the small intestine. Some cases of chronic intestinal pseudoobstruction have associated bladder dysfunction or autonomic or peripheral neuropathy.

In most patients, other causes of constipation should be excluded. Blood testing for thyroid chemistries and calcium levels screen for hypothyroidism and hyperparathyroidism. Serologic testing for rheumatologic conditions and for paraneoplastic dysmotility syndromes is considered in selected cases. The colon is structurally evaluated to exclude mechanical obstruction. Barium enema radiography excludes blockage and can detect colonic dilation, loss of haustra, and crudely quantify prolongation of contrast retention. For patients older than age 45 to 50, colonoscopy is performed to screen for colon cancer, especially if symptoms are of recent onset. Deep rectal biopsy can help diagnose amyloidosis if this is a clinical consideration. Barium upper gastrointestinal radiography can demonstrate slow transit or lumenal dilation if diffuse intestinal pseudoobstruction is present. Radiography of the urinary tract may be abnormal in other cases of intestinal pseudoobstruction. In some patients, surgical full-thickness biopsy specimens of the small intestine are needed to confirm a diagnosis of chronic intestinal pseudoobstruction. After structural causes of constipation are eliminated as diagnostic possibilities, many patients with presumed slow transit constipation may be treated empirically with fiber supplements, osmotic laxatives, isotonic electrolyte solutions that contain polyethylene glycol, or prokinetic drugs (tegaserod). Functional testing is performed for those individuals who do not respond to laxative therapy to determine if alternate therapies may provide symptom relief.

Quantification of colonic transit using radiographic assessment of evacuation of radiopaque markers defines the presence and severity of slow transit constipation. Furthermore, the technique can estimate regional transit to determine if motor function is diffusely or locally impaired. Some centers use colonic transit scintigraphy, which assesses regional and total colonic transit of an orally ingested or intestinally perfused radioisotope; however, there is little data to suggest that this method is superior to marker techniques. If slow transit constipation is confirmed, more potent colonic stimulants including colchicine and the prostaglandin E analog misoprostol can be tried. When all drug therapy is unsuccessful and all other remediable causes of constipation are excluded, subtotal colectomy with ileorectal anastomosis may be considered. The long-term results from surgery are generally good, with improvement in defecation frequency and stool consistency. Other symptoms including pain and bloating may not decrease. Patients with megarectum may undergo rectal resection with possible coloanal anastomosis. If there is clinical suspicion of a generalized dysmotility syndrome such as chronic intestinal pseudoobstruction, gastric emptying scintigraphy may demonstrate gastroparesis, or gastroduodenal manometry can define the presence of visceral neuropathy or myopathy. Such findings represent contraindications to subtotal colectomy.

Other tests can characterize anorectal outlet dysfunction as a cause of chronic constipation. Loss of the rectoanal inhibitory reflex on anorectal manometry, as demonstrated by a failure of internal anal sphincter relaxation with rectal balloon inflation, raises concern for Hirschsprung disease. Defecography is a videofluoroscopic technique in which thick barium paste is placed in the rectum and the process of defecation is recorded. This technique identifies structural problems (e.g., rectoceles, rectal prolapse and intussusception, pelvic floor abnormalities) or functional disorders (e.g., rectosphincteric dyssynergia) that may manifest as constipation. Patients with pelvic floor or anal sphincter dysfunction may respond to biofeedback techniques that retrain coordinated defecation. Some structural abnormalities are treated surgically.

Maintaining adequate nutrition is an important goal in treating chronic intestinal pseudoobstruction. Oral antibiotics may produce immediate dramatic improvement in patients with small intestinal bacterial overgrowth. Prokinetic drugs have generally produced disappointing results in treating chronic intestinal pseudoobstruction, although octreotide may reduce symptoms in some individuals either when given alone or with erythromycin. When propulsion cannot be restored or if bacterial overgrowth cannot be eradicated, some patients will require prolonged total parenteral nutrition at home, which carries long-term risks of infection and liver disease. In patients with localized pseudoobstruction, surgical bypass may produce symptomatic improvement (e.g., duodenojejunostomy for megaduodenum). Venting enterostomies may provide relief of gaseous distention and bloating in selected patients who depend on total parenteral nutrition.

HIRSCHSPRUNG DISEASE

Etiology and Pathogenesis

Aganglionosis is caused by arrested migration of cells caudad from the neural crest. In Hirschsprung disease, the aganglionic segment always extends from the internal anal sphincter for a variable distance proximally. The aganglionic region remains permanently contracted, causing proximal dilation. Involvement of the entire colon or extension into the small intestine is very rare. The disease is characterized by the absence of ganglion cells in the myenteric and submucosal plexuses. In contrast, nerve fibers are hypertrophic with abundant thickened bundles. The defect occurs in 1 in 5000 live births and exhibits some familial tendencies. There are associations with Down syndrome, hydrocephalus, ventricular septal defect, kidney deformities, cryptorchidism, bladder diverticula, imperforate anus, Meckel diverticula, the Laurence-Moon-Bardet-Biedl syndrome, and congenital central hypoventilation syndrome.

Clinical Features, Diagnosis, and Management

Hirschsprung disease is suspected if an infant does not pass meconium at birth and if there is abdominal distention, which are relieved by inserting a rectal tube. In 20% of patients, diarrhea results from pseudomembranous enterocolitis because of the obstruction. Older individuals, including some adults, report a lifelong history of severe constipation and recurrent fecal impaction. In older children and adults, aganglionic segments usually are very short. Diagnosis is suggested by barium enema radiography, which shows a narrowed distal colon with proximal dilation. Diagnosis is suspected by loss of the rectoanal inhibitory reflex on anorectal manometry. Deep rectal biopsy demonstration of the presence of submucosal ganglia excludes a diagnosis of classical Hirschsprung disease. Specific histological examinations of full thickness rectal biopsies obtained surgically may be needed to diagnose Hirschsprung disease definitively in some infants. Definitive surgical cure is the treatment of choice. Several operations are performed to remove or counterbalance the obstructing aganglionic segment, with good long-term results. Ten percent to 20% of patients experience postoperative soiling.

ACUTE COLONIC PSEUDOOBSTRUCTION AND ACUTE MEGACOLON

Etiology and Pathogenesis

Acute colonic pseudoobstruction may result from transient electrolyte disturbances, overwhelming infection, hypotension, multisystem failure, spinal injury, recent surgery, or medications. Acute megacolon occurs in patients with fulminant inflammatory bowel disease, severe infectious colitis, or with colonic infarction.

Clinical Features, Diagnosis, and Management

Most patients with acute colonic pseudoobstruction are middle-aged or older and present with abdominal distention and reduced bowel sounds. Fever, peritoneal signs, and leukocytosis usually are absent. Abdominal radiography typically shows gaseous colonic distention, which is maximal in the cecum. In such cases, oral feedings should be stopped, intravenous fluids are started, a nasogastric tube is inserted, all nonessential medications are discontinued, and any underlying metabolic abnormality is corrected. When colonic obstruction is a consideration, a diatrizoate (Hypaque) enema can be diagnostic and can further stimulate colonic evacuation. Colonic decompression also is accomplished by passing a rectal tube or by frequent tap water enemas. In some cases, intravenous neostigmine may evoke prompt gas evacuation. However, because of the profound cardiovascular complications associated with neostigmine administration, this drug should be given only with careful cardiac monitoring. When the cecal diameter is more than 11 cm, colonoscopic decompression is attempted to aspirate intralumenal gas. Tube cecostomy may be effective for patients who are refractory to medical and colonoscopic management and who exhibit persistent cecal dilation of more than 11 cm. Exploratory laparotomy is indicated for patients manifesting fever, leukocytosis, or peritoneal signs. In these settings, the right colon may already be nonviable or perforated. Toxic megacolon from inflammatory or ischemic conditions usually is an indication for prompt surgery.

COLONIC DYSMOTILITY IN OTHER CONDITIONS

In some cases of idiopathic diarrhea, transit through the proximal and transverse colon may be accelerated, leading to increased fecal evacuation. In carcinoid syndrome, transit through the small intestine, ascending colon, and transverse colon is markedly accelerated, which contributes to diarrhea. Postprandial colonic tone is increased, and carcinoid syndrome potentially reduces the capacity of the colon. Many of the therapies that reduce diarrhea act by inhibiting motor activity, including opiates, which retard transit in the colon and small intestine; anticholinergics and calcium channel antagonists, which blunt increases in postprandial colonic motility; and the somatostatin analog octreotide, which delays transit in the small intestine in addition to exerting antisecretory effects.

Other conditions have secondary effects on colonic motor activity, contributing to symptoms in affected patients. In malabsorptive conditions, fat delivery to the cecum and ascending colon induces vigorous high-amplitude contractions and rapid aboral transit. Ulcerative colitis is associated with loss of haustral folds and reduced fasting phasic contractions. In these individuals, colonic transit is rapid perhaps reflecting the lack of retarding pressure waves. Conversely, ulcerative proctitis is associated with high-amplitude rectal contractions, which may elicit tenesmus. Numerous medications accelerate (laxatives and prokinetics) or delay (opiate antidiarrheals) colonic transit.

CHAPTER 45

Bacterial Infections of the Colon

INFECTION WITH *SHIGELLA* SPECIES

Incidence and Epidemiology

About 15,000 cases of shigellosis occur annually in the United States. Most infections (69%) occur in children younger than 5 years. The organism is transmitted by the fecal-oral route; via infected food or water, or in chronic care facilities, day-care centers, or nursing homes. Shigellosis is highly contagious; it requires only small inoculums (180 organisms) to establish infection. Ninety percent of infections occur from *Shigella sonnei* or *Shigella flexneri*, although *Shigella dysenteriae* has been associated with pandemic disease.

Etiology and Pathogenesis

Shigella species are aerobic, nonmotile, glucose-fermenting, gram-negative rods. Four species have been identified: *Shigella boydii*, *Shigella dysenteriae*, *Shigella flexneri*, and *Shigella sonnei*. The primary method by which *Shigella* species cause disease is by direct invasion and destruction of colonic epithelium; however, the bacteria also produce enterotoxins. *Shigella* toxin has an A-B subunit structure that binds to specific cell receptors. After binding, the toxin is internalized, where it inhibits cellular protein synthesis and elicits fluid secretion. Serum and secretory antibodies to *Shigella* organisms produced after exposure to the organism offer some protection from subsequent clinical attacks. Host resistance factors include gastric acidity and normal colonic microflora.

Clinical Features

Shigella infection is characterized by the acute onset of bloody diarrhea with mucus, accompanied by fever and abdominal pain. After a 1-day to 3-day incubation period, symptomatic disease generally persists for 5 to 7 days in adults and 2 to 3 days in children. The illness may have two phases: an initial small bowel phase of severe watery diarrhea, followed by a dysenteric phase with smaller volumes of blood-tinged mucus or blood clots. Symptoms may be severe in malnourished children or debilitated adults, whereas some healthy individuals may note only mild diarrhea. Physical examination may reveal lower abdominal tenderness with normal or increased bowel sounds. Dehydration may occur in some cases, but peritoneal findings are rare and should suggest other diagnoses. The infection most severely affects the rectosigmoid colon, but 15% of cases exhibit pancolitis.

Complications of *Shigella* infection include bacteremia, Reiter syndrome, and the hemolytic uremic syndrome. Bacteremia has a 20% mortality rate as a result of

349

renal failure, hemolysis, thrombocytopenia, gastrointestinal hemorrhage, and shock. Reiter syndrome, a triad of arthritis, urethritis, and conjunctivitis, occurs most commonly in men between ages 20 and 40 and presents 2 to 4 weeks after infection with *Shigella* species (or certain strains of *Salmonella*, *Yersinia*, or *Campylobacter*). Eighty percent of patients who develop Reiter syndrome are HLA-B27 positive. The arthritic manifestations, which are distributed asymmetrically, often are chronic and relapsing and require management with NSAIDs. Although hemolytic uremic syndrome is most often associated with enterohemorrhagic *Escherichia coli* infection, it may complicate infections with *Shigella*. The syndrome is characterized by microangiopathic hemolytic anemia, thrombocytopenia, and renal failure. It has been postulated that hemolytic uremic syndrome results from the systemic effects of Shiga toxin. The syndrome has a mortality rate of less than 10%.

Findings on Diagnostic Testing

Examination of stool will identify leukocytes and erythrocytes. The laboratory diagnosis of infection with Shigella species is made by identification in stool culture.

Management and Course

Antibiotics reduce the duration and severity of symptoms in shigellosis, shorten the period of fecal excretion of the organism, and are recommended for all patients with diarrhea, except those with mild symptoms (Table 45-1). Ciprofloxacin is the drug of choice, or azithromycin in case of fluoroquinolone resistance. As for other diarrheal illness, oral or intravenous rehydration should be administered. Antidiarrheal agents are contraindicated because they may prolong symptoms and delay clearance of the organism. Oral vaccines against infection with *Shigella* are being developed.

TABLE 45-1
Antibiotic Treatment Regimens for Adults with *Shigella* Infection

Mild, self-limited cases	Supportive care and hydration
Moderate clinical smyptoms (non–*S dysenteriae* type 1)	Ciprofloxacin 1 g orally for 1–2 d
Severe clinical symptoms	Ciprofloxacin, 500 mg orally bid for 5 d
Infection with *S dysenteriae* type 1	
Treatment failures of short-course therapy	
Ciprofloxacin-resistant stains	Azithromycin, 500 mg orally on d 1; 250 mg orally each day for 4 d
Shigella bacteremia	Ciprofloxacin, 500 mg orally bid for 5 d
TMP-SMZ or ampicillin-sensitive strains	TMP-SMZ, 160 mg/800 mg orally bid for 5 d; Ampicillin, 500 mg orally qid for 5 d

TMP-SMX, trimethoprim-sulfamethoxazole.

INFECTION WITH *CAMPYLOBACTER* SPECIES

Incidence and Epidemiology

Campylobacter species (*Campylobacter jejuni* and *Campylobacter coli*) are the most common cause of bacterial diarrhea in the United States. The Centers for Disease Control and Prevention estimate that *Campylobacter* is responsible for 2 million illnesses per year. Seasonal variation of infection exists, and the peak incidence is during the summer. The organism is transmitted by ingesting contaminated poultry, unpasteurized milk, or contaminated water, or by exposure to infected pets. Children younger than 5 years are most susceptible to infections caused by *Campylobacter*.

Etiology and Pathogenesis

Campylobacter organisms are curved, gram-negative rods that possess oxidase and catalase activity. *C jejuni* and *C coli* produce disease by four mechanisms: motility, adherence, invasion, and generation of toxins. The first three factors allow the organism to damage or destroy intestinal epithelial cells, whereas the toxins enhance cell death and increase intestinal fluid secretion. Acute infection with *Campylobacter* species confers short-term immunity to subsequent infection.

Clinical Features

The incubation period of *Campylobacter* is 18 hours to 8 days. A prodrome of fever, headache, malaise, and myalgia may precede symptoms of watery and bloody diarrhea with abdominal pain. Other reported symptoms include nausea, vomiting, and weight loss. Although the disease usually resolves within 1 week, some patients experience a relapsing course similar to ulcerative colitis. Physical examination may reveal localized tenderness suggestive of appendicitis. Complications of infections with *Campylobacter* species include bacteremia, hemorrhage, toxic megacolon, Reiter syndrome, erythema nodosum, urticaria, cholecystitis, pancreatitis, abortion, Guillain-Barré syndrome, and hemolytic uremic syndrome.

Findings on Diagnostic Testing

Laboratory studies may show evidence of volume depletion and peripheral leukocytosis. Stool examination usually reveals leukocytes and erythrocytes. The diagnosis is confirmed by positive stool cultures. Rapid detection methods that use DNA probes and polymerase chain reaction (PCR) are being developed.

Management and Course

The mainstay of therapy for infections with *Campylobacter* species is fluid and electrolyte replacement. By the time a diagnosis is confirmed, most patients will have experienced a decrease in their symptoms, obviating the need for treatment. For severe dysentery, relapsing symptoms, systemic infection, or immunosuppression, antibiotic therapy can effectively eradicate the organism. Erythromycin (500 mg, twice daily, or 250 mg, four times daily, for 5 days) is efficacious, but there is no evidence that the antibiotics reduce the duration or severity of symptoms. Ciprofloxacin is an alternate choice, but quinolone-resistant strains have been described. Azithromycin (500 mg daily for 3 days) is effective in areas of quinolone resistance. Adding an aminoglycoside is recommended for cases of systemic infection.

ENTEROCOLITIS INDUCED BY CLOSTRIDIUM DIFFICILE

Incidence and Epidemiology

Clostridium difficile is the most common cause of nosocomial diarrhea. The inpatient incidence is 20 to 60 cases per 100,000 patient-days; however, the incidence among outpatients is only 7.7 cases per 100,000 person-years. *C difficile* may be isolated from the stool of only 3% of healthy individuals, whereas the prevalence among hospitalized patients is 20%. The major risk factors for symptomatic *C difficile* infection are exposure to antimicrobials, hospitalization, and host susceptibility. The antibiotics most commonly used for treatment include clindamycin, ampicillin, and cephalosporins. *C difficile* is prevalent in chronic care facilities, nursing homes, newborn nurseries, and neonatal intensive care units. To reduce transmission of *C difficile*, hospital personnel should wear disposable gloves when handling stool or linen, and they should wash their hands after patient contact. Incontinent patients with diarrhea caused by *C difficile* should be placed in isolation. Bleach solutions may be effective against environmental contamination.

Etiology and Pathogenesis

C difficile is a gram-positive, obligate anaerobic rod. Colonic damage is mediated by the release of two potent toxins, A and B. These toxins inactivate Rho proteins, leading to collapse of the cell cytoskeleton, increased tight junction permeability, and fluid secretion. An intense inflammatory response is initiated by the toxins and mediated by nuclear factor–κB (NF-κB), which in turn increases production of interleukin-8 (IL-8), tumor necrosis factor–α (TNF-α), prostaglandin E_2, and leukotriene B_4.

Clinical Features

C difficile is associated with a wide spectrum of disease ranging from, in order of decreasing severity, pseudomembranous colitis, antibiotic-associated colitis without pseudomembranes, to antibiotic-associated diarrhea. Pseudomembranous colitis presents with diarrhea and cramps generally within the first week of antibiotic therapy, although delays in symptom onset of up to 6 weeks have been reported. Associated symptoms include fever, nausea, vomiting, tenesmus, and dehydration. Physical findings may include abdominal distention and diffuse tenderness. Peripheral leukocytosis usually is present. Occult fecal blood loss is common but hematochezia is rare. Complications of pseudomembranous colitis include toxic megacolon, perforation, and peritonitis. Findings that suggest a fulminant course include fever, tachycardia, localized abdominal tenderness with guarding, ascites, decreased bowel sounds, and signs of toxemia. In these cases of toxic megacolon, striking leukocytosis (white blood cell count of up to 40,000–80,000 cells/μL), and hypoalbuminemia, caused by protein-losing enteropathy, may be present.

Antibiotic-associated colitis without pseudomembranes follows a more benign course, with insidious development of fecal urgency, cramps, watery diarrhea, malaise, fever, and abdominal tenderness. Antibiotic-associated diarrhea without colitis is characterized by the absence of systemic findings and by diarrhea that resolves when antibiotics are stopped.

Infection with *C difficile* can also complicate the course of inflammatory bowel disease. A stool toxin assay is recommended for patients with Crohn's disease or ulcerative colitis who have unexplained relapses, especially after recent exposure to antibiotics.

Findings on Diagnostic Testing

Stool examination reveals leukocytes in 50% of patients with pseudomembranous colitis, but fecal leukocytes are less common with milder infections caused by *C difficile*. The gold standard for diagnosing *C difficile* intestinal infection is the stool cytotoxin assay. If a stool specimen submitted for testing contains toxin, cellular rounding or detachment of cultured human fibroblasts is observed after an incubation of 24 to 48 hours. The cytotoxin assay is positive in 95% to 100% of patients with pseudomembranous colitis and in 60% to 75% of patients with colitis without pseudomembranes. Enzyme-linked immunosorbent assays that detect *C difficile* toxins are also commercially available. Although less sensitive than the cell culture assay, results are available the same day and are highly specific for infection. *C difficile* stool cultures do not differentiate asymptomatic carriers from patients with colitis and thus are of limited clinical use.

Sigmoidoscopy is not necessary to diagnose infection with *C difficile*; however, endoscopic evaluation may be considered for very ill, hospitalized patients for whom reliance on stool toxin assays may delay initiating appropriate therapy. Endoscopic diagnosis hinges on the presence of pseudomembranes, which appear as yellow-white raised plaques 2 to 5 mm in diameter. Histological examination of the pseudomembrane reveals a summit lesion, which is composed of fibrin, mucus, and inflammatory cells erupting from an epithelial microulceration.

Management and Course

The initial step in management should be to discontinue the inciting antimicrobial, which effectively resolves symptoms in 15% to 23% of patients. In patients who do not respond, metronidazole and vancomycin have proven efficacy in eradicating infection. Oral metronidazole (250 mg, four times daily, or 500 mg, three times daily, for 10 days) is the recommended initial course for treating pseudomembranous colitis. In patients with ileus, intravenous metronidazole (500 mg every 6 hours) is an alternate therapy. Oral vancomycin (125 mg, four times daily for 10 days) can effectively eradicate *C difficile* after 1 week. Opiate antidiarrheals (e.g., loperamide, diphenoxylate with atropine) are not recommended for treating severe colitis but may be useful in mild cases.

Fifteen percent to 20% of patients with pseudomembranous colitis relapse after successful antibiotic treatment, usually 1 to 2 weeks after completing therapy. Possible etiologies for relapse include persistence of spores or vegetative forms of the organism or reinfection from environmental sources. There is little antimicrobial resistance to *C difficile* eradication; therefore a repeated course of the initial antibiotic regimen is recommended. Various strategies are available for multiple relapses (Table 45-2). Prolonged courses of antibiotics with a tapering dose have had therapeutic success, as have regimens combining oral vancomycin and rifampicin or vancomycin and an anion exchange resin (e.g., cholestyramine, colestipol) that binds the *C difficile* toxins. Because resins also bind the antibiotics used for therapy, they should be administered at least 1 hour before or after the antibiotic. More novel eradication strategies include oral administration of nonpathogenic organisms (e.g., *Saccharomyces boulardii*) that inhibit the growth of *C difficile*, rectal infusions of feces, or intravenous infusions of immunoglobulin.

TABLE 45-2
Suggested Approach to Recurrent *Clostridium difficile* Diarrhea and Colitis

First relapse
Symptomatic treatment only if diarrhea is mild
10- to 14-day course of metronidazole or vancomycin if symptoms are more severe or persistent

Second relapse:
Vancomycin taper
125 mg/6 h for 7 d
125 mg/12 h for 7 d
125 mg/d for 7 d
125 mg every other day for 6 d (i.e., 3 doses)
125 mg every 3 days for 9 d (i.e., 3 doses)

Other reported treatments for multiple relapses:
Vancomycin in tapering dose, as above, plus cholestyramine 4 g bid
Oral *Saccharomyces boulardii* in combination with metronidazole or vancomycin
Vancomycin, 125 mg qid, and rifampicin, 600 mg bid, for 7 days
Intravenous immunoglobulin

Reprinted with permission from Kelly CP, LaMont TJ. *Clostridium difficile* infection. *Annu Rev Med* 1998;49:375.

COLITIS INDUCED BY *ESCHERICHIA COLI*

Enteroinvasive Escherichia coli

Etiology and Pathogenesis

Enteroinvasive *Escherichia coli* (EIEC) is a rare cause of traveler's diarrhea. The pathogenesis initiates with attachment and invasion of colonocytes by the organism, which proliferates within cells and finally destroys the host cell. EIEC possesses a virulence plasmid identical to that possessed by *Shigella*.

Clinical Features, Diagnosis, and Management

The clinical presentation of EIEC includes fever, malaise, anorexia, abdominal cramps, and watery diarrhea, followed by passage of blood-tinged stool or mucus. Fecal blood and leukocytes are present in many but not all patients. Laboratory confirmation of EIEC in clinical practice requires serotyping *E coli* O and H antigens. The disease usually is self-limited and uncomplicated. Treatment should concentrate on fluid and electrolyte replacement. The role of antibiotic therapy in EIEC infection is undefined, but it is reasonable to give patients with dysentery a 5-day course of either trimethoprim-sulfamethoxazole (160 mg/800 mg, twice daily), ampicillin (500 mg, four times per day), or ciprofloxacin (500 mg, twice daily).

Enterohemorrhagic Escherichia coli

Etiology and Pathogenesis

Infection with enterohemorrhagic *Escherichia coli* (EHEC) is caused by the O157:H7 strain, which is transmitted to humans in poorly cooked ground beef, unpasteurized dairy products or fruit juices, and fecally contaminated water. The highest incidence of infection occurs in children younger than 5 years, although elderly patients are also affected. Outbreaks are clustered in schools, day-care centers, and nursing homes. Factors that enhance EHEC virulence include adhesins that provide attachment to host cells, plasmid-encoded hemolysin, and two Shiga-like toxins that cause damage through thrombus formation and vasculitis leading to ischemia and hemorrhage.

Clinical Features, Diagnosis, and Management

After an incubation of 3 to 9 days, EHEC-associated hemorrhagic colitis manifests watery diarrhea and abdominal cramping pain, followed by bloody diarrhea 2 to 5 days later. The severity of blood loss ranges from blood-tinged mucus to passage of large clots. Vomiting is present in three fourths of patients, whereas fever is generally absent. Complications of infection with EHEC include hemolytic uremic syndrome and intestinal hematoma causing intestinal obstruction, rhabdomyolysis, and pancreatic necrosis with subsequent development of diabetes mellitus. Fecal leukocytes are typically not present. *E coli* O157:H7 can be identified by culturing on sorbitol-MacConkey medium and agglutination with O157 and H7 antiserum. The most important goal of treatment is replacement of fluid and electrolytes. Recovery without sequelae is the usual outcome, although patients with hemolytic uremic syndrome may have long-term renal failure or neurological deficits. Antibiotics are not recommended for this infection because they do not diminish the duration of symptoms or prevent complications and may increase the risk of developing hemolytic uremic syndrome. Novel therapies for treating *E coli* O157:H7 include reagents that bind the Shiga-like toxins to prevent interaction with host cell receptors.

SEXUALLY TRANSMITTED COLORECTAL PATHOGENS

Gonorrheal Proctitis

Although most anorectal infection with *Neisseria gonorrhoeae* is asymptomatic, purulent or bloody discharge may be present, along with pruritus ani, tenesmus, or constipation. Complications of *N gonorrheae* proctitis include perirectal abscesses, fistulae, strictures, and sepsis. Sigmoidoscopy reveals rectal mucosal erythema, friability, and superficial erosions. The diagnosis of gonococcal proctitis is based on positive results of cultures obtained from rectal swabs. Rectal gonorrhea should be treated with ceftriaxone, 250 mg intramuscularly, which eradicates 98% of infections. Alternative regimens include a single oral dose of ciprofloxacin (500 mg) or norfloxacin (800 mg), or a single intramuscular dose of spectinomycin (2 gm), cefotaxime (1 gm), or ceftizoxime (500 mg). Doxycycline should be given to cover potential coinfection with *Chlamydia* species.

Proctitis Caused by Chlamydia trachomatis

Infection with *Chlamydia trachomatis*, the causative agent of lymphogranuloma venereum, is the most common etiology of bacterial sexually transmitted illness in the United States. The clinical presentation may vary from asymptomatic carriage to granulomatous proctitis. The latter has symptoms of bloody diarrhea, mucopurulent discharge, and, less commonly, rectal pain, tenesmus, constipation, and fistulae. Physical examination may reveal lower abdominal tenderness as well as tender, enlarged inguinal lymph nodes. Sigmoidoscopic findings include friable mucosa with multiple ulcerations. Biopsy specimens show granulomatous inflammation with giant cells; inflammation with neutrophils, eosinophils, and crypt abscesses; and organisms visible by Giemsa staining. The diagnosis of *C trachomatis* proctitis is confirmed by culture of rectal swabs. The treatment of choice is tetracycline 500 mg, four times daily, or doxycycline 100 mg, twice daily, for 21 days, although less severe infections may respond to courses of 7 to 10 days or a single 1-g dose of azithromycin.

Proctitis Caused by Herpes Simplex Virus

Herpes simplex virus (HSV) type 2 is responsible for 90% of anorectal cases of herpes. Infection is characterized by recurrent symptoms of anal pain, tenesmus, pruritus ani, constipation, inguinal adenopathy, sacral and posterior thigh paresthesias, and urinary retention. Anoscopic or sigmoidoscopic examination during active infection may show vesicles and ulcers. Biopsy specimens of the lesions show acute and chronic inflammation, microabscesses, and superficial ulcerations. HSV proctitis is diagnosed by viral cultures or by PCR detection of HSV DNA. Mild flares may respond to stool softeners, sitz baths, and analgesics. Acyclovir (400 to 800 mg per day) decreases both the duration of symptoms and viral shedding.

Anorectal Syphilis

Anorectal syphilis is caused by the spirochete *Treponema pallidum*. Primary syphilis may produce indurated chancres in the anal canal or rectum that are 1 to 2 cm in diameter. These lesions are generally asymptomatic. Secondary syphilis presents as condyloma lata, which develops 6 weeks to 6 months after the initial exposure. Characteristic lesions are smooth, wartlike lesions in the rectum. Colitis may also be present, usually limited to the distal 15 to 20 cm of the colon. Symptoms of these lesions include pain, discharge, and tenesmus. Only rarely is tertiary syphilis diagnosed in anorectal disease, although rectal gumma has been reported. Biopsy specimens exhibit a chronic inflammatory process with a predominance of lymphocytes, histiocytes, and plasma cells. Dark-field microscopic examination of the exudates may reveal spirochetes. The diagnosis of syphilis is confirmed by serologic testing, although false-negative tests are common in early disease. Anorectal syphilis is treated with a single intramuscular injection of benzathine penicillin (2.4 million units), or doxycycline (100 mg, twice daily), or tetracycline (500 mg, four times daily) for 2 weeks (primary syphilis) or 4 weeks (latent syphilis).

Human Papillomavirus

Anal warts or condyloma acuminata appear as verrucous, papilliform skin lesions resulting from infection with human papilloma virus. Warts occur on the glans penis in men and on the labia, vulva, and cervix in women. Transmission is usually through anal intercourse or autoinoculation to the perianal area and anus. Symptoms may be absent or may include rectal discharge, bleeding, or pruritus ani. Complications of infection include strictures, discharge, and bleeding. Human papillomavirus infection has been associated with the development of neoplasia, such as cervical and anal cancer. The diagnosis is made clinically after excluding anorectal syphilis and squamous cell cancer. Although cure generally is not possible, lesions may be treated with podophyllin (20% solution in tincture of benzoin), cryotherapy, and surgical fulguration. Recurrences and posttherapy anal strictures are common.

CHAPTER 46

Inflammatory Bowel Disease

INCIDENCE AND EPIDEMIOLOGY

Chronic inflammatory bowel diseases (IBD) include ulcerative colitis, a disorder in which inflammation affects the mucosa and submucosa of the colon, and Crohn's disease, in which inflammation is transmural and may involve any or all segments of the gastrointestinal tract. The incidence and prevalence of ulcerative colitis are 2 to 10 and 35 to 100, respectively, per 100,000 population in the United States. The incidence and prevalence of Crohn's disease are 1 to 6 and 10 to 100 per 100,000. There is an increased incidence of IBD in relatives of patients with IBD, indicating a genetic predisposition. Both conditions are more prevalent in Jews (especially Ashkenazi Jews) and less common in African Americans. The peak age of onset of both diseases is between 15 and 25 years, and a second peak is sometimes observed between 55 and 65 years. Most series report similar incidences of the two disorders in men and women. Ulcerative colitis is more common than Crohn's disease in children younger than 10 years. Among patients with ulcerative colitis, the incidence of tobacco smoking is lower than that in the general population, whereas the incidence of smoking among patients with Crohn's disease patients is as high or higher than that in the general population. Appendectomy appears to protect against the development of ulcerative colitis, especially if done before age 21.

ETIOLOGY AND PATHOGENESIS

Genetics

Fifteen percent of IBD patients have first-degree relatives who also have IBD. The lifetime risks of developing IBD among first-degree relatives of IBD patients are 8.9% for offspring, 8.8% for siblings, and 3.5% for parents. The incidence of ulcerative colitis is higher in relatives of Crohn's disease patients. Similarly, the predisposition to develop either disease increases in relatives of ulcerative colitis patients, suggesting that the two diseases are related. Monozygotic twins have a higher concordance rate than dizygotic twins. There is no increase in IBD in spouses of affected patients, indicating that environmental factors do not determine the incidence of IBD in families. The HLA-DR1/DQw5 and DRB3*0301 haplotypes are associated with Crohn's disease, and HLA-DR2 is associated with ulcerative colitis. In ulcerative colitis, HLA DRB1*0103 and allele 2 of the interleukin-1 receptor antagonist are associated with extensive disease. The IBD1 susceptibility locus on chromosome 16 is associated with Crohn's disease, whereas the IBD2 locus on chromosome 12 is associated with both conditions. The NOD2 gene associated with IBD1 encodes for a cytosolic protein in monocytes that is an intracellular receptor for bacterial lipopolysaccharide. Fifteen percent of patients with Crohn's disease have NOD2 mutations. Increases in intestinal permeability are observed in asymptomatic first-degree relatives of persons with Crohn's disease. Similarly, clinically healthy relatives of patients with ulcerative colitis have an increased incidence of antineutrophil cytoplasmic antibody positivity, suggesting that the autoantibody is more than just a marker of colonic inflammation.

Potential Triggers

There is evidence of immune activation in IBD, with infiltration of the lamina propria with lymphocytes, macrophages, and other cells, although the antigenic trigger is unknown. Various viruses and bacteria (e.g., measles virus, *Mycobacterium paratuberculosis*) have been proposed as triggers, but there is little support for any specific infectious cause of IBD. A second hypothesis is that a dietary antigen or normally nonpathogenic microbial agent activates an abnormal immune response. As a result of failed normal suppressor mechanisms, immune activation in IBD may be inappropriately vigorous and prolonged in response to a normal lumenal antigen. In mouse models of colitis, genetic defects in T-cell function or cytokine production elicit uncontrolled immune responses to normal colonic flora. A third hypothesis is that the trigger in IBD is an autoantigen expressed on the patient's intestinal epithelium. In this theory, the patient mounts an initial immune response against a lumenal antigen, which then persists and may be amplified because of antigenic similarity between the lumenal antigen and host proteins. This autoimmune hypothesis involves destruction of the epithelial cells by antibody-dependent cellular cytotoxicity or direct cell-mediated cytotoxicity. The detection of anticolon antibodies in the sera of ulcerative colitis patients supports this theory. However, these antibodies are also found in conditions with no intestinal involvement. Antibodies directed against tropomyosin also are observed in ulcerative colitis.

Immune Factors

Various immune system mechanisms are altered in IBD. Class II molecules on intestinal epithelial cells participate in antigen processing in the intestinal immune compartment. Enhanced staining of the class II molecule HLA-DR occurs in active ulcerative colitis and Crohn's colitis. Cell-mediated immune responses also may be involved in the pathogenesis of IBD. There is increased antibody secretion by intestinal mononuclear cells in IBD, especially of the IgM and IgG classes that fix complement. Ulcerative colitis is associated with increased production of IgG1 (by Th2 lymphocytes) and IgG3, subtypes that respond to proteins and T-cell-dependent antigens. Crohn's disease is associated with increased IgG2 production (by Th1 lymphocytes), which responds to carbohydrates and bacterial antigens. There is also increased production of proinflammatory cytokines (IL-1, IL-6, IL-8, and tumor necrosis factor–α[TNF-α]), most likely in activated macrophages in the lamina propria. IL-8 promotes neutrophil infiltration, IL-1 activates T cells, IL-1 and TNF-α stimulate adhesion molecule expression, and interferon-γ enhances intestinal permeability. Other cytokines (IL-10, TGF-β) down-regulate the immune response. Defective production of these cytokines leads to chronic inflammation. Cytokines also are involved in wound healing and fibrosis. The efficacy of infliximab, a chimeric antibody to TNF-α, in Crohn's disease supports the key role of cytokines in IBD pathogenesis. Other immune factors in the generation of IBD include production of superoxide and other reactive oxygen species by activated neutrophils, soluble mediators that increase permeability and induce vasodilation, leukotriene neutrophil chemotactic compounds, and nitric oxide that promotes vasodilation and edema.

Animal models provide insight into IBD pathogenesis. In mice, disruption of genes for IL-2, IL-10, and TNF-β produces colitis. HLA-B27 transgenic rats exhibit colitis as well as arthritis and gastritis. In severe combined immunodeficient mice, repletion with $CD4^+$ helper cells promotes development of colitis, indicating the importance of T-cell factors in IBD. The ability of antibodies to TNF-α and interferon-γ to prevent this response raises the possibility that intestinal damage from unrestrained T-cell activation is mediated by these two molecules. Adoptive transfer of bacterial antigen-activated $CD4^+$cells from C3H/HeJBir mice, which spontaneously develop colitis, to severe combined immunodeficient mice induces colitis, emphasizing the pathogenic importance of enteric flora.

CLINICAL FEATURES

Ulcerative Colitis

The dominant symptom in ulcerative colitis is diarrhea, which is often bloody. Bowel movements may be frequent but of low volume as a result of rectal inflammation. Abdominal pain (usually lower quadrant or rectal), fever, malaise, and weight loss may also be reported. Localized rectal involvement may be characterized only by bloody diarrhea, with or without urgency, tenesmus, pain, or incontinence. Elderly patients rarely report constipation as a result of rectal spasm. Patients with ulcerative colitis can be classified according to disease severity, which helps direct disease management (Table 46-1). Diarrhea and rectal bleeding are the only complaints of mild disease, which is often associated with a normal physical examination. Most patients with ulcerative proctitis have mild disease. Moderate disease, which occurs in 27% of patients, is characterized by five or six bloody stools per day, abdominal pain, abdominal tenderness, low-grade fever, and fatigue. Nineteen percent of patients exhibit severe ulcerative colitis, which is characterized by frequent episodes of bloody diarrhea (>6 stools per day), profound weakness, weight loss, fever, tachycardia, postural hypotension, significant abdominal tenderness,

---

TABLE 46-1
Classification of Ulcerative Colitis

Severe

Diarrhea: six or more bowel movements per day, with blood
Fever: mean evening temperature >37.5°C or >37.5°C on at least 2 of
    4 days at any time of day
Tachycardia: mean pulse rate higher than 90 beats/min
Anemia: hemoglobin of <7.5 g/dL, allowing for recent transfusions
Sedimentation rate: >30 mm/hr

Mild

Mild diarrhea: fewer than four bowel movements per day, with only small
    amounts of blood
No fever
No tachycardia
Mild anemia
Sedimentation rate: <30 mm/hr

Moderately severe

Intermediate between mild and severe

hypoactive bowel sounds, and anemia and hypoalbuminemia on laboratory investigation. Abdominal distention with severe disease raises the possibility of toxic megacolon.

Most cases of ulcerative colitis begin indolently and gradually worsen over several weeks, but some cases exhibit an initial attack of fulminant disease. At initial presentation, colitis extending to the cecum is present in 20% of patients, whereas 75% have no disease proximal to the sigmoid colon. Fifteen percent of the patients with initial proctitis extend their disease more proximally within 10 years. More than 90% of persons with mild disease go into remission after the first attack. Patients with initially severe disease often require colectomies. In most individuals, the disease follows a chronic intermittent course; long quiescent periods are interspersed with acute attacks lasting weeks to months. In some, however, the disease is continuously active. Older patients are more likely to report long periods of disease quiescence. For those with severe disease at initial presentation, 50% will need a colectomy within 2 years, whereas less than 10% of patients with mild disease or proctitis require surgery after 10 years. Relapse may be triggered by noncompliance with maintenance medications to suppress colonic inflammation, use of nonsteroidal antiinflammatory drugs or antibiotics, intercurrent colonic infection, and cessation of smoking.

Severe ulcerative colitis can cause life-threatening complications. If the inflammatory process extends beyond the submucosa into the muscularis, the colon dilates, producing toxic megacolon. Clinical criteria suggestive of toxic megacolon include a temperature higher than 38.6°C, a heart rate higher than 120 beats per minute, a neutrophil count of more than 10,500 cells/μL, dehydration, mental status changes, electrolyte disturbances, hypotension, abdominal distention, tenderness (with or without rebound), and hypoactive or absent bowel sounds. Toxic megacolon usually occurs in patients with pancolitis, often early in the course of their disease. Medications that impair colonic motor function may initiate or exacerbate megacolon. Perforation of the colon may complicate toxic megacolon or may occur in cases of severe ulcerative colitis without megacolon. Strictures are uncommon, but lumenal narrowing is observed in 12% of patients after 5 to 25 years of disease, usually in the sigmoid colon and rectum. Strictures present as increases in diarrhea or new fecal incontinence and may mimic malignancy on endoscopic or radiographic evaluation.

Crohn's Disease

There are three main patterns of disease distribution in Crohn's disease: (1) involvement of the ileum and cecum (40% of patients); (2) disease confined to the small intestine (30%); and (3) disease of only the colon (25%), which is pancolonic in two thirds and segmental in one third. Less commonly, the disease affects the proximal gastrointestinal tract. Predominant symptoms in Crohn's disease include diarrhea, abdominal pain, and weight loss. They may exist for months to years before a diagnosis is made (Table 46-2). With colonic disease, diarrhea may be of small volume with urgency and tenesmus, whereas, if disease is extensive, small intestinal involvement produces larger stool volumes with steatorrhea. Diarrhea from small intestinal disease occurs from loss of mucosal absorptive surface area (producing bile salt–induced or osmotic diarrhea), bacterial overgrowth from strictures, and enteroenteric or enterocolonic fistulae. Pain results from intermittent partial obstruction or serosal inflammation. Commonly, pain and distention from terminal ileal disease are reported in the right lower quadrant. Weight loss occurs in most patients because of malabsorption and reduced oral intake; 10% to 20% of patients lose more than 20% of their body weight. Gastroduodenal involvement

TABLE 46-2
Frequency of Clinical Features in Crohn's Disease

FEATURE	ILEITIS (%)	ILEOCOLITIS (%)	COLITIS (%)
Diarrhea	~ 100	~ 100	~ 100
Abdominal pain	65	62	55
Bleeding	22	10	46
Weight loss	12	19	22
Perianal disease	14	38	36
Internal fistulae	17	34	16
Intestinal obstruction	35	44	17
Megacolon	0	2	11
Arthritis	4	4	16
Spondylitis	1	2	5

in Crohn's disease produces epigastric pain, nausea, and vomiting secondary to stricture or obstruction. Fatigue, malaise, fever, and chills are constitutional symptoms that contribute to the morbidity of Crohn's disease. When the disease is active, the patient may appear chronically ill, exhibiting pallor; temporal and interosseous wasting; abdominal tenderness; and a sensation of abdominal fullness or a mass secondary to thickened bowel loops, mesenteric thickening, or an abscess. The Crohn's Disease Activity Index assigns numerical scores to stool frequency, abdominal pain, sense of well-being, systemic manifestations, the use of antidiarrheal agents, abdominal mass, hematocrit, and body weight and has been used as a quantitative measure of disease activity in clinical studies.

Crohn's disease is a relapsing and remitting disease that spontaneously improves without treatment in 30% of cases. Patients in remission can expect to remain in remission for 2 years in 50% of cases. However, 60% of patients require surgery within 10 years of diagnosis. Of patients who undergo surgical resection, 45% will eventually require reoperation. Crohn's disease can produce significant disability, and 50% of patients make significant changes in employment to accommodate decreased working hours and leaves of absence.

Crohn's disease often is associated with gastrointestinal complications. Abscesses and fistulae result from extension of a mucosal breach through the intestinal wall into the extraintestinal tissue. Abscesses occur in 15% to 20% of patients and most commonly arise from the terminal ileum, but they may occur in iliopsoas, retroperitoneal, hepatic, and splenic regions, and at anastomotic sites. Abscesses present with fever, localized tenderness, and a palpable mass. Infection usually is polymicrobial (e.g., *Escherichia coli*, *Bacteroides fragilis*, *Enterococcus*, and α-hemolytic *Streptococcus* species). Twenty percent to 40% of patients with Crohn's disease have fistulous disease. Fistulae may be enteroenteric, enterocutaneous, enterovesical, or enterovaginal. They develop when disease is active and may persist after remission. Large enteroenteric fistulae produce diarrhea, malabsorption, and weight loss. Enterocutaneous fistulae produce persistent drainage that usually is refractory to medical therapy. Rectovaginal fistulae lead to foul-smelling vaginal discharge, and enterovesical fistulae produce pneumaturia and recurrent urinary infection. Obstruction, especially of the small intestine, is a common complication caused by mucosal thickening, muscular hyperplasia and scarring from prior inflammation, or adhesions. Perianal disease, including anal ulcers, abscesses, and fistulae, can also affect the groin, vulva, or scrotum and is a complication that often is difficult to treat. Fistulae drain serous or mucous material, whereas perianal abscesses cause fever; redness; induration; and pain that is exacerbated by defecation, sitting, and walking.

Extraintestinal Features

Extraintestinal manifestations of IBD are divided into two groups: those in which clinical activity follows activity of bowel disease and those in which clinical activity is unrelated to bowel activity. Extraintestinal disease is more common with ulcerative colitis and Crohn's colitis than with ileal Crohn's disease. Colitic arthritis is a migratory arthritis of the knees, hips, ankles, wrists, and elbows that usually lasts a few weeks, rarely produces joint deformity, and usually responds to treatment of bowel inflammation. In contrast, the activities of sacroiliitis and ankylosing spondylitis do not follow the course of the bowel disease and do not respond to the therapy for intestinal inflammation. Sacroiliitis often is asymptomatic and is found incidentally by radiography. The prevalence of ankylosing spondylitis, which is characterized by morning stiffness, low back pain, and stooped posture, increases 30-fold with ulcerative colitis. It is associated with the HLA-B27 phenotype. Unlike colitic arthritis, ankylosing spondylitis can be relentlessly progressive and unresponsive to medications.

Hepatobiliary complications of IBD include steatosis, pericholangitis, chronic active hepatitis, cirrhosis, sclerosing cholangitis, and gallstones. Pericholangitis, histologically defined by lymphocytic and eosinophilic inflammation of the portal tract and degeneration of the bile ductules, produces asymptomatic elevations of alkaline phosphatase levels. Sclerosing cholangitis is a chronic cholestatic disease marked by fibrosing inflammation of the intrahepatic and extrahepatic bile ducts; it occurs in 1% to 4% of patients with ulcerative colitis and in lesser numbers of patients with Crohn's disease. Conversely, the prevalence of IBD is so high in patients with sclerosing cholangitis that colonoscopy should be performed even on those without intestinal symptoms. Early in the course of sclerosing cholangitis, liver biopsy specimens show portal tract enlargement, edema, and bile duct proliferation, which progress to fibrosis and cirrhosis in advanced disease. Patients may be asymptomatic at first, but as the disease progresses, fever, right upper quadrant pain, jaundice, or even death may occur. Cholangiocarcinoma develops in 10% to 15% of patients with IBD who have long-standing sclerosing cholangitis. Cholesterol gallstones develop in patients with Crohn's disease because of the bile salt depletion that occurs with ileal disease or resection.

Complications of IBD may involve other organ systems. Osteoporosis or osteopenia occurs in up to half of IBD patients from malabsorption, malnutrition, smoking, persistent inflammation, and steroid use. Oxalate renal stones form with ileal Crohn's disease because of intralumenal calcium binding by malabsorbed fatty acids. Other urologic complications include urinary tract infection resulting from fistulae, ureteral obstruction caused by localized inflammation, and renal amyloidosis. Pyoderma gangrenosum, a discrete ulcer with a necrotic base usually found on the lower extremities, occurs in 1% to 5% of patients with ulcerative colitis and less frequently in Crohn's disease. Lesions almost always develop during a bout of acute colitis. Erythema nodosum appears as raised, tender nodules found usually over the anterior surface of the tibia, and is particularly common in children with Crohn's disease. The lesions respond well to treatment of the intestinal disease. Sweet syndrome (acute febrile neutrophilic dermatosis) also is associated with IBD. Uveitis is an inflammation of the anterior eye chamber resulting in blurred vision, headache, eye pain, photophobia, and conjunctival irritation. Episcleritis is characterized by scleral injection and burning eyes. Deep vein thrombosis, pulmonary emboli, and intracranial and intraocular thromboembolic events may result from clotting factor activation and thrombocytosis.

FINDINGS ON DIAGNOSTIC TESTING

Laboratory Studies

Laboratory studies that reflect disease activity in ulcerative colitis are hemoglobin level, leukocyte count, electrolytes, serum albumin, and erythrocyte sedimentation rate. Such values usually are normal in mild to moderate disease, although mild anemia and elevation in the sedimentation rate may be seen. Anemia, hypoalbuminemia, hypokalemia, and metabolic alkalosis may be prominent in severe disease. As part of the initial evaluation, infectious colitis should be excluded. Stool should be inspected for leukocytes, and cultures should be obtained for *Campylobacter*, *Shigella*, *Salmonella*, *Yersinia*, and other organisms. For watery diarrhea, stools are examined for *Giardia lamblia*. If antibiotics have been taken recently, stool should be tested for *Clostridium difficile* toxin. The role of microbes in exacerbating disease is controversial, although viral and bacterial organisms (especially *Clostridium difficile*) have been implicated in some cases. In immunosuppressed patients, consideration is given to possible cytomegalovirus colitis, which has a presentation similar to that of ulcerative colitis.

Laboratory findings in Crohn's disease are nonspecific. Anemia results from chronic disease; blood loss; and iron, folate, and vitamin B_{12} deficiency. Active Crohn's disease elevates leukocyte counts and sedimentation rate, but marked increases suggest abscess formation. Hypoalbuminemia may indicate severe disease, malnutrition, or protein-losing enteropathy. For patients with diarrhea, testing of stools for infection is indicated as for ulcerative colitis. Measurement of fecal fat, either qualitatively (Sudan stain) or quantitatively, can provide evidence of ileal disease.

Complications and extraintestinal manifestations of IBD can be suggested by selected laboratory studies. Profound leukocytosis with a neutrophil predominance in ulcerative colitis is worrisome for perforation or toxic megacolon. Pericholangitis and sclerosing cholangitis produce liver chemistry abnormalities, especially elevations of alkaline phosphatase. Pyuria in a patient with Crohn's disease suggests a possible enterovesical fistula, whereas hematuria raises concern for renal stones.

Serologic markers have been promoted to diagnose and differentiate ulcerative colitis from Crohn's disease; however, their utility must be confirmed in prospective studies. Perinuclear antineutrophil cytoplasmic antibodies (pANCA) are found in 60% of ulcerative colitis patients but in only 10% of individuals with Crohn's disease. pANCA-positive Crohn's disease patients appear to have ulcerative colitis-like, left-sided colonic disease. Anti–*Saccharomyces cerevisiae* antibodies (ASCA) are found in 60% of Crohn's disease patients but in only 10% of individuals with ulcerative colitis.

Endoscopy

Colonoscopy at the initial presentation of a patient with suspected IBD can establish the diagnosis and define the extent of disease. However in some cases, distinguishing between acute infectious colitis and the presenting flare of IBD may be difficult. Thus, subsequent endoscopic evaluations may be needed to confirm the presence of IBD in a patient with chronic symptoms. With severe disease, sigmoidoscopy may provide enough information to initiate therapy without the

TABLE 46-3
Colonoscopic Findings in Inflammatory Bowel Disease

FEATURE	ULCERATIVE COLITIS	CROHN'S DISEASE
Inflammation		
Distribution		
Colon		
Contiguous	+++	+
Symmetric	+++	+
Rectum	+++	+
Friability	+++	+
Topography		
Granularity	+++	+
Cobblestoned	+	+++
Ulceration		
Location		
Colitis	+++	+
Ileum	0	++++
Discrete lesion	+	+++
Features		
Size >1 cm	+	+++
Deep	+	++
Linear	+	+++
Aphthoid	0	++++
Bridging	+	++

Specificity index range: 0 (not seen) to ++++ (diagnostic)

risks of perforation associated with colonoscopy in this setting. Deep ulcerations or suspected toxic megacolon are contraindications to lower endoscopy. In ulcerative colitis, the inflammation begins in the rectum and extends proximally to the point where visible disease ends without skipping any areas (Table 46-3). Mild disease is characterized by superficial erosions, loss of vascularity, granularity, exudation, and friability. In severe disease, large ulcers and denuded mucosa may dominate. With chronic disease, the mucosa flattens and inflammatory polyps (pseudopolyps) develop. Pseudopolyps are not premalignant and do not need to be resected. Crohn's colitis exhibits a different appearance in many but not all cases. Aphthous ulcers predominate in early or mild disease, whereas severe disease is characterized by cobblestoning and large, deep, linear or serpiginous ulcers. With gastroduodenal Crohn's disease, antral aphthous and linear ulcers may be seen on upper endoscopy. Unlike ulcerative colitis, mucosal involvement in Crohn's disease is not contiguous; patches of colon are often relatively disease free (areas skipped), and the rectum may or may not be involved. Ileal disease is common in Crohn's disease. The ileum is normal in most ulcerative colitis patients, although backwash ileitis is seen in 10% to 20% of the cases of pancolitis. Capsule endoscopy has been used in some cases to exclude subtle small intestinal Crohn's disease in patients without obstruction. Strictures are more common with Crohn's disease, as is perianal involvement. Strictures and mass lesions in patients with long-standing IBD

(>10 years) strongly suggest malignancy. In addition to its diagnostic capability, colonoscopy has therapeutic potential (e.g., pneumatic dilation) in patients with colonic strictures.

Specialized endoscopy can help assess the extraintestinal manifestations of IBD. Endoscopic retrograde cholangiopancreatography (ERCP) can diagnose sclerosing cholangitis and cholangiocarcinoma and can be used to dilate or stent biliary strictures in sclerosing cholangitis, possibly reducing pruritus and other manifestations of obstructive jaundice.

Radiography

Findings of radiographic evaluation complement those of endoscopy in patients with IBD. Plain abdominal radiography may be normal or show colonic dilation in toxic megacolon, air-fluid levels from intestinal obstruction in Crohn's disease, or pneumoperitoneum with perforation. Barium enema radiographs are normal in early or mild ulcerative colitis but show a narrowed, shortened, and tubular lumen with loss of haustra in severe or long-standing disease. Mucosal texture is granular with mild ulcerative colitis but nodular with severe disease. The presacral space (i.e., the distance from the sacrum to the rectal lumen) increases to more than 2 cm with severe proctitis. A dilated and irregular terminal ileum suggests backwash ileitis. Mild Crohn's disease exhibits multiple aphthous ulcers, which enlarge, deepen, and interconnect to form the characteristic cobblestone appearance of more severe disease. Barium enema radiography is superior to endoscopy for detecting fistulae and strictures. However, barium enema radiography may miss malignancy in some IBD patients and is not the preferred test for this diagnosis. Strictures, mucosal irregularities, and bowel loop fixation may be apparent from small intestinal barium radiography. Such features usually are prominent in the ileum. Antral and duodenal mucosal abnormalities, strictures, or fistulae indicate proximal involvement in Crohn's disease.

Other tests are useful in selected cases. Computed tomography (CT) and ultrasound detect abscesses (including those that are perianal) and fluid collections and may assist in their percutaneous drainage. CT may also characterize obstruction and fistulae in Crohn's disease. Magnetic resonance imaging may have a role in defining perianal disease. Scintigraphic scans have been used to localize and characterize areas of intestinal inflammation or abscess.

Imaging studies are useful in characterizing complications and extraintestinal manifestations of IBD. Spine radiography shows squaring of the vertebrae, straightening of the spine, and lateral and anterior syndesmophytes in ankylosing spondylitis, whereas pelvic radiographs of the pelvis in sacroiliitis reveal blurring of the margins of the sacroiliac joints, with patchy sclerosis. Ultrasound and biliary scintigraphy are performed on patients with suspected biliary colic or cholecystitis secondary to gallstones in Crohn's disease. Magnetic resonance cholangiopancreatography and percutaneous transhepatic cholangiography are used in some cases to screen for sclerosing cholangitis or cholangiocarcinoma. Intravenous pyelography or CT may demonstrate enterovesical fistulae or renal stones.

Pathology

Histological evaluation of colonic biopsy specimens may distinguish ulcerative colitis from Crohn's disease and both forms of IBD from acute colitis in some but not all cases. Distortion and atrophy of the crypts, acute and chronic inflammation of the lamina propria, and a villous mucosal surface are more common with ulcerative colitis than with acute, self-limited colitis. The presence of granulomas provides the best histological distinction between the two diseases. In one series, granulomas were found in 60% of Crohn's disease patients versus 6% of patients with ulcerative colitis. Crypt atrophy, neutrophilic infiltration, and surface erosions are more common in ulcerative colitis than in Crohn's disease. Despite these variations, histological discrimination between the two forms of chronic IBD cannot be made in 15% to 25% of cases.

Histology also is performed to characterize extrahepatic manifestations of IBD. Liver biopsy specimens may show characteristic findings of pericholangitis, although findings in sclerosing cholangitis may be indistinguishable from those in pericholangitis. In such settings, biliary imaging can distinguish the two possibilities. Skin biopsy can diagnose pyoderma gangrenosum.

Ulcerative colitis and Crohn's disease exhibit characteristic findings on gross surgical specimens. Findings in ulcerative colitis are generally limited to the mucosa and submucosa; the muscularis propria is involved only in fulminant disease. Conversely, the bowel wall is thickened and stiff and the mesentery is thickened, edematous, and contracted in Crohn's disease because of transmural involvement. Adipose tissue creeps over the serosal surface, and intestinal loops may be matted together. Lymphoid aggregates may be observed involving the submucosa and occasionally the muscularis propria. Granulomas are found in many surgically resected intestinal, lymph node, mesentery, peritoneal, and liver specimens in Crohn's disease. Axonal necrosis of autonomic nerves is considered characteristic of Crohn's disease.

MANAGEMENT AND COURSE

Nutritional Management

In most cases, the only nutritional therapy required is a well-balanced diet. Some patients with small intestinal Crohn's disease have secondary lactase deficiency and should restrict lactose intake or use supplemental lactase. Patients with strictures should avoid high residue foods. Oral or parenteral iron supplements may be indicated for significant blood loss. Specific calcium, magnesium, zinc, vitamin B_{12}, vitamin D, or vitamin K supplements may be required to counter clinical or biochemical evidence of deficiency caused by Crohn's enteritis. Extensive terminal ileal resections (>100 cm) promote vitamin B_{12}, fat, and bile salt malabsorption. Steatorrhea may be reduced by consuming a low-fat diet. The bile salt–binding resin cholestyramine can reduce bile salt diarrhea, but this agent may worsen fat malabsorption. Medium-chain triglycerides, which are absorbed in the proximal intestine and do not require bile salts, are substituted for conventional long-chain triglycerides in some cases. Fish oil supplements may reduce steroid requirements in some IBD patients, although this is controversial. When oral intake is inadequate, enteral feedings may be provided through nasogastric, gastrostomy, or jejunostomy tubes. Elemental feedings that consist of amino acids, monosaccharides, vitamins, minerals, and essential fatty acids offer theoretical benefits in improving absorption and reducing the antigenic load to the distal intestine, but there is no convincing evidence that such feedings alter the course of disease. Severe IBD exacerbations or extensive small intestinal resections with Crohn's disease may warrant initiating total parenteral nutrition. Parenteral nutrition also is helpful in improving the nutritional status of patients with ulcerative colitis before colectomy.

Medication Therapy

5-Aminosalicylate Preparations

Drugs that contain 5-aminosalicylate (5-ASA) are a mainstay of therapy for mild to moderate IBD. The mechanisms of the beneficial actions of 5-ASA are unknown, although inhibition of local lipoxygenase pathways and free-radical scavenging and modulation of cytokine production have been proposed. Sulfasalazine consists of sulfapyridine and 5-ASA joined by a diazo bond, which is cleaved by colonic bacteria, releasing the active 5-ASA molecule and the inert antibiotic moiety. This promotes exposure of the colonic mucosa to high levels of 5-ASA, whereas very little drug is absorbed systemically. Sulfasalazine is started at low doses and is gradually increased to 4 g per day, as tolerated, in mild to moderate ulcerative colitis. After remission is achieved, doses can be tapered to 2 g per day for long-term maintenance therapy, which reduces relapses from 75% to 20% at 1 year. Sulfasalazine is also useful for Crohn's colitis and has been used to maintain remission in Crohn's colitis, although there are limited data to support this practice. Sulfasalazine has little effect in Crohn's disease limited to the small intestine. Dose-related side effects of sulfasalazine stem from the sulfapyridine component and include nausea, vomiting, headache, dyspepsia, abdominal discomfort, and hemolysis. Enteric-coated preparations may reduce sulfasalazine-induced abdominal discomfort. Hypersensitive dose-independent reactions include rash, fever, aplastic anemia, agranulocytosis, and autoimmune hemolysis. Other side effects of sulfasalazine include reduced sperm counts (which recover 3 months after stopping the drug), folate deficiency (caused by inhibition of intestinal folate conjugase), and rarely, bloody diarrhea (caused by the 5-ASA component).

Other 5-ASA preparations are commonly prescribed in selected IBD subsets. Enemas that contain 4 g 5-ASA are effective for treating distal ulcerative colitis and induce remission in 93% of patients. 5-ASA suppositories (500 mg) are useful in ulcerative proctitis. Oral 5-ASA (mesalamine) preparations (Asacol, Pentasa) are increasingly used because of their efficacy and favorable side-effect profiles. Asacol is coated with a methacrylic acid copolymer (Eudragit-S) that releases 5-ASA in the terminal ileum and colon at pH of 7 or higher. Pentasa uses a semipermeable membrane that more prominently releases 5-ASA at pH of 6 or higher in the small intestine and proximal colon. In addition to treating colitis in IBD, these drugs may be effective in patients with ileal Crohn's disease and can maintain remission in both ulcerative colitis and Crohn's disease. Olsalazine consists of two 5-ASA molecules covalently bound by an azo bond. Balsalazide is composed of 5-ASA linked via a diazo bond to the inert carrier 4-aminobenzoyl-β-alanine. Both agents are cleaved by enteric flora in the colon and are indicated for treating colitis. All 5-ASA products exhibit potential nephrotoxicity; thus caution should be exercised when using these drugs in patients with renal dysfunction. Olsalazine causes small intestinal chloride secretion, producing watery diarrhea in 5% to 10% of patients.

Corticosteroids

Corticosteroids are effective in inducing remission in ulcerative colitis and Crohn's disease. These agents block the early (enhanced vascular permeability, vasodilation, and neutrophil infiltration) and the late (vascular proliferation, fibroblast activation, and collagen deposition) stages of the inflammatory process. Oral prednisone is effective in moderate ulcerative colitis and produces improvement within 3 weeks. Intravenous methylprednisolone is useful for inpatients with more severe ulcerative colitis. Corticosteroids also produce remission in 60% to 92% of cases of Crohn's disease within 7 to 17 weeks; however, the presence of an abscess should be excluded to minimize the risk of sepsis on therapy. Maintenance steroid therapy is ineffective in preventing recurrences in ulcerative colitis and Crohn's disease. Steroid enemas are effective in treating left-sided ulcerative colitis reliably up to the level of the mid-descending colon. Systemic absorption of steroid enemas is significant and increases the risks of long-term use.

The side effects of corticosteroids may limit their use in IBD. Prednisone at a dose of 10 mg or more taken for longer than 3 weeks may suppress the hypothalamic-pituitary-adrenal axis for 1 year after therapy is discontinued. Individuals thus treated should receive supplemental steroids for surgery or severe illness. Common side effects of steroid therapy include increased appetite, centripetal obesity, moon facies, acne, insomnia, depression, psychosis, growth retardation (in children), increased infections, hypertension, glucose intolerance, cataracts, irreversible glaucoma, and (in rare cases) blindness. Avascular necrosis of the femoral head can produce permanent disability. Osteoporosis is a devastating side effect that can occur with prednisone doses as low as 8 to 10 mg per day. Patients on long-term steroid therapy should receive supplemental calcium and vitamin D and should undergo periodic bone densitometry studies. More aggressive therapies including bisphosphonates, calcitonin, and hormonal treatments may be indicated in some cases.

Budesonide is a steroid whose systemic toxicity is diminished by rapid first-pass metabolism in the liver. It is formulated with a Eudragit-S coating to direct its absorption to the distal ileum and proximal colon and has been approved for treating Crohn's disease. Although observed less frequently than with prednisone, budesonide does suppress plasma cortisol levels. The drug is useful for inducing remission of Crohn's disease but has an undefined role in maintaining remission.

Immunomodulators

Azathioprine and 6-mercaptopurine (6-MP) are useful in certain clinical settings, including disease refractory to steroid therapy, as steroid sparing agents when long-term therapy is needed, or if steroid side effects are prominent. Immunosuppressants also are beneficial in healing fistulae in Crohn's disease. In contrast, these agents are less effective for acute IBD exacerbations because clinical responses may not be observed for 3 to 4 months after initiating therapy. Blood counts are monitored frequently because of the bone marrow–suppressive effects of these agents (especially leucopenia). Liver chemistry levels also are monitored to detect possible hepatotoxicity. Other side effects of azathioprine and 6-MP include pancreatitis (3.3%), infections (7%), and allergic reactions (2%). The therapeutic efficacy and toxicity of these drugs relate to their metabolites. These drugs are metabolized by thiopurine methyltransferase (TPMT) to the active agents, 6-thioguanine (6-TG) and 6-methylmercaptopurine ribonucleotides, and the inactive metabolite, 6-methylmercaptopurine (6-MMP). The therapeutic efficacy and hematologic toxicity of 6-MP and azathioprine relate to serum 6-TG levels, whereas elevated 6-MMP levels correlate with other side effects. TPMT genotyping can identify individuals predisposed to drug toxicity. There is a theoretical risk of malignancy with these medications; however, case series have observed no clear increase in neoplasms with long-term therapy. One analysis suggested that the enhanced life expectancy from successfully treating Crohn's disease exceeded the decrease in life span from rare cases of lymphoma.

Intravenous cyclosporine is effective for severe ulcerative colitis refractory to steroid therapy. These individuals are then started on oral cyclosporine plus 6-MP when remission is achieved. It is unclear if this approach prevents the ultimate need for colectomy in many patients; however, it may defer surgery to a time when the procedure can be elective. Oral cyclosporine has not shown convincing efficacy in Crohn's disease. The side effects of cyclosporine include renal insufficiency, hypertension, paresthesias, tremor, and headache. Methotrexate is considered an effective alternative to 6-MP and azathioprine if these agents are not tolerated. Prominent side effects of methotrexate include nausea, bone marrow suppression, elevated liver chemistry levels, and a long-term risk for development of cirrhosis.

Antibiotics

Broad-spectrum antibiotics are important in treating suppurative complications of Crohn's disease, including abscesses and perianal disease, as well as small intestinal bacterial overgrowth from stasis proximal to a stricture. Metronidazole has efficacy for perianal Crohn's disease and may reduce disease activity in Crohn's colitis. The mechanism of action of metronidazole is unknown. Side effects include peripheral neuropathy, a bad taste in the mouth, and disulfiram-like reactions. Ciprofloxacin has also shown efficacy in some patients with mild to moderate Crohn's disease, especially of the colon. One trial demonstrated the efficacy of adding ciprofloxacin to conventional therapy of ulcerative colitis with prednisone and mesalamine.

Infliximab

Infliximab is a mouse-human chimeric monoclonal IgG1 antibody directed against TNF. The drug has demonstrated impressive efficacy in treating refractory flares of Crohn's disease. Infliximab also is useful for closing fistula secondary to Crohn's disease and is increasingly used as maintenance therapy for patients with Crohn's disease who do not respond to or who have unacceptable toxicity from other immunosuppressive agents. Toxicity increases with repeated dosing of infliximab and includes hypersensitivity reactions (rash, fever, myalgias, and arthralgias) and infectious complications (varicella-zoster virus, *Candida esophagitis*, tuberculosis). Responses may also diminish with time in some patients secondary to development of antibodies. Infliximab may increase the risk of lymphoma.

Miscellaneous Agents

Antidiarrheal agents (e.g., loperamide, diphenoxylate with atropine) may reduce defecation frequency and fecal urgency in patients with mild IBD. Similarly, anticholinergic drugs can reduce pain, cramps, and fecal urgency, especially after meals. These drugs, as well as opiate analgesics, should be avoided in severe disease because of the risk of toxic megacolon. Nicotine patches may reduce symptoms in some patients with ulcerative colitis.

Medical Management of Ulcerative Colitis

The medical management of ulcerative colitis depends on the extent and severity of disease. 5-ASA (or steroid) enemas are given nightly for 2 to 3 weeks for mild disease extending to 60 cm of the distal colon. If the patient responds, the frequency of enemas can be tapered to alternate nights, then to every third night to minimize disease recurrences. 5-ASA suppositories or corticosteroid foam may be used for proctitis. Oral 5-ASA preparations also can be used for mild distal ulcerative colitis, but responses are slower with these agents than with rectal therapy. Patients with refractory disease or severe distal colitis may respond to corticosteroids or 6-MP therapy, whereas those with very mild disease may need only antidiarrheal agents. Maintenance therapy for proctitis may include oral 5-ASA preparations or 5-ASA enemas every other night.

Mild cases of pancolitis are usually treated with an oral 5-ASA compound. Patients who have more than five to six bowel movements per day or those in whom a therapeutic response is desired in less than 3 to 4 weeks should receive oral prednisone, which will produce a response in a few days to 3 weeks. Patients with severe diarrhea, bleeding, or systemic symptoms are initially given 40 mg per day. After symptoms are controlled, the dose is reduced by 5 mg every 1 to 2 weeks while the patient is switched to a 5-ASA preparation for maintenance. If steroids cannot be withdrawn and the patient continues to take more than 15 mg prednisone per day for 6 months, 6-MP or azathioprine therapy or colectomy should be considered.

The mainstays for treating severe ulcerative colitis are bed rest, intravenous hydration, blood transfusions as needed, parenteral antibiotics for signs of infection, and intravenous steroids. If ileus is present, the patient is given nothing by mouth and nasogastric suction is initiated. Total parenteral nutrition is provided if oral nutrition is to be withheld for a prolonged period. If there is no response within 7 to 10 days, continuous intravenous cyclosporine can be given for 7 days, with doses aimed at obtaining serum levels of 100 to 400 ng/mL. Patients who respond to cyclosporine are switched to oral cyclosporine (8 mg/kg per day), whereas those who do not improve are referred for colectomy.

Medical Management of Crohn's Disease

It is difficult to provide generally applicable guidelines for managing Crohn's disease because of the varied clinical presentations. For mild to moderate colonic or ileocolonic disease, an oral 5-ASA preparation is reasonable initial therapy. Because of its relatively greater release in the small intestine, Pentasa may be a better choice for ileitis or ileocolitis. Oral budesonide may be useful for ileal flares of Crohn's disease that respond poorly to 5-ASA preparations. Oral prednisone is used for more active disease and for patients who have failed to respond to 5-ASA compounds. Severe flares of Crohn's disease are managed with intravenous steroids. Infliximab is given for acute flares unresponsive to steroids, often with additional initiation of 6-MP or azathioprine to maintain disease control. Chronic use of immunosuppressive agents is indicated for patients with prolonged disease or disease refractory to steroids and for patients who have side effects from steroid therapy. If effective, immunosuppressants are usually continued for 1 to 3 years. Chronic infliximab therapy is offered for steroid-resistant individuals who do not tolerate other immunosuppressives. Fistulae and perianal disease are treated with metronidazole, immunosuppressants, or infliximab. Maintaining remission with 5-ASA preparations is recommended for those brought into remission by steroids or surgery. Maintenance with immunosuppressives is recommended for those brought into remission on those drugs. Maintenance therapy has increased importance for patients who have undergone multiple surgical resections.

Surgical Management

Twenty percent to 25% of patients with ulcerative colitis eventually undergo colectomy, which cures the colonic disease and many but not all of the extraintestinal manifestations. Urgent indications for colectomy in ulcerative colitis include toxic megacolon, perforation, refractory fulminant colitis in the absence of dilation, and severe hemorrhage. Nonurgent indications include failure of medical therapy, severe drug side effects that prevent adequate medication regimens, dysplasia, and carcinoma. Uveitis, pyoderma gangrenosum, and colitic arthritis usually respond to colectomy, whereas ankylosing spondylitis and sclerosing cholangitis do not.

The ileal pouch–anal canal anastomosis is the procedure of choice for most patients with uncomplicated ulcerative colitis who undergo colectomy because it preserves normal continence. In this operation, the colon is completely removed, and the mucosa and submucosa are dissected from the rectum. A pouch is constructed from the distal 30 cm of ileum and sewn to the dentate line. A temporary diverting ileostomy may be needed until the anastomosis heals. Postoperatively, defecation frequency decreases after 1 year to five to six daily bowel movements. Complications include incontinence, intractable diarrhea, infection, or anastomotic breakdown. In severely ill and some very old patients, a Brooke ileostomy may be performed with proctocolectomy in a one-stage or two-stage (colectomy and ileostomy followed by proctectomy) procedure. A disadvantage of this procedure is the need to wear an appliance to collect the ileal discharge. Complications of the Brooke ileostomy include stomal prolapse, retraction, herniation, and stenosis. The Kock continent ileostomy involves constructing an ileal valve that can be periodically drained with a rubber catheter; this obviates the need to wear an external bag. This operation has largely been replaced by the ileal pouch–anal canal anastomosis.

In contrast to ulcerative colitis, surgery does not cure Crohn's disease. Thus, the extent and frequency of resections should be minimized. Indications for surgery in Crohn's disease include disease intractability, failure of medical therapy, obstruction, fistulae, and abscess formation. Approximately 60% of patients with Crohn's disease require surgery within 10 years of diagnosis. Of these, 50% need a repeat operation within 10 years. Even in those who do not require reoperation, disease recurrences are frequent (>70%) postoperatively. Stricturoplasty represents an alternative to resection for Crohn's strictures. For extensive colitis with rectal involvement, total proctocolectomy with Brooke ileostomy is the procedure of choice. Subtotal colectomy with ileoproctostomy is only for patients with absolutely normal rectums. Ileal pouch–anal canal anastomosis is not appropriate for patients with Crohn's colitis.

Management of Complications and Extraintestinal Manifestations

For some cases of toxic megacolon, medical therapy may lead to improvement and obviate the need for surgery. Nasogastric suction is initiated, intravenous steroids are given, and broad-spectrum antibiotics often are administered in anticipation of peritonitis. Fluid and electrolyte replacement should be aggressive because electrolyte disturbances may contribute to impaired colonic motor function. A successful medical response is defined by improvement within 24 to 48 hours in signs of toxicity and reduction in colonic diameter on abdominal radiography. If there is no improvement within 48 hours, colectomy should be performed because of the high risk of perforation. Broad-spectrum antibiotics are indicated for abscesses in Crohn's disease, in addition to percutaneous or surgical drainage. After the abscess has been drained and the inflammation subsides, resection of the affected bowel usually is required. Surgical excision also is required for fistulae that are proximal to strictures.

Specific therapies are indicated for selected extraintestinal manifestations of IBD. Colitic arthritis usually responds to corticosteroid therapy. NSAIDs can reduce pain from arthritic complications of IBD but may exacerbate bowel inflammation. Pruritus secondary to sclerosing cholangitis may respond to cholestyramine. Ursodeoxycholic acid decreases liver chemistry abnormalities in sclerosing cholangitis but does not alter the outcome of this complication. Sclerosing cholangitis has become a common indication for liver transplantation. Pyoderma gangrenosum and erythema nodosum usually abate if the intestinal disease is controlled with corticosteroids. Pyoderma gangrenosum also reportedly responds to cyproheptadine, dapsone, cyclosporine, azathioprine, infliximab, and direct local corticosteroid injection or topical tacrolimus application. Uveitis may respond to local steroids and atropine. Topical steroids also are beneficial for episcleritis.

Surveillance for Colonic Neoplasia

Patients with ulcerative colitis have an increased likelihood of developing colon carcinoma, with a lifetime risk of 3% to 5%. Risk factors for colon cancer in ulcerative colitis include duration and extent of disease, sclerosing cholangitis, backwash ileitis, and a family history of colon cancer. For pancolitis, the risk is appreciable 8 to 10 years after diagnosis. Patients with left-sided disease are at less risk. In contrast to the normal population, development of colon cancer in ulcerative colitis does not follow the standard progression of adenoma to carcinoma. Moreover, multicentric tumors, which are rare in the general population (2% to 3%), account for up to 26% of cancers in ulcerative colitis. Thus, surveillance programs are designed to detect premalignant dysplasia in mucosal areas that appear no different from surrounding regions. Dysplasia is defined by nuclear stratification, loss of nuclear polarity, and nuclear and cellular pleomorphism. Areas of special concern are dysplasia-associated lesions or masses (DALM), which are nodular, or raised colonic regions that are malignant in 40% of cases. The usual approach to surveillance of pancolitis is colonoscopy every 1 to 3 years beginning 7 to 10 years after diagnosis and taking four biopsy specimens every 10 cm of colon. If high-grade dysplasia is found and confirmed by an experienced pathologist, colectomy should be performed. The approach to low-grade dysplasia should probably be the same as that for high-grade dysplasia, although some investigators have advocated confirming dysplasia with a repeat colonoscopy. For left-sided colitis, some have recommended deferring surveillance until 15 to 20 years after diagnosis.

The incidence of colon cancer in patients with Crohn's colitis is clearly higher than that in the general population. The risk for extensive Crohn's colitis appears to be similar to that of ulcerative pancolitis; thus a surveillance strategy similar to that for ulcerative colitis has been advocated for extensive Crohn's colitis. There is an increased risk of developing adenocarcinoma of the small intestine in ileal Crohn's disease.

INFLAMMATORY BOWEL DISEASE IN SPECIAL PATIENT POPULATIONS

Pregnancy and Inflammatory Bowel Disease

Most pregnant women with IBD deliver healthy babies, although the incidence of spontaneous abortion is slightly higher than that in the general population. Active disease may lead to a slight increase in rates of prematurity and spontaneous abortion. Prior colectomy or ileostomy is not an impediment to successful completion of pregnancy. Sulfasalazine use has not been shown to adversely affect the outcome of pregnancy; thus there is no need to discontinue the drug. However, folate supplements should be given to prevent fetal deficiencies secondary to sulfasalazine. Similarly, the risk of fetal complications is not increased by corticosteroid use. If possible, women should use the minimal dose or delay pregnancy until the disease is quiescent and medications can be withdrawn. Azathioprine and 6-MP are potentially teratogenic, retard growth, and increase the risk of prematurity. These drugs should be withdrawn unless required to control the disease. Metronidazole also induces abortion and should be avoided if possible. In general, quiescent IBD at conception remains inactive throughout pregnancy, but active ulcerative colitis may worsen. The course of active Crohn's disease is less consistent during pregnancy. Fertility in women with IBD is normal or only minimally impaired.

Inflammatory Bowel Disease in Childhood and Adolescence

In general, ulcerative colitis that presents in childhood is similar to disease in adults. Diagnosing Crohn's disease may be delayed in children because of differences in abdominal pain that suggest functional disease and prominence of extraintestinal manifestations. Growth failure, retarded bone development, and delayed sexual maturation also are prevalent in children with Crohn's disease. In this age group, corticosteroids can contribute to growth failure. Nutritional supplementation is important in children with IBD and should provide more calories (50 to 93 kcal/kg per day) than would normally be required. The principles of medication therapy for children with IBD are similar to those for adults, and dose is adjusted for body weight. The indications for surgery are the same for children and adults. The success of surgical resection in reversing growth retardation is disappointing.

CHAPTER 47

Miscellaneous Inflammatory and Structural Disorders of the Colon

COLLAGENOUS AND LYMPHOCYTIC COLITIS

Etiology and Pathogenesis

Microscopic colitis is a term that describes a spectrum of disorders in which the colonic mucosa appears intact despite histological evidence of inflammation. Two distinct types of microscopic colitis—collagenous colitis and lymphocytic colitis—are both characterized by chronic watery diarrhea. Both disorders exhibit infiltration of the mucosal lamina propria with mononuclear cells, epithelial cell damage, preserved crypt architecture without cryptitis, and an increased number of intraepithelial lymphocytes. Collagenous colitis is histologically differentiated from lymphocytic colitis by a linear subepithelial collagen band that is 10 to 100 μm thick (normal, <4 μm). This thickened collagen layer is most prominent beneath the surface epithelium between the crypts, preferentially involves the cecum and transverse colon (82% and 83% of cases, respectively), and is least likely to be seen in a biopsy specimen of the rectum, which is affected in 72% of cases. The mean age at presentation is 60 to 65, and most patients are women.

The pathogenesis of collagenous and lymphocytic colitis is not completely defined but appears to be immune-mediated. The disorders share an epidemiological association with celiac sprue, as well as with arthritis and other autoimmune disorders. NSAIDs are used more frequently by patients with microscopic colitis than by control populations, which suggests an etiologic role for these medications. Other proposed causes include a genetic predisposition, bile salt malabsorption, and ingestion of injurious agents such as L-tryptophan. Defective sodium and chloride absorption and chloride/bicarbonate exchange, as well as active colonic chloride secretion, cause diarrhea in lymphocytic colitis.

Clinical Features, Diagnosis, and Management

The clinical presentation of collagenous and lymphocytic colitis consists of chronic nonbloody diarrhea (300 to 1700 g per day) associated with nocturnal stools, fecal incontinence, cramping, nausea, weight loss, and abdominal distention. Diarrhea usually abates with fasting. Laboratory abnormalities are unusual, although anemia, hypoalbuminemia, elevations in sedimentation rate, and, rarely, steatorrhea may occur. A colonoscopy with biopsy is usually sufficient to diagnose these disorders. Several specimens must be taken from different colonic regions, concentrating on proximal sites. The results of the biopsy studies will be positive in 82% of patients in a single sampling if specimens from the rectum, sigmoid colon, and descending colon are pooled. Careful histological analysis should exclude other causes of diarrhea including acute infectious colitis, inflammatory bowel disease, radiation colitis, ischemia, amyloidosis, and eosinophilic gastroenteritis. Clinical symptoms of collagenous and lymphocytic colitis may spontaneously remit, sometimes after NSAIDs are discontinued. Placebo-controlled clinical trials have shown that prednisone and bismuth subsalicylate effectively induce symptom remission. Anecdotal data support the efficacy of 5-aminosalicylate (5-ASA), sulfasalazine, antibiotics, and immunosuppressive drugs (Table 47-1). Celiac disease should be excluded in patients with disease refractory to antiinflammatory drugs, and antihistamines may be considered for patients with large numbers of mast cells in biopsy specimens.

TABLE 47-1
Sequential Approach to Treating Microscopic Colitis

	TOXICITY
1. *Symptomatic*: loperamide, diphenoxylate with atropine, fiber	+
2. *Binding agents*: bismuth subsalicylate, cholestyramine	++
3. *5-aminosalicylate*: sulfasalazine, mesalamine	+++
4. *Antibiotics*: metronidazole, ciprofloxacin, erythromycin, tetracycline	++++
5. *Corticosteroids*: budesonide, prednisone	+++++
6. *Immunosuppressives*: 6-mercaptopurine/azathioprine, methotrexate	++++++
7. *Antisecretory*: octreotide	+++++++
8. *Surgery*: colectomy, diverting ileostomy	++++++++

DIVERSION COLITIS

Etiology and Pathogenesis

Diversion colitis is inflammation that develops in the distal bypassed colon within Hartmann pouches or mucous fistulae after excluding the fecal stream. Histological findings include diffuse follicular lymphoid hyperplasia with germinal centers. Early in its course, diversion colitis is characterized by infiltration of the mucosa with lymphocytes, plasma cells, neutrophils, and reactive epithelial cells. More advanced lesions include crypt abscesses, mild crypt distortion, Paneth cell metaplasia, and, rarely, mucin granulomas. Severe involvement produces diffuse nodularity and small ulcerations. The pathogenesis of diversion colitis is unclear, but it has been postulated that fecal diversion abolishes the supply of short-chain fatty acids that provide fuel to the colonocytes. This hypothesis is supported by the observation that short-chain fatty acid enemas improve clinical, endoscopic, and histological variables in some patients with diversion colitis. However, involvement of other factors, such as lumenal growth factors, dietary constituents, and bacterial metabolic products, must be considered. The incidence of the disorder is higher if surgery is performed for inflammatory bowel disease (89%) than for carcinoma (23%), which suggests that preexisting disease also plays an important role in the development of diversion colitis.

Clinical Features, Diagnosis, and Management

One third of patients will develop mucoid discharge, rectal bleeding, and pain in 1 to 9 months after surgical diversion. Endoscopic findings include erythema, granularity, friability, aphthous ulcers, and exudate. Biopsy specimens show lymphoid follicular hyperplasia, neutrophilic infiltration, and crypt inflammation. The clinical, endoscopic, and histological manifestations of diversion colitis resolve when the fecal stream is restored. Because most patients are asymptomatic or have only mild symptoms, therapy is rarely needed. Short-chain fatty acid enemas (acetate, 60 mmol/L; propionate, 30 mmol/L; and butyrate, 40 mmol/L) may induce remission of severe diversion colitis. 5-ASA enemas have been successful; however, corticosteroid enemas usually are ineffective.

ENDOMETRIOSIS

Etiology and Pathogenesis

Endometriosis, the presence and growth of endometrial glands and stroma outside the uterus, occurs in 15% of menstruating women (usually ages 32 to 41); 37% of them have intestinal implants. Postmenopausal women may experience symptomatic endometriosis if they are taking estrogen replacements. Most patients have rectosigmoid involvement (95%); other locations such as the appendix (10%) and ileum (5%) are less common. Bluish-gray peritoneal or serosal implants may invade the bowel wall, resulting in muscular hypertrophy and fibrosis; mucosal involvement is rare. Mucosal biopsy specimens infrequently show crypt distortion, crypt abscesses, or ulceration.

The cause of endometriosis is unknown. Peritoneal seeding may be caused by retrograde menstruation with ectopic implantation of viable uterine tissue. Hematogenous and lymphatic spread may account for remote implants such as rarely occur in pleural, pericardial, and lymph node endometriosis. Alternatively, it may be that peritoneal cells undergo metaplastic transformation to endometrial epithelial cells. Finally, shed endometrium in the abdomen and pelvis may induce endometrial metaplasia of peritoneal cells.

Clinical Features, Diagnosis, and Management

Patients with endometriosis may present with abdominal pain, constipation, diarrhea, rectal bleeding, localized abdominal tenderness, palpable nodules on rectal examination, or even appendicitis. Most patients (80%) experience pelvic symptoms such as dysmenorrhea, dyspareunia, infertility, and dysfunctional uterine bleeding. Surprisingly, few patients report a temporal association of their intestinal symptoms with their menstrual cycle. Barium enema radiography and colonoscopic findings may be normal in the presence of serosal implants. Obstructing lesions can produce extrinsic compression or smooth strictures with overlying normal mucosa. Endoscopic evaluation with biopsy may be diagnostic in patients with rectal bleeding caused by mucosal invasion. Endoscopic ultrasound may detect colonic wall invasion. Computed tomographic (CT) and magnetic resonance imaging scans rarely are useful. Definitive diagnosis often requires laparoscopy or laparotomy.

Superficial serosal implants can be treated with hormonal therapy or nonresective surgery. Danazol, medroxyprogesterone, and gonadotropin-releasing hormone analogs (e.g., leuprolide) have been shown to reduce pain and diminish the size of pelvic endometrial nodules. Anterior rectal and rectovaginal septal implants may be ablated with a laparoscopic laser. Segmental colectomy usually is required to treat partial colonic obstructions because of poor response to medications or the inability to exclude malignancy.

CHEMICAL-INDUCED COLONIC INJURY

Etiology and Pathogenesis

A variety of chemicals and therapeutic agents have been shown to cause colonic injury (Table 47-2). Enemas, laxatives, NSAIDs (both nonselective and selective cyclooxygenase-2 inhibitors), and oral contraceptives have been implicated in the pathogenesis of chemical-induced colitis. Soap-induced colitis produced by detergent enemas may cause liquefaction necrosis of the colonic mucosa, similar to alkaline-associated esophageal injury. Diarrhea may be mild and watery or severe and bloody. Corresponding endoscopic appearances range from mucosal edema with loss of vascularity to mucosal sloughing and ulceration as deep as the muscularis propria. Hyperosmolar water-soluble contrast media (e.g., Gastrografin,

TABLE 47-2
Therapeutic Agents That Induce Colonic Injury

Enemas	Soap, water-soluble contrast media, hydrogen peroxide
Laxatives	Melanosis coli, cathartic colon
Drugs associated with bowel ischemia	Oral contraceptives, vasopressin, ergotamine, alosetron, cocaine, dextroamphetamine, neuroleptics, digitalis
Miscellaneous	NSAIDs, selective cyclooxygenase-2 inhibitors, penicillamine, gold, isotretinoin, antibiotics, chemotherapy, methyldopa, flucytosine, glutaraldehyde

Hypaque, and Renografin 76) can induce colitis, ranging from minimal inflammation to severe colitis with necrosis and perforation. The pathogenesis may be related to decreased blood flow to the colon. Hydrogen peroxide enemas, historically used to relieve fecal impaction, treat meconium ileus, and reduce intestinal gas, can cause ischemic damage to the mucosa, submucosa, and muscularis as a result of the penetration of gas into the bowel vasculature, which reduces blood flow. Colitis has also been reported after ethanol, hydrofluoric acid, and vinegar enemas.

Clinical Features, Diagnosis, and Management

Patients with chemical-induced colonic injury present with abdominal pain, bloody or nonbloody diarrhea, tenesmus, fever, rectal and abdominal tenderness, and possible peritoneal signs. Leukocytosis is often present. Colonoscopic findings are nonspecific. Perianal excoriations may suggest the diagnosis. Treatment involves intravenous fluids, bowel rest, and possibly intravenous antibiotics or surgery.

LAXATIVE EFFECTS ON THE COLON

Etiology and Pathogenesis

Melanosis coli is easily recognized during colonoscopy by the characteristic pigmentation, which results from using anthraquinone laxatives (cascara, aloe, rhubarb, senna, frangula). Melanosis usually develops 9 months after initiating anthraquinone laxatives and can disappear within 9 months after withdrawing them. The condition affects mainly the cecum and rectum, although the entire colon may be involved. It is associated with increases in brown, pigment-laden macrophages in the lamina propria. The source of the pigment is unknown.

Cathartic colon results from the chronic use (>15 years) of irritating laxatives, such as anthraquinones. Laxative use leads to hypertrophy of the muscularis mucosae, thinning of the muscularis propria, submucosal fat deposition, loss of myenteric plexus neurons, and replacement of ganglia by Schwann cells. Anthraquinones may produce other toxic effects on the colonic myenteric nerves that lead to the development of cathartic colon.

Clinical Features, Diagnosis, and Management

Melanosis coli is a benign condition without symptoms. Its presence implies chronic anthraquinone use; therefore, the physician should question any such patient concerning the use of these potentially harmful laxatives. Patients with cathartic colon complain of bloating, fullness, pain, and incomplete fecal evacuation, although some surreptitious users may present with chronic unexplained diarrhea or protein-losing enteropathy. Electrolyte and volume abnormalities may include hypokalemia and hypovolemia. Therapy for cathartic colon centers on withdrawing irritant laxatives, which is accomplished with bulking agents, a high-fiber diet, and a bowel retraining program that may involve using nonstimulant cathartics such as osmotic laxatives or Fleet enemas. A subtotal colectomy may be necessary if the condition is severe or refractory, but this option should be a last resort because many cases of cathartic colon are reversible.

MEDICATIONS THAT PRODUCE COLONIC ISCHEMIA

Etiology and Pathogenesis

Oral contraceptive use is associated with hypercoagulability, vasospasm, and endothelial proliferation; all contribute to the development of ischemic colitis. Vasopressin causes colonic ischemia by reducing blood flow, whereas cocaine and dextroamphetamine evoke intense mesenteric vasospasm. Ergot preparations produce colonic vasospasm, and ergotamine suppositories can cause rectal ulcers with obliteration of small blood vessels, endothelial proliferation, and thickening of the vascular wall. Ischemic colitis has also been associated with the use of neuroleptics and tricyclic antidepressants. Digitalis is associated with colonic ischemia, in part because of the underlying disease states (e.g., congestive heart failure) that produce colonic hypoperfusion. This drug additionally produces mesenteric vasoconstriction in animal models, and thus may directly contribute to consequent ischemia. Alosetron, a 5-hydroxytryptamine 3 receptor antagonist, was released as a drug for diarrhea-predominant irritable bowel syndrome; however, its prescription has been severely limited because of reports of associated ischemic colitis.

Clinical Features, Diagnosis, and Management

The principal symptoms of medication-induced colonic ischemia include abdominal pain, bloody or nonbloody diarrhea, tenesmus, nausea, vomiting, and fever. Leukocytosis may be present, and abdominal radiography may show thumbprinting consistent with bowel wall edema. Colonoscopy may reveal friability, edema, erythema, granularity, ulceration with or without pseudomembranes, and necrosis.

MISCELLANEOUS MEDICATION-INDUCED COLITIDES

Etiology and Pathogenesis

The prevalence of NSAID use is such that an estimated 10% of newly diagnosed cases of colitis are related to their use. Offending drugs include mefenamic and flufenamic acid, diclofenac, indomethacin, enteric-coated aspirin, ibuprofen, phenylbutazone, naproxen, and piroxicam. The colitis usually resolves with NSAID withdrawal, although steroids and sulfasalazine have been shown to have therapeutic potential. Relapse of quiescent inflammatory bowel disease, especially ulcerative colitis, has also been associated with NSAID use. NSAIDs reportedly cause segmental colonic ischemia, diverticular perforation or hemorrhage, proctitis, eosinophilic and collagenous colitis, and diaphragm-like strictures of the colon.

A variety of other drugs have been associated with colonic injury. Gold salts produce colitis, probably because of their local toxic effects. Isotretinoin, a vitamin A analog used in treating acne, causes acute colitis and may reactivate quiescent inflammatory bowel disease. Hemorrhagic colitis has been reported after use of ampicillin, amoxicillin, and erythromycin. Chemotherapeutic agents for treating cancer, such as cytosine arabinoside, methotrexate, cyclophosphamide, and 5-fluorouracil, may induce colonic injury. Methyldopa has been associated with colitis, and the antifungal agent, flucytosine, produces colonic inflammation that resembles ulcerative colitis. Sodium phosphate bowel preparations may cause focal colitis, which generally resolves spontaneously within 1 to 8 weeks.

Clinical Features, Diagnosis, and Management

Patients with NSAID-induced colonic injury present with diarrhea, occult or gross gastrointestinal bleeding, weight loss, and fever. Laboratory studies may show anemia, leukocytosis, or an elevated sedimentation rate. Colonoscopic findings include proctitis, patchy inflammation, thin strictures or membranes, focal ulcerations, and severe ulcerative pancolitis. Gold salt–induced colitis presents with bloody diarrhea, pain, tenesmus, fever, and leukocytosis. Colonoscopic findings may include ulceration and friability, most often in the rectosigmoid region, although the colitis may be diffuse. In most instances, withdrawing the offending medication leads to improvement in the drug-induced colitis. Some patients with gold salt–induced colitis require medical therapy with steroids, sulfasalazine, British anti-Lewisite, or oral cromolyn, and rarely, surgical resection.

COLONIC ULCERS

Isolated Nonspecific Colonic Ulcer

Etiology and Pathogenesis

Isolated nonspecific colonic ulcers are most often located in the cecum (67% of cases). Almost all lesions are found on the antimesenteric aspect of the lumen. The patient population exhibits a slight female predominance and a mean age of 45 at presentation. Most ulcers are round or oval and solitary (0.5 to 6.5 cm in diameter) and on histological examination, exhibit nonspecific inflammatory changes. The etiology of nonspecific ulcers is uncertain, although vascular factors, changes in local acid-base balance, foreign body trauma, infection, neurological stress, toxins, and medications (NSAIDs, corticosteroids, oral contraceptives) are possible causes.

Clinical Features, Diagnosis, and Management

The symptoms of nonspecific colonic ulcers include right lower quadrant abdominal pain, hematochezia, occult blood loss, perforation, abdominal mass, obstruction, fever, and leukocytosis. Colonoscopy is the diagnostic procedure of choice. CT scanning is useful for detecting perforation or abscess complications, whereas angiography may be needed to locate a briskly bleeding ulcer that cannot be seen by endoscopy. Conservative management is recommended for uncomplicated disease. Follow-up colonoscopy is recommended after 4 to 6 weeks to document healing. Surgery to oversew or excise an ulcer or right hemicolectomy is recommended for ulcer perforation, significant hemorrhage, or abscess formation.

Dieulafoy-type Colonic Ulcer

Etiology and Pathogenesis

Dieulafoy-type ulcers of the colon are rare. Similar to a gastric Dieulafoy ulcer, the lesion consists of a solitary mucosal defect with erosion of a submucosal large-caliber artery (Fig. 47-1). The cause of this disorder is unknown.

Clinical Features, Diagnosis, and Management

Patients present with massive painless hematochezia. Mesenteric angiography usually is necessary for diagnosis because the magnitude of hemorrhage precludes endoscopic visualization. Although surgical resection has been regarded as the

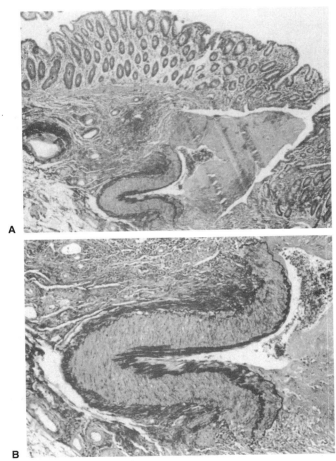

A

B

FIGURE 47-1. Dieulafoy-type ulcer of the colon. A: Low magnification shows a thick-walled, tortuous muscular artery just below the muscularis mucosa, with fresh ulceration overlying the artery at the site of bleeding. B: Higher magnification reveals details of the site of bleeding at the apex of the artery's curve toward the mucosa. (From Barbier P, Luder P, Triller J, et al. Colonic hemorrhage from a solitary minute ulcer. Report of three cases. *Gastroenterology* 1985;88:1065.)

definitive therapy, endoscopy is increasingly being used. Endoscopic methods include electrocoagulation and injection or heater probe thermocoagulation.

Stercoral Ulcer

Etiology and Pathogenesis

Colonic ulceration may result from ischemic pressure necrosis caused by a large stercoral (fecal) mass. Risk factors for stercoral ulceration include chronic constipation, confinement to a chronic care facility or nursing home, renal failure, transplantation, hypothyroidism, colonic strictures, foreign bodies, and use of constipating medications. Stercoral ulceration may lead to perforation, usually on the antimesenteric side of the lumen of the sigmoid or rectosigmoid colon, and peritonitis.

Clinical Features, Diagnosis, and Management

Affected patients have abdominal pain often accompanied by peritoneal signs. A palpable abdominal or rectal mass, rectal bleeding, and leukocytosis may also be present. Abdominal radiography may reveal pneumoperitoneum, marked fecal retention, and calcific fecaliths. Surgical resection is the definitive therapy for perforated and nonperforated stercoral ulcers. Resecting the perforation with an end colostomy and Hartmann pouch or mucous fistula have the lowest mortality rates of the surgical options.

Solitary Rectal Ulcer Syndrome

Etiology and Pathogenesis

Solitary rectal ulcer syndrome affects young adults; the mean age is 20 to 30. The endoscopic appearance is variable. The classic lesion consists of a single ulcer less than 5 cm in diameter on the anterior rectal wall, 6 to 10 cm proximal to the anal verge; however, there may be multiple ulcers, polypoid lesions, or a flat region of rectal erythema. Histological criteria for diagnosis include replacement of the lamina propria by fibroblasts, smooth muscle, and collagen, with associated hypertrophy and disorganization of the muscularis mucosae, erosion of the mucosa, displacement of the mucosal glands, and the presence of submucosal cystic glands. Proposed causes of solitary rectal ulcers include self-digitation, congenital rectal wall abnormalities, localized inflammatory bowel disease, or infection; however, a combination of rectal prolapse with high fecal voiding pressure that induces mucosal trauma or ischemia is the most likely etiology.

Clinical Features, Diagnosis, and Management

Patients present with constipation, tenesmus, incomplete evacuation, straining on defecation, lower abdominal pain, rectal bleeding, passing of mucus, fecal incontinence, and rectal prolapse. Patients with polypoid lesions may respond to bowel retraining, bulk laxatives, and reassurance. Antiinflammatory drugs such as salicylates, sucralfate, and corticosteroids have successfully treated solitary rectal ulcers. Surgery (i.e., abdominal rectopexy) is advised for patients with rectal prolapse who respond poorly to medical therapy. Rarely, more extensive resection or a diverting colostomy is needed.

Typhlitis

Etiology and Pathogenesis

Typhlitis, an acute necrotizing colitis primarily of the cecum, typically occurs in immunosuppressed patients with leukemia, but it also occurs in immunosuppressed patients undergoing cancer chemotherapy; in patients with drug-induced granulocytopenia, aplastic anemia, or periodic neutropenia; in renal transplant recipients or autologous bone marrow transplant recipients; and in persons with AIDS. Involved segments of the intestinal tract may exhibit ulcers, wall thickening, edema, hemorrhagic necrosis, and lumenal dilation. Histological findings include submucosal edema, mucosal necrosis without inflammation, and bacterial infiltration of small blood vessels. It has been proposed that typhlitis results from sequential destruction of the colon wall beginning with failure to maintain an intact epithelial barrier, followed by bacterial invasion and intramural proliferation, production of bacterial endotoxins, necrosis, hemorrhage, perforation, and sepsis.

Clinical Features, Diagnosis, and Management

Typhlitis must be considered in a febrile, neutropenic patient with abdominal pain, nausea, vomiting, distention, diarrhea, and associated stomatitis and pharyngitis. Peritoneal signs suggest perforation. Blood cultures positive for *Pseudomonas, Candida,* or other enteric organisms suggest sepsis. Abdominal radiographs may show a distended fluid-filled cecum, a dilated small intestine, diminished colonic gas, thumbprinting, a soft tissue mass, or cecal pneumatosis. CT scans reveal cecal thickening with pericecal fluid or a soft tissue mass. Ultrasound may show the target or halo sign of a solid mass with an echogenic center. Barium enema radiography and colonoscopy are relatively contraindicated because of the risk of perforation, but gentle sigmoidoscopy may be performed to exclude other forms of colitis. Medical therapy includes nasogastric suction, intravenous hydration, and broad-spectrum antibiotics that cover *Pseudomonas* organisms. Antimotility drugs should be avoided. Amphotericin B is added to the regimen to treat possible fungal infection if fever persists for more than 72 hours. Indications for surgery include free intraperitoneal perforation, severe hemorrhage, uncontrolled sepsis, and refractory disease. Regardless of therapy, typhlitis has a high mortality rate (40% to 50%). There is a high rate of recurrence during subsequent chemotherapy among patients who develop typhlitis during induction chemotherapy and who are medically treated.

COLITIS CYSTICA PROFUNDA

Etiology and Pathogenesis

Colitis cystica profunda is a benign disease characterized by large, submucosal, mucus-filled cysts, usually in the rectum. The lesions can be solitary or multiple in a localized, segmental, or diffuse distribution. The pathogenesis is not known. One theory describes a congenital origin related to a weakened muscularis mucosae, whereas other theories implicate inflammation and mucosal trauma. Colitis cystica profunda may be one manifestation of a spectrum of disease states, including solitary rectal ulcer syndrome and rectal prolapse. Localized disease is likely to be caused by ischemia secondary to trauma induced by rectal prolapse.

Clinical Features, Diagnosis, and Management

The mean age at presentation is 30. The most common symptoms include bloody or mucous rectal discharge, diarrhea, abdominal or rectal pain, tenesmus, and obstruction. Rectal examination may reveal palpable smooth masses, rectal wall thickening, and stenosis. Endoscopic findings include obvious cysts with overlying mucosa that may be normal, or they may show erythema, edema, friability, ulceration, mass effect, prolapse, or stricture. The lesions usually are located on the anterior rectal wall within 12 cm of the anal verge. Barium enema radiography may reveal thickened valves of Houston, an increased presacral space, filling defects, stricture, and prolapse. Definitive diagnosis is based on histological findings obtained by surgical excision. The findings include enlargement of the submucosa with benign cysts; replacement of the lamina propria with collagen and smooth muscle cells; and adjacent mucosal edema, ulceration, inflammation, pseudomembranes, and crypt distortion. Most cases follow a chronic, stable course. Although not a premalignant lesion, adenocarcinoma may be adjacent to areas of colitis cystica profunda. If symptoms are minimal, reassurance and dietary fiber supplementation are appropriate therapy. Local surgical and endoscopic procedures for more symptomatic patients (i.e., those with hemorrhage, obstruction, pain, and stenosis) include transanal cyst excision, posterior proctectomy, electrocautery, and injection sclerosis. Despite therapy, recurrence is common. Diverting colostomy is reserved for the most disabled patients.

PNEUMATOSIS CYSTOIDES INTESTINALIS

Etiology and Pathogenesis

Pneumatosis cystoides intestinalis is characterized by multiple, thin-walled, noncommunicating, gas-filled cysts that range in size from a few millimeters to several centimeters in the wall of the small intestine or colon. The cysts, which do not have an epithelial lining, contain hydrogen gas and are found in the submucosa or subserosa. Inflammation with neutrophils, eosinophils, plasma cells, lymphocytes, and epithelioid granulomas may be observed. The pathogenesis may be linked to the mechanical introduction of gas into the bowel wall, invasion of the bowel wall by gas-producing bacteria, and trapping of excess intralumenal gas produced by bacterial carbohydrate fermentation within the bowel wall. The condition is associated with chronic obstructive pulmonary disease, intestinal obstruction, rheumatologic disease (scleroderma), bowel infarction, pseudomembranous colitis, and necrotizing enterocolitis. The lesions may also be of iatrogenic origin after surgery or endoscopy.

Clinical Features, Diagnosis, and Management

Many patients with pneumatosis cystoides intestinalis are asymptomatic, and they are diagnosed after routine radiography or endoscopy. Symptomatic manifestations include diarrhea, abdominal discomfort, distention, hematochezia, mucus discharge, or weight loss. Complications include volvulus, pneumoperitoneum, obstruction, intussusception, tension pneumoperitoneum, hemorrhage, and perforation. Abdominal radiography may reveal linear or cystic bowel wall lucencies, pneumoperitoneum, or retroperitoneal air. CT scans are more sensitive than barium radiography in detecting intramural air and portal or mesenteric gas. The colonoscopic appearance of pneumatosis cystoides intestinalis consists of multiple, pale blue, rounded, soft masses. Cysts usually resolve with treatment of the underlying medical condition, but some patients benefit from high-flow oxygen or even hyperbaric oxygen therapy. Antibiotics (metronidazole, ampicillin) and elemental diets have been used to resolve cysts in some patients. Surgery is reserved for severe refractory symptoms or complications. Postoperative cyst recurrence is common.

MALAKOPLAKIA

Etiology and Pathogenesis

Malakoplakia is a granulomatous inflammatory disorder characterized by yellow, soft plaques or nodules (1 to 20 mm) on the mucosal surface anywhere in the gastrointestinal tract. The rectum, sigmoid colon, and descending colon are the most common sites of involvement; other organs that may be affected include the urinary tract, genitals, skin, lung, bone, and brain. A bimodal age distribution exists, with higher prevalence in children younger than 13 years and middle-aged adults. Predisposing conditions include chronic *Escherichia coli* infection, sarcoidosis, tuberculosis, immunosuppression, and hypogammaglobulinemia. Up to one half of patients have synchronous malignancies, including colorectal cancer in one third of patients. The pathogenesis may relate to a defect in the phagocytic or digestive activity of macrophages.

Clinical Features, Diagnosis, and Management

Patients may be asymptomatic, or they may have diarrhea, abdominal pain, rectal bleeding, obstruction, an intestinal mass, weight loss, or a fistula. The diagnosis is confirmed by biopsy, which reveals a diffuse histiocytic infiltrate with periodic acid–Schiff (PAS)-positive eosinophilic cytoplasm (von Hansemann cell) containing basophilic, laminated cytoplasmic calculospherules (Michaelis-Gutmann bodies). A patient with a diagnosis of malakoplakia should be evaluated for associated malignancy or infection. Localized disease can be excised or fulgurated, whereas diffuse involvement can be treated with antituberculosis medications, antibiotics (e.g., trimethoprim-sulfamethoxazole, ciprofloxacin), or cholinergic agonists (e.g., bethanechol).

CHAPTER 48

Colonic Polyps and Polyposis Syndromes

A *polyp* is any protrusion above the mucosal surface. Polyps of the colon are classified into three types: epithelial neoplastic, epithelial nonneoplastic, and submucosal (Table 48-1). The clinical significance of polyps relates both to their potential for malignant transformation in colorectal cancer and to the opportunity to decrease the incidence of colorectal cancer by removing polyps.

ADENOMATOUS POLYPS

Incidence and Epidemiology

Three fourths of the polyps detected by colonoscopy are adenomas. The prevalence of adenomas is subject to wide geographic variation, ranging from less than 5% in some areas of South America to more than 50% among Hawaiians of Japanese descent. The age-adjusted prevalence of polyps is 30% higher in men than in women,

TABLE 48-1
Classification of Colorectal Polyps

EPITHELIAL		SUBMUCOSAL
Neoplastic	*Nonneoplastic*	**SUBMUCOSAL**
Premalignant (adenomas)	**Mucosal**	Lymphoid Collection
Tubular	**Hyperplastic**	Pneumatosis cystoides
Tubulovillous	**Inflammatory**	intestinalis
Villous	Pseudopolyp	Colitis cystica profunda
Low-grade dysplasia		Lipoma
High-grade dysplasia	**Hamartoma**	Carcinoid
(intramucosal carcinoma)	Juvenile	Metastatic lesions
	Peutz-Jeghers	Leiomyoma
Malignant (carcinomas)	**Other**	Hemangioma
Carcinomatous		Fibroma
Malignant polyp		Endometriosis
		Other

and the prevalence increases with age. The overall prevalence of adenomas in the United States is about 40%.

Etiology and Pathogenesis

Histopathology

Adenomatous polyps are benign neoplasms that result from disordered cell proliferation and differentiation. In normal colonic crypts, proliferation is limited to cells in the lower third of the crypts. In adenomas, however, cell proliferation extends to the upper portion of the crypts. All adenomas exhibit varying degrees of dysplasia. The dysplasia is characterized by enlarged hyperchromatic nuclei; an increase in the number of mitotic cells; and a decrease in cellular mucin, cytoplasmic volume, stroma, and apoptosis. These features differentiate adenomas from hyperplastic polyps.

Nonpolypoid or flat adenomas are an important clinical condition that may represent an early phase of adenomas in the hereditary nonpolyposis colorectal cancer (HNPCC) syndrome. They have been identified in familial clusters and are characterized by localized dysplasia and minimal, if any, elevation of the mucosal surface. More than one third of flat adenomas have foci of high-grade dysplasia.

Adenoma-to-Carcinoma Sequence

The progression from adenoma to carcinoma is an accepted model of malignant transformation. Mutations in the adenomatous polyposis coli (*APC*) gene and DNA methylation appear to be early events that induce epithelial cell hyperproliferation. Subsequent mutations in the K-*ras* oncogene and deletions of the p53 and *DCC* (deleted in colon cancer) tumor suppressor genes result in an increase in cellular atypia and eventually in the development of malignancy. In general, the severity of polyp dysplasia correlates with the number of genetic alterations. In contrast to polyposis syndromes and sporadic colon cancer, the HNPCC, or Lynch, syndrome is based on mutations in a different molecular pathway. HNPCC develops from instability in microsatellite DNA sequences caused by defects in DNA mismatch repair. Instead of alterations of K-*ras*, *p53*, or *DCC*, germline mutations of *MLH2*, *MSH1*, *MSH6*, or *PMS2* are present.

Morphologic studies of adenomatous polyps support the adenoma-to-carcinoma model. Large adenomas often have small foci of adenocarcinomas, whereas small de novo carcinomas are rarely found. Moreover, the chance of finding adenocarcinoma increases with polyp size, greater degrees of cellular atypia, and higher proportions of villous architecture. Finally, studies confirm that removal of adenomatous polyps reduces the risk of colon cancer.

Risk Factors

Both genetic and environmental factors influence the risk of adenomas and colorectal cancer. Although hereditary factors play a primary role in cancer development in patients with familial adenomatous polyposis (FAP) and HNPCC, these disorders account for only a small minority of adenomas and colon cancers. Environmental factors associated with the risk of polyps and cancers include components of diet, exercise, and smoking. Epidemiologic studies show that a diet high in fat and low in fiber increases the risk of developing colonic adenomas and carcinoma. This may be due to the effects of dietary fats on increasing synthesis and delivery of bile acids to the colon, some of which have cancer-promoting properties. One exception to the proposed model implicating dietary fat is that fish oil intake inversely correlates with colorectal cancer incidence. Fermentation of ingested fiber releases short-chain fatty acids that may inhibit the development of neoplasia. Unfortunately, most prospective studies examining the independent effects of fiber supplementation or a low-fat diet do not show an associated decrease in adenoma incidence; however, a controlled trial of a low-fat diet combined with a wheat bran supplement conducted in Australia showed decreased adenoma incidence in the active arm. Other micronutrients such as vitamins A, C, beta carotene, and calcium have been shown to decrease the incidence of metachronous adenomas. Conversely, ingestion of heterocyclic amines (formed in high-temperature cooking) and *N*-nitroso compounds (derived from meat) are associated with increased cancer risk. Obesity and lack of physical exercise correlate with adenoma and colorectal cancer risk, perhaps from the trophic effects of obesity-related insulin resistance.

Development of colonic adenomas has been linked to several extraintestinal disorders. Patients with acromegaly have a twofold to sixfold increased risk of developing colonic adenomas, and current recommendations include colonoscopic surveillance of this population. An increased rate of adenomas and carcinomas occurs among patients who have undergone ureterosigmoidostomy. There is also an association between *Streptococcus bovis* infection and colon cancer, but this is likely due to mucosal disruption caused when the malignancy provides a portal of entry for the bacterium, rather than a carcinogenic effect of the organism. Other diseases that have inconsistently been associated with colonic adenomas include breast cancer, prior cholecystectomy, atherosclerosis, and diverticular disease.

Clinical Features

Adenomatous polyps generally do not cause symptoms unless they are larger than 1 cm; consequently most polyps are detected during screening examinations or during evaluation for symptoms unrelated to the polyps. When symptomatic, the most common manifestations include rectal bleeding (overt and occult), change in bowel habits, abdominal pain, and rectal prolapse. Polyps smaller than 1.5 cm rarely bleed. Large villous adenomas may be associated with a syndrome of profuse watery diarrhea and volume depletion. Polyps will occasionally autoamputate, which causes rectal bleeding. The physical examination of a patient with colonic adenomas is often unrevealing. Digital rectal examination may detect polyps in the distal 7 to 10 cm of the rectum.

Findings on Diagnostic Testing

Laboratory Studies

The results of laboratory studies usually are normal in patients with colonic adenomas. Intermittent bleeding from large polyps may produce a positive result on a fecal occult blood test or may lead to iron deficiency anemia. Large secreting villous adenomas may cause electrolyte abnormalities.

Endoscopic Studies

Colonoscopy is the procedure of choice if the clinical presentation suggests that a patient has a colonic polyp. Colonoscopy possesses the highest sensitivity and specificity of any diagnostic modality for detecting adenomatous polyps (95% and 99%, respectively), and it also allows for biopsy and removal of polyps, thereby fulfilling a therapeutic role. Tubular adenomas generally appear as smooth erythematous polyps on endoscopy. In contrast, villous adenomas have a lobular appearance, and they are large and often friable. However, it is not possible to reliably distinguish polyp histology by endoscopic appearance; thus biopsy or polypectomy is essential in establishing the histological subtype.

Histological Evaluation

Adenomas are classified by their dominant histology. Tubular adenomas are the most common (85%); tubulovillous adenomas (10%), villous adenomas (5%), and serrated adenomas (hyperplastic intermingled with adenomatous features, 1%) account for the remainder. The cellular atypia of any adenoma may be graded as mild, moderate, or severe. Severe focal atypia implies that a carcinomatous focus is present that does not interrupt the basement membrane. When malignant cells invade the basement membrane but do not penetrate the muscularis mucosae, the lesion is termed *intramucosal carcinoma*. In general, the risk of high-grade dysplasia or invasive adenocarcinoma correlates with the size of the polyp and the degree of villous architecture.

Radiographic Studies

Research shows that double-contrast barium enema radiography detects only 50% of colonic polyps with a specificity of 85%. Air insufflation enhances mucosal detail and exposes polyps, which appear as intralumenal protrusions coated with barium or as discrete rings with barium collected at their bases or along the stalks of pedunculated polyps. The rectosigmoid region is often difficult to visualize, even by experienced radiologists. Therefore, flexible or rigid sigmoidoscopy is necessary for complete evaluation of the colon. Barium enema radiography does not afford the capability to obtain histological specimens; thus colonoscopy is required when a barium study suggests the presence of a colonic polyp.

Management and Course

Natural History

Although colonic adenomas are premalignant lesions, the proportion that progresses to adenocarcinoma is unknown. Older literature reporting the long-term follow-up of patients with polyps that had been identified but not removed suggested that the risk of developing adenocarcinoma from a 1-cm polyp was 3% at 5 years, 8% at 10 years, and 24% at 20 years after diagnosis. Both the rate of growth and the malignant potential of individual polyps vary substantially. Serial examinations over several years illustrate that many polyps remain stable or even regress. The difference between the mean age at diagnosis of colonic adenoma and at diagnosis of adenocarcinoma leads to an estimate of the mean time of progression from adenoma to colorectal cancer of about 7 years. Other epidemiologic studies suggest that adenomatous polyps with severe atypia progress to cancer in an average of 4 years, whereas those manifesting mild atypia require 11 years to progress.

Therapy

Chemoprevention. NSAIDs including aspirin have been associated with reduced mortality from colorectal cancer. Several NSAIDs including sulindac and celecoxib have been shown to effectively decrease the incidence of recurrent adenomas in patients with FAP. Epidemiologic data show lower cancer risk among NSAID users at average risk of colorectal cancer; however, direct evidence supporting the use of aspirin and other NSAIDs to prevent sporadic colorectal cancer is lacking.

Endoscopy and surgery. Most adenomatous polyps can be removed by endoscopic polypectomy. Diminutive (<5 mm) polyps can be excised with cautery biopsy or bipolar electrocoagulation. Cautery biopsy enhances hemostasis and facilitates polyp obliteration, but residual adenomatous tissue may be left behind in up to 20% of cases. Occasionally, numerous diminutive polyps are encountered, particularly in the rectum, rendering endoscopic differentiation of adenomatous and hyperplastic polyps impossible. In this setting, several polyps should be sampled for histological examination, and polypectomy performed later if any of the polyps are adenomatous. In general, polyps larger than 5 mm in diameter and all pedunculated polyps should be excised with snare electrocautery. Most polyps can be completely removed in a single resection, and the intact polyp can be examined histologically to confirm the absence of adenomatous tissue at the resection margin. Large, broad-based, sessile polyps may require several sessions of saline injection with piecemeal snare resection.

Although all colonic adenomas have malignant potential, the decision to proceed with polypectomy is based on the patient's clinical status. As a general rule, patients with a life expectancy of 10 years or more should have adenomatous polyps removed. The risk is small for a diminutive polyp to progress to malignancy over a 3- to 5-year interval. Therefore, if patients have severe life-limiting illnesses or if endoscopic obliteration poses extreme risks, endoscopic removal of asymptomatic polyps can be deferred. Contraindications to colonoscopic polypectomy include severe coagulopathy, recent myocardial infarction, uncontrolled cardiopulmonary symptoms, pregnancy, abdominal perforation, and recent colonic surgery. In general, polypectomy is safe; the complication rate is less than 3%.

If endoscopic removal of large or multiple polyps is not possible, laser ablation, argon plasma coagulation, or surgical resection may be necessary. Nd:YAG laser ablation can effectively remove clusters of diminutive adenomatous polyps. However, the technique carries a 5% rate of hemorrhage or stenosis. Argon plasma coagulation is limited to a penetration depth of 3 to 5 mm; the complication rate is somewhat lower than that of laser techniques. Both ablative procedures preclude retrieval of the intact polyp for histological examination. The safe removal of large, sessile polyps sometimes requires surgery.

Principles of screening and surveillance programs. Most sporadic colorectal cancers (except in inflammatory bowel disease) derive from polyps. Controlled trials have shown that screening with fecal occult blood testing decreases mortality from colorectal cancer. Case-control studies of screening sigmoidoscopy have also shown mortality benefit. Screening colonoscopy appears to have the greatest potential to reduce the incidence of and mortality from colorectal cancer based on case-control and prospective cohort studies; however, randomized controlled trials confirming the mortality benefit of sigmoidoscopy or colonoscopy have yet to be completed. At this time, screening average-risk populations for the presence of adenomas and colorectal cancer is recommended, starting at age 50, and extending at least to age 80, or to such time that life expectancy is at least 10 years. The most efficacious or cost-effective strategy has not been defined; thus screening using annual fecal occult blood testing, sigmoidoscopy every 5 years, a combination of fecal occult blood testing and sigmoidoscopy, or colonoscopy every 10 years are equally advocated. Despite a paucity of evidence to support its use, barium enema radiography at 5- to 10-year intervals has also been recommended for screening.

Because synchronous polyps are common (50%) in patients with adenomatous polyps, a patient with a documented colonic adenoma should undergo a colonoscopic examination of the entire colon. Similarly, the prevalence of recurrent (metachronous) polyps warrants a surveillance program of follow-up colonoscopies to detect the development of new polyps before they progress to adenocarcinoma. The data from the National Polyp Study suggest that the recurrence rate for metachronous polyps is about 10% per year. Polyps with high-grade atypia and multiple polyps have a higher recurrence rate. Current recommendations advise surveillance colonoscopy every 3 years if three or more adenomas are removed. A 5-year interval is appropriate if one to two small (<1 cm diameter) polyps are found. More frequent surveillance is advised when there is doubt about the adequacy of the polyp resection, if the polyps removed contain high-grade dysplasia, or if the patient has multiple neoplasms.

Malignant polyps.   Colonic adenomas with severe atypia or noninvasive carcinoma do not metastasize because there are no lymphatic channels above the muscularis mucosae. These lesions are cured by colonoscopic polypectomy. The distinction between noninvasive and invasive carcinoma requires meticulous histological examination by an experienced pathologist. When malignant cells penetrate the muscularis mucosae, the polyp is considered an invasive carcinoma. In this case, the decision to perform colonoscopic resection only or surgical resection is based on the characteristics of the malignant polyp. Poor prognostic features include the presence of incomplete endoscopic resection, a poorly differentiated carcinoma, a carcinoma within 2 mm of the polypectomy margin, venous or lymphatic invasion, sessile (not pedunculated) morphology, or extension beyond the base of the polyp stalk (Table 48-2). Surgical resection of the underlying bowel is recommended if one or more of these features is present. Pedunculated polyps that can be completely resected and that lack all high-risk features may be treated with polypectomy alone. All patients with malignant polyps who are treated with

---

TABLE 48-2
Poor Prognostic Features of Malignant Polyps

Incomplete endoscopic resection
Poorly differentiated carcinoma
Cancer within 2 mm of polypectomy margins
Venous or lymphatic invasion
Sessile lesion
Cancer larger than one half of polyp volume
Large polyp (>2 cm)

polypectomy alone should have surveillance colonoscopy within 1 to 3 months and at 1 year.

NONADENOMATOUS POLYPS

Hyperplastic Polyps

Hyperplastic polyps are composed of elongated glands with epithelial infoldings and increased mucus, which give a serrated appearance to the mucosa. Cellular proliferation and differentiation are normal; thus, hyperplastic polyps are nonneoplastic and have no malignant potential. Hyperplastic polyps account for more than 15% of all polyps and for more than half of the diminutive polyps reported in case series. They appear by endoscopy as small, sessile protrusions of pale epithelium and usually are found in the rectum. Hyperplastic polyps rarely exceed 1 cm and are almost universally asymptomatic. Some studies have suggested that patients with hyperplastic polyps have a higher incidence of adenomatous polyps, but this association remains controversial. Although no treatment or surveillance is recommended for hyperplastic polyps, they are often removed because it is difficult to distinguish them visually from adenomatous polyps.

Inflammatory Polyps

Chronic inflammatory conditions of the colon can induce the formation of two types of mucosal polyps. Pseudopolyps are islands of residual intact colonic mucosa surrounded by excavated or denuded mucosa. Inflammatory polyps are areas of regenerating mucosa and granulation tissue that form in response to chronic inflammation. These polyps are common in inflammatory bowel disease but are also associated with amebiasis, strongyloidiasis, tuberculosis, schistosomiasis (polyps harbor eggs or adult worms), solitary rectal ulcer syndrome, ischemic colitis, and diverticular disease. Inflammatory polyps may become large and pedunculated, and occasionally they may produce symptoms of hemorrhage or obstruction. The major challenge in diagnosing inflammatory polyps is to differentiate them from adenomatous polyps. This is particularly important in inflammatory bowel disease, given the high risk of colonic adenocarcinoma with long-standing ulcerative colitis. If a patient with ulcerative colitis has numerous polyps, biopsy specimens of several should be obtained to exclude adenomatous changes before labeling them as pseudopolyps.

Juvenile Polyps

Juvenile polyps, or retention polyps, most commonly occur in children between the ages of 1 and 10 years, but occasionally they are observed in adults. They have been reported in 2% of asymptomatic children and in 30% of children examined for symptoms of rectal bleeding. Juvenile polyps account for 97% of all polyps found in children younger than 15 years. The most common presenting symptom is hematochezia, which results from spontaneous sloughing of the polyp. Prolapse of the polyp through the rectum may also occur. On colonoscopy, juvenile polyps appear as single, pedunculated, smooth, cherry-red polyps. They often are friable or ulcerated. The histological appearance of a juvenile polyp is that of a hamartoma with distended, mucin-filled cystic glands, edematous lamina propria, and prominent vasculature. Isolated juvenile polyps have no malignant potential; however, familial juvenile polyposis is associated with an increased risk of adenomas and carcinomas of the gastrointestinal tract. Three genes, *PTEN, SMAD4/DPC4,* and *BMPR1A,* are associated with familial juvenile polyposis.

Submucosal Masses

Because polyps represent intralumenal projections of mucosa, any submucosal mass may mimic a mucosal polyp. Lymphoid hyperplasia in the lamina propria is characterized by discrete, white polypoid lesions smaller than 5 mm. Diffuse nodular lymphoid hyperplasia (submucosal lymphoid follicles) appears as diffuse polyposis, but biopsy specimens reveal normal mucosa or focal submucosal lymphocyte collections. In most cases, lymphoid hyperplasia is found incidentally, and no specific treatment is necessary.

Pneumatosis cystoides intestinalis is characterized by multiple air-filled cystic structures within the submucosa of the colon or small intestine. The air-filled cysts appear as multiple polypoid lesions by endoscopy and are easily distinguished from solid lesions by radiography. Most patients with pneumatosis intestinalis are asymptomatic; however, these lesions can be associated with ischemia, necrotizing enterocolitis, infarction, and pneumoperitoneum, and consequently patients may present with symptoms appropriate for these disorders.

Lipomas may appear as submucosal masses, most commonly in the right colon near the ileocecal valve. Superficial lipomas have a distinctive yellow appearance. Other less common benign lesions include fibromas, neurofibromas, leiomyomas, myoblastomas, hemangiomas (such as the blue rubber bleb nevus syndrome), and endometriosis. The colon is rarely the site of metastasis for malignant submucosal lesions, including melanoma, lymphoma, Kaposi sarcoma, adenocarcinomas, plasma cell leukemia, and malignant carcinoids.

FAMILIAL ADENOMATOUS POLYPOSIS

Incidence and Epidemiology

Familial adenomatous polyposis (FAP), also known as adenomatous polyposis coli (APC) or familial polyposis coli, is an autosomal dominant disease characterized by the early onset of hundreds or thousands of intestinal polyps with an inevitable progression to colon cancer (Table 48-3). Three adenomatous polyposis syndromes are variants of FAP: Gardner syndrome, attenuated adenomatous polyposis coli (attenuated FAP), and Turcot syndrome. Gardner syndrome is characterized by polyposis and extraintestinal benign tumors, including osteomas, desmoids, and epidermoid cysts. Attenuated FAP is a less aggressive form of FAP. Turcot syndrome is characterized by colonic polyposis and central nervous system malignancies.

About 0.07% to 0.5% of all colon carcinomas are associated with FAP. Worldwide, the prevalence of FAP ranges from 1 in 7000 to 1 in 30,000 persons. There is no gender preference and little geographic variation. Adenomatous polyps develop in adolescence or young adulthood, and colonic adenocarcinoma develops at a mean age of 39. In attenuated FAP, the age of presentation is about 10 years later.

Etiology and Pathogenesis

FAP results from a germline mutation of the *APC* gene, which has been localized to chromosome 5. The APC protein controls cell growth through the Wingless and Wnt signaling pathway mediated by β-catenin. In FAP, the normal degradation of

TABLE 48-3
Polyposis Syndromes

SYNDROME	GENE MUTATION	RISK FOR COLORECTAL CANCER	HISTOLOGY	DISTRIBUTION	EXTRAINTESTINAL FEATURES
Familial adenomatous polyposis	APC (regulator of Wnt signaling)	100%	Adenomatous	Stomach, small intestine, colon	Desmoid tumors, epidermoid cysts, fibromas, osteomas, CHRPE, dental abnormalities
Peutz-Jeghers syndrome	STK11 (LKB1) (regulator of apoptosis through p53)	39%	Hamartomatous	Stomach, small intestine, colon	Orocutaneous melanin pigment, other malignancies (pancreatic, breast, ovarian, uterine, lung)
Juvenile polyposis	SMAD4 (DPC4), BMPR1A (regulators of TGF-beta signaling)	9%–68%	Hamartomatous	Stomach, small intestine, colon	Macrocephaly, hypertelorism
Cowden syndrome	PTEN (regulator of cell cycling, translation, and apoptosis)	Minimal	Juvenile, lipoma, inflammatory, ganglioneuroma, lymphoid hyperplasia	Esophagus, stomach, small intestine, colon	Facial trichilemmomas, oral papillomas, multinodular goiter, fibrocystic breast, other malignancies (thyroid, breast, uterine)
Hereditary mixed polyposis syndrome	chromosome 6	Unknown	Atypical juvenile, adenomatous, hyperplastic	Colon	None
Gorlin syndrome	PTCH (regulator of TGF-beta and Wnt signaling)	Unknown	Hamartoma	Gastric	Mandibular bone cysts, pits of palms and soles, macrocephaly, basal cell carcinoma

CHRPE, congenital hypertrophy of the retinal pigment epithelium.

β-catenin is disrupted, which results in upregulation of numerous genes, including c-*myc*, cyclin D1, matrilysin, c-*jun*, *FOSL1* (fos-like antigen 1), *PLAUR* (plasminogen activator receptor, urokinase-type), and *PPARD* (peroxisome proliferator–activated receptor–delta), leading to cell growth and suppression of apoptosis. In addition, the APC protein itself appears to bind to microtubules, which may directly interfere with normal cellular migration through the crypt.

The colonic epithelium in patients with FAP is characterized by increased proliferation along the crypts, which increases the susceptibility to subsequent mutations or deletions of genes such as K-*ras*, *p53*, and *DCC* that are critical in neoplastic transformation and carcinogenesis in both FAP as well as in sporadic colorectal cancers. One third of FAP cases appear to be the result of a new, spontaneous *APC* mutation. The colonic polyps in FAP are primarily tubular adenomas, sometimes so numerous that they carpet the entire colon. Histologically, adenomas in FAP are indistinguishable from sporadic tubular adenomas. Microadenomas, which are foci of adenomatous epithelium within a single crypt, are a distinctive feature of FAP.

The mutations in Gardner syndrome are identical to those in FAP, although other genetic alterations may be responsible for development of mesenchymal tumors in this syndrome. Most patients with Turcot syndrome also have truncating mutations of the *APC* gene. Turcot syndrome appears to be genetically heterogeneous, however, some patients have mutations in the genes responsible for HNPCC as their primary germline defect.

Clinical Features

Gastrointestinal Polyposis

Patients with FAP usually develop adenomatous polyps in adolescence or young adulthood, but colonic adenomas have been reported as early as age 4 and as late as age 40. Polyps often carpet the colon and number in the hundreds to thousands, but they rarely produce symptoms until late in the course of disease. Patients not previously identified as having FAP may present with rectal bleeding, diarrhea, and abdominal pain in the third and fourth decades, at which time they likely harbor colon cancer. Cancer is diagnosed at the mean age of 39, and more than 90% of patients develop cancer by age 50. Patients with attenuated FAP often have fewer polyps, and the onset of adenomas and progression to adenocarcinoma is delayed by 10 years. Differentiating these patients from patients with HNPCC may be difficult, but the presence of duodenal polyps or extraintestinal features of FAP may be helpful clues.

Gastric polyps are present in 23% to 100% of patients with FAP. If present, they usually are numerous, asymptomatic, located in the proximal fundus or body, and have a hamartomatous (nonneoplastic, fundic gland) histology. Adenomatous polyps of the stomach occur in 10% of patients with FAP, usually in the antrum but occasionally in the body or fundus.

Duodenal polyps occur in 50% to 90% of patients with FAP, and in contrast to gastric polyps, they usually are adenomatous. These polyps tend to be multiple, developing in the periampullary region, where they may rarely cause biliary obstruction or pancreatitis. The lifetime risk of developing cancer from duodenal adenomas is 3% to 5%. Cancer develops most commonly in the periampullary region and is one of the most common causes of death in patients with FAP who have undergone prophylactic colectomy. Adenomas may also develop in the jejunum (50%) and ileum (20%), but malignant transformation is rare.

Extraintestinal Manifestations

Gardner syndrome is a subtype of FAP with characteristic extraintestinal manifestations. Desmoid tumors are benign mesenchymal neoplasms that occur throughout the body but frequently in the mesentery and other intra-abdominal regions. These masses may infiltrate adjacent structures or compress adjacent visceral organs or blood vessels, producing abdominal pain. Abdominal examination may demonstrate a mass lesion. Osteomas are benign bony growths that occur throughout the skeletal system but most commonly involve the skull and mandible. They have no malignant potential and generally do not cause symptoms. Dental abnormalities include dental cysts, unerupted teeth, supernumerary teeth, and odontomas. These lesions are benign and generally cause no symptoms.

Cutaneous lesions associated with FAP include epidermoid cysts, sebaceous cysts, fibromas, and lipomas. Epidermoid cysts are located on the extremities, face, and scalp. Fibromas most commonly occur on the scalp, shoulders, arms, and back. Infected cysts may cause symptoms.

Congenital hypertrophy of the retinal pigment epithelium (CHRPE), or pigmented ocular fundus lesions, affects 60% to 85% of patients with FAP. This retinal abnormality is characterized by hamartomas of the retinal epithelium, which appear as multiple, discrete, round or oval areas of hyperpigmentation. Although the pathogenesis of CHRPE remains unknown, the presence of multiple lesions in both eyes is essentially pathognomonic for FAP.

Turcot syndrome is characterized by adenomatous polyposis in association with central nervous system malignancies, such as medulloblastomas, astrocytomas, and ependymomas, which usually manifest within the first two decades of life. Neurological surveillance may be indicated for persons at risk of developing FAP, especially in families with Turcot syndrome. Two thirds of persons with Turcot syndrome have *APC* mutations, but the remaining one third appears to have a variant of HNPCC. Cerebellar medulloblastoma develops in persons with the HNPCC-like form at a rate 90 times higher than that in the general population.

Findings on Diagnostic Testing

Screening and Surveillance

Genetic testing for FAP is performed to confirm a suspected diagnosis of FAP, to identify the mutation in a patient with known FAP, and to screen relatives of a proband with established FAP. The laboratory methods include protein truncation testing, which identifies truncated APC protein in vitro, DNA sequencing, and linkage testing, which uses DNA markers to track the segregation of proposed mutations through affected families. Children who carry mutated genes should be screened by endoscopy. Because polyps are distributed throughout the colon in FAP, flexible sigmoidoscopy is considered an adequate screening procedure. Screening should begin at age 10 to 12 and continue every 1 to 2 years until age 35. After that, the examination interval can be increased to 3 years. If genetic testing is unsuccessful or unavailable, all relatives should be screened by endoscopy. If the diagnosis of FAP is established, patients should be screened every 1 to 3 years for synchronous duodenal adenomatous polyps, supplementing a forward-viewing endoscope with a side-viewing duodenoscope to assess the periampullary region.

Relatives of a proband with attenuated FAP require screening by colonoscopy because this syndrome produces fewer polyps that may spare the colon examined by sigmoidoscopy. Screening for these persons should be initiated at an age 10 years younger than the earliest age at which colon cancer is diagnosed within the family.

Radiographic Studies

Radiological tests are not recommended for imaging the colon of patients with suspected FAP. However, bone radiography may be required to document the sclerotic lesions characteristic of osteomas to establish a diagnosis of Gardner syndrome. Patients with Gardner syndrome who complain of abdominal pain or in whom a palpable mass is detected are best examined by computed tomographic (CT) scanning to evaluate for intra-abdominal desmoid tumors. CT or magnetic resonance imaging scans of the brain can identify malignancies in the central nervous system of patients with Turcot syndrome.

Management and Course

Therapy for Colonic Polyposis

Patients with FAP may initially have only a few polyps, but the number and size of adenomas gradually increase over several years. Left untreated, patients with FAP invariably develop colon adenocarcinoma at a mean age of 39, and more than 90% develop cancer by age 50. After the diagnosis of FAP is established, elective surgery to remove the colon is recommended. Sulindac, which promotes polyp regression in a subset of patients, may be useful if surgery is delayed. Before surgery, all patients should undergo colonoscopy to survey the colon for gross evidence of malignancy. In addition, upper gastrointestinal endoscopy with a side-viewing duodenoscope and barium radiography of the small intestine should be performed to exclude concurrent malignancy in the small intestine and to remove accessible small polyps.

The surgical options for FAP include total proctocolectomy with ileostomy, total colectomy with ileal pouch–anal canal anastomosis, and subtotal colectomy with ileorectal anastomosis. In the last procedure, the rectal stump remains at risk of developing adenomatous polyps and cancer, and surveillance sigmoidoscopy is required every 3 to 6 months. Sulindac may slow the progression of adenomatous polyps in the retained rectal mucosal segment but does not obviate the need for surveillance and endoscopic ablation of incident rectal adenomas. Up to 30% of patients who undergo subtotal colectomy eventually require completion of the rectal resection because of the inability to control polyps or to prevent progression to cancer. This has prompted many clinicians to consider a continence-sparing colectomy with ileal pouch–anal canal anastomosis as the procedure of choice.

Therapy for Duodenal Neoplasms

Progression of duodenal adenoma to adenocarcinoma, particularly periampullary cancer, occurs in 3% to 5% of patients with FAP, usually at an age later than colonic malignancy (mean age at diagnosis is between 45 and 52). The optimal treatment for adenomatous duodenal polyps is undefined. Large villous adenomas should be considered for surgical resection, given the high risk for coexisting malignancy. Smaller tubular adenomas can be treated safely with endoscopic ablation, and successful ablation of papillary adenomas has been reported. It is not known if sulindac alters the natural course of duodenal adenomas.

Therapy for Extraintestinal Manifestations

Occasionally, extraintestinal tumors are a source of symptoms in patients with FAP. Desmoid tumors in Gardner syndrome invade or compress blood vessels, nerves, and hollow viscera, and account for 10% of deaths in FAP. Patients with small asymptomatic lesions should be observed, but patients with enlarging or symptomatic desmoids should be given tamoxifen or sulindac. Failure of this conservative treatment may necessitate chemotherapy, radiation therapy, or surgery.

HAMARTOMATOUS POLYPOSIS SYNDROMES

Peutz-Jeghers Syndrome

Etiology and Pathogenesis

Peutz-Jeghers syndrome is an uncommon autosomal dominant disorder characterized by intestinal hamartomatous polyposis and mucocutaneous pigmentation. The prevalence is estimated at 1 in 120,000 persons. The mucocutaneous lesions consist of brown or black melanin spots 1 to 5 mm in diameter that involve mainly the perioral and buccal areas, but also occur on the face, palms, soles, and digits, and rarely on the intestinal mucosa. There is an elevated risk of gastrointestinal and extraintestinal malignancies, including breast, cervical, and ovarian tumors in females; testicular tumors in males; and pancreatic tumors in both sexes. Almost all women with Peutz-Jeghers syndrome have benign ovarian tumors.

Clinical Features, Diagnosis, and Management

In contrast to the polyps in FAP, polyps in Peutz-Jeghers syndrome are hamartomatous and fewer in number (10 to 20). They usually appear in the first decade of life and are found in the stomach, small intestine, and colon. Large polyps, which usually do not manifest until young adulthood, may cause symptoms of hemorrhage or intestinal obstruction. The distinctive histological appearance of a Peutz-Jeghers polyp is that of branching glands of normal epithelium surrounded by smooth muscle.

A small percentage of Peutz-Jeghers polyps follows an adenomatous progression, thus raising the risk of gastrointestinal malignancies. For this reason, a person with Peutz-Jeghers syndrome should have a screening colonoscopy every 3 years beginning at age 25. Because of the risk of gastric and small intestinal malignant transformation, upper gastrointestinal endoscopy and small intestinal radiography are recommended every 2 years beginning at age 10. In addition, endoscopic or abdominal ultrasonography to screen for pancreatic malignancy is suggested every 1 to 2 years, starting at age 30. Endoscopic removal of all gastric, duodenal, and colonic polyps is recommended. Small intestinal polyps that are not accessible to endoscopic therapy should be observed until they are symptomatic or larger than 1.5 cm in diameter, at which time surgical removal is suggested. In addition to screening for gastrointestinal malignancies, breast or testicular examinations should be performed routinely.

Juvenile Polyposis

Etiology and Pathogenesis

Juvenile polyposis is a rare disorder that is transmitted as an autosomal dominant trait. Diagnosis is confirmed by any of the following criteria: (1) at least 5 juvenile polyps in the colon or rectum, (2) juvenile polyps throughout the gastrointestinal tract, or (3) any number of juvenile polyps in a person with a known family history of juvenile polyps. Other inherited syndromes with juvenile polyps such as Cowden disease, Bannayan-Riley-Ruvalcaba syndrome, and Gorlin syndrome should be ruled out. The prevalence of juvenile polyposis is about 1 in 100,000 persons.

Clinical Features, Diagnosis, and Management

Colonic polyps are most common, but polyps may occur throughout the gastrointestinal tract. Symptoms usually develop in the first two decades of life and include hematochezia, abdominal pain, intussusception, and even passage of polyp tissue with bowel movements. Although hamartomas are not believed to possess malignant potential, juvenile polyposis, especially in the familial form, appears to undergo adenomatous transformation thereby resulting in increased cancer risk. The estimated incidence of colonic adenocarcinoma varies widely to include 9% to 68% of persons with juvenile polyposis with a mean age of 34 at diagnosis. In addition to colorectal cancer, juvenile polyposis is associated with increased risk of gastric, duodenal, pancreatic, and biliary malignancy. Juvenile polyposis is also associated with congenital anomalies, including macrocephaly and hypertelorism.

Genetic testing for *PTEN*, *SMAD4/DPC4*, and *BMPR1A* is available and recommended for juvenile polyposis, especially for the familial form. Upper gastrointestinal endoscopy and colonoscopy should be performed in persons who carry the mutation (and in relatives if isolation of the mutation in the proband fails), beginning in the late teenage years and earlier if symptoms develop. These tests should be repeated at 3-year intervals. Barium radiography of the small intestine may also be used to identify lesions beyond the reach of endoscopic instruments. Colonoscopic polypectomy can remove a small number of polyps, but unlike sporadic juvenile polyps, the polyps in juvenile polyposis often recur. When the number of polyps exceeds 10 to 20, a colectomy should be considered. The increased awareness of the risk of cancer in patients with juvenile polyposis has made prophylactic colectomy a viable alternative to long-term endoscopic surveillance.

Cowden Disease

Cowden disease, or multiple hamartoma syndrome, is an autosomal dominant condition characterized by diffuse hamartomas of the skin, gastrointestinal tract, and mucous membranes. Hamartomas are found in the esophagus, stomach, duodenum, and colon. The cardinal feature of the condition is multiple facial trichilemmomas, which are keratotic papules that appear in adolescence. Additional extraintestinal manifestations include verrucous lesions of the face and limbs, papillomatosis of the gingival and buccal mucosa, and hyperkeratotic papules involving the hands and feet. Unlike other polyposis syndromes, these polyps rarely cause symptoms and do not increase the risk of gastrointestinal malignancy. However, patients with Cowden disease have an increased incidence of breast, thyroid, and endometrial malignancies.

Bannayan-Riley-Ruvalcaba Syndrome

This syndrome is characterized by macrocephaly, delayed psychomotor development, lipomatosis, hemangiomatosis, pigmented macules of the glans penis, and intestinal juvenile polyps. Both Bannayan-Riley-Ruvalcaba syndrome and Cowden disease are believed to be derived from mutations in the *PTEN* gene.

Gorlin Syndrome

Nevoid basal cell carcinoma syndrome, or Gorlin syndrome, is an autosomal dominant disorder. The prevalence is about 1 in 55,600 persons, and it is caused by mutations of the *PTCH* gene on chromosome 9q. Manifestations include multiple basal cell carcinomas, mandibular bone cysts, pits in the skin of the palms and soles, intracranial calcification, large head circumference, and congenital skeletal anomalies. Gastrointestinal findings include gastric hamartomas.

ACQUIRED POLYPOSIS SYNDROMES

Cronkhite-Canada Syndrome

Etiology and Pathogenesis

Cronkhite-Canada syndrome is a rare noninherited disorder characterized by generalized gastrointestinal juvenile polyposis, cutaneous hyperpigmentation, hair loss, and nail atrophy. Hundreds of polyps may develop in the stomach, small intestine, and colon. Adenomatous transformation may occur, resulting in an increased risk of colon cancer. About 12% to 15% of persons with Cronkhite-Canada syndrome eventually develop colon cancer.

Clinical Features, Diagnosis, and Management

Signs include cutaneous hyperpigmentation, hair loss, onychodystrophy, gastrointestinal hemorrhage, and skin changes. The hyperpigmentation consists of dark brown macules that range in size from 2 mm to 10 cm in diameter and occur over the extremities, face, palms and soles, back and chest, and scalp. Hypogeusia may be a dominant symptom. Diarrhea and weight loss may develop as a result of a protein-losing enteropathy caused by excess mucous secretion by crypt cells. The prognosis of Cronkhite-Canada syndrome is variable. Some patients progress rapidly to death, usually because of complications of malnutrition, whereas others experience spontaneous remission. Case reports have suggested that clinical improvement may result from administration of corticosteroids, antibiotics, and total parenteral nutrition. Surgery may be necessary to treat complications of bleeding, malignancy, intussusception, or protein-losing enteropathy. Colonoscopic surveillance is recommended to evaluate for adenomatous changes and colon cancer.

Hyperplastic Polyposis Syndrome

There are case reports of patients with hundreds of hyperplastic polyps throughout the colon, a condition that mimics FAP. These patients can be treated conservatively with periodic colonoscopy to exclude adenomas and to remove larger lesions.

CHAPTER 49

Malignant Tumors of the Colon

ADENOCARCINOMA

Incidence and Epidemiology

Colorectal cancer is the second leading cause of death from cancer in the United States. More than 150,000 cases of colorectal cancer are diagnosed annually in the United States, resulting in nearly 60,000 deaths per year. Geographic variation in the global incidence of colorectal cancer is considerable; the United States and Eastern and Northern Europe have a higher incidence than developing countries. Environmental factors are likely to play a major role in this variation because emigrants to a high-risk region develop cancer at the rate of their new location, even though their country of origin was a low-risk region. Although specific gene mutations have been identified for both sporadic and familial development of colorectal cancer, dietary patterns associated with increased risk have also been confirmed.

Etiology and Pathogenesis
Environmental Factors

Micronutrient and macronutrient dietary constituents are associated with the risk of colorectal cancer. Epidemiologic studies show that animal fats, particularly from red meat sources, contribute to an increased risk of developing colon cancer. Animal models used to study the pathogenesis of this association show that high-fat intake increases colonocyte proliferation and tumor formation. This cell transformation appears to be mediated by increased colonic concentrations of bile acids, which are known cancer promoters. In addition, populations with low fiber intake have an increased incidence of colon cancer. Frequent ethanol use may produce a two-to threefold increase in colon cancer. In contrast, societies in which the dietary intake of marine fish is high have markedly lower rates of colorectal cancer. Higher levels of dietary folate are also associated with lower risk for colon cancer. Although the antioxidant vitamins A, E, and C have been postulated to lower the risk for malignancy, a large prospective placebo-controlled trial failed to detect a decrease in the incidence of recurrent adenomatous polyps among patients treated with supplements of these vitamins.

Genetic Factors

Many inherited disorders are associated with increased risk for colonic adenocarcinoma, including the polyposis syndromes discussed in Chapter 48. However, the polyposis syndromes account for less than 1% of all colorectal cancers, whereas hereditary nonpolyposis colorectal cancer (HNPCC, or Lynch syndrome) accounts for 2% to 3% of colorectal cancers. Colorectal cancer develops as a result of genetic alterations at loci involved in the control of cell growth. The progression from normal colonocytes to adenomatous tissue and finally to colon carcinoma involves a stepwise accumulation of mutations, each of which provides a growth advantage to affected cells. Two different pathways leading to genomic instability result in colorectal cancer: *chromosomal instability* (loss of heterozygosity) and *microsatellite instability*. Most colon cancers stem from the former, which involves an uneven distribution of genetic material among daughter cells, resulting in aneuploidy. Microsatellite instability is caused by the loss of DNA mismatch repair activity and is the mechanism for cancer development in HNPCC.

Chromosomal instability. The initial events in colorectal cancer development appear to involve somatic mutations in the adenomatous polyposis coli (APC) gene. Alteration of *APC* is a key to the formation of both sporadic and familial colorectal cancers such as familial adenomatous polyposis. The *APC* gene regulates cell death and mutation of this gene, provides increased proliferative capacity to affected cells, and leads to the formation of adenomas. Subsequent mutations in the K-*ras* cellular protooncogene, which occur in most large colonic adenomas, lead to further growth dysregulation. The transition from adenoma to carcinoma appears to be the result of mutation of the tumor suppressor gene *p53*. The protein product of the *p53* gene normally halts cellular proliferation in cells with damaged DNA. Mutations of *p53* result in uninhibited replication of cells with damaged DNA, permitting these cells to accumulate even more severe genetic damage. Replication of these defective cells can result in loss of chromosomal segments containing several alleles (i.e., loss of heterozygosity). This can lead to deletions of other tumor suppressor genes, including *DCC* (deleted in colon cancer), a late event in the transformation to malignancy. Eventually, the cells acquire the capability to invade, or metastasize, at which point the neoplasm is considered malignant. Colonic malignancies need not contain all of these mutations, and there are likely to be other genetic alterations vital to carcinogenesis that have not been discovered. However, this sequential mutation model of carcinogenesis does provide a conceptual framework for understanding the final common pathway leading to colorectal cancer.

Microsatellite instability and hereditary nonpolyposis colorectal cancer. HNPCC is an autosomal dominant disorder characterized by the occurrence, within a family, of multiple cases of colorectal cancer in the absence of polyposis. As opposed to sporadic colorectal cancers, in which losses, gains, and structural rearrangements of chromosomes occur (i.e., chromosomal instability), HNPCC results from microsatellite instability whereby mutations in mismatch repair genes, which normally correct errors in DNA replication, result in cancer formation. Protein products of mismatch repair genes recognize and repair DNA replication errors in postmitotic cells. Cells without mismatch repair activity accumulate random mutations and therefore are more likely to acquire mutations responsible for carcinogenesis. Because all colonic cells of affected persons have one intact copy of the gene, a second somatic mutation of this gene is required before mismatch repair function is lost. This "second hit" mechanism explains the absence of polyposis in HNPCC because damage to both alleles occurs in only a small portion of colonic cells. To date, five mismatch repair genes have been identified (*hMSH2*, *hMLH1*, *hPMS1*, *hPMS2*, and *hMSH6*). HNPCC is distinguished from sporadic colorectal cancer by the early onset of colorectal cancer (mean age at diagnosis is 40), a higher risk for synchronous tumors (18% versus 6%), right-sided tumors (60% to 80% versus 25%), and more frequent mucinous tumors (35% versus 20%). HNPCC is divided into two variants: Lynch syndromes I and II. Lynch syndrome I is isolated, early-onset colorectal cancer, whereas Lynch syndrome II manifests as the early occurrence of carcinoma at other sites as well (e.g., endometrium, ovaries, genitourinary tract, stomach, and small intestine).

Additional genetic factors.   There are familial factors that increase susceptibility to colorectal cancer that are not transmitted in a standard Mendelian pattern. A history of colorectal cancer in a first-degree relative increases the risk of colorectal cancer (age-adjusted relative risk (RR) 1.72; 95% CI 1.34 to 2.19). This effect is amplified if the affected relative is age 45 or younger (RR 5.37; 95% CI 1.98 to 14.6) or if there are multiple affected family members (RR 2.75; 95% CI 1.34 to 5.63). Identification of the genetic factors responsible for this familial risk may further clarify the molecular mechanisms of carcinogenesis. Parents and siblings of patients with adenomatous polyps are also at increased risk of colorectal cancer (RR 1.78; 95% CI 1.18 to 2.67), and if a patient has both a parent with colorectal cancer and a sibling with adenomatous polyps, the risk is even greater (RR 3.25; 95% CI 1.92 to 5.52).

Diseases Associated with Increased Risk of Colorectal Cancer

Several clinical disorders have been associated with an increased risk of colonic adenocarcinoma. Inflammatory bowel disease, particularly ulcerative colitis, is associated with an increased incidence of colorectal cancer. The risk of cancer depends on the duration and extent of disease. The risk of developing cancer increases by about 1% per year 8 to 10 years after diagnosis of ulcerative pancolitis. Patients with proctitis, left-sided ulcerative colitis, or Crohn's disease that does not involve the entire colon have a lower risk. Patients with pelvic irradiation for cervical cancer or ureterosigmoidostomy for bladder cancer have increased risks of developing colon adenocarcinoma, although the onset may be delayed by decades. Other clinical conditions associated with colon cancer include group D *Streptococcus* bacteremia, infection with *Schistosoma haematobium*, and acromegaly.

Adenoma-to-Carcinoma Sequence

Epidemiologic evidence supports the model of an adenoma-to-carcinoma sequence. The mean age at diagnosis of adenomatous polyps is 7 years younger than the mean age at diagnosis of colonic adenocarcinoma. In addition, the prevalence of colorectal cancer in populations correlates well with the prevalence of adenomatous polyps. Pathological analyses of surgically excised colorectal carcinomas often reveal adjacent adenomatous tissue, and larger colorectal adenomas often exhibit cellular atypia with microscopic foci of invasive carcinoma. Finally, the most convincing evidence that adenocarcinomas arise from adenomas comes from the National Polyp Study, which confirms that removal of adenomatous polyps lowers the incidence of colorectal malignancy.

Clinical Features

Most colorectal cancers are diagnosed in patients older than age 50. Colorectal cancer generally grows slowly, and symptoms or signs are due to complications of obstruction, hemorrhage, local invasion, or cancer cachexia. Colonic obstruction develops most commonly in the transverse, descending, and sigmoid colons where lumenal diameters are smaller than the proximal colon. Incomplete colonic obstruction may present initially with intermittent abdominal pain. However, as obstruction becomes complete, nausea, vomiting, distention, and obstipation may occur.

Colorectal adenocarcinomas bleed as a result of tumor friability and ulceration. Although most bleeding is occult, hematochezia occurs in a minority of patients. Patients with tumors in the distal colon are more likely to have hematochezia or a positive result on a fecal occult blood test (FOBT) as the presenting feature, whereas patients with right-sided colonic lesions are more likely to present with iron deficiency anemia.

Local invasion of tumor into adjacent structures may produce tenesmus (rectum), or pneumaturia, recurrent urinary tract infections, and ureteral obstruction (bladder). A patient may present with an acute abdomen if the tumor causes colonic perforation. Fistulae may develop between the colon and stomach or small intestine. Malignant ascites results from local tumor extension through the serosa, with peritoneal seeding. Advanced metastatic disease to the liver may be characterized by abdominal pain, jaundice, and portal hypertension.

A wasting syndrome consisting of anorexia with muscle and weight loss may occur that appears to be out of proportion to tumor burden. The cause of this metabolic disorder may stem from the systemic effects of mediators such as tumor necrosis factor.

Findings on Diagnostic Testing

Diagnostic testing for colorectal cancer should be separated into the evaluation of patients with symptoms or signs consistent with colorectal cancer, including patients with positive results on FOBTs, and the more controversial topic of screening asymptomatic populations to decrease mortality from colorectal cancer.

Evaluation of Symptomatic Patients

Laboratory studies. Results of laboratory tests may be normal or may indicate an iron deficiency anemia. Liver chemistry abnormalities raise the possibility of hepatic metastases. The serum level of carcinoembryonic antigen (CEA) is elevated in most but not all cases of colorectal adenocarcinomas. A baseline CEA level should be obtained in a patient diagnosed with colorectal cancer as a reference for comparison with levels obtained after treatment to assess for incomplete tumor resection or recurrence. However, because many conditions cause nonspecific elevations of CEA, measuring the CEA level is not reliable as a primary screening test.

Endoscopic studies. Patients with symptoms suggestive of colonic obstruction, bleeding, or invasion should undergo diagnostic evaluation to exclude colorectal cancer. Colonoscopy is the procedure of choice because of its superior accuracy in detecting colonic neoplasms and because biopsies and endoscopic polypectomy can also be performed. The sensitivity of colonoscopy for detecting small malignancies is superior to barium enema radiography, and its sensitivity approaches 100% for neoplasms larger than 1 cm. If colorectal cancer is diagnosed in the distal colon, it is imperative to visualize the entire colon because there is a 5% incidence of synchronous malignancies. The complication rate (perforation and hemorrhage) of colonoscopy is less than 5 per 1000 cases.

Radiographic studies. Double-contrast barium enema radiography can detect most colon cancers if performed by experienced personnel. Technical limitations may preclude adequate imaging of the rectosigmoid region; therefore, if barium enema radiography is chosen to evaluate a patient with suspected colonic adenocarcinoma, flexible sigmoidoscopy should be performed to exclude a neoplasm in this region. The sensitivity of barium enema radiography is highly dependent on the skill of the radiologist; diagnostic misinterpretation is common in inexperienced hands. In addition, many patients cannot comply with the changes in body position necessary for an adequate examination. When colorectal malignancy is diagnosed, an abdominal computed tomographic scan is recommended to exclude hepatic metastases. Similarly, chest radiography may be required to exclude pulmonary dissemination.

Management and Course

Prognosis

The prognosis in colorectal cancer can be estimated by the tumor stage. The most widely used staging classification is the modified Dukes classification, although TNM and Astler-Coller systems are also used (Table 49-1). Malignant lesions in the mucosa that do not penetrate the muscularis mucosae are considered intramucosal carcinoma and are cured with adequate endoscopic or surgical resection. Dukes stage A refers to invasive cancer confined to the submucosa. Stage B is subdivided into stage B1, which includes tumors invading the muscularis propria, and stage B2, which includes tumors extending into the surrounding serosa. Stage C is defined by regional lymph node involvement, which can be subdivided into stages C1 (one to four nodes involved) and C2 (more than four nodes involved). Stage D disease is defined by the presence of any distant metastatic disease. The age-adjusted 5-year survival rates for colorectal adenocarcinoma by stage are Dukes A, 95% to 100%; Dukes B, 80% to 85%; Dukes C, 50% to 70%; and Dukes D, 5% to 15%.

Other features correlate with the natural history of patients with colonic adenocarcinoma. Poorly differentiated and mucinous tumors are associated with a poor 5-year survival rate, and each comprises about 20% of all colonic adenocarcinomas. Flow cytometry can be used to identify aneuploid malignancies, which are characterized by cell populations with irregular DNA content as a result of genetic instability. Aneuploid tumors are associated with a poorer prognosis than diploid tumors. Despite the predictive value of tumor stage, there is no evidence that the size of the tumor mass is an independent predictor of survival.

Therapy

Except for colonoscopic removal of malignant polyps with favorable prognostic features (see Chapter 48), the only reliable method for curing colorectal adenocarcinoma is surgical resection. A right hemicolectomy is indicated for tumors in the cecum, ascending colon, and transverse colon; lesions in the splenic flexure and descending colon are treated with a left hemicolectomy. Sigmoid and proximal rectal malignancies can be removed with a low anterior resection. Localization and staging of rectal tumors is critical because lesions that invade the muscularis propria require an extensive abdominoperineal resection with colostomy, whereas lesions confined to the submucosa may be amenable to a sphincter-sparing transanal resection. Transrectal ultrasound can be used to determine the depth of invasion. The operative mortality rate for colon cancer surgery is 5%, although emergency operations carry a higher rate of mortal complications. Solitary hepatic metastasis or a small number of lesions localized to one hepatic lobe may also be surgically removed. Aggressive surgical resection of hepatic metastases can result in a 25% to 35% 5-year disease-free survival rate. It is not known if resecting a solitary pulmonary metastasis improves survival.

Adjuvant Therapy

One third of patients who undergo surgical resections with curative intent will develop recurrent disease. Adjuvant chemotherapy is used in an attempt to reduce the postoperative recurrence of colorectal cancers. Patients with Dukes stage A cancer

TABLE 49-1
Pathological Classifications of Colorectal Cancer

AJCC/UICC Staging Classification
Primary tumor

Tx	Primary tumor cannot be assessed
T0	No evidence of cancer in specimen (postpolypectomy)
Tis	Carcinoma in situ
T1	Submucosal invasion
T2	Muscularis propria invasion
T3	Subserosa invaded (for rectal cancer, perirectal tissues invaded)
T4	Adjacent organs invaded or peritoneum perforated (for rectal cancer, pelvic organs invaded)

Regional lymph nodes (RLN)

Nx	RLN status not assessed
N0	No RLN involvement
N1	1–3 RLN metastases
N2	$\geq$4 RLN metastases
N3	Metastasis to apical nodes or nodes along a major vascular trunk

Distant metastasis

Mx	Metastatic status not assessed
M0	No distant metastasis
M1	Distant metastasis

Dukes Stages vs. TNM Stages
Dukes A = T1 or T2, N0, M0
Dukes B = T3 or T4, N0, M0
Dukes C = T1–4, N1 or 2, M0
Dukes D = M1

Astler-Coller Stages vs. TNM Stages
A = T1, N0, M0
B_1 = T2, N0, M0
B_2 = T3 or 4, N0, M0
B_3 = T4, N0, M0
C_1 = T2, N1 or 2, M0
C_2 = T3, N1 or 2, M0
C_3 = T4, N1 or 2, M0

AJCC, American Joint Commission on Cancer; TNM, tumor-node-metastasis; UICC, International Union Against Cancer.

rarely develop recurrent disease and adjuvant therapy is not recommended for this group. For patients with Dukes stage C colon cancer, 1 year of adjuvant therapy with levamisole and 5-fluorouracil significantly increases the disease-free interval and overall survival rate. Adjuvant chemotherapy does not improve outcomes for patients with Dukes stage B disease.

Based on its location beneath the peritoneal reflection, rectal cancer is considered separately with regard to the need for adjuvant therapy. Several studies have reported decreased pelvic recurrences and improved survival with adjuvant therapy for rectal carcinoma. In contrast to more proximal tumors, both Dukes stage B2 and Dukes stage C rectal tumors benefit from this therapy. Also in contrast to more proximal colon cancers, the most efficacious adjuvant therapy for rectal cancer combines postoperative radiation therapy with chemotherapy (5-fluorouracil with or without semustine). Preoperative radiation therapy for patients with unresectable rectal tumors may sufficiently decrease the tumor size to make resection possible.

Management of Unresectable Disease

Despite the presence of distant metastatic disease, palliative resection should be considered for patients with colonic lesions because untreated colonic adenocarcinoma is associated with a high incidence of obstruction. If resection is deferred until symptoms of obstruction develop, operative morbidity and mortality can be excessive. Nd:YAG laser photocoagulation may palliate rectal cancer in patients who are not operative candidates, but a high risk of perforation precludes laser palliation of lesions located above the peritoneal reflection. Newer palliative techniques such as endoscopic placement of self-expanding metal endoluminal stents may eclipse traditional therapies.

Therapy for patients with extensive metastatic disease in the liver and other sites is limited. No systemic chemotherapeutic regimen has been demonstrated that improves survival rates. Most regimens include 5-fluorouracil and produce response rates of 15% to 20%. Delivery of 5-fluorouracil into the hepatic artery has resulted in an 80% response rate (reduction in tumor size). However, surgery is required for catheter placement, and side effects including ischemic gastroduodenal ulcers and biliary strictures have been reported in 80% of patients. This therapy has not been demonstrated to improve survival.

Principles of Screening Programs

Colorectal cancer is a prevalent condition possessing an identifiable precursor lesion (adenomatous polyp) that, when treated, alters the natural history of the disease. Thus, development of colorectal cancer is a process ideal for screening. Screening strategies include the FOBT, flexible sigmoidoscopy, combinations of FOBT with sigmoidoscopy, barium enema radiography, colonoscopy, and computed tomographic or magnetic resonance colonography ("virtual colonoscopy"). The most accessible screening test is the FOBT. There are several assays to detect occult blood, but the guaiac-based Hemoccult II is most widely used. Colorless guaiac is converted to a pigmented quinone in the presence of peroxidase activity and hydrogen peroxide. Because hemoglobin contains peroxidase activity, the addition of hydrogen peroxide to the guaiac reagent transforms the slide to a blue color. The sensitivity of Hemoccult II for detecting colorectal malignancy ranges from 50% for a single test to 70% for six tests performed over 3 days. Although the false-positive rate is less than 1%, the low prevalence of colonic adenocarcinoma in healthy populations reduces the positive predictive value to less than 10%. Rehydration of slides that have dried out improves the sensitivity to about 90% but produces a higher false-positive rate and lowers the positive predictive value of the FOBT to less than 5%. This translates into a larger number of unnecessary diagnostic evaluations, which dramatically increase the cost of screening.

These performance characteristics can be modified by dietary factors. Ingestion of red meats or peroxidase-containing legumes may increase the false-positive rate, particularly with rehydrated slides. Although iron supplements do not result in activating the color indicator, the dark color of the stool may be misinterpreted as a positive test by an inexperienced processor. High doses of antioxidants (e.g., vitamin C) may interfere with guaiac oxidation to quinone. For these reasons, patients should be counseled to avoid ingesting red meats, peroxidase-containing legumes, and vitamin C several days before testing.

Manufacturers have attempted to improve the accuracy of FOBTs. Hemoccult SENSA is the next generation hemoccult card, whereas HemeSelect uses a specific antibody to detect human hemoglobin but requires laboratory processing. Hemoccult SENSA and HemeSelect have high sensitivity for detecting colonic adenocarcinoma, 94% and 97%, respectively, but both are associated with a high false-positive rate. HemoQuant provides a quantitative measure of the fecal hemoglobin level; however, it also requires laboratory processing. The role of these newer FOBTs in colorectal cancer screening programs must be clarified by population-based studies.

Prospective controlled studies have confirmed the efficacy of an annual FOBT in reducing the mortality of colorectal adenocarcinoma. A 33% reduction in colon cancer mortality among subjects screened annually with a FOBT was seen in a large trial. Unfortunately, patient adherence to screening programs using FOBTs is less than 40%. Case-control studies have reported that screening with sigmoidoscopy results in about 30% reduced mortality from colorectal cancer. Prospective cohort and retrospective case-control studies estimate that screening colonoscopy reduces the incidence of colorectal cancer by 76% to 90% and decreases mortality from colorectal cancer by about 60%. These studies estimate that the protective effect of endoscopic procedures lasts up to 10 years.

The sensitivity of computed tomographic or magnetic resonance colonography, otherwise known as virtual colonoscopy, for detecting colonic lesions varied widely when compared to conventional colonoscopy in several large prospective studies. It is likely that variation in the methods of performing virtual colonoscopy, including the colonic preparation, use of contrast agents, and interpretation based on primary two-dimensional or three-dimensional reconstruction form the basis of the discrepancy. Widespread use of virtual colonoscopy to screen for colorectal neoplasia cannot be recommended until standard techniques for performing it are developed and evidence is established that the mortality from colorectal cancer may be reduced by implementing it.

Recommendations for Screening Average-Risk Asymptomatic Populations

The American Cancer Society, the National Cancer Institute, the U.S. Preventive Services Task Force, the American Gastroenterological Association, and other advisory groups have recommended that screening for colorectal neoplasia in adults with average risk begin at age 50. Despite variation in the specific modalities recommended by each group, the following strategies have been advocated: (1) annual FOBT, (2) sigmoidoscopy every 5 to 10 years, (3) combination of annual FOBT plus sigmoidoscopy every 5 to 10 years, (4) barium enema radiography every 5 to 10 years, and (5) colonoscopy every 10 years. Patients with positive screening results obtained through noncolonoscopic strategies should be further evaluated by colonoscopy to diagnose neoplasia and perform polypectomy. A diagnosis of adenomatous polyps mandates surveillance.

Principles of Surveillance Programs

As opposed to screening, which is defined as the use of tests to detect prevalent disease in an average-risk population, patients at high risk of developing adenocarcinoma of the colon undergo surveillance, which is defined as the use of repeated tests to detect incident disease in a high-risk population. The guidelines for surveillance of patients with adenomatous polyps and persons at risk of polyposis syndromes are discussed in Chapter 48.

Surveillance should be considered for first-degree relatives of a patient diagnosed with HNPCC. The clinical criteria for HNPCC (Amsterdam criteria) are that at least *three relatives develop colorectal cancer*, that cancer occurs in at least *two generations* where one person is a first-degree relative of the other two, and that at least *one individual is diagnosed before age 50*. Although the test is not widely available, patients may be diagnosed with HNPCC by detecting mutations of the mismatch repair genes *hMSH2*, *hMLH1*, *hPMS1*, *hPMS2*, or *hMSH6* in circulating lymphocytes or in tumor cells. Therefore, even if the Amsterdam criteria are not fulfilled, detection of the familiar clustering of colon cancers or other Lynch syndrome II malignancies should prompt consideration of molecular genetic testing of the affected patient to identify relatives who should undergo surveillance colonoscopy. The initial colonoscopy in such relatives should be performed at age 25 or 5 years earlier than the youngest age at which colorectal cancer developed in a family member. If no polyps are found, colonoscopy should be repeated every 2 years; if polyps are found, the surveillance interval should be reduced to 1 year. If a cancer is found, subtotal colectomy with ileorectal anastomosis is the appropriate therapy, followed by annual surveillance of the rectal stump. The role of genetic testing for detecting mismatch repair gene mutations in relatives of affected patients is undefined.

Patients with a family history of colorectal cancer in a single first-degree relative have a 75% to 80% increase in the risk of cancer, compared to patients who have no history of colorectal cancer. There is no consensus on the appropriate surveillance interval for this population. Persons with multiple first-degree relatives or with one first-degree relative younger than age 55 with colon cancer are at higher risk and should be considered for surveillance colonoscopy 5 years earlier than the earliest age at onset of colon cancer in the family. The subsequent surveillance procedures and intervals are then tailored according to the extent of the family history. Patients with a single affected relative may be surveyed at the same interval as average-risk populations, whereas patients with a family history that suggests HNPCC or attenuated familial adenomatous polyposis may require annual or biennial colonoscopy.

Patients who survive curative therapy for colorectal adenocarcinoma should undergo periodic colonoscopic surveillance. In the first postoperative year, colonoscopy is performed 3 to 6 months after surgery and again at 12 months to evaluate for anastomotic recurrence. Subsequently, the surveillance program is no different from that for individuals with prior adenoma (i.e., colonoscopy every 3 years).

The high risk of developing colon cancer in patients with long-standing ulcerative colitis has prompted the suggestion that patients with pancolitic involvement of more than 8 to 10 years duration should undergo surveillance colonoscopy every 2 years. Multiple biopsy specimens should be obtained randomly from four quadrants in all segments of the colon and from any polypoid, plaquelike, or masslike lesion. The implications of findings of morphologic dysplasia are discussed in Chapter 46.

COLONIC LYMPHOMA

Etiology and Pathogenesis

Primary colonic lymphomas comprise less than 0.5% of all colonic malignancies. There is an increased incidence among patients with rheumatoid arthritis, Sjögren syndrome, Wegener granulomatosis, systemic lupus erythematosus, congenital immune deficiency syndromes, and acquired immunodeficiency syndrome (AIDS), as well as in organ transplant recipients treated with immunosuppressive therapy.

TABLE 49-2
Distribution of 3000 Gastrointestinal Carcinoid Tumors

ORGAN	PERCENTAGE OF TOTAL	PERCENTAGE WITH METASTASIS
Stomach	3	18
Duodenum	1	16
Jejunum	2	35
Ileum	28	35
Appendix	47	3
Colon	2	60
Rectum	17	12

The most common gastrointestinal sites of involvement include the stomach (41%), small intestine (32%), and ileocecal region (11%); only 9% occur in the colon and 2% in the appendix.

Clinical Features, Diagnosis, and Management

Patients usually present with nonspecific abdominal pain, weight loss, constipation, and gastrointestinal hemorrhage. On colonoscopy, tumors appear as discrete masses or, less commonly, as diffuse infiltrative lesions. Most gastric and colonic lesions can be diagnosed by biopsy. Although the optimal treatment has not been defined, most regimens include chemotherapy and radiation therapy. Surgery may be effective for localized disease, but the overall 2-year survival rate is only 40%.

CARCINOID TUMORS

Carcinoids are part of the amine precursor uptake and decarboxylation family of tumors and are most common in the appendix, where they usually are diagnosed incidentally. The ileum is the second most common site. Hemorrhage affects 25% of patients with rectal carcinoid tumors. Neither appendiceal nor rectal carcinoids commonly metastasize (Table 49-2). Carcinoid tumors are rare in other regions of the colon; however, tumors in the proximal colon, appendix, and ileum may hemorrhage, and they may metastasize to the liver and produce the carcinoid syndrome that consists of abdominal pain, diarrhea, flushing, wheezing, and cutaneous changes. Because of the malignant potential of colonic carcinoids, surgical resection is the treatment of choice.

CHAPTER 50

Anorectal Diseases

HEMORRHOIDS

Etiology and Pathogenesis

Hemorrhoids occur in up to 50% of adults in the United States and result from dilation of the superior and inferior hemorrhoidal veins that form the physiological hemorrhoidal cushion. Internal hemorrhoids arise above the dentate line in three locations—right anterior, right posterior, and left lateral—and are covered by columnar epithelium. External hemorrhoids arise below the mucocutaneous junction and are covered by squamous epithelium. Skin tags are redundant folds of skin arising from the anal verge. They may be residua of resolved, thrombosed, external hemorrhoids. The pathogenesis of hemorrhoids is believed to involve deterioration of the supporting connective tissue of the hemorrhoidal cushion, causing hemorrhoidal bulging and descent. Internal hemorrhoids are similar to arteriovenous malformations and exhibit high levels of oxygen saturation. Some investigators have suggested that anal sphincter hypertrophy may predispose an individual to hemorrhoidal enlargement. Although widely believed that constipation is an important risk factor for hemorrhoids, recent studies suggest a more prominent role for diarrheal disorders.

Clinical Features, Diagnosis, and Management

Patients with internal hemorrhoids may exhibit gross but not occult bleeding (rarely requiring transfusion), discomfort, pruritus ani, fecal soiling, and prolapse. First-degree hemorrhoids do not protrude from the anus. Second-degree hemorrhoids prolapse with defecation but spontaneously reduce. Third-degree hemorrhoids prolapse and require digital reduction, and fourth-degree hemorrhoids cannot be reduced and are at risk of strangulation. Most patients with new-onset bleeding should be evaluated with sigmoidoscopy or colonoscopy to confirm that the source of hemorrhage is hemorrhoidal. Most first-degree and second-degree hemorrhoids can be managed with a high-fiber diet, adequate fluid intake, possible use of bulking agents, sitz baths twice daily, and good anal hygiene. Suppositories, ointments, and witch hazel may relieve discomfort in some cases. Rubber band ligation, injection sclerotherapy with sodium morrhuate or 5% phenol, liquid nitrogen cryoprobes, electrocoagulation, or photocoagulation with lasers or infrared light are effective in treating selected patients with bleeding or other symptoms caused by first-degree, second-degree, and selected third-degree internal hemorrhoids. Surgical hemorrhoidectomy is the treatment of choice for most third-degree hemorrhoids, all fourth-degree hemorrhoids, and other hemorrhoids refractory to nonsurgical therapy. In patients with high resting anal sphincter pressures, lateral internal sphincterotomy may achieve results comparable with those of rubber band ligation.

Thrombosis of an external hemorrhoid can produce severe pain and bleeding. Most thrombosed external hemorrhoids can be managed with sitz baths, bulking agents, stool softeners, and topical anesthetics; resolution occurs after 48 to 72 hours. If surgical evacuation or excision is required, it should be performed within 48 hours of symptom onset. Symptoms of skin tags include sensation of a growth and difficulty with anal hygiene. Treatment is conservative, and surgical resection is rarely needed.

ANORECTAL VARICES

Etiology and Pathogenesis

Anorectal varices are unrelated to hemorrhoids and are a consequence of portal hypertension in 45% of patients with cirrhosis. Anorectal varices appear as discrete, serpentine, submucosal veins that compress easily and extend from the squamous portion of the anal canal into the rectum.

Clinical Features, Diagnosis, and Management

Massive, life-threatening bleeding may occur from the anal or rectal portion of the varix. Injection sclerotherapy, cryotherapy, rubber band ligation, and hemorrhoidectomy can all produce torrential hemorrhage. Treatment by underrunning the variceal columns with an absorbable suture controls bleeding in most cases. Inferior mesenteric vein embolization and ligation have been used. Surgical or transjugular intrahepatic portosystemic shunting may ultimately be required.

ANAL FISSURE

Etiology and Pathogenesis

An anal fissure is a painful linear ulcer in the anal canal, usually located in the posterior midline (90%) and less often in the anterior midline. Lateral fissures suggest a predisposing illness such as inflammatory bowel disease (usually Crohn's disease), proctitis, leukemia, carcinoma, syphilis, or tuberculosis. Fissures are caused by traumatic tearing of the posterior anal canal during passage of hard stool. They may become chronic from high resting anal sphincter tone, which promotes a relative ischemia that prevents fissure healing. Reflex overshoot anal contraction after defecation contributes to spasm and pain.

Clinical Features, Diagnosis, and Management

Severe pain with scant red bleeding is the hallmark of an anal fissure. The fissure is best identified by simple inspection after spreading the buttocks. An acute anal fissure is a small, linear tear perpendicular to the dentate line. Chronic anal fissures appear as the triad of a fissure, a proximal hypertrophic papilla, and a sentinel pile at the anal verge. Patients usually respond to a high-fiber diet, the addition of bulking agents, stool softeners, topical anesthetics (e.g., benzocaine, pramoxine), and warm sitz baths. When these measures fail, agents that reduce anal pressure and increase anal blood flow, including topical nitroglycerin or diltiazem ointments, or intramuscular injection of botulinum toxin may promote fissure healing. Surgical lateral subcutaneous internal anal sphincterotomy may be necessary for some patients with chronic fissures.

ANORECTAL ABSCESS AND FISTULA

Etiology and Pathogenesis

An anorectal abscess is an undrained collection of perianal pus, whereas an anorectal fistula is an abnormal communication between the anorectal canal and the perianal skin. Diseases associated with these disorders include hypertension, diabetes, heart disease, inflammatory bowel disease, and leukemia. Infection, most commonly with *Escherichia coli*, *Enterococcus* species, or *Bacteroides fragilis*, results from obstruction of anal glands as a result of trauma, anal eroticism, diarrhea, hard stools, or foreign bodies. Abscess and fistula formation may occur without primary glandular infection in patients with Crohn's disease, anorectal malignancy, tuberculosis, actinomycosis, lymphogranuloma venereum, radiation proctitis, leukemia, and lymphoma. Abscesses are classified by site of origin and potential pathways of extension. Fistulae are divided into intersphincteric, transsphincteric, suprasphincteric, and extrasphincteric types.

Clinical Features, Diagnosis, and Management

Swelling and acute pain, exacerbated by sitting, movement, and defecation, are the main symptoms of an anorectal abscess. Malaise and fever are common. A foul-smelling discharge suggests that the abscess is spontaneously draining through the primary anal orifice. Inspection reveals erythema, warmth, swelling, and tenderness, although intersphincteric abscesses may produce only localized tenderness. Anal ultrasound and magnetic resonance imaging (MRI) can determine the location of an abscess relative to the sphincters. Anorectal abscesses require surgical drainage to prevent necrotizing infection, which carries a 50% mortality rate. Superficial perineal or ischiorectal abscesses may be drained under local anesthesia, but other abscesses require surgery in an operating room. Antibiotics usually are not necessary and may mask signs of underlying suppurative infection. Broad-spectrum antibiotics are indicated for patients with diabetes, immunosuppression, leukemia, valvular heart disease, or extensive soft tissue infection. Warm sitz baths, stool-softening agents, and analgesics can minimize disease recurrence postoperatively.

Anorectal fistulae produce chronic, purulent drainage, pain on defecation, and pruritus ani. Examination may reveal a red, granular papule that exudes pus. Patients who are neutropenic may exhibit point tenderness and poorly demarcated induration. These patients have high mortality rates from disseminated infection. Multiple perineal openings suggest the possibility of Crohn's disease or hidradenitis suppurativa. Anoscopy and sigmoidoscopy are performed to locate the primary orifice at the level of the dentate line and to exclude proctitis. MRI findings predict the clinical outcome. The presence of an anorectal fistula is an indication for surgery, which involves removing the primary orifice and opening the fistulous tract with conservation of the external sphincter. Patients with Crohn's disease who have chronic fistulae may benefit from immunosuppressive therapy or antibiotics such as metronidazole or ciprofloxacin. Inflixamab, a chimeric monoclonal antibody to tumor necrosis factor, is effective against many refractory anal fistulae secondary to Crohn's disease. Local surgery or diversion of the fecal stream is necessary in some cases. Postoperative care is the same as that for anorectal abscesses.

RECTAL PROLAPSE

Etiology and Pathogenesis

Rectal prolapse is protrusion of the rectum through the anal orifice. The prolapse may be complete (all layers visibly descend), occult (internal intussusception without visible protrusion), or mucosal (protrusion of distal rectal tissue but not the entire circumference). Rectal prolapse in children may be idiopathic or secondary to spina bifida, meningomyelocele, or cystic fibrosis. In adults, the condition is associated with poor pelvic tone, chronic straining, fecal incontinence, pelvic trauma, and neurological disease. Defects that result from rectal prolapse include weakened endopelvic fascia, levator ani diastasis, loss of the normal horizontal rectal position, an abnormally deep pouch of Douglas, a redundant rectosigmoid colon, a weak anal sphincter, denervation of the striated muscle, and loss of the anocutaneous reflex. Disturbed sphincter function and innervation may explain the frequent reports of fecal incontinence after surgical correction of rectal prolapse.

Clinical Features, Diagnosis, and Management

Patients report prolapse of tissue as well as defecatory straining, incomplete evacuation, tenesmus, and incontinence. On examination, the prolapse may be obvious when the patient is asked to sit and strain. Endoscopy or barium enema radiography excludes malignancy but may reveal a concomitant solitary rectal ulcer. Defecography is the best test to demonstrate occult prolapse. Persistently prolapsed tissue must be promptly reduced manually with or without intravenous sedation to avoid strangulation, ulceration, bleeding, or perforation. Complete rectal prolapse should be treated surgically (anterior sling rectopexy or Ripstein procedure, abdominal proctopexy with or without sigmoid resection). Perineal exercises or buttock strapping can be suggested to patients who refuse or who cannot undergo surgery. Perineal or extraabdominal rectosigmoidectomy or diverting colostomy may be performed for elderly or debilitated patients. Occult prolapse is treated surgically if incontinence or solitary rectal ulcer is present; otherwise, conservative therapy is recommended.

ANAL STENOSIS

Etiology and Pathogenesis

Anal stenosis results from malignancy (anal carcinoma, rectal carcinoma, invasion by urogenital malignancy) or benign conditions (prior rectal surgery, trauma, inflammatory bowel disease, laxative abuse, chronic diarrhea, radiation injury, tuberculosis, actinomycosis, lymphogranuloma venereum, congenital causes).

Clinical Features, Diagnosis, and Management

Patients present with small caliber stools, painful or resistant defecation, and bleeding. Mild strictures may respond to periodic dilation and dietary fiber supplementation; severe stenosis may require surgical anoplasty with or without lateral internal sphincterotomy.

SOLITARY RECTAL ULCER

Etiology and Pathogenesis

Solitary rectal ulcer results from prolonged straining and difficulty initiating defecation. Ninety percent of patients have associated rectal prolapse, which is likely to be an important pathogenic factor. Patients also have higher anal pressures and thicker rectal walls that lead to increased transmural pressures during defecation.

Clinical Features, Diagnosis, and Management

Patients present with fecal mucus and blood, altered bowel habits, and anorectal pain. On sigmoidoscopy, a variety of findings are seen that range from localized erythema or nodularity to multiple shallow ulcers. Typically, lesions are noted on the anterior rectal wall 7 to 10 cm from the anal verge. Conservative management with treatments to reduce straining and improve bowel habits is initiated. Refractory cases may benefit from surgical rectopexy or biofeedback therapy.

FECAL INCONTINENCE

Etiology and Pathogenesis

Fecal incontinence is the loss of rectal contents against one's wishes. Women, elderly individuals, and institutionalized persons are affected most often. Traumatic obstetric and surgical injuries, rectal or hemorrhoidal prolapse, and neuropathic disease may impair anal sphincter function and lead to incontinence (Table 50-1). Traumatic or neuropathic injury that leads to abnormal straightening of the anorectal angle can also cause incontinence. Other factors that predispose to fecal incontinence include loss of anal or rectal sensation secondary to neuropathy; poor rectal distention with ulcerative proctitis, radiation proctitis, or ischemia; and overwhelming diarrhea. Hypersensitivity to distention and abnormal rectal motility probably account for the incontinence often seen in patients with irritable bowel syndrome.

Clinical Features, Diagnosis, and Management

Partial incontinence is defined as minor soiling and poor flatus control. The elderly and those with internal anal sphincter deficiency, fecal impaction, and rectal prolapse are prone to partial incontinence. Some "leakers" have near normal sphincter pressures and experience soiling secondary to hemorrhoids or fissures. Major incontinence is the frequent loss of large amounts of stool. It is caused by neurological disease, traumatic injury, and surgical damage. Examination may reveal anal deformity, tumors, infections, fistulae, prolapsing hemorrhoids, loss of anal tone, and absence of the anal wink. The anorectal angle and puborectalis function are crudely assessed by palpating this muscle in the posterior midline during rest and voluntary squeeze.

Several tools assess the mechanisms of continence. Sigmoidoscopy excludes malignancy and proctitis. Anorectal manometry defines resting and maximal anal pressures, rectal compliance, and rectal sensitivity to distention. Advances in

TABLE 50-1
Causes of Fecal Incontinence

Diarrhea

Fecal impaction

Irritable bowel syndrome

Anal diseases
  Anal carcinoma
  Congenital abnormalities
  Protruding internal hemorrhoids
  Rectal prolapse
  Perianal infections
  Fistulae
  Injury (e.g., surgical, obstetric, accidental)

Rectal diseases
  Rectal carcinoma
  Rectal ischemia
  Proctitis (e.g., inflammatory bowel disease, radiation therapy, infection)

Neurological diseases
  Central nervous system (e.g., cerebrovascular accident, dementia, toxic or metabolic
    disorders, spinal cord injury or tumors, multiple sclerosis, tabes dorsalis)
  Peripheral nervous system (e.g., diabetes, cauda equina lesions)

Miscellaneous
  Childbirth injury
  Chronic constipation
  Descending perineum
  Advanced age

manometric technology include ambulatory monitoring and topographic characterization of sphincter pressures. Rectal compliance and sensitivity are quantified using rectal balloon inflation. Miniature probes measure thermal and electrical sensitivity of the anal canal. Electromyography assesses external sphincter and puborectalis muscle activity. Anorectal ultrasound and endoanal MRI measure sphincter muscle thickness and detect muscle defects from trauma or surgical injury. Defecography demonstrates the evacuation of a simulated barium stool and provides static and dynamic measurements of the anorectal angle, pelvic floor, and puborectalis function. Continence is tested by measuring leakage of rectally infused saline or resistance to evacuation of a solid object.

Fecal incontinence often responds to a combination of interventions. Fiber therapy or opiate antidiarrheals are indicated for treating diarrhea. Anticholinergics may blunt the gastrocolonic response and reduce meal-associated incontinence. Fecal impactions are removed with enemas or by manual disimpaction. For individuals who fail these conservative measures, anal biofeedback produces success rates as high as 70% in appropriate patients. With this technique, the patient associates external anal contractions with visual cues such as manometric contractions or electrical discharges on electromyography. Similarly, biofeedback can be used to improve rectal sensation in patients with underlying neuropathy. Conditions that respond poorly to biofeedback therapy include severe organic disease with reduced rectal sensation, irritable bowel syndrome, anterior rectal resection, and prior posterior anal sphincterotomy. Surgery is generally reserved for patients with major incontinence. Prior anal injury may be repairable with external anal sphincter repair; posterior proctopexy may be performed for complex sphincter injury, pelvic neuropathy, and loss of the normal anorectal angle. Anterior reefing procedures may be useful for women with anterior sphincter defects. Gracilis muscle transposition with or without electrical stimulation may benefit a patient with a destroyed sphincter or a congenital pelvic floor abnormality. Artificial sphincters may be implanted. Recently, sacral nerve stimulators have shown promise in reducing incontinent episodes in a range of clinical conditions. As a last resort, placing a colostomy should be considered.

PRURITUS ANI

Etiology and Pathogenesis

Pruritus ani is an itchy sensation of the anus and perianal skin that may result from perianal disease (fissures, fistulae, hemorrhoids, malignancy) or from residual fecal material. *Candida albicans* and dermatophyte infections appear as localized erythematous rashes but may also be present on apparently normal skin. Pinworm (*Enterobius vermicularis*) causes nocturnal pruritus ani in children and in adults exposed to infected children. Scabies (*Sarcoptes scabiei*) and pubic lice produce pruritus ani that may be associated with genital itching. Sexually transmitted diseases associated with the condition include herpes simplex, gonorrhea, syphilis, condyloma acuminatum, and molluscum contagiosum. Generalized skin conditions (e.g., psoriasis) as well as local irritants, allergens, and chemicals may produce perianal itching. Clinical experience suggests that certain dietary products such as coffee, cola, beer, tomatoes, chocolate, tea, and citrus fruits may be causative. Idiopathic pruritus ani results from a combination of perianal fecal contamination and trauma.

Clinical Features, Diagnosis, and Management

Most cases of pruritus ani are successfully managed. If identified, dermatologic, infectious, and anorectal disorders should receive specific treatment (Table 50-2). A diagnosis of pinworms can be confirmed by detecting eggs on adhesive cellophane tape applied to the perianal skin early in the morning. Foods that predispose to diarrhea or pruritus should be eliminated. The key to management in most cases rests on keeping the anal area clean and dry while minimizing trauma induced by wiping and scratching. The perianal skin should be cleansed with a moistened pad after defecation. Witch hazel or lanolin preparations can soothe irritated tissues. The area should be dried with a blow dryer or with a soft tissue using a blotting motion. Thin cotton pledgets may be needed for those with fecal discharge. Excess perspiration can be controlled with baby powder and loose cotton clothing. Healing can be facilitated by applying 1% hydrocortisone cream twice daily for no more than 2 weeks (because of atrophic effects on the skin) and zinc oxide ointment. Nocturnal pruritus may benefit from oral antihistamines (e.g., diphenhydramine). Intractable symptoms may respond to intracutaneous injections of methylene blue.

TABLE 50-2
Causes of Pruritus Ani

Anorectal diseases
Diarrhea
Fecal incontinence
Hemorrhoids
Anal fissures
Fistulae
Rectal prolapse
Anal malignancy

Infections
Fungal (e.g., candidiasis, dermatophytes)
Parasitic (e.g., pinworms, scabies)
Bacterial (e.g., *Staphylococcus aureus*)
Venereal (e.g., herpes, gonorrhea, syphilis, condyloma acuminatum)

Local irritants
Moisture, obesity, perspiration
Soaps, hygiene products
Toilet paper (e.g., perfumed, dyed)
Underwear (e.g., irritating fabric, detergent)
Anal creams and suppositories
Dietary (e.g., coffee, beer, acidic foods)
Medications (e.g., mineral oil, ascorbic acid, quinidine, colchicine)

Dermatologic diseases
Psoriasis
Atopic dermatitis
Seborrheic dermatitis

RECTAL FOREIGN BODIES AND TRAUMA

Etiology and Pathogenesis

A variety of foreign bodies can become lodged in the rectum after insertion for medical treatment, concealment, assault, and eroticism. Foreign bodies are classified as low-lying if they are in the rectal ampulla and high-lying if they are at or proximal to the rectosigmoid junction. Rectal trauma may result from penetrating injury (e.g., gunshot), blunt trauma (e.g., motor vehicle collisions), impalement (e.g., assault), sexual activities (e.g., fist fornication), and iatrogenic injury (e.g., endoscopy, enemas, surgery).

Clinical Features, Diagnosis, and Management

Anteroposterior and lateral radiographs may define the location of a foreign body and detect pneumoperitoneum, if present. Small, low-lying objects can be removed through an anoscope, whereas larger objects (e.g., vibrators) may require regional anesthesia, anal dilation, and a grasping forceps. Large, bulky items may be removed by inflating Foley catheters in the colon proximal to the object, followed by gentle traction on the catheters for careful extraction. High-lying foreign bodies are removed using spinal anesthesia and the lithotomy position. Gentle pressure on the abdomen pushes the object within the reach of forceps directed through a rigid sigmoidoscope. Laparotomy is indicated for objects that cannot be delivered distally, if abdominal distress develops, or if broken glass is present. Surgical procedures required for some cases of major rectal trauma include a diverting colostomy, presacral drain placement, rectal irrigation, and sphincter preservation.

ANAL MALIGNANCIES

Etiology and Pathogenesis

Several histological types of anal carcinoma have been described, including squamous cell (70% to 80%), basaloid or cloacogenic (20% to 30%), mucoepidermoid (1% to 5%), and small-cell anaplastic (<5%) types. Patients present at a mean age of 60. Risk factors include receptive anal intercourse in men; genital or anal warts in both sexes; smoking; human immunodeficiency virus (HIV) infection, multiple sexual partners, cervical dysplasia, and immunosuppression. A causal role has been proposed for human papilloma virus infection, particularly type 16. Anal adenocarcinoma may arise in anorectal fistulae. Extramammary Paget disease is a perianal glandular tumor that appears in the seventh decade as an erythematous, well-demarcated eczematoid plaque. Anal melanomas typically are large (>4 cm), nonpigmented in one third of cases, and tend to metastasize early. Survival rates are poor. Basal cell carcinoma of the anus is characterized by rolled skin edges with central ulceration. Bowen disease is a slow-growing, squamous cell carcinoma in situ that manifests as red-brown scaly or crusted plaques.

Clinical Features, Diagnosis, and Management

Bleeding, pain, pruritus, or palpable lymphadenopathy may be the presenting symptoms of anal cancer, although many patients are asymptomatic until the disease is detected in routine examination. At presentation, 15% to 30% of patients have lymph node involvement, and 10% have liver or lung metastases. The diagnosis is made by biopsy. Lesions arising from the anal canal are more aggressive, whereas those originating from the anal margin are more differentiated and less malignant. Findings that confer a poor prognosis include squamous cell tumors larger than 2 cm, basaloid or anaplastic carcinomas, sphincteric invasion, and nodal spread. Radiation therapy plus chemotherapy with 5-fluorouracil and mitomycin C cause complete tumor regression in most cases of small, noninfiltrating anal cancers, with a 5-year survival rate of 70% and preservation of sphincter function. Cisplatin-based regimens may prove superior to those containing mitomycin. Wide local excision remains a therapeutic option for some patients, although anal canal adenocarcinoma typically recurs despite resection. Surgical treatment of extramammary Paget disease includes wide local excision or radical abdominoperitoneal resection with ipsilateral groin dissection for advanced disease with nodal involvement. Surgery rarely cures anal melanoma. Resection or radiation therapy provides excellent results in treating basal cell carcinoma. Resection cures Bowen disease.

PROCTALGIA FUGAX AND LEVATOR ANI SYNDROME

Etiology and Pathogenesis

Proctalgia fugax is characterized by sudden, brief episodes of severe rectal pain and is associated with irritable bowel syndrome and psychogenic disorders. In most cases, the cause is unknown. A familial internal anal sphincter myopathy has been described that causes proctalgia fugax and difficulty with defecation. The levator ani syndrome refers to aching rectal pain due to tenderness and spasm of the levator ani muscle group (ileococcygeus, pubococcygeus, puborectalis).

Clinical Features, Diagnosis, and Management

Attacks of proctalgia fugax are described as intense stabbing or aching midline pain above the anus, lasting seconds to minutes, associated with an urge to expel flatus, a desire to lie on one side with hips flexed, cold sweats, syncope, and priapism. Often the attacks occur at night. Frequently, no clear precipitating cause is identified. Unproven local therapies include rectal massage, firm perineal pressure, and warm soaks or baths. Anecdotal reports claim that various medications, including amyl nitrate, nitroglycerin, salbutamol, clonidine, and diltiazem, reduce symptoms.

The pain of the levator ani syndrome is more chronic, aching, and pressure-like than that of proctalgia fugax. Defecation and prolonged sitting precipitate the pain. On examination, palpable tenderness and spasm of the levator muscles may be elicited. Treatment includes reassurance, local heat, rectal massage, muscle relaxants, electrogalvanic stimulation, and biofeedback training.

MISCELLANEOUS CONDITIONS

Coccygodynia is a sharp or aching pain in the coccyx that may radiate to the rectal region or buttocks and can be caused by traumatic arthritis, dislocation or fracture, difficult childbirth, or prolonged sitting. Manipulating the coccyx on examination reproduces the pain. Therapies include warm soaks, analgesics, local corticosteroid injection, and, rarely, coccygectomy. Other causes of anorectal pain include cauda equina tumors, pelvic tumors, perianal endometriosis, intermittent enteroceles, and retrorectal tumors and cysts.

Pilonidal disease is an acquired condition of the midline coccygeal skin in which small skin pits precede development of a draining sinus or abscess. In contrast to anorectal fistula or hidradenitis suppurativa, there is no communication with the anorectum. Patients, usually young men, present with a painful swelling and drainage. Definitive treatment usually is surgical. Squamous cell carcinoma may complicate the course of pilonidal disease.

Hidradenitis suppurativa is a suppurative condition of apocrine glands in the axilla and inguinoperineal regions that manifests in adolescence and young adulthood. Risk factors include obesity, acne, perspiration, and mechanical trauma. Repeated inflammation and healing produce fibrosis and draining sinus tracts, including anal and rectal fistulae. Warm, wet compresses are applied, and antibiotics are administered topically and systemically, but surgery is usually necessary.

CHAPTER 51

Structural Anomalies and Hereditary Diseases of the Pancreas

EMBRYOLOGY AND ANATOMY OF THE PANCREAS

The pancreas develops from two separate outpouchings of the duodenum. The ventral pancreas forms at the base of the hepatobiliary diverticulum and is drained by the duct of Wirsung, which usually shares a common channel with the distal common bile duct before emptying into the duodenum. The dorsal pancreas is an elongated structure that is drained by the duct of Santorini directly into the duodenum. In the second month of gestation, the ventral pancreas rotates to the left of the duodenum and migrates with the distal common bile duct to lie below the dorsal pancreas. Fusion of the duct of Wirsung and the distal portion of the duct of Santorini forms the main pancreatic duct. Most pancreatic secretions drain out the duct of Wirsung through the ampulla of Vater. The duct of Santorini usually drains only a small proportion of the pancreatic secretions. It is an accessory duct that drains into the duodenum through the minor papilla. It often regresses or ends blindly in the duodenal wall.

The adult pancreas is a 12- to 20-cm-long, flattened, transversely oriented gland without a fibrous capsule that lies behind the peritoneum of the posterior abdominal wall. The pancreatic head is adjacent to the duodenal sweep. The pancreatic neck, a constricted part of the gland 3 to 4 cm wide, extends from the head of the pancreas to the left. In front of the aorta in the midline, the pancreatic body continues to the left, posterior to the gastric antrum and body. The midline portion of the body is pushed forward by the L1 and L2 vertebral bodies to lie relatively fixed in location closest to the anterior abdominal wall and most vulnerable to blunt abdominal injuries. The pancreas terminates in the tail, which is adjacent to the hilum of the spleen. The sphincter of Oddi consists of circular smooth muscle that surrounds the common channel of the common bile duct and the main pancreatic duct.

The arterial blood supply to the pancreas originates from the celiac and superior mesenteric arteries. The pancreatic head and the duodenum have a common blood supply from the anterior and posterior pancreaticoduodenal arteries. The body and tail of the pancreas derive their blood supply from branches of the splenic artery. The general pattern of venous drainage of the pancreas is the same as that of the arterial supply; blood from the pancreas ultimately drains into the portal vein. The duodenum and pancreatic head have a common lymphatic drainage. Lymph eventually flows into the celiac and superior mesenteric groups of the paraaortic lymph nodes. The lymphatics of the pancreatic tail pass to the splenic nodes, and those of the body pass upward to the pancreaticosplenic nodes. The sympathetic efferent innervation of the pancreas derives from the greater, lesser, and least splanchnic nerves, whereas the parasympathetic innervation derives from the vagus nerves. Intrapancreatic ganglion cells are observed within the pancreatic interlobular tissues; unmyelinated fibers pass to exocrine and endocrine cells.

The pancreas is a lobulated organ with lobular subunits consisting of acini. The acini are rounded or tubular and are lined by single rows of epithelial cells. The acinar lumen connects with intralobular ducts to form the interlobular ducts, which ultimately coalesce to form the main pancreatic duct. Ductules are lined by columnar, goblet, and occasional argentaffin cells. Acinar cells contain highly basophilic cytoplasm reflective of the numerous ribosomes that are involved in protein production. The endocrine portion of the pancreas consists of 1 million islets of Langerhans. The islets are diffusely distributed throughout the gland, except in the tail, where they are relatively concentrated. The insulin-secreting B cells comprise 75% to 80% of the cells in the islets. The remaining cells are A, D, EC, and PP cells, which produce glucagon, somatostatin, 5-hydroxytryptamine, and pancreatic polypeptide, respectively.

PANCREAS DIVISUM

Incidence and Epidemiology

Pancreas divisum is the most common congenital structural anomaly of the pancreas. Autopsy series suggest a prevalence of 5% to 10%, but endoscopic series report a prevalence of 2% to 4%. Pancreas divisum is found in 16% to 25% of patients with idiopathic pancreatitis, which suggests that the condition may be an important cause of pancreatitis. Although pancreas divisum is a congenital anomaly, it usually is not detected until adulthood.

Etiology and Pathogenesis

Pancreas divisum results when the ventral (Wirsung) and dorsal (Santorini) pancreatic ducts fail to fuse during the second month of embryonic development. In some cases there is a thin ductal stricture joining the two large ducts, an anomaly termed *incomplete pancreas divisum*. In pancreas divisum, most of the pancreas is drained by the accessory duct rather than by the proximal main pancreatic duct. It is postulated that increased resistance and ductal hypertension caused by the smaller caliber of the accessory duct and the minor papilla may induce pancreatitis.

Clinical Features

Most patients with pancreas divisum are asymptomatic and experience no significant clinical sequelae from the condition. It is not uncommon for the diagnosis to be made incidentally by endoscopic retrograde cholangiopancreatography (ERCP). In some patients, however, pancreas divisum is believed to be the cause of recurrent attacks of acute pancreatitis. As with pancreatitis induced by other causes, steady, severe epigastric pain, often radiating to the back, nausea, vomiting, and ileus are the dominant symptoms. Some patients report complete resolution of symptoms between attacks, whereas others have chronic abdominal pain and steatorrhea from chronic pancreatitis. Some patients experience only subtle episodic abdominal discomfort, which may represent a mild episode of pancreatitis. Patients with pancreatitis associated with pancreas divisum may experience any of the sequelae and complications found with acute or chronic pancreatitis secondary to other causes.

Findings on Diagnostic Testing

Laboratory Studies

Laboratory findings in patients with pancreatitis associated with pancreas divisum are similar to findings in patients with pancreatitis from other causes.

Structural Studies

Endoscopic retrograde pancreatography (ERP) is the definitive means for diagnosing pancreas divisum. Injection of contrast medium into the pancreatic duct through the major papilla reveals a short, narrow, arborizing duct in the pancreatic head that tapers to a blind end; the neck, body, and tail of the pancreas do not fill with contrast. In some patients, cannulation of the duct of Wirsung is not possible because of its small size. The diagnosis is confirmed by dye injection of the minor papilla, which demonstrates filling of a separate duct of Santorini all the way to the tail of the pancreas. In patients with recurrent acute pancreatitis, this duct may appear normal or slightly dilated. Patients with chronic pancreatitis usually have other ductal changes: ductal dilation and ectasia, dilated and blunted secondary radicals, intraductal stones, and possibly, pseudocysts.

Management and Course

Patients with recurrent attacks of acute pancreatitis attributable to pancreas divisum may benefit from endoscopic sphincterotomy of the minor papilla, after which a temporary pancreatic stent may be placed across the papilla to protect the duct from edema and inflammation caused by the sphincterotomy. Although this therapy seems to decrease the episodes of acute pancreatitis, minor sphincterotomy is not effective for patients with chronic pancreatitis. Medical therapy with enzyme supplements and analgesics should always be the initial treatment for patients with chronic pancreatitis. Patients with refractory pain or pseudocysts may require surgical intervention.

ANNULAR PANCREAS

Etiology and Pathogenesis

Annular pancreas is a congenital disorder that is characterized by a band of pancreatic tissue that encircles the second portion of the duodenum. The annulus probably results from tethering a portion of the ventral pancreas as the ventral and dorsal pancreas rotate around the duodenum in the first 2 months of embryological development. Annular pancreas is associated with other congenital defects, including Down syndrome, Meckel diverticulum, intestinal malrotation, tracheoesophageal fistulae, imperforate anus, and cardiac abnormalities.

Clinical Features, Diagnosis, and Management

Most patients present in the first year of life with vomiting and failure to thrive as a result of duodenal stenosis. Occasionally, annular pancreas is diagnosed in adulthood when patients complain of postprandial fullness or bloating and some develop gastrointestinal hemorrhage and acute pancreatitis. In infants, abdominal radiography may show the double bubble sign of duodenal obstruction. Upper gastrointestinal barium radiography demonstrates a concentric narrowing, 0.5 to 5.0 cm in length, of the second portion of the duodenum. ERCP or magnetic resonance pancreatography may be used to visualize the ductal system and can confirm a diagnosis of annular pancreas. Symptomatic patients require a surgical bypass of the obstructed segment. Division of the annulus is not recommended because of the high rate of developing postoperative pancreatic fistulae.

HETEROTOPIC PANCREAS

Etiology and Pathogenesis

Aberrant rests of pancreatic tissue can occur anywhere in the gastrointestinal tract but rarely in extraabdominal sites such as the lung. The probable cause is abnormal differentiation of pluripotent endodermal stem cells. The incidence is 0.6% to 15%, but most cases are subclinical.

Clinical Features, Diagnosis, and Management

Seventy-five percent of pancreatic rests occur in the submucosa of the stomach and small intestine. Upper gastrointestinal endoscopy or upper gastrointestinal barium radiography shows a 2- to 4-cm submucosal nodule that often has a central depression. Heterotopic pancreas is usually an asymptomatic condition, although patients may present with pain, nausea, vomiting, and gastric outlet obstruction. The lesions occasionally ulcerate, producing gastrointestinal hemorrhage. Because a pancreatic rest contains the full histological complement of normal pancreatic tissue, there is an extremely small risk that adenocarcinoma, islet cell tumors, or pseudocysts will develop within the rest itself. Asymptomatic rests need no treatment, but symptomatic pancreatic rests should be surgically excised.

AGENESIS OR HYPOPLASIA OF THE PANCREAS

Agenesis of the pancreas is a rare congenital anomaly that results in absolute endocrine and exocrine insufficiency. In hypoplasia of the pancreas, also known as *lipomatous pseudohypertrophy of the pancreas*, the islets of Langerhans are intact, but the acinar cells are replaced by fatty tissue. Although the mechanisms for development remain unclear, an intrauterine infection may be the primary insult that disrupts embryological development of the exocrine gland.

CONGENITAL CYSTS

Congenital pancreatic cysts are usually solitary and sporadic, but some hereditary disorders such as polycystic kidney disease, cystic fibrosis, and von Hippel–Lindau syndrome manifest multiple pancreatic cysts. Most congenital cysts are diagnosed in infancy as abdominal masses, which may cause symptoms related to gastroduodenal or biliary obstruction. Some congenital cysts are not detected until adulthood, and they must be differentiated from pseudocysts, cystadenomas, and cystadenocarcinomas. Nonresectional drainage procedures are effective for chronic pseudocysts, whereas cystic neoplasms should be removed. Asymptomatic lesions require no therapy.

CYSTIC FIBROSIS

Incidence and Epidemiology

Cystic fibrosis, an autosomal-recessive disease with an incidence of 1 in 3200 live births in white populations, is the most common hereditary disease of the exocrine pancreas and the most common lethal genetic defect in white populations. The gene frequency may be as high as 5% among persons of Northern European ancestry, but the disease may occur in any social or ethnic group. In the United States, there are more than 7 million asymptomatic heterozygotes and 30,000 affected homozygotes.

Etiology and Pathogenesis

The cystic fibrosis gene is located on chromosome 7q32 and encodes a chloride channel termed the *cystic fibrosis transmembrane conductance regulator* (CFTR). Major mutations in *both* alleles result in complete loss of CFTR function and typical cystic fibrosis. About 1000 different mutations and sequence variations have been identified in the human *CFTR* gene, although a three base-pair deletion at codon 508 accounts for about 70% of the mutations in white patients. The mutation of this gene results in the loss of a single amino acid, phenylalanine, which prevents transport of the CFTR protein to the cell surface. Under normal conditions, chloride secretion through the CFTR activates a chloride-bicarbonate exchange and promotes transcellular movement of sodium and water. A defect of CFTR function impairs apical bicarbonate secretion as well as transcellular sodium and water secretion. This defective dilution and alkalinization leads to inspissation of protein-rich pancreatic secretions and ultimately to ductal obstruction and acinar disruption. As the disease progresses, pancreatic autodigestion contributes to the pancreatic injury, which culminates in diffuse fibrosis and cystic degeneration. Although islet cells are spared in the early stages of the disease, insulin production may be compromised in the late stages. Defective CFTR function is also responsible for obstructive secretions in the lungs, genital tract, and biliary tract, where focal biliary cirrhosis may result.

Clinical Features

The pancreatic manifestations of cystic fibrosis are apparent by age 5 years in 85% of patients, although 8% of patients are older than 10 years when the disease is diagnosed (Table 51-1). The earliest complication is meconium ileus, which occurs in 15% of cases and presents in the first week of life as abdominal distention, bilious vomiting, and delayed passage of meconium. The inspissated meconium becomes impacted in the small intestine. Some patients may have associated atresia of the small intestine or volvulus, which may be complicated by peritonitis.

The most common clinical presentation of pancreatic insufficiency consists of poor weight gain and growth retardation despite adequate caloric intake. In the first few months of life, stools are watery, but later in the first year, the stools are bulky and greasy, characteristic of steatorrhea. Frequent passage of bulky stools,

TABLE 51-1
Presenting Features in Patients with Cystic Fibrosis

FEATURE	PERCENT
Acute or persistent respiratory symptoms	50.5
Failure to thrive, malnutrition	42.9
Steatorrhea	35.0
Meconium ileus	18.8
Family history	16.8
Electrolyte imbalance	5.4
Rectal prolapse	3.4
Neonatal screening	2.3
Nasal polyps	2.0
Genotype	1.2
Hepatobiliary disease	0.9
Other	1.2

chronic coughing, and decreased muscle mass contribute to the development of rectal prolapse in 20% of patients. Older children and adults may present with bowel obstruction or intussusception caused by inspissated stool or partially digested food. Deficiencies of fat-soluble vitamins A, D, E, and K may occur at any age with significant steatorrhea. A patient with cystic fibrosis who does not have exocrine insufficiency may rarely present with acute pancreatitis. This complication is more common in older individuals, with a frequency of 2.4% in patients older than 30 years. These patients often have a compound heterozygous genotype and may have the cystic fibrosis phenotype with abnormal sweat chloride levels and pulmonary disease. Diabetes mellitus affects 10% to 15% of young adults with cystic fibrosis and concomitant exocrine insufficiency.

Hepatobiliary disorders (e.g., gallbladder cysts and gallstones) are common in patients with cystic fibrosis, but the most clinically significant disease is focal biliary cirrhosis, which occurs in 5% of young children and adults. Inspissation of bile in intrahepatic bile ducts leads to periportal inflammation and fibrosis and bile duct proliferation. Patients may present with asymptomatic alkaline phosphatase elevations, jaundice, splenomegaly, and complications of portal hypertension. Patients with cystic fibrosis have an increased incidence of pancreatic and intestinal cancers compared with control populations, and they have an increased risk of gastroesophageal reflux disease and gastrointestinal bleeding, presumably due to unbuffered gastric acid.

Findings on Diagnostic Testing

Laboratory Studies
Patients with cystic fibrosis exhibit several laboratory abnormalities. Hypoproteinemia may result from chronic catabolism and malabsorption. Minimal elevations in serum amylase and lipase levels may reflect low-grade pancreatitis, whereas a rare patient with acute pancreatitis may have marked enzyme elevations. Hepatic involvement is characterized by nonspecific elevations in liver chemistry levels, with a disproportionate increase in alkaline phosphatase levels. Deficiencies of vitamin K or vitamin B_{12} may manifest as prolongation of prothrombin time or

macrocytic anemia. Chronic pulmonary infections and malnutrition cause other nonspecific abnormalities, including anemia, leukocytosis, and low serum nitrogen levels.

Evaluation of Exocrine Function

Patients with pancreatic exocrine insufficiency usually have steatorrhea, which is assessed best by a quantitative 72-hour fecal fat assay. Testing pancreatic exocrine function by administering secretin or cholecystokinin, followed by measuring pancreatic bicarbonate or enzyme output, frequently reveals diminished secretory capacity before clinically significant maldigestion is detected. ERP is rarely necessary, but if performed, the ductal structures may display a range of nonspecific changes similar to those in chronic pancreatitis.

Sweat Testing

The gold standard for confirming the diagnosis of cystic fibrosis is the sweat test. When performed in an experienced laboratory, analyses of sodium and chloride concentrations in sweat are 99% sensitive for detecting affected homozygotes. Sodium and chloride concentrations in the sweat of patients with cystic fibrosis typically exceed 77 and 74 mEq/L, respectively, because of the diminished water content of sweat. False-positive assays may occur with dehydration, edema, congestive heart failure, malnutrition, adrenal insufficiency, diabetes insipidus, and after taking some medications.

Genetic Testing

When the sweat test result is equivocal or prenatal screening is desired, genetic analysis may be useful if the patient has one of the common *CFTR* mutations. A mutation in a single amino acid at a nucleotide binding site accounts for 70% of the mutant alleles. However, the sensitivity of genetic screening is limited, and as many as 2% to 15% of patients may have one or two unidentified mutations.

Management and Course

The natural course of cystic fibrosis is dominated by recurrent pulmonary infections, impaired growth, and malnutrition. Improvement in the median survival time to about age 30 is the result of recent therapeutic advances and earlier diagnosis. The clinical severity of cystic fibrosis varies widely; some patients have relatively uncomplicated courses of disease and live into their fourth and fifth decades. This variability may be caused by different *CFTR* mutations and corresponding defects in chloride channel function.

Although the pulmonary complications of cystic fibrosis are the most common cause of hospitalization and mortality, gastrointestinal complications may contribute significantly to morbidity, and specific therapeutic intervention is often warranted. Pancreatic enzyme replacement improves steatorrhea and corrects nutritional deficiencies. Large enzyme doses and acid suppression with H_2 receptor antagonists ensure adequate delivery of intact enzymes to the small intestine. Doses can be adjusted according to the fat content of the meal. Enzyme bioequivalence may vary by manufacturer. Patients deficient in vitamins A, D, E, and K should receive supplements. If severe protein and calorie malnutrition persist despite these measures, enteral or parenteral nutrition may be necessary.

Obstruction of the small intestine by meconium or an impacted, partially digested food bolus may be confirmed with a meglumine (Gastrografin) enema. The high osmolarity of this water-soluble contrast stimulates lumenal water secretion, which may disrupt the impaction. The mucolytic agent, *N*-acetylcysteine, given orally or rectally, also helps to relieve obstruction. If conservative therapy fails or signs of peritonitis develop, surgical exploration is necessary and has long-term survival rates approaching 100%.

HEREDITARY PANCREATITIS

Etiology and Pathogenesis

About two thirds of families with hereditary pancreatitis have gain-of-function mutations in the cationic trypsinogen gene *PRSS1*, and one third have unidentified mutations. The cationic trypsinogen R122H and N291 mutations are the most prevalent; the former affects about two thirds of families, and the latter about one third. *PRSS1* mutations are thought to induce a conformational change in the trypsin molecule, which results in an inaccessible autolysis site resistant to hydrolysis and a persistently active, unregulated, trypsin molecule.

Clinical Features

Hereditary pancreatitis is an autosomal dominant syndrome with about 80% penetrance, characterized by recurrent attacks of pancreatitis that progress to chronic pancreatitis in about 50% of cases. The mean age at onset is 10 years. With long-standing disease, the pancreas becomes calcified, and large calcium stones in the pancreatic ducts are common. Patients with hereditary pancreatitis develop maldigestion, chronic pain, pancreatic pseudocysts, splenic vein thrombosis, and distal bile duct strictures. Patients with hereditary pancreatitis have an increased incidence of pancreatic cancer beginning 30 to 40 years after the onset of pancreatitis, with an estimated accumulated risk of 40% at age 70. Tobacco smoking increases this risk.

Diagnosis and Management

Genetic testing for the R122H and N291 mutations of the cationic trypsinogen gene *PRSS1* is available but should be approached with caution because the results may have broad implications for the patient's future health, family, employment, and insurability. Common indications for genetic testing include recurrent (two or more) attacks of otherwise unexplained acute pancreatitis, idiopathic chronic pancreatitis, and a family history of pancreatitis in a symptomatic patient. No specific treatment for hereditary pancreatitis exists, although vitamins, antioxidant therapy, and enzyme supplements may be helpful. Patients should be counseled regarding the increased risk of pancreatic cancer, and tobacco smoking should be strongly discouraged. The role of endoscopic ultrasonography as a screening tool in this high-risk population is being explored, and prophylactic pancreatectomy is being studied at select academic centers.

PANCREATIC SECRETORY TRYPSIN INHIBITOR (SPINK1) GENE MUTATION–ASSOCIATED PANCREATITIS

The *SPINK1* gene codes for an acinar-secreted protein that regulates activated trypsin by blocking trypsin's active catalytic site. Associations between *SPINK1* mutations and early-onset idiopathic and familial pancreatitis, the fibrocalculous form of tropical pancreatitis, and alcohol-associated pancreatitis have been described.

SHWACHMAN-DIAMOND SYNDROME

The Shwachman-Diamond syndrome is an autosomal recessive disorder characterized by pancreatic exocrine insufficiency, neutropenia, metaphyseal dysostosis, and eczema. With an incidence of 5 in every 100,000 live births, it is the second most common cause of pancreatic insufficiency in children after cystic fibrosis. Neutropenia is classically cyclical and may be associated with anemia and thrombocytopenia. Infectious complications resulting from neutropenia are the most common cause of death. Remarkably, patients who survive into adulthood often experience improvement in pancreatic exocrine function.

CHAPTER 52

Acute Pancreatitis

INCIDENCE AND EPIDEMIOLOGY

Acute pancreatitis is a clinical syndrome of sudden-onset abdominal pain and elevations in the levels of serum pancreatic enzymes caused by an acute necroinflammatory response in the pancreas. The hospitalization rates for acute pancreatitis vary among communities because of the demographic differences in the causes of acute pancreatitis (Table 52-1). In the United States, more than 80% of the cases of acute pancreatitis are caused by binge drinking of ethanol or by biliary stones. In urban settings, most cases are associated with alcohol use, whereas in suburban or rural settings, gallstones tend to be the predominant cause. In contrast, infection with *Ascaris lumbricoides* is the cause of pancreatitis in 10% to 20% of patients in Asian populations.

ETIOLOGY AND PATHOGENESIS

Pathogenic Mechanisms

Although the mechanisms responsible for pancreatitis are not well defined, the fundamental defects appear to be breakdowns in the normal exocrine function and cellular defenses of the pancreas. Premature activation of intrapancreatic zymogens by trypsinogen autoactivation or the lysosomal enzyme cathepsin B is the pivotal derangement and may result from intracellular retention and impaired cellular transport of zymogen granules. The normal zymogen granule has protective levels of pancreatic trypsin inhibitor, which may be quantitatively reduced or functionally

TABLE 52-1
Differential Diagnosis of Acute Pancreatits

Ethanol

Gallstones
 Choledocholithiasis
 Biliary sludge
 Microlithiasis

Mechanical/structural injury
 Sphincter of Oddi dysfunction
 Pancreas divisum
 Trauma
 Post–endoscopic retrograde cholangiopancreatography
 Pancreatic malignancy
 Peptic ulcer disease
 Inflammatory bowel disease

Medications
 Azathioprine/6-mercaptopurine
 Dideoxyinosine
 Pentamidine
 Sulfonamides
 L- Asparaginase
 Thiazide diuretics

Metabolic
 Hyperlipidemia
 Hypercalcemia

Infectious
 Viral
 Bacterial
 Parasitic

Vascular
 Vasculitis
 Atherosclerosis

Genetic mutations
 Cationic trypsinogen (hereditary) (serine protease-1, *PRSS1*)
 Serine protease inhibitor, Kazal-type 1 (*SPINK1*)
 Cystic fibrosis transmembrane conductance regulator (*CFTR*)

Miscellaneous
 Scorpion bite
 Idiopathic pancreatitis
 Cystic fibrosis
 Coronary bypass
 Tropical pancreatitis

defective in acute pancreatitis. Excessive cholinergic stimulation may also contribute to pancreatic injury. Once intrapancreatic zymogen activation is initiated, a cascade of inflammatory cells and chemical mediators potentiates cellular destruction, increases vascular permeability, and promotes local ischemia. Although the causes of acute pancreatitis are diverse, intracellular zymogen activation followed by a necroinflammatory response of variable severity appears to be the final common pathway.

Risk Factors

Gallstones and biliary sludge induce pancreatitis by transient obstruction of the main pancreatic duct. Patients with gallstones have a 12- to 20-fold increased risk of pancreatitis, but the overall incidence of pancreatitis is less than 0.2% per year in this patient population. Microlithiasis, microscopic crystals of cholesterol monohydrate or calcium bilirubinate, as well as ultrasonographically visible biliary sludge, also increase the risk of pancreatitis, presumably by mechanisms similar to those for gallstones. Microlithiasis and biliary sludge may account for up to two thirds of the cases of idiopathic pancreatitis.

Ethanol induces pancreatitis by several mechanisms: main pancreatic duct obstruction resulting from altered sphincter of Oddi function, small ductule obstruction by concretions of secreted protein, altered fluidity of the pancreatic cell membrane, direct toxic effects, and ethanol-induced hypertriglyceridemia. Ethanol sensitizes the acinar cell to cholecystokinin (CCK)-stimulated intracellular zymogen proteolysis and stimulates CCK release from the small intestine. Pancreatitis usually occurs in the setting of long-standing alcohol abuse or binge drinking, but only 5% of heavy drinkers develop clinical pancreatitis. Most patients with ethanol-induced acute pancreatitis have underlying chronic pancreatitis. This finding is consistent with the observation that initial pancreatitis attacks almost always present after years of significant alcohol intake.

Obstruction of pancreatic secretion is a less common cause of acute pancreatitis. Sphincter of Oddi dysfunction occurs mostly in patients who have had cholecystectomies. It is associated with increases in sphincter pressure (>40 mm Hg above basal duodenal pressure) caused by increased smooth muscle tone or fibrotic stricturing. Pancreas divisum results when the ventral (Wirsung) and dorsal (Santorini) ducts fail to join during fetal development. The small accessory duct of Santorini and minor papilla may produce a relatively high outflow resistance. Sphincter of Oddi dysfunction or pancreas divisum is observed in more than 25% of patients with idiopathic pancreatitis in some series. Whether this represents a causal or coincidental association in any individual patient is difficult to discern.

Other disease processes are associated with pancreatitis. Ten percent of patients with pancreatic adenocarcinoma manifest acute pancreatitis. Penetrating duodenal ulcers may extend into the pancreas and produce focal pancreatitis. Hypercalcemia and hyperlipidemia are two metabolic disturbances that can trigger acute pancreatitis. Hyperlipidemia also may be a consequence of the fat necrosis in acute pancreatitis resulting from any cause, but levels of serum triglycerides of more than 1000 mg/dL have been reliably defined as a precipitant of pancreatitis. Pancreatic infarction resulting from atherosclerotic disease or vasculitis is a rare cause of acute pancreatitis. Infections with mumps, coxsackie B virus, and cytomegalovirus may be complicated by pancreatitis. Infection with *A lumbricoides* causes up to 20% of cases of acute pancreatitis in Asia. Patients infected with the human immunodeficiency virus (HIV) may develop pancreatitis from HIV involvement of the pancreas, HIV medications, opportunistic infections with organisms such as cytomegalovirus or *Mycobacterium avium* complex, or from neoplasms (Kaposi sarcoma and lymphoma). Mutations in the trypsinogen gene (*PRSS1*) lead to amplified trypsin activity and a form of familial pancreatitis, whereas mutations in the trypsin inhibitor gene (*SPINK1*) impair the body's natural defense mechanism against intracellular activation of pancreatic enzymes and predispose to pancreatitis. Heterozygous mutations in the cystic fibrosis transmembrane conductance regulator gene (*CFTR*) increase in patients with acute and chronic pancreatitis. Patients with inflammatory bowel disease may experience pancreatitis, precipitated by medications, due to duodenal involvement of Crohn's disease, or in association with sclerosing cholangitis. The increased incidence of gallstones in Crohn's disease may further increase the risk of pancreatitis.

Trauma or manipulation of the pancreatic duct can cause pancreatitis. Endoscopic retrograde cholangiopancreatography (ERCP) is the most common iatrogenic cause of pancreatitis; about 5% of patients develop the complication. Sphincterotomy, underlying sphincter of Oddi dysfunction, excessive dye injection into the pancreas (acinarization), and hyperosmolar contrast increase the risk of pancreatitis, which can be as high as 20% in select groups. Blunt abdominal trauma can cause pancreatitis, usually by disrupting the main pancreatic duct as it crosses over the vertebral body. Postoperative pancreatitis occurs most often after upper abdominal procedures. Other surgical procedures, especially coronary bypass surgery, have been associated with hyperamylasemia, but clinical pancreatitis is unusual. Percutaneous biopsies of the pancreas and lithotripsy reportedly induce pancreatitis.

Medications are common causes of pancreatitis (see Table 52-1). Of the patients taking azathioprine or 6-mercaptopurine, 3% develop acute pancreatitis, almost always in the first month of therapy. Pentamidine, even in aerosol form, produces pancreatitis. The onset of pancreatitis associated with 2′,3′-dideoxyinosine may occur several months after drug initiation. Medications that have been less convincingly associated with pancreatitis include sulfonamides, 5-aminosalicylates, furosemide, thiazides, estrogens, tetracyclines, and cimetidine. The etiologic role of corticosteroids remains uncertain. Except for estrogens, which may produce pancreatitis by inducing hypertriglyceridemia, the mechanism of drug-induced pancreatitis is unknown.

CLINICAL FEATURES

The initial symptom of acute pancreatitis is almost always abdominal pain, which is described as a deep, visceral pain that develops over several hours in the epigastric and umbilical region. Pain persists for hours to days and may radiate to the middle to lower back. Patients often are restless. Increased pain when supine prompts many patients to sit leaning forward in an effort to minimize discomfort. However, 5% of patients with acute pancreatitis present without abdominal pain.

Nausea and vomiting are present in most patients. Low-grade fever is commonly observed in uncomplicated pancreatitis, but high fever and rigors suggest coexisting infection. In some cases of severe pancreatitis, the diagnosis is overlooked because of the patient's inability to report pain because of delirium, hemodynamic instability, or extreme respiratory distress.

Physical examination of a patient with pancreatitis may reveal several findings. Abdominal tenderness with guarding is common and usually most pronounced in the epigastric region. Bowel sounds are diminished as a result of superimposed ileus. Tachycardia may be secondary to severe pain, but hypovolemia is common, and severe cases may be complicated by hypotension from extravasation of fluids or hemorrhage in the retroperitoneum. Rare patients present with periumbilical

Cullen sign) or flank (Grey Turner sign) ecchymoses. Ethanol-induced pancreatitis is occasionally accompanied by signs or symptoms of alcoholic liver disease, including jaundice, hepatomegaly, ascites, and encephalopathy. It is estimated that 1% of alcoholics will have both pancreatitis and liver disease. Gallstone pancreatitis may be accompanied by jaundice caused by a retained common bile duct stone, although any severe cause of pancreatitis may be associated with jaundice that is caused by biliary obstruction from an edematous pancreas or associated fluid collection.

FINDINGS ON DIAGNOSTIC TESTING

Laboratory Studies

Elevated serum amylase and lipase levels are the most common abnormalities seen in laboratory studies of patients with acute pancreatitis and result from increased release and decreased renal clearance of the enzymes. Elevations greater than five-fold are virtually diagnostic of pancreatitis, but disease severity does not correlate with the degree of enzyme elevation. Total serum amylase is composed of pancreatic and salivary isoforms. Salivary amylase levels increase with salivary gland disease, chronic alcoholism without pancreatitis, cigarette smoking, anorexia nervosa, esophageal perforation, and several malignancies. The pancreatic amylase isoform may also be elevated in cholecystitis, intestinal perforation, renal failure, and intestinal ischemia. Five percent to 10% of episodes of acute pancreatitis produce no increases in serum amylase and lipase levels, which are most common in underlying chronic alcoholic pancreatitis, long-term glandular destruction, and fibrosis with loss of functional acinar tissue. Hyperamylasemia has been reported in up to 40% of patients with AIDS; yet clinical disease occurs in less than 10%. Macroamylasemia is characterized by persistent elevation of serum amylase levels because of decreased renal excretion of a high molecular weight macroamylase. The disorder is benign. Differentiation from pathological hyperamylasemia relies on calculating the amylase-to-creatinine clearance ratio (ACCR), which equals (serum creatinine × urine amylase)/(urine creatinine × serum amylase) × 100. An ACCR less than 1% suggests macroamylasemia.

Serum lipase is reportedly a more specific marker of pancreatitis, but mild elevations are observed in other conditions (e.g., renal failure and intestinal perforation). In pancreatitis, lipase levels may remain elevated for several days after amylase levels have normalized. Therefore, if the diagnosis is delayed, hyperlipasemia may be the only abnormal laboratory finding. A lipase-to-amylase ratio higher than 2 is reportedly specific for alcoholic pancreatitis; however, this should not replace the history and physical examination as the primary means for discerning the cause of pancreatitis.

Patients often have other laboratory abnormalities. Leukocytosis can result from inflammation or infection. An increased hematocrit may signal decreased plasma volume caused by extravasation of fluid; a decreased hematocrit may be caused by retroperitoneal hemorrhage. Pancreatic necrosis develops in about half of the patients whose hematocrit is higher than 44% when admitted to the hospital or if the hematocrit fails to decrease 24 hours after admission. Electrolyte disorders are common, particularly hypocalcemia, which in part is caused by sequestration of calcium salts as saponified fats in the peripancreatic bed. Patients with underlying liver disease or choledocholithiasis may have abnormal liver chemistry levels. Bilirubin levels higher than 3 mg/dL suggest a biliary cause of pancreatitis.

Structural Studies

Ultrasound is the most sensitive noninvasive means for detecting gallstones, biliary tract dilation, and gallbladder sludge. Intralumenal gas may obscure images of the pancreas in 30% to 40% of patients, however, rendering ultrasound an insensitive technique for detecting the changes associated with pancreatitis. Computed tomographic (CT) scanning is superior to ultrasound for imaging the peripancreatic bed. In mild cases, the pancreas may appear edematous or enlarged. More severe inflammation may extend into surrounding fat planes, producing a pattern of peripancreatic fat streaking. CT scanning also is optimal for defining inhomogeneous pancreatic phlegmons with ill-defined margins or well-defined pseudocysts. A dynamic arterial phase CT scan can identify areas of tissue necrosis, which are at significant risk of subsequent infection. The magnitude of pancreatic necrosis predicts the prognosis. Given its high cost and the limited yield in evaluating mild disease, CT scanning should be reserved for patients with severe disease. Once pancreatitis has resolved, CT scanning may have a role in excluding pancreatic cancer as a cause of pancreatitis in older patients. Magnetic resonance cholangiopancreatography, which is considerably more expensive than ultrasound or CT scanning, has a sensitivity higher than 90% for detecting bile duct stones. Endoscopic ultrasound is a sensitive test for detecting persistent biliary stones and can be used to distinguish patients who may benefit from treatment with ERCP. Endoscopic ultrasound also is useful for detecting small pancreatic or ampullary tumors, pancreas divisum, and chronic pancreatitis.

ERCP is primarily a therapeutic tool in acute biliary pancreatitis; it has no role in diagnosing acute pancreatitis. After an acute attack has resolved, ERCP should be considered if the cause of the pancreatitis is unclear.

MANAGEMENT AND COURSE

Prognosis

The most common prognostic criteria used to assess acute pancreatitis are the Ranson criteria, which are observations made at admission and at 48 hours after admission, and the simplified Glasgow criteria, which are variables measured at any time during the first 48 hours after admission (Table 52-2). The prognostic accuracy of the two scales is similar. Although the Ranson criteria were developed to assess alcoholic pancreatitis, they are frequently applied to pancreatitis from other causes. If two signs or fewer are present, mortality is less than 1%; three to five signs predict a mortality rate of 5%; and six or more signs increase the mortality rate to 20%. Other factors associated with a poor prognosis include obesity and extensive pancreatic necrosis. A CT-based scoring system, measurement of serum levels of the trypsinogen activation peptide, and the APACHE II score have also been used to assess the severity of acute pancreatic damage.

Complications

Patients with severe pancreatitis may develop peripancreatic fluid collections or pancreatic necrosis; either can become infected. The role of prophylactic antibiotics in patients with severe pancreatitis is controversial, although two meta-analyses have concluded that prophylaxis decreases sepsis and mortality in patients with necrosis. If administered, imipenem-cilastatin, cefuroxime, and a combination of a quinolone

TABLE 52-2
Prognostic Criteria for Acute Pancreatitis

RANSON CRITERIA	SIMPLIFIED GLASGOW CRITERIA
At admission	**Within 48 hr of admission**
Age >55	Age >55
Leukocyte count >16,000/μL	Leukocyte count >15,000/μL
Lactate dehydrogenase >350 IU/L	Lactate dehydrogenase >600 IU/L
Glucose >200 mg/dL	Glucose >180 mg/dL
Aspartate aminotransferase >250 IU/L	Albumin <3.2 g/dL
	Calcium <8 mg/dL
	Arterial PO_2 <60 mm Hg
	Serum urea nitrogen >45 mg/dL
48 hr after admission	
Hematocrit decrease >10%	
Serum urea nitrogen increase >5 mg/dL	
Calcium <8 mg/dL	
Arterial PO_2 <60 mm Hg	
Base deficit >4 meq/L	
Estimated fluid sequestration >6 L	

Adapted from Agarwal N, Pitchumoni CS, Sivaprasad AV. Evaluating tests for acute pancreatitis. *Am J Gastroenterol* 1990;85:356; and Marshall JB. Acute pancreatitis: a review with an emphasis on new developments. *Arch Intern Med* 1993;153:1185.

with metronidazole are most effective for preventing infectious complications. Infections in the first 1 to 2 weeks usually involve peripancreatic fluid collections or pancreatic necrosis and are characterized by florid symptoms. More indolent courses are characteristic of pancreatic abscesses, which can arise several weeks after a bout of pancreatitis in well-defined pseudocysts or areas of resolving pancreatic necrosis. Gram stain and culture of fluid obtained by CT-guided aspiration is mandatory if infection is suspected. Polymicrobial, gram-negative enteric bacteria, and anaerobic organisms are most often identified. Infected necrotic tissue and pancreatic abscesses require immediate surgical debridement, although some well-defined abscesses may be drained percutaneously. Sterile pancreatic necrosis should be managed with supportive medical care unless symptomatic or if significant clinical deterioration occurs.

Pseudocysts develop in 10% of patients with acute pancreatitis, most commonly in patients with alcoholic pancreatitis. Pseudocysts can persist for several weeks, causing pain, compressing adjacent organs, and eroding into the mediastinum. Cysts more than 5 to 6 cm in diameter have a 30% to 50% risk of complications, including rupture, hemorrhage, and infection. Although most pseudocysts spontaneously resolve or decrease in size, persistent (>6 weeks) large cysts or rapidly expanding cysts should be drained using surgical, endoscopic, or percutaneous procedures. Percutaneous drainage may be complicated by formation of a pancreaticocutaneous fistula. Administration of the somatostatin analog octreotide may lower the risk of fistula formation by decreasing pancreatic secretions. Endoscopic drainage may be achieved by transpapillary stent placement or transgastric placement of a cystenterostomy. The use of endoscopic ultrasound in endoscopic drainage can decrease the risk of hemorrhage and free perforation. Rarely, pseudocysts may erode into the splenic artery and present as hemosuccus pancreaticus, a life-threatening event.

Pancreatitis may be complicated by several pulmonary processes. Mild hypoxemia is present in most patients with pancreatitis. Chest radiography may demonstrate increased interstitial markings or pleural effusions, which usually are left-sided and small but occasionally are large enough to compromise respiration. The interstitial edema occurs in the setting of normal cardiac function; the etiology is unclear. Severe adult respiratory distress syndrome requires artificial respiratory support. Multisystem organ failure develops in about 50% of patients with pancreatic necrosis and is an independent predictor of mortality.

Other systemic complications of severe pancreatitis include stress gastritis, renal failure, coagulopathy, hypocalcemia, delirium, and disseminated fat necrosis (involving bones, joints, and skin). Extension of the inflammatory process into the peripancreatic bed may produce splenic vein thrombosis, which may be complicated by development of splenomegaly, gastric varices, and gastrointestinal hemorrhage.

Therapy

Therapy for most cases of acute pancreatitis is supportive, although severe cases may require massive volume repletion with crystalloids and colloids. Growing evidence suggests that enteral feeding beyond the ligament of Treitz is safe even for patients with moderately severe pancreatitis; compared to parenteral nutrition, it is less expensive and may decrease infectious complications. Total parenteral nutrition should be considered for patients with pronounced ileus. Parenteral meperidine is preferred over morphine as an analgesic because of the risk of morphine-induced sphincter of Oddi spasm. Nasogastric suctioning is useful primarily for intractable vomiting, but it is not needed in all cases. There is no evidence to support the routine use of antibiotics or somatostatin. The decision to reinitiate feeding should not be based on serum enzyme levels but rather on the clinical status of the patient. Resolution of pain and emergence of hunger reliably indicate that the patient is ready to eat.

Gallstone pancreatitis is managed differently than acute pancreatitis from other causes. Emergency ERCP with sphincterotomy and stone extraction reduces the complication rate and shortens the hospital stay for patients with severe gallstone pancreatitis. These procedures should be reserved for patients with severe disease or for those who fail to improve with conservative treatment. ERCP does not significantly worsen pancreatitis. Patients with mild gallstone pancreatitis should be treated conservatively; ERCP is performed after recovery to assess for retained bile duct stones. The risk of recurrent gallstone pancreatitis is up to 33%; therefore, all patients should undergo expeditious and definitive surgical therapy. For patients who are poor operative risks, endoscopic sphincterotomy without cholecystectomy is an acceptable therapeutic option.

CHAPTER 53

Chronic Pancreatitis

INCIDENCE AND EPIDEMIOLOGY

Chronic pancreatitis causes irreversible morphologic and functional damage to the pancreas. In many cases, there are intermittent flares of acute pancreatitis. The clinical distinction between acute recurrent pancreatitis, with restoration of normal pancreatic function and structure between attacks, and chronic pancreatitis may be difficult. Ethanol use accounts for most cases of chronic pancreatitis in the United States, whereas in Asia and Africa, malnutrition is the major cause (Table 53-1). The prevalence of chronic pancreatitis in autopsy series is 0.04% to 5.0%, although it may be as high as 45% among alcoholics. Most cases are probably subclinical; only 5% to 10% of heavy ethanol users develop clinical pancreatitis.

ETIOLOGY AND PATHOGENESIS

Ethanol Use

Intake of alcohol is the cause of up to 80% of cases of chronic pancreatitis in Western societies. Alterations in pancreatic secretion appear to play a pathogenic role in ethanol-induced chronic pancreatitis. Alcohol consumption increases the sensitivity of the pancreas to cholecystokinin (CCK), resulting in increased enzyme secretion. The resultant high-protein, high-viscosity output of the pancreas provides the substrate for protein plug formation in secondary ductules. Ethanol may further promote ductal precipitates by decreasing the production of lithostatin, a pancreatic protein that inhibits the formation of calcium stones. The main cause of pancreatic injury and dysfunction is the blockage of small ductules and eventually the main pancreatic duct by protein plugs and stones.

There does not seem to be a threshold level of alcohol consumption below which there is no risk of pancreatitis. Persons who consume as little as one ethanol-containing beverage per day have a higher risk of developing chronic pancreatitis than persons who abstain. The risk increases with increased mean daily consumption and duration of ethanol use, but the type of alcohol and pattern of drinking do not influence the risk. Alcohol consumption alone does not appear to be sufficient to induce pancreatitis, given that fewer than 10% of chronic, heavy alcohol users ever manifest clinical disease. Other triggering factors such as genetic susceptibility, environmental exposure, and diet are likely to interact with ethanol to produce chronic pancreatitis.

Malnutrition

Malnutrition-induced (or tropical) pancreatitis is the most prevalent form of chronic pancreatitis in developing Asian and African countries. Consumption of cassava, a plant indigenous to these regions, may contribute to pancreatic injury by increasing

TABLE 53-1
Causes of Chronic Pancreatitis

Ethanol (70%)

Idiopathic (including tropical) (20%)

Other (10%)
   Hereditary
   Hyperparathyroidism
   Hypertriglyceridemia
   Obstruction
   Trauma
   Cystic fibrosis
   Autoimmune pancreatitis
   Pancreas divisum

serum thiocyanate levels, which subsequently increases cellular free radical production. Ingesting a diet deficient in micronutrients and antioxidants then exposes the pancreas to injury by unopposed free radicals. Pancreatic calculi and ductular obstruction also contribute to ongoing injury, as seen in alcoholic pancreatitis.

Other Causes

Disorders that produce long-standing obstruction of the main pancreatic duct are associated with chronic pancreatitis, including tumors, traumatic strictures, and pancreas divisum. The association of sphincter of Oddi dysfunction with chronic pancreatitis remains controversial. A small percentage of patients with hyperparathyroidism develop pancreatic duct stones and calcific pancreatitis from increased pancreatic calcium secretion. Hereditary pancreatitis is caused by a missense mutation in the cationic trypsinogen gene (*PRSS1*) that codes for a trypsin molecule that is resistant to the normal mechanisms of inactivation. Hereditary pancreatitis manifests in childhood or young adulthood and is transmitted in an autosomal dominant manner. In Western countries, idiopathic chronic pancreatitis is the second most common form of the disease after alcoholic chronic pancreatitis. A bimodal age distribution in adolescents and the elderly suggests that there may be two distinct pathophysiological causes. Autoimmune pancreatitis is characterized by increased immunoglobulin G levels, diffuse enlargement of the pancreas, and irregular narrowing of the main pancreatic duct. Patients often present with biliary obstruction and respond to treatment with steroids. Cystic fibrosis is a common cause of chronic pancreatic insufficiency in children. Cigarette smoking accelerates the progression of chronic pancreatitis, particularly calcific pancreatitis.

CLINICAL FEATURES

Abdominal pain and malabsorption are the most common clinical features of chronic pancreatitis. Pain, which is present in 85% of patients, is likely to be caused by noxious stimulation of peripancreatic afferent nerves or increased intraductal pressure. Morphologic studies show that the pancreatic nerves are larger and more numerous in patients with chronic pancreatitis. Pain typically is felt in the upper quadrants and may radiate to the back. It often is less intense while sitting forward. Patients may report steady, unremitting pain or several days of pain with pain-free intervals. Food ingestion increases the intensity of pain, leading to a fear of eating (sitophobia), which is the main cause of weight loss in early chronic pancreatitis.

Malabsorption in late chronic pancreatitis results from inadequate secretion of pancreatic enzymes. Maldigestion is the physiological defect that occurs when the exocrine function is less than 10% of normal. Steatorrhea is the initial manifestation of malabsorption; azotorrhea occurs in more advanced disease. Because the mucosal absorptive capacity is intact, voluminous diarrhea is unusual; most patients complain of bulky or greasy stools. A pattern of steatorrhea and weight loss in the absence of abdominal pain is common in idiopathic chronic pancreatitis.

Most patients eventually develop symptomatic hyperglycemia. Although insulin often is required to control symptoms, most patients are not prone to ketosis. Patients with ethanol-induced chronic pancreatitis may have symptoms of liver disease, including ascites, encephalopathy, variceal bleeding, and jaundice. Jaundice can also result from compression or stricturing of the intrapancreatic portion of the common bile duct.

Physical examination findings may be normal or there may be marked abdominal tenderness. Patients may have stigmata of chronic alcoholism including gonadal atrophy, gynecomastia, and palmar erythema. A midline mass suggests the presence of a pseudocyst or complicating neoplasm. Patients rarely have pancreatic ascites. Marked deficiencies of fat-soluble vitamins (A, D, E, and K) are seldom seen.

FINDINGS ON DIAGNOSTIC TESTING

Laboratory Studies

The findings of laboratory evaluation are often normal in chronic pancreatitis. Patients rarely exhibit hyperbilirubinemia and abnormal liver chemistry levels as a result of concurrent alcoholic liver disease or common bile duct stricture. Acute flares of pancreatitis may be accompanied by leukocytosis. Macrocytic anemia occurs in a rare patient with vitamin B_{12} deficiency. Coagulopathy may result from vitamin K malabsorption or alcoholic liver disease. Because azotorrhea occurs only in advanced disease, serum albumin levels usually are normal despite profound weight loss. Serum amylase and lipase levels may be slightly elevated, but marked elevations, as observed in acute pancreatitis, are unusual. If exocrine function is severely impaired, serum lipase levels may be low, whereas serum amylase levels usually are normal in this setting because salivary amylase production is normal.

Assessment of Pancreatic Exocrine Function

Numerous methods for assessing pancreatic enzyme output are available. The simplest tests are those that detect increased fat in the stool, which develops if exocrine secretion is less than 10% of normal. Steatorrhea may be detected by qualitative fecal fat tests (Sudan stain) or quantitative 72-hour fecal fat measurements. In severe cases, the amount of fat excreted in the feces may approach the amount of fat ingested, which is indicative of profound reductions in pancreatic enzyme output. Such high degrees of steatorrhea are rarely observed with mucosal disease of the small intestine.

Pancreatic exocrine function is more accurately assessed by pancreatic stimulation tests after injecting secretin or CCK, or after ingesting a high protein meal, with simultaneous collection of pancreatic secretions through a catheter positioned in the distal duodenum. The collected fluid is assayed for bicarbonate (for secretin stimulation) or lipase and trypsin (for CCK stimulation). Chronic pancreatitis is characterized by decreased secretory output in response to these stimulants. Pancreatic stimulation tests may yield false-positive results in diabetes mellitus, cirrhosis, and after Billroth II gastrojejunostomy. Incomplete duodenal recovery of pancreatic juice or gastric acid inactivation of enzymes may lead to underestimation of pancreatic function. The sensitivity of pancreatic function tests for detecting chronic pancreatitis is 70% to 95%, which includes most patients with only mild to moderate pancreatic insufficiency.

The findings from a Schilling test are abnormal in chronic pancreatitis because of impaired cleavage of R protein, which prevents the binding of vitamin B_{12} to intrinsic factor. Expanding this test to include vitamin B_{12} bound to intrinsic factor can differentiate the maldigestion of R protein from the malabsorption of the vitamin B_{12}–intrinsic factor complex. Ingestion of the triglyceride ^{14}C-olein with subsequent measurement of breath $^{14}CO_2$ excretion assesses triglyceride digestion and absorption.

Structural Studies

Confirming the diagnosis of chronic pancreatitis usually requires imaging studies of the pancreas. Abdominal radiography demonstrates the diagnostic finding of pancreatic calcifications in 30% to 40% of patients with chronic pancreatitis. This obviates the need for more expensive imaging procedures. Ultrasound has a sensitivity of 70% and a specificity of 90% for detecting chronic pancreatitis. If abdominal radiography and ultrasound fail to confirm the diagnosis, a computed tomographic (CT) scan demonstrates the architectural changes of chronic pancreatitis with a sensitivity of 80% and a specificity of 90%. Findings may include duct dilation, calcifications, and cystic lesions. CT scans can also be useful in differentiating chronic pancreatitis from pancreatic carcinoma, and they can reveal splenomegaly and venous collaterals resulting from splenic vein thrombosis. Endoscopic retrograde pancreatography (ERP) provides the most detailed anatomic assessment of the pancreatic ducts. In the absence of a histological specimen, ERP is the gold standard for diagnosing chronic pancreatitis. The main pancreatic duct is normal in early pancreatitis, but the side branches may be dilated. Patients at this stage often have normal secretory function, but occasionally the exocrine function is reduced out of proportion to the ERP findings. With more advanced disease, dilation and an irregular contour of the main pancreatic duct may be observed. Although pancreatic cancer may produce a discrete stricture of the main pancreatic duct, chronic pancreatitis often leads to multiple ductal strictures and filling defects as a result of stone formation. Brush cytology specimens obtained under fluoroscopic guidance may be used to distinguish benign strictures from malignant strictures. Endoscopic ultrasound (EUS) has emerged as a means for obtaining detailed images of the pancreas. Several reports suggest that this technique is equivalent to ERP; both tests exhibit sensitivities and specificities higher than 90%. Unlike ERP, EUS has no risk of inducing pancreatitis. EUS-guided fine-needle aspiration can differentiate chronic pancreatitis from malignancy. ERP and EUS are costly invasive procedures that should be used only when less invasive procedures fail to substantiate the diagnosis of chronic pancreatitis or if a diagnostic finding such as a stricture, ductal dilation, or intraductal calculus will alter management. Advances in magnetic resonance (MR) imaging and MR cholangiopancreatography allow detailed examination of the pancreatic and biliary ducts without exposure to radiation or the use of oral or intravenous contrast agents. These techniques also can be used to direct endoscopic therapy.

MANAGEMENT AND COURSE

Medical Therapy

Medical therapy for chronic pancreatitis focuses on relief of pain and repletion of digestive enzymes. If the patient has symptoms of maldigestion, pancreatic enzyme supplements should be taken before all meals. Although some preparations are specifically designed to release enzymes into the duodenum (Table 53-2), there is little evidence to suggest that encapsulated preparations are superior to standard supplements. Steatorrhea usually is more difficult to treat than azotorrhea. At least 25,000 to 30,000 units of lipase per meal are necessary to provide adequate lipolysis; therefore, patients will need to take 2 to 10 pills with each meal, depending on the preparation. Gastric acid can destroy pancreatic enzymes, necessitating the administration of enteric-coated preparations or acid suppressants (e.g., H_2 receptor antagonists or proton pump inhibitors) to some patients.

Enzyme replacement therapy may also decrease the pain associated with chronic pancreatitis. A decrease in enzyme secretion increases the CCK level, which in turn produces pancreatic hyperstimulation. By interrupting the feedback upregulation of CCK release, enzyme replacements reduce hormonal stimulation of the pancreas, thereby decreasing intraductal pressures. Non–enteric-coated preparations are the only supplements that reliably deliver enzymes to the proximal duodenum where feedback regulation begins. Patients with chronic pancreatitis of nonalcoholic pathogenesis, who have constant rather than intermittent pain and only mild to moderate pancreatic insufficiency, respond best to enzyme therapy.

Analgesics remain the primary means of controlling the pain of chronic pancreatitis. An initial trial of acetaminophen or NSAIDs is preferable. Patients should be cautioned about excessive doses of acetaminophen. Severe cases require

TABLE 53-2
Pancreatic Enzyme Preparations

PREPARATION	DELIVERY*	CONTENTS (UNITS)		
		Lipase	Amylase	Protease
Cotazyme	Capsule	8000	30,000	30,000
Cotazyme-S	Enteric-coated microsphere	5000	20,000	20,000
Creon 10	Enteric-coated microsphere	10,000	33,200	37,500
Ilozyme	Uncoated tablet	11,000	30,000	30,000
Ku-Zyme HP	Enteric-coated microsphere	8000	30,000	30,000
Pancrease MT-4	Enteric-coated microtablet	4000	12,000	12,000
Pancrease MT-10	Enteric-coated microtablet	10,000	30,000	30,000
Pancrease MT-16	Enteric-coated microtablet	16,000	48,000	48,000
Protilase	Enteric-coated microsphere	4000	20,000	25,000
Viokase	Uncoated tablet	8000	30,000	30,000
Viokase	Powder	16,800	70,000	70,000
Zymase	Enteric-coated microsphere	12,000	24,000	24,000

*Enteric-coated microspheres and microtablets are encased in a cellulose capsule.
Source: Adapted from Berardi RR, Dunn-Kucharski VA. Pancreatitis and cholelithiasis. In DiPiro JT, Talbert RL, Hayes PE, et al. (eds), *Pharmacotherapy: A Pathophysiologic Approach*. Norwalk, CT: Appleton & Lange, 1993;614.

administering opiate analgesics. Concerns over addiction should not interfere with the goal of pain relief; a strong patient-physician relationship may prevent abuse of prescribed narcotics.

The somatostatin analog octreotide inhibits pancreatic secretion and has visceral analgesic effects; thus, it might be expected to decrease pain in chronic pancreatitis. Octreotide may also have a role in managing refractory pancreatic fistulae or pseudocysts.

Nonmedical Therapy

A small percentage of patients are refractory to medical measures and require more invasive procedures to control pain. Although celiac plexus neurolysis has been effective for pain control in patients with pancreatic adenocarcinoma, results in patients with chronic pancreatitis have been disappointing. Most patients experience only transient relief. Endoscopic pancreatic stone extraction, occasionally performed in conjunction with extracorporeal shock wave lithotripsy, reduces pain in 50% to 80% of cases. Patients with tight strictures may obtain pain relief after endoscopic balloon dilation and stent placement.

For severe debilitating pain unresponsive to medical therapy, surgical therapy is a legitimate means of restoring the quality of life to a patient with chronic pancreatitis. Patients with dilation of the main pancreatic duct are optimal candidates for pancreaticojejunostomy (modified Puestow procedure), a procedure with initial success rates of 80%. Unfortunately, many patients develop recurrent pain several years postoperatively. Patients without significant ductal dilation may require partial or subtotal pancreatectomy according to the extent of parenchymal disease. One half of patients experience pain relief. Ketosis-prone diabetes invariably complicates subtotal pancreatectomy. Pancreatic islet cell autotransplantation at the time of the operation may prevent postoperative diabetes.

Complications

Patients with chronic pancreatitis who report severe refractory pain or worsening of pain should be evaluated for the development of a pseudocyst. Ultrasound detects many pseudocysts, but a CT scan is the definitive diagnostic procedure. Pseudocysts in chronic pancreatitis usually are found in the body of the gland. They may rupture, bleed, or become infected; the risk of these complications is much lower than the corresponding risk of complications from acute pseudocysts. Cysts larger than 6 cm rarely resolve and require internal drainage using surgical or endoscopic techniques. EUS can be used to direct endoscopic drainage of mature cysts that impinge on the gastric or duodenal walls. Percutaneous CT-guided catheter drainage has proved successful in some cases, although a persistent pancreaticocutaneous fistula may develop.

CHAPTER 54

Pancreatic Adenocarcinoma

DUCTAL ADENOCARCINOMA

Incidence and Epidemiology

With 29,000 deaths yearly, pancreatic adenocarcinoma is the fifth leading cause of death from cancer in the United States. More than 80% of patients present after age 60. The incidence of this cancer has more than doubled since 1930, with especially prominent increases in women. The annual incidence of pancreatic adenocarcinoma is 12 per 100,000 in men and slightly less in women. Urban populations have a higher incidence than age-matched rural populations. Advanced age and other severe diseases contribute to the poor outcome for patients with pancreatic adenocarcinoma.

Etiology and Pathogenesis

Pathogenic Mechanisms

Many advances in understanding pancreatic cancer have occurred at the genetic level. Similarly to adenocarcinoma of the colon, pancreatic neoplasia appears to arise from the transformation of normal ductal epithelium to papillary lesions without atypia, to papillary lesions with atypia, and ultimately to invasive adenocarcinoma. Each step in the pathogenic process is likely to be mediated by cumulative genetic mutations. Four genetic mutations commonly appear in temporal sequence in pancreatic cancer. Point mutations in the oncogene Ki-*ras* are present in 90% of adenocarcinomas and are likely to occur at an early stage of carcinogenesis. Similarly, 50% to 70% of tumors harbor a defect in the tumor suppressor gene *p53*, which seems to be induced by hypoxia, a condition that is especially profound in pancreatic cancer. Inactivation of tumor suppressor gene *p16* in 80% to 90% of tumors leads to the loss of regulation of cell growth. A third tumor suppressor gene *SMAD4* (formerly known as *DPC4*) is deleted or mutated in 50% of pancreatic carcinomas, an event that is thought to occur relatively late in the process of ductal transformation.

Risk Factors

Several environmental exposures increase the risk of developing pancreatic adenocarcinoma (Table 54-1). Cigarette smoking is associated with a twofold increase in the rate of pancreatic cancer; it manifests at least 10 years before similar neoplasia in nonsmokers. The dietary content of fat also correlates with the incidence of pancreatic carcinoma. Canada and the United States, with mean dietary fat intakes of more than 120 g per day, have twice the rates of pancreatic cancer of Japan and Italy, where mean fat intakes range from 40 to 80 g per day. An increased risk of pancreatic cancer in obese patients with body mass indexes higher than 30 kg/m^2 is thought to be due to abnormal glucose metabolism, insulin resistance, and hyperinsulinemia. Exposure to industrial chemicals and petroleum derivatives such as

---

TABLE 54-1
Risk Factors for Pancreatic Adenocarcinoma

Advanced age
Men older than 40
Urban location
Diabetes mellitus
Hereditary pancreatitis
Tobacco smoking
High-fat diet
Occupational exposure to carcinogens (chemical, petroleum industries)

---

aminobenzene, methylnitrosourethane, and β-naphthylamine coal tar derivatives have been associated with pancreatic adenocarcinoma, but the magnitude of this risk is unclear. Preliminary reports have linked pancreatic cancer with excessive coffee and alcohol consumption, but further analyses have refuted these claims.

Pancreatic adenocarcinoma may develop in patients who have other pancreatic disease. Although pancreatic cancer induces glucose intolerance in up to 60% of affected patients, preexisting diabetes mellitus has been postulated to predispose to pancreatic cancer. Twenty percent of patients with diabetes have had their diseases longer than 2 years before being diagnosed with pancreatic carcinoma. This suggests that the biochemical or pathological consequences of diabetes may promote tumor formation in small numbers of persons. Patients with chronic pancreatitis also are at increased risk of developing pancreatic adenocarcinoma. The two diseases share numerous clinical and imaging similarities. The risk increases with the duration of pancreatitis; it is 2% at 10 years and 4% at 20 years of disease. Hereditary pancreatitis carries a 40% lifetime risk of pancreatic cancer. The mechanism of tumor promotion in long-standing diabetes and chronic pancreatitis remains unclear.

Clinical Features

Most patients experience abdominal pain that often radiates to the back. The indolent onset of the pain contrasts with the acute severe pain of acute pancreatitis and cholangitis. Careful questioning of the patient often reveals that pain developed up to 3 months before the onset of jaundice. The pain of pancreatic cancer results from ductal obstruction or malignant perineural invasion. It usually is poorly localized and constant. Persistent severe pain often reflects unresectability and is associated with perineural invasion. As with other forms of pancreatic pain, the severity may be increased by lying supine and decreased by leaning forward while sitting.

Seventy percent of pancreatic adenocarcinomas occur in the head of the pancreas, and virtually all of these lesions produce obstructive jaundice. Cancers in the body or tail of the gland only rarely cause jaundice because of the anatomic spacing between the tumors and the common bile duct that courses posterior to the head of the pancreas. Jaundice in patients with tumors in the pancreatic body or tail usually results from adenopathy in the porta hepatis or extensive liver metastasis. Pruritus and pale-colored stools are common with jaundice, owing to impaired bile excretion caused by an extrahepatic biliary obstruction.

The loss of more than 10% of body weight almost invariably occurs with pancreatic cancer. Weight loss usually results from anorexia and inadequate caloric intake. Sixty percent of patients with pancreatic adenocarcinoma have delayed gastric emptying, most often in the absence of mechanical gastroduodenal obstruction. Gastroparesis may be secondary to infiltration of the local splanchnic neural network and disruption of the neurohumoral mechanisms responsible for coordinated gastroduodenal motility. Reduced secretion of pancreatic enzymes with consequent maldigestion can also contribute to weight loss. Maldigestion is particularly prominent with tumors of the pancreatic head because obstruction of the pancreatic duct in this location results in nearly total loss of pancreatic enzyme secretion.

Diabetes mellitus is present in more than 60% of patients with pancreatic adenocarcinoma. Most patients first experience glucose intolerance within 2 years of the diagnosis of pancreatic cancer, which suggests that the malignancy causes diabetes. Enhanced secretion of islet amyloid peptide from the islets of Langerhans adjacent to the tumor is the purported cause. Elevated serum levels of this peptide produce marked insulin resistance and relative glucose intolerance.

Acute pancreatitis is the initial manifestation in 5% to 10% of pancreatic tumors. Adenocarcinoma of the pancreas should be considered in any older adult with acute pancreatitis unrelated to gallstones or ethanol. Duodenal obstruction caused by local invasion of the pancreatic mass occurs in 10% of patients. Obstruction is rarely a presenting feature, and it is almost always a preterminal event. Other uncommon complications include gastric variceal hemorrhage resulting from splenic vein thrombosis, major depression, and migratory superficial thrombophlebitis (Trousseau syndrome).

The physical examination of patients with pancreatic adenocarcinoma often reveals jaundice and evidence of significant weight loss. The chest and extremities may have extensive excoriations and lichenification from constant scratching because of the effects of jaundice. Tumors in the body and tail may be detected as palpable masses because they grow to enormous size before causing symptoms. With long-standing biliary obstruction, the gallbladder may become markedly distended and palpable, defining the classic Courvoisier sign.

Findings from Diagnostic Testing

Laboratory Studies

At the time of clinical presentation, patients often have several laboratory abnormalities, but none are specific for the diagnosis of pancreatic adenocarcinoma. Serum amylase and lipase levels may be mildly elevated, but this finding is not universal, and normal levels should not preclude further testing. There may be mild elevations of liver chemistry levels and disproportionate increases in alkaline phosphatase levels. Hematologic abnormalities include anemia caused by nutritional deficiencies or blood loss and thrombocytopenia caused by splenomegaly associated with splenic vein thrombosis. The tumor markers carcinoembryonic antigen (CEA) and CA19-9 are elevated in 75% to 85% of patients with pancreatic adenocarcinoma. Assays of these serum markers lack the specificity necessary for a reliable diagnosis and the search for better diagnostic markers is ongoing.

Imaging Studies

Ultrasound has a sensitivity of 70% for identifying pancreatic cancer, but overlying intralumenal gas and excess adipose tissue often compromise image quality. Even if examination of the pancreas is incomplete, ultrasound may demonstrate ancillary findings of pancreatic cancer, including dilation of the biliary tract and enlargement of the gallbladder. Computed tomography (CT) is superior to ultrasound and provides a sensitivity of 80% for detecting pancreatic masses. CT can define the tumor stage using dynamic contrast-enhanced imaging and can identify unresectable lesions with a positive predictive value of 98%. False-positive results may occur in the presence of focal pancreatitis or if normal anatomical variants are mistaken for tumors. Spiral or helical CT represents an advance in tomographic technology; image resolution is improved and imaging during the arterial and venous phases of contrast enhancement is possible. Ongoing studies should clarify whether spiral CT is superior to standard dynamic CT for detecting and staging pancreatic masses. Ultrasound and CT are used to guide needle biopsy of a pancreatic mass; however, anecdotal reports of tumor seeding along the needle track have prompted concern about performing these procedures in patients with potentially resectable tumors.

Endoscopic retrograde cholangiopancreatography (ERCP) has a sensitivity and specificity of 90% in diagnosing pancreatic malignancy. Abrupt obstruction of both a dilated common bile duct and a dilated pancreatic duct is termed the *double-duct sign*. This finding is virtually diagnostic of pancreatic cancer and is usually indicative of an advanced tumor in the pancreatic head. Less advanced lesions and cancers in the body or tail more often produce discrete pancreatic duct strictures. Cytologic samples of a pancreatic stricture can be obtained at the time of ERCP, but the yield is limited and the sensitivity is only 30% to 40%.

Endoscopic ultrasound (EUS) has a sensitivity of 90% for detecting pancreatic tumors. It is more sensitive than CT or ultrasound for detecting tumors smaller than 2 cm. EUS is the most accurate imaging test for staging the local extent of pancreatic tumors and is particularly useful for detecting invasion of the major splanchnic vessels. EUS-guided fine-needle aspiration of the mass can establish a cytologic diagnosis of adenocarcinoma, with a sensitivity of 80% to 90%. Because the needle track is confined to the area of surgical resection, there is no concern for tumor seeding outside the field of resection.

Management and Course

Staging

Curative surgical resection provides the only chance for long-term survival to patients with pancreatic adenocarcinoma. Unfortunately, more than 85% of patients have unresectable disease at presentation. Preoperative staging of pancreatic cancer is essential to establish the prognosis and to plan the optimal treatment strategy. As with many other cancers of the gastrointestinal tract, pancreatic tumors are staged on the basis of the TNM classification system (Table 54-2). The staging system

---

TABLE 54-2
TNM Classification of Pancreatic Cancer

Primary Tumor (T)

T1	Tumor ≤2 cm, limited to pancreas
T2	Tumor ≥2 cm, limited to pancreas
T3	Tumor extends beyond the pancreas but does not involve the celiac axis or the superior mesenteric artery
T4	Tumor involves the celiac axis or superior mesenteric artery (unresectable primary tumor)

Regional Lymph Nodes (N)

N0	No regional lymph node metastasis
N1	Regional lymph node metastasis

Distant Metastasis (M)

M0	No distant metastasis
M1	Distant metastasis

continues to evolve and now allows for attempted curative resection in patients with superior mesenteric and even portal vein invasion (T3). Only those primary tumors involving the celiac axis and superior mesenteric artery (T4) are deemed unresectable. Most tumors involving the major splanchnic vessels cannot be resected for cure. Because splenectomy and hence splenic vein resection are often performed at the time of pancreatic cancer resection, invasion of the splenic vein does not preclude complete excision of the tumor. Although metastasis to regional lymph nodes (N1) does not preclude complete surgical excision, patients with these tumors have an unfavorable prognosis relative to patients without lymph node metastasis. Several complementary procedures are used to define the stage of pancreatic cancer. Contrast-enhanced CT scanning is the best noninvasive means for detecting liver metastasis. Invasion of the large splanchnic vessels can be detected with a sensitivity of 30% to 50%. Angiography detects vascular invasion with a sensitivity of 75%. EUS has emerged as the most accurate means of detecting vascular invasion, with a sensitivity and specificity approaching 90%. As with angiography, EUS is not a reliable method for detecting distant metastatic disease; hence the optimal staging strategy combines CT and EUS studies. Magnetic resonance imaging has been refined to improve the definition of the vascular anatomy of the peripancreatic bed. Ongoing studies will define the staging role of this imaging method.

Surgical Therapy

Surgical exploration to perform curative resection should be attempted in all patients who have apparently resectable disease. An initial staging laparoscopy should be part of the planned resection to inspect the peritoneum and liver for evidence of distant metastases not detected on CT scans. Even when all staging procedures, including laparoscopy, indicate a resectable tumor, unresectable disease is found in 10% to 20% of patients after surgical dissection. Cancers localized to the pancreatic head require a pancreaticoduodenectomy—the Whipple procedure. Lesions in the body or tail can be treated with distal pancreatectomy. Alternative procedures, including total pancreatectomy and the pylorus-sparing Whipple procedure, have no proven advantage relative to standard operations. In the past, operative mortality rates for curative resection averaged 10% to 20%, but specialized centers are reporting mortality rates of 2% to 5%. The poor overall prognosis for pancreatic cancer is underscored by 5-year survival rates of 10% to 25% for patients who undergo surgical resection. The long-term survival of patients with T1 cancers is only 35% to 40%; most deaths result from recurrent disease. Unfortunately, survival for 5 years does not guarantee a cure from this disease; 40% of these persons eventually die of recurrent pancreatic adenocarcinoma. Lymph node metastasis, poorly differentiated histology, and tumors larger than 2.5 cm are all associated with a poor prognosis.

Palliative Therapy

Because most patients with pancreatic cancer have unresectable disease at presentation and have an expected survival of 6 months, palliation of symptoms is the primary goal. Correction of nutritional deficiencies and control of pain can be achieved with supportive measures. Malabsorptive symptoms can be alleviated with adequate pancreatic enzyme supplementation. Adequate protein and caloric intake may require enteral nutrition, given the high rate of malnutrition in these patients. NSAIDs and acetaminophen may be adequate for pain control, but if pain is severe, narcotics should be administered. Narcotics may have constipating effects, necessitating the concomitant use of osmotic or stimulant laxatives. For relief of tumor-associated refractory pain, surgical or radiologically guided percutaneous injection of alcohol into the celiac ganglion is 90% effective.

Obstructive jaundice and pruritus may be treated by surgical biliary bypass or by endoscopic or percutaneous placement of a biliary stent. Endoscopic stent placement and surgical bypass are more than 90% successful in relieving biliary obstruction, but surgical therapy is associated with longer hospitalizations, higher morbidities, and higher periprocedural mortality rates. Percutaneous stent placement for distal common bile duct malignant strictures has a higher morbidity and mortality relative to endoscopic stent placement because of the hemorrhage and bile leaks associated with transhepatic puncture. Therefore, endoscopic placement is preferred. Unfortunately, 40% of biliary stents become obstructed with debris and sludge 5 to 6 months after placement. As a prophylactic measure, plastic stents often are replaced every 3 to 6 months to prevent cholangitis secondary to stent occlusion. Expandable metallic biliary stents have shown lower occlusion rates, but high cost precludes routine use. Further studies are needed to define the optimal roles of metallic versus plastic stents in patients with pancreatic adenocarcinoma.

In contrast to biliary obstruction, symptomatic duodenal obstruction is best managed surgically. This complication occurs in 10% of patients with pancreatic cancer. Gastrojejunostomy is the procedure of choice. Unfortunately, duodenal obstruction is often preterminal, and surgical intervention may be contraindicated because of the overall poor clinical status of the patient.

The role of chemotherapy and radiation therapy for patients with pancreatic cancer is limited. Combined radiation and chemotherapy may prolong survival by 2 to 4 months, but there is often significant therapeutically induced toxicity. The chemotherapeutic agent gemcitabine slightly improves survival, reduces pain, and improves the quality of life; it may provide greater benefit than fluorouracil-based regimens.

OTHER MALIGNANT AND PREMALIGNANT DISEASES OF THE PANCREAS

Cystic Neoplasms

Cystic neoplasms of the pancreas may be benign or malignant. These lesions must be differentiated from the pseudocysts that often complicate the course of acute and chronic pancreatitis. Cystadenomas are classified as mucinous, also termed *macrocystic adenomas*, and serous, also termed *microcystic adenomas*. The distinction is critical because serous cystadenomas have almost no malignant potential, whereas mucinous cystadenomas have a high incidence of progression to cystadenocarcinoma. Both lesions occur more commonly in women; serous lesions usually are diagnosed in elderly patients, and mucinous lesions usually are diagnosed in middle-aged patients. Because mucinous lesions are larger, abdominal pain, weight loss, and vomiting are common presenting symptoms. Serous lesions are usually smaller than 4 to 6 cm and contain many small cysts smaller than 1 to 2 cm in diameter. One third of serous lesions exhibit a characteristic stellate "sunburst" calcification, sometimes evident on abdominal radiography. In contrast, mucinous cystadenomas contain a few large cysts, and a curvilinear calcification of the cyst capsule may occur. Despite these characteristic anatomic features, distinguishing the two neoplasms on the basis of imaging alone is difficult. Although increases in cyst fluid viscosity and CEA levels may favor the diagnosis of a mucinous neoplasm, only surgical biopsy can confirm the diagnosis. Asymptomatic serous lesions require no further therapy, but all mucinous lesions and symptomatic serous lesions require surgical resection. In comparison with the poor survival rate of ductal adenocarcinoma, patients with mucinous cystadenomas and cystadenocarcinomas have a 5-year survival rate higher than 50% after surgical resection.

Solid and Papillary Epithelial Neoplasms

Solid and papillary epithelial neoplasms arise from the epithelium of ductules, usually in the tail of the pancreas. Most patients are adolescent girls or women in their early twenties. Tumors are often larger than adenocarcinomas and frequently exhibit a cystic appearance on CT or ultrasound studies as a result of liquefaction necrosis. Despite their large size, many tumors remain localized. Resection is associated with long-term survival.

Mucinous Ductal Ectasia

Mucinous ductal ectasia, also referred to as a mucin-producing cystic tumor, is a premalignant lesion of the pancreatic duct. The etiology is unknown, but studies suggest that it is being recognized in increasing numbers. Massive dilation of the pancreatic duct is characteristic. Patients present with abdominal pain, weight loss, and steatorrhea. By endoscopic examination, the ampulla of Vater may be seen to release copious amounts of viscous mucus into the duodenum. Papillary projections of dysplastic mucosa and intraductal collections of mucinous debris often produce diffuse filling defects on ERCP. At presentation, patients often have coexisting adenocarcinoma, which suggests that mucinous ductal ectasia is a variant of mucinous cystadenocarcinoma. Surgical excision is curative if the lesion is detected before carcinoma develops. Because the lesion often involves the entire pancreatic duct, pancreatectomy is the procedure of choice.

CHAPTER 55

Endocrine Neoplasms of the Pancreas

INCIDENCE AND EPIDEMIOLOGY

Pancreatic endocrine neoplasms are rare; they have an estimated prevalence of 10 per 1 million people. Insulinomas and gastrinomas are the most common, whereas tumors that secrete vasoactive intestinal polypeptide (VIPomas) or glucagon are much less common. Only a small number of cases of symptomatic somatostatinomas have been reported, and the incidence of tumors that secrete growth hormone releasing factor (GRFomas) is unknown. Tumors that secrete pancreatic polypeptide (PPomas) and nonfunctional tumors do not generally produce clinical syndromes related to excess circulating hormone, but may account for one third of all pancreatic endocrine tumors.

ETIOLOGY AND PATHOGENESIS

Endocrine tumors of the pancreas are neoplastic proliferations of small round cells with immunohistochemical features characteristic of APUDomas (amine precursor uptake and decarboxylation [APUD]). Other members of this tumor family include medullary carcinoma of the thyroid, pheochromocytoma, melanoma, and carcinoids. Pancreatic endocrine tumors are subclassified on the basis of the clinical and pathophysiological consequences of excess hormone production. Although immunohistochemical staining of these tumors often demonstrates the presence of more than one hormone, the clinical features are almost invariably defined by the hypersecretion of only one hormone. Up to 20% of pancreatic endocrine tumors do not secrete hormones. Symptoms from these nonfunctional tumors are caused by local mass effects. A variable percentage of each tumor subtype is associated with the autosomal dominant syndrome, multiple endocrine neoplasia (MEN) type I. The *MEN1* gene, which maps to chromosome 11q13, was identified by positional cloning and is thought to encode a tumor suppressor protein that mediates growth inhibition via transforming growth factor β. Eighty percent of patients with MEN I syndrome have pancreatic endocrine tumors, which are more often multicentric than sporadic tumors. Other inherited disorders associated with pancreatic endocrine tumors include von Recklinghausen disease, von Hippel Lindan syndrome, and tuberous sclerosis.

CLINICAL FEATURES

Insulinoma

Patients with insulinomas almost invariably present with symptoms of hypoglycemia. Symptoms of neuroglycopenia include confusion, lightheadedness, syncope, visual disturbances, and behavioral changes. In some patients, the reactive sympathetic response dominates the presentation, producing tremor, irritability, malaise, and palpitations. Symptoms may be present for years before a diagnosis is established, and patients may be incorrectly diagnosed with psychiatric disorders. Unlike other types of neuroendocrine tumors that can occur in extrapancreatic locations, insulinomas occur almost exclusively in the pancreas. They usually are smaller than 2 cm, and only 10% are malignant. Insulinomas occur sporadically in 95% of cases; the remaining 5% are associated with MEN I. The average age of presentation is between 40 and 50, and there is a slight female predominance.

VIPoma

VIPoma, also termed *Verner-Morrison syndrome* or the *WDHA* (watery diarrhea, hypokalemia, and achlorhydria) *syndrome,* produces secretory diarrhea that results from activation of adenylate cyclase and leads to increased net sodium and chloride secretion. Diarrhea may be intermittent in the early phase, but eventually it is profuse and watery despite fasting, and is often described as resembling weak tea. Hypokalemia is the result of potassium losses in the stool, and achlorhydria or hypochlorhydria results from VIP inhibition of gastric acid secretion.

Other symptoms include glucose intolerance, which is secondary to VIP-mediated glycogenolysis; flushing caused by VIP-induced vasodilation; and hypercalcemia, which develops by unknown pathways. Similar to insulinomas, VIPomas in adults are almost invariably localized to the pancreas. VIPomas often are larger than 5 cm and up to 60% are malignant. VIPoma is only rarely associated with the MEN I syndrome. The sporadic form can occur at any age.

Glucagonoma

Glucagonomas produce a syndrome of dermatitis, weight loss, anemia, and glucose intolerance, most often in persons age 50 to 60. Many clinicians assume that all patients with glucagonoma are glucose intolerant, but up to 15% of patients are euglycemic. In fact, other catabolic effects of glucagon such as weight loss and hypoaminoacidemia are more consistently associated with these tumors. The classic cutaneous finding is necrolytic migratory erythema, which begins as erythematous patches in the intertriginous and perioral regions. As lesions expand, they become confluent, raised, and bullous. Chronic lesions become hyperpigmented. Correction of hypoaminoacidemia may improve the rash. The anemia is normochromic and normocytic and develops by unknown mechanisms. Other less common features of glucagonoma include thromboembolic phenomena, diarrhea, and steatorrhea. Tumors are large and located almost exclusively in the pancreas; 50% are malignant.

Somatostatinoma

Most symptoms of the somatostatinoma syndrome result from the inhibitory effects of somatostatin on the secretion of other gastrointestinal hormones. Inhibition of cholecystokinin (CCK) and gastrin release results in decreased pancreatic enzyme and gastric acid secretion. The decrease in pancreatic exocrine function may be sufficient to cause maldigestion and steatorrhea. Somatostatin also decreases the intestinal transit time and inhibits intestinal absorption. Therefore, development of diarrhea and steatorrhea is probably multifactorial. A decrease in circulating CCK leads to gallbladder stasis, which fosters sludge and gallstone formation. Inhibition of insulin release results in glucose intolerance or overt diabetes mellitus. The net catabolism and malabsorption caused by the somatostatin-secreting tumor leads to weight loss in most patients. Tumors usually are large, and most are malignant. Forty percent to 50% of somatostatinomas originate in the intestine. Diabetes, weight loss, diarrhea, and gallbladder disease are less common in patients with intestinal somatostatinomas.

GRFoma

GRFomas stimulate excessive growth hormone secretion and produce clinical manifestations identical to those of acromegaly. The incidence of these tumors is unknown. GRFomas usually are larger than 6 cm and most are extrapancreatic. In 30% of cases, the tumors are malignant. One third of patients with a GRFoma have MEN I.

PPoma and Nonfunctional Tumors

Excess circulating pancreatic polypeptide does not produce significant symptoms; therefore, PPomas are clinically indistinguishable from nonfunctional tumors. Symptoms of PPomas and nonfunctioning endocrine tumors are caused by the local and regional effects of the mass. Patients may report abdominal pain, back pain, or weight loss. Tumors usually are larger than 5 cm, and most are metastatic at the time of diagnosis.

FINDINGS ON DIAGNOSTIC TESTING

Laboratory Studies

Confirming the diagnosis of pancreatic endocrine neoplasms rests on demonstrating inappropriately elevated levels of the relative hormone as well as localization of the tumor. Several provocative tests can establish unregulated insulin secretion, but the most accepted assay relies on documenting an increase in serum insulin concentration during fasting-induced hypoglycemia. Patients fast as inpatients for up to 72 hours. Blood glucose and insulin levels are monitored every 2 to 4 hours or more frequently if the blood sugar level decreases to less than 50 mg/dL. The test is terminated if blood glucose levels are persistently less than 40 mg/dL or if neuroglycopenic symptoms develop. With hypoglycemia, an insulin-to-glucose ratio higher than 0.3 or failure of serum insulin levels to decrease to less than 6 μU/mL is consistent with the diagnosis of insulinoma. More than 90% of insulinomas are detected with this assay, but alternative diagnoses such as surreptitious use of insulin or sulfonylureas should be considered (Table 55-1). Therefore, serum should also be assayed to determine levels of C-peptide (elevated in

---

TABLE 55-1
Differential Diagnosis of Fasting Hypoglycemia

Endogenous mediators
  Insulinoma
  Nesidioblastosis
  Spontaneous autoimmune anti-insulin antibody syndrome
  Autoantibodies to insulin receptor
  Noninsulin tumor–associated hypoglycemia

Reduced hepatic glucose output
  Deficient gluconeogenesis or glycogen storage
  Hormonal deficiencies (e.g., adrenal insufficiency)
  Enzyme defects (e.g., glucose-6-phosphatase deficiency)
  Ethanol consumption and poor nutrition
  Severe liver disease

Medication or other pharmacological causes
  Sulfonylureas or biguanides
  Insulin administration
  Ingestion of ackee fruits (i.e., hypoglycin)
  Other medications (e.g., aspirin, pentamidine)

Sources: Modified from Boden G. Glucagonomas and insulinomas. *Gastroenterol Clin North Am* 1989;18:831; and Comi RJ, Gorden P, Doppman JL. Insulinoma. In: Go VLW, DiMagno EP, Gardner JD, et al. eds. *The Pancreas: Biology, Pathobiology, and Disease.* 2nd ed. New York: Raven Press; 1993;979.

insulinoma, decreased in surreptitious use of insulin), sulfonylureas, and antibodies to insulin.

Except for gastrinomas, other endocrine tumors of the pancreas do not require provocative testing to document unregulated hormone secretion. Glucagonoma is suggested by marked elevations of serum glucagon levels (>500 pg/mL), which may also occur with severe stress, renal insufficiency, or hepatic dysfunction but typically not to the levels seen with tumor presence. Similarly, the diagnoses of VIPoma, somatostatinoma, GRFoma, and PPoma require documenting elevated serum levels of the corresponding peptides.

Structural Studies

Imaging procedures are required to characterize nonfunctional tumors. Imaging studies also play a critical role in localizing and establishing the extent of actively secreting pancreatic endocrine neoplasms. The sensitivities of ultrasound, computed tomography, and magnetic resonance imaging depend on the size of the tumor. These tests detect up to 80% of tumors larger than 3 cm but fail to identify 90% of tumors smaller than 1 cm. Glucagonomas, VIPomas, PPomas, and nonfunctional tumors usually are detected as large pancreatic masses, which renders these imaging methods well suited for identifying them. However, ultrasound and computed tomography identify only 10% to 40% of gastrinomas and insulinomas; specialized procedures usually are required to localize small tumors precisely.

Endocrine tumors are typically hypervascular. Selective angiography demonstrates a characteristic vascular mass in 60% to 70% of cases and may also identify hepatic metastases. Provocative angiographic studies may localize small insulinomas and gastrinomas. Selective portal vein sampling for insulin involves transhepatic placement of a catheter into the portal vein. Serum insulin measurements taken from various locations along the splenic, superior mesenteric, and portal veins permit successful localization of insulinomas in 77% to 90% of patients. One technique uses selective injection of calcium into arterial tributaries of the pancreas, followed by measurement of serum insulin levels from the hepatic veins. This method of venous sampling for insulin avoids the risks associated with transhepatic puncture of the portal vein and accurately defines the pancreatic location of 90% to 100% of insulinomas. A similar technique of selective intraarterial injection of secretin followed by hepatic vein measurement of gastrin levels successfully localizes 75% of gastrinomas.

Endoscopic ultrasonography (EUS) is particularly useful for defining insulinomas. Accuracy approaches 100% when performed in experienced centers. EUS is helpful in localizing pancreatic gastrinomas, but its sensitivity for detecting extrapancreatic gastrinomas is about 50%. Except for insulinomas, most endocrine tumors contain somatostatin receptors. Nuclear scintigraphic techniques using radiolabeled analogs of somatostatin have been shown to detect a large subset of endocrine tumors and may be particularly useful in identifying distant metastatic disease. Due to its sensitivity and its ability to image the entire body in one study, somatostatin receptor scintigraphy has largely replaced more invasive studies such as angiography. It is recommended as the initial imaging study in all cases of known or suspected pancreatic endocrine tumors, except insulinoma. Somatostatin receptor scintigraphy fails to detect up to 50% of insulinomas because of a lack of somatostatin receptor expression. Intraoperative ultrasound, palpation of the pancreas, and examination of the small intestine are the most direct means of identifying endocrine tumors.

MANAGEMENT AND COURSE

Surgical Therapy

All patients with pancreatic endocrine neoplasia without evidence of metastatic disease on angiography, somatostatin receptor scintigraphy, computed tomography, or magnetic resonance imaging studies should undergo exploratory laparotomy by a surgeon who has extensive experience in evaluating and treating gastrointestinal endocrine tumors. If imaging studies fail to identify a tumor, exploratory surgery along with intraoperative ultrasound should be performed to search for the primary tumor. Complete surgical excision is curative for more than 90% of cases of insulinoma. It usually involves simple enucleation or distal pancreatectomy because the tumors are rarely malignant. Multicentric or metastatic disease is present in the majority of the other endocrine tumors; complete surgical resection is possible in some patients. If complete resection is achieved, the 10-year survival rate is 90%, whereas the corresponding survival rate for unresectable tumors is 20%. The presence or absence of liver metastases is the single most important prognostic factor. The only reliable means of determining the malignant nature of an endocrine tumor is the presence of metastases; therefore, all localized tumors should be resected unless severe illness precludes surgical intervention. Resection of the primary tumor has been shown to decrease the rate of liver metastases significantly. Because of the favorable prognosis and slow growth rate of neuroendocrine tumors relative to other cancer types, some centers have advocated liver transplantation for young patients with metastatic disease confined to the liver.

Medical Therapy

Patients awaiting surgical excision and patients with inoperable disease as a result of metastatic spread or other severe illness usually require medical therapy for tumor-associated symptoms. Nutritional deficits, hypovolemia, and electrolyte disorders should be corrected. Although patients with symptomatic insulinomas should have expeditious surgery, control of hypoglycemia may be difficult in the preoperative period. Many patients avoid symptoms by eating frequent meals, but occasionally, refractory hypoglycemia requires more aggressive therapy. Large amounts of parenteral glucose may produce hypokalemia from intracellular sequestration of potassium. Diazoxide inhibits insulin release and stimulates glycogenolysis; it is useful in controlling refractory hypoglycemia in preoperative patients and in patients with unresectable disease.

The somatostatin analog octreotide is a potent inhibitor of hormone release from gastrinomas, VIPomas, glucagonomas, and GRFomas, but it is a less effective suppressor of insulin secretion (Table 55-2). Octreotide improves skin rash, diarrhea, and weight loss in patients with glucagonoma, but it has little effect on glucose intolerance. The somatostatin analog improves diarrhea in patients with gastrinoma by inhibiting gastric acid secretion. It corrects diarrhea in patients with VIPoma by inhibiting VIP secretion. Initial doses range from 50 to 150 μg subcutaneously, three times daily. Escalating doses, up to 750 μg three times daily, may be required if tachyphylaxis develops. Synthetic somatostatin analogs now available have greatly simplified long-term treatment. Whether octreotide has tumoricidal effects is controversial, but a small percentage of patients experience reductions in tumor size. Side effects (e.g., steatorrhea, gallstones) are common with high doses and after prolonged use. Glucose intolerance may develop or worsen, and a small percentage of patients experience nausea, vomiting, and crampy abdominal pain. Somatostatin receptor–mediated radiotherapy exploits the high densities of

TABLE 55-2
Effects of Octreotide in Patients with Pancreatic Endocrine Tumors

	TUMOR TYPE			
	Insulinoma	*VIPoma*	*Glucagonoma*	*GRFoma*
Number of patients treated	48	29	16	8
Number of patients treated >1 month	10	26	14	8
Symptoms improved (%)	31	86	81	100
Marker hormone level reduced (%)	41	86	75	100
Dose range (μg/day)	50–1500	100–450	100–2250	100–1500
Decrease in tumor size (% of patients)	22	0	0	16

GRFoma = tumor that secretes excess growth hormone releasing factor; VIPoma = tumor that secretes excess vasoactive intestinal polypeptide.

somatostatin receptors present on almost all neuroendocrine tumors and may offer effective treatment, but further testing of its efficacy is required.

Several chemotherapy regimens have been evaluated in patients with metastatic pancreatic endocrine neoplasms. Streptozocin in combination with doxorubicin or 5-fluorouracil has shown response rates of 12% to 70%. Streptozocin plus doxorubicin is the regimen of choice because it may also provide a survival advantage. Chlorozotocin, an analog of streptozocin that has fewer adverse effects, may prove superior to streptozocin. High-dose interferon (human leukocyte, α-interferon) produces variable response rates, but most reports suggest that it is minimally effective. Hepatic artery chemoembolization reduces the size of liver metastases and improves symptoms in most patients, but procedure-related morbidity is common.

CHAPTER 56

Structural Anomalies, Tumors, and Diseases of the Biliary Tract

EMBRYOLOGY AND ANATOMY OF THE BILIARY TRACT

The biliary tract and liver originate near the junction of the foregut and the midgut as a ventral diverticulum. Shortly after it develops, this diverticulum divides into the cranial bud, which develops into the liver and intrahepatic bile ducts, and the caudal bud, which develops into the gallbladder and cystic duct. The stalk of the diverticulum forms the extrahepatic bile ducts. These primordial buds are initially composed of solid cords of endodermal cells, which later vacuolize, forming the patent lumen of the biliary tract.

The gallbladder lies in a depression on the inferior surface of the liver at the boundary between the right and left lobes. The area of the gallbladder not attached to the liver is covered by the peritoneum and is in contact with the duodenum, pancreatic head, and hepatic flexure of the colon. The fundus is the rounded end of the gallbladder that projects beyond the liver. The body is the largest part of the gallbladder. It is connected to the liver on one side and covered by peritoneum on the free surface. The infundibulum is the transitional area between the body and neck of the gallbladder, an S-shaped structure in the deepest part of the cystic fossa. The arterial supply of the gallbladder is derived from the cystic artery. Venous drainage is by multiple small veins directly into the liver or toward the cystic duct. The lymphatic drainage parallels that of the venous drainage. Sympathetic innervation originates in the celiac plexus, whereas the parasympathetic supply is through branches of both vagal nerves. The gallbladder mucosa has many folds that increase the surface contact with bile. The well-developed muscularis is covered by an almost avascular connective tissue layer and the serosa.

The intrahepatic segmental bile ducts coalesce to form the right and left hepatic ducts, which merge to form the common hepatic duct. The lengths of the right and left hepatic ducts vary from 0.5 to 2.5 cm. They join outside the liver in 95% of cases. The cystic duct, which is 0.1 to 0.4 cm in diameter and 0.5 to 8.0 cm long, connects the gallbladder neck to the common hepatic duct. The spiral valves of Heister are projections of the cystic duct mucosa that prevent excessive distention or collapse of the gallbladder. The common bile duct is 5 to 17 cm long, with a diameter of 0.3 to 1.1 cm. It consists of scanty circular muscle covered by a fibroareolar coat. The lumen is lined by columnar epithelium that is continuous with that of other biliary structures. The lumens of the common bile duct and main pancreatic duct usually join to form the ampulla of Vater, although these ducts drain separately in 30% of cases. A complex system of circular and longitudinal smooth muscle, known as the sphincter of Oddi, surrounds the intraduodenal segment of the common bile duct and the ampulla of Vater.

DEVELOPMENTAL ANOMALIES OF THE BILIARY TRACT

Etiology and Pathogenesis

Failure of vacuolization of the primordial hepatic buds can result in intrahepatic or extrahepatic biliary atresia or congenital absence of the gallbladder. Incomplete vacuolization can lead to a septated gallbladder or biliary hypoplasia with stenosis. Abnormal migration of the caudal bud into the cranial bud may produce an intrahepatic gallbladder. Inadequate caudal migration leads to a free-floating gallbladder.

Clinical Features, Diagnosis, and Management

Biliary atresia is the most frequent cause of death from liver disease in children. It occurs in 1 in 10,000 to 15,000 live births. Infants who develop biliary atresia rarely are jaundiced at birth and frequently have bile-stained meconium. With biliary atresia, jaundice is evident several weeks after birth. Treatment requires definitive surgical drainage (i.e., a Kasai procedure). Even after adequate drainage, 5-year survival is only 50%, and liver transplantation may be necessary.

BILIARY CYSTS

Incidence and Epidemiology

Cystic anomalies occur throughout the biliary system. The incidence of biliary cysts is highest in Japan where one half to two thirds of all reported cases have occurred; they are far less common in Western countries, including the United States. Except for choledochoceles, which occur with equal frequency in males and females, biliary cysts are more common in females. Many patients (40% to 60%) are diagnosed before age 10; up to one third presents after age 20.

Etiology and Pathogenesis

Five types of biliary cysts are described by the Todani classification. Type I cysts are characterized by saccular dilation of the common bile duct and are the most common type; they account for 75% to 85% of biliary cysts. Type II cysts are diverticula of the extrahepatic ducts and are rare; they account for 2% to 3% of cases. Type III cysts (termed choledochoceles) represent a dilated, prolapsed segment of the intraduodenal portion of the common bile duct. Choledochoceles are further classified into type A, which are saccular dilations of the intraduodenal portion of the common bile duct, and type B, which are diverticula of the intraduodenal portion of the common bile duct. Type IV cysts are diffuse cystic dilations in the intrahepatic and extrahepatic biliary tract. Type V cystic dilations are limited to the intrahepatic biliary system (also known as Caroli disease). A sixth type of biliary cyst involving isolated cystic dilation of the cystic duct has been proposed but few cases have been reported.

Several mechanisms are likely in the formation of biliary cysts. Theories on their origins include abnormal embryogenesis with unequal proliferation of the endodermal cell cords. Other investigators suggest that biliary cysts are acquired because of the insertion of the pancreatic duct high into the common bile duct; an anomaly observed in many patients with biliary cysts. Long-term exposure to pancreatic juice may result in chronic inflammation, edema, fibrosis, and obstruction of the bile ducts, with subsequent dilation of the common bile duct. The presence of an abnormal distal muscle segment, similar to the colonic abnormalities of Hirschsprung disease, has also been suggested as a possible cause. Studies suggest that viral infection (reovirus), genetic mutations, and impaired protein glycosylation (in Caroli disease) may be pathogenetic.

Clinical Features

Patients with type I choledochal cysts typically present in infancy with jaundice and failure to thrive, although 20% of patients present after age 2 with intermittent abdominal pain and recurrent jaundice. Patients rarely remain asymptomatic. Cirrhosis and portal hypertension are frequent complications, particularly if the cysts present in infancy. Patients with type II cysts classically present with obstruction of the common bile duct. Seventy-five percent of patients with choledochoceles (type III cysts) present after age 20 with pain and obstructive jaundice. Pancreatitis is a complication in 30% to 70% of cases of choledochocele. Patients with type IV and type V cysts typically have recurrent cholangitis, liver abscesses, and portal hypertension. Caroli disease may be associated with medullary spongy kidney, which should be distinguished from autosomal dominant polycystic kidney disease. The latter disease is characterized by hepatic cysts, which are pathologically distinct from biliary cysts. Unlike biliary cysts, hepatic cysts do not communicate with the biliary tract

Findings on Diagnostic Testing

Imaging with ultrasound or computed tomography (CT) may detect biliary cysts. However, direct visualization of the biliary system with endoscopic retrograde cholangiopancreatography (ERCP) or percutaneous transhepatic cholangiography (PTC) has long been the standard for diagnosing biliary cysts. Advances in magnetic resonance imaging have made magnetic resonance cholangiopancreatography (MRCP) useful for diagnosis. Because the test is noninvasive, MRCP has replaced ERCP and PTC for initial evaluation of these patients. ERCP and PTC offer a therapeutic advantage over MRCP if stones or potentially malignant disease is suspected. Endoscopic ultrasound can provide detailed images of cyst structure, and intraductal ultrasound can evaluate malignant transformation.

Management and Course

Small intraduodenal choledochoceles are best treated by endoscopic sphincterotomy, but all other biliary cysts require surgical therapy. For extrahepatic cysts, excision and drainage is preferable to drainage alone because of the risks of recurrent cholangitis and malignant transformation. Resection is the preferred treatment for localized intrahepatic cysts The patient with diffuse intrahepatic cysts may require hepatic transplantation if hepatic failure or portal hypertension develops. Chronic antibiotic therapy may reduce the risk of recurrent cholangitis, particularly in Caroli disease.

In addition to cholangitis, pancreatitis (type III), biliary cirrhosis, and liver abscesses may complicate the course of disease in patients with biliary cysts. Cyst rupture during pregnancy or labor has prompted the recommendation that pregnant women with symptomatic cysts deliver by cesarean section. The most feared complication is malignant degeneration. This risk is particularly high for adult patients, as 15% develop carcinoma. Carcinoma may occur throughout the biliary tract and pancreas, including the gallbladder and sites uninvolved by the cysts. The prognosis of these tumors is dismal. Almost all patients die soon after diagnosis.

SCLEROSING CHOLANGITIS

Incidence and Epidemiology

Bile duct injury characterized by inflammation, fibrosis, thickening, and stricture formation is termed *sclerosing cholangitis*. Primary sclerosing cholangitis (PSC) refers to bile duct injury not attributable to other causes, in contrast to secondary sclerosing cholangitis, which has a known cause (Table 56-1).

PSC is a disease that affects mostly young men. Two thirds of cases are diagnosed in individuals younger than 45, and the male-to-female ratio is 2:1. PSC is associated with many disorders that involve immune dysregulation (Table 56-2). Fifty percent to 75% of patients with PSC have associated ulcerative colitis. Less than 5% have Crohn's disease. Conversely, only 3% to 5% of patients with chronic ulcerative colitis are diagnosed with PSC, and there is no relationship between the severity and duration of ulcerative colitis and the risk of developing PSC.

Etiology and Pathogenesis

The etiology of PSC remains unknown, but the distinctive pattern of disease associations has generated several theories. Most patients with PSC have circulating immune complexes and autoantibodies. The most prevalent autoantibodies are characterized by immunoreactivity in the perinuclear region of neutrophils and are called *perinuclear antineutrophil cytoplasmic antibodies* (pANCAs). Although their etiologic role remains unclear, the presence of pANCAs in 50% to 80% of patients with ulcerative colitis and 90% of patients with PSC raises the possibility of a common pathogenetic link for these disorders. Other putative pathogenetic mechanisms in PSC include portal venous bacteremia with subsequent periductal

---

TABLE 56-1
Causes of Secondary Sclerosing Cholangitis

Operative trauma

Choledocholithiasis

Chronic pancreatitis

Ischemic cholangiopathy
  Liver allograft rejection
  Hepatic arterial infusion of chemotherapy
  Surgical trauma

Histiocytosis X

Cholangiocarcinoma

TABLE 56-2
Disorders Associated with Primary Sclerosing Cholangitis

DISORDER	PREVALENCE (%)
Inflammatory bowel disease	
Chronic ulcerative colitis	50–75
Crohn's disease	<5
Immunodeficiency syndromes	Rare
Angioimmunoblastic lymphadenopathy	
Acquired immunodeficiency syndrome	
Familial immunodeficiency syndromes	
Miscellaneous	
Recurrent pancreatitis	4–25
Antiphospholipid antibody syndrome	Rare
Sjögren syndrome	Rare
Rheumatoid arthritis	Rare
Retroperitoneal fibrosis	Rare

inflammation; occult infection with cytomegalovirus; and a genetic predisposition, suggested by the association of the disease with HLA-B8 and -DR3.

The mechanisms of injury in secondary sclerosing cholangitis are specific to the precipitating condition (see Table 56-1). Ischemia is the cause of bile duct injury in patients undergoing hepatic artery catheter–delivered chemotherapy and after liver allograft rejection. Gallstone-induced biliary sclerosis results from direct, repetitive traumatic damage to the bile duct.

Clinical Features

The onset of PSC is insidious, and it can be diagnosed when asymptomatic elevations in serum liver biochemistry values are detected. Alternatively, symptomatic patients may have progressive fatigue, pruritus, weight loss, and jaundice for an average of 2 years before a diagnosis is made. Cholangitis is uncommon and often indicates the presence of superimposed choledocholithiasis or bile duct carcinoma. Patients with associated inflammatory bowel disease are more likely to have both intrahepatic and extrahepatic ductal disease. Isolated involvement of the extrahepatic ducts is more common in patients without inflammatory bowel disease (38%) than in patients with inflammatory bowel disease (7%). A small percentage of patients with PSC have other associated immune disorders (e.g., Sjögren syndrome, hereditary acquired immunodeficiency syndromes, or the antiphospholipid antibody syndrome) (see Table 56-2). PSC should be differentiated from other causes of chronic cholestasis, including primary biliary cirrhosis, autoimmune hepatitis, and recurrent pyogenic cholangitis (oriental cholangiohepatitis).

Findings on Diagnostic Testing

Most patients have at least a twofold elevation of alkaline phosphatase levels, which is out of proportion to the elevations of serum bilirubin levels. Aminotransferase levels are only mildly increased. The standard technique for diagnosis is ERCP, which is preferred over PTC because of the technical difficulties of cannulating strictured intrahepatic ducts. The characteristic cholangiographic features include multifocal strictures, usually in the intrahepatic and extrahepatic ducts, with intervening normal or dilated ductal segments that produce a "string of beads" pattern. This pattern is not specific for PSC and may be seen in patients with metastatic cancer to the liver, primary biliary cirrhosis, allograft ischemic injury, and the diffuse form of cholangiocarcinoma. Differentiating cholangiocarcinoma from PSC can be difficult, especially because bile duct cancer is a potential complication of PSC. Magnetic resonance imaging is used more often in the initial evaluation of patients with suspected PSC. Liver biopsy is required for staging disease severity and determining prognosis, but it is rarely diagnostic.

Management and Course

PSC usually follows a slow, progressive course. A small subset of patients has stable disease for decades, but over years, most patients with PSC progress to portal hypertension and death caused by liver failure. The 5-year survival rate is 60% to 70%. Patients who present with symptomatic disease have significantly worse prognoses. Cholangiocarcinoma complicates the course of disease in 7% to 15% of patients with PSC; it can be difficult to diagnose in view of the cholangiographic abnormalities observed in PSC. The mean age at diagnosis of cholangiocarcinoma in these patients is 42, compared with the mean age of 66 for the general population.

The treatment of PSC patients is primarily supportive. Orthotopic liver transplantation is reserved for patients with end-stage disease, recurrent cholangitis despite medical therapy, or uncontrolled peristomal variceal bleeding. No immunosuppressive regimen has been demonstrated to slow the progression of the disease. Although ursodeoxycholic acid (ursodiol) may relieve pruritus and improve biochemical profiles, it fails to halt disease progression. Prophylactic colectomy in patients with ulcerative colitis does not alter the natural course of PSC nor does it prevent the complication of cholangiocarcinoma. Dominant symptomatic strictures may be treated with endoscopic balloon dilation and stenting. Surgical resection and biliary reconstruction may be necessary for selected patients with refractory strictures or for those who may have bile duct carcinoma.

CARCINOMA OF THE BILE DUCTS

Incidence and Epidemiology

Cholangiocarcinoma is a rare tumor that generally occurs in middle-aged persons. The relatively young median age of onset results in part from the association with PSC and biliary cysts. Unlike gallbladder tumors, there are minimal racial and geographic differences in the incidence of bile duct carcinoma.

Etiology and Pathogenesis

No specific causes have been identified for bile duct cancer, but there are several disease associations. The high incidence of these tumors in Southeast Asia may be the result of chronic infestation with the liver fluke, *Clonorchis sinensis.* However, this infection does not have a proven pathogenetic role. Other disease associations include PSC and biliary cysts. There have also been reports of an increased incidence of cholangiocarcinoma in patients and relatives of patients with hereditary nonpolyposis colon cancer. Cholangiocarcinoma has not been linked to cirrhosis, gallstone disease, carcinogens, or drug exposures.

Clinical Features

Nonspecific symptoms of anorexia and weight loss are common in patients with cholangiocarcinoma. Jaundice develops if the extrahepatic ducts become obstructed. Pain and cholangitis are not typical symptoms unless the patient has had prior surgery or superimposed choledocholithiasis. Fifty percent of extrahepatic tumors involve the hilum of the right and left hepatic ducts (i.e., Klatskin tumor), and the other 50% involve the common hepatic duct or common bile duct. Ten percent of tumors spread diffusely throughout the biliary tract and may mimic PSC. Bile duct tumors tend to invade locally, and patients generally do not present with widely metastatic disease.

Findings on Diagnostic Testing

Initially, ultrasound should be used to evaluate patients suspected of having bile duct tumors. Intrahepatic bile duct dilation with no evidence of extrahepatic dilation suggests an extrahepatic bile duct tumor. A CT scan is more accurate in defining distal common bile duct lesions and is more sensitive than ultrasound in detecting intrahepatic lesions. The definitive imaging procedure is cholangiography by PTC or ERCP. If a CT scan or ultrasound suggests obstruction in the hilar region, PTC is the preferred procedure for further evaluation. Contrast-enhanced CT, angiography, and magnetic resonance imaging can define vascular invasion.

Histological confirmation of malignancy can be obtained by transhepatic or endoscopic cytologic brushings. These tests have sensitivities of only 30% to 50% but show specificities approaching 100%. Because of this, cytology is useful if results are positive but of little value if negative. The addition of forceps biopsy to cytologic testing increases the diagnostic yield to 70%. Many tumors are well differentiated and occur in PSC, making diagnosis very difficult without surgical resection.

Management and Course

Surgical resection is the only option for long-term survival. At diagnosis, 20% to 30% of proximal duct tumors and 60% to 70% of distal duct tumors are resectable. Involvement of both the right and left hepatic lobes or invasion of the portal vein or hepatic artery indicates unresectability. The median survival time for patients who successfully undergo resection with tumor-free margins is 3 years, compared with 1 year for patients who have unresectable tumors.

Jaundiced patients with unresectable tumors should be considered for palliative biliary-enteric anastomosis. If the patient is a poor operative candidate, placement of a biliary stent during ERCP or PTC usually provides adequate drainage. Radiation therapy may also palliate symptoms and improve survival. Hepatic transplantation prolongs survival, but the high incidence of recurrent disease in these patients suggests that transplantation should be done only in the setting of a research protocol.

CARCINOMA OF THE GALLBLADDER

Incidence and Epidemiology

Carcinoma of the gallbladder is a disease of the elderly. It is three times more common in women than in men. The female predominance has been attributed to a strong association with gallstones, which are present in 80% of patients with gallbladder tumors. There is a marked ethnic and geographic variation in the incidence of this tumor. It is the most common gastrointestinal malignancy in Native

Americans. It is also prevalent among Latin American women, Japanese women, and Northern Europeans.

Etiology and Pathogenesis

The strong association of gallbladder carcinoma with gallstone disease has led to speculation that the bacterial and chemical microenvironment in association with cholelithiasis is carcinogenic, but the mechanisms involved are unknown. The duration of gallstone disease is important because patients with cholelithiasis for more than 40 years have a higher incidence of gallbladder carcinoma than those with stones for a shorter period. Despite this increased risk, the very low incidence of gallbladder cancer does not warrant prophylactic cholecystectomy in patients with asymptomatic stones. Other factors associated with a high risk of gallbladder cancer include calcification of the gallbladder wall (porcelain gallbladder), biliary cysts, and *Salmonella typhi* carriage. Although the carcinogens are unknown, workers in the textile, rubber, and automotive industries have higher incidences of gallbladder malignancies.

Clinical Features

The signs and symptoms of gallbladder carcinoma are nonspecific. Only 10% to 20% of patients have the diagnosis established preoperatively. Pain is the most common complaint, but the pattern is variable. Jaundice occurs in 30% to 60% of patients and is a poor prognostic sign, usually indicative of an unresectable tumor. Other symptoms include nausea, vomiting, anorexia, and weight loss. Cholecystenteric fistulae are rare complications of gallbladder tumors.

Management and Course

Most patients with gallbladder tumors have stage IV or unresectable disease. The median survival time for these patients is 5 months. Patients with noninvasive stage I tumors limited to the gallbladder can be cured by simple cholecystectomy. Stage II and stage III tumors have a small chance of cure with a radical cholecystectomy, which involves wedge resection of the liver and regional lymphadenectomy. The role of chemotherapy and radiation therapy has not been defined for treating gallbladder tumors.

CHAPTER 57

Biliary Tract Stones and Postcholecystectomy Syndrome

GALLSTONES

Incidence and Epidemiology

Gallstone-related conditions are among the most common gastrointestinal disorders requiring hospitalization. Prevalence varies widely among ethnic groups. Pima Indians, Chileans, and whites in the United States manifest the highest rates. Asians in Singapore and Thailand have exceptionally low incidences of gallstone disease. The composition of stones also varies among cultures. Cholesterol stones account for 75% of gallstones in Western countries, whereas pigment or bilirubinate stones predominate in Africa and Asia. Gallstones are more prevalent in females across all age and ethnic groups.

Etiology and Pathogenesis

Biliary tract stones are divided into two general categories: cholesterol stones and pigment stones. This classification results from distinct pathophysiological alterations in bile composition and the disparate clinical associations and risk factors (Table 57-1). Cholesterol stones are predominantly composed of cholesterol monohydrate with small amounts of calcium salts and glycoproteins. Cholesterol gallstones may form whenever the tightly regulated process of cholesterol secretion in bile is disturbed. Bile may become supersaturated with cholesterol if bile acid secretion decreases or if free cholesterol secretion increases. Because phospholipids help solubilize cholesterol into micelles, any decrease in bile phospholipid content also promotes stone formation. Stone formation is also fostered by stasis within the gallbladder. Several nucleation factors, including gallbladder mucin, make the gallbladder a fertile environment for stone formation.

Pigmented biliary tract stones are subclassified into black and brown stones based on differences in chemical composition and associated clinical features (see Table 57-1). Both are composed of calcium bilirubinate. Black stones contain polymers of bilirubinate, whereas brown stones contain monomers of bilirubinate as well as cholesterol and fatty acid salts. β-Glucuronidase from bacteria and, to a lesser extent, from biliary mucosal sources deconjugates bilirubin glucuronides. In gallbladder stasis, the unconjugated bilirubin then precipitates as calcium bilirubinate crystals, which subsequently accumulate to form pigment stones.

TABLE 57-1
Risk Factors and Conditions Associated with Gallstone Formation

Cholesterol stones
  Age
  Female sex
  Estrogens
  Pregnancy
  Diabetes mellitus
  Obesity
  Hypertriglyceridemia
  Prolonged fasting
  Rapid weight loss
  Ileal disease or resection
  Cystic fibrosis

Black pigment stones
  Chronic hemolysis
  Cirrhosis
  High-protein diet

Brown pigment stones
  Biliary infections
  Foreign bodies (e.g., sutures)
  Low-protein diet

Clinical Features

Gallbladder stones produce a wide spectrum of clinical presentations, including episodic biliary colic, acute cholecystitis, and chronic cholecystitis. Passage of a gallstone through the common bile duct may lead to acute cholangitis or acute pancreatitis. Despite the high incidence of these complications in the general population, more than two thirds of patients with gallstones will never develop symptoms.

Biliary Colic

Most patients with symptomatic cholelithiasis present with biliary colic. This is a visceral pain that is caused by transient gallstone obstruction of the cystic duct. The pain typically is severe and episodic and lasts 30 minutes to several hours. The term *biliary colic* is a misnomer because the pain is steady and does not fluctuate in intensity. It is usually epigastric and is often referred to the right shoulder or interscapular region. During attacks, patients are restless and may have associated diaphoresis and vomiting. The interval between attacks is highly variable and may be days to years. There is no convincing evidence that ingesting fatty foods precipitates an attack of biliary colic.

Acute Cholecystitis

When a biliary colic attack lasts longer than 3 hours or if localized right upper quadrant tenderness and fever develop, the diagnosis of acute cholecystitis should be entertained. The pain of acute cholecystitis may wane, but the tenderness usually increases. A Murphy sign, the abrupt cessation in inspiration in response to pain on palpation of the right upper quadrant, is a classic finding observed in 60% to 70% of patients. High fever, hemodynamic instability, and peritoneal signs suggest gallbladder perforation, which is a complication in 10% of patients with acute cholecystitis. Ten percent to 15% of patients develop jaundice, which is a symptom that may be caused by gallstone obstruction of the common bile duct, or by Mirizzi syndrome, which is an obstruction of the common hepatic duct caused by edema and inflammation at the origin of the cystic duct. Most patients with acute cholecystitis have had previous attacks of biliary pain.

Chronic Cholecystitis
Patients with chronic cholecystitis usually have gallstones and have had repeated attacks of biliary pain or acute cholecystitis, which results in a thickened and fibrotic gallbladder. It is uncommon for the gallbladder to be palpable during an attack of pain. In fact, patients may have few symptoms referable to the gallbladder itself, presenting instead with complications such as cholangitis and gallstone pancreatitis.

Acalculous Cholecystitis
There is no evidence of cholelithiasis in 5% to 10% of patients with acute cholecystitis. Acalculous cholecystitis occurs in critically ill patients, often with multiorgan failure, extensive burn injuries, major surgery, and trauma. Perforation is more common and the course is more fulminant.

Findings on Diagnostic Testing
Laboratory Studies
Most patients with acute cholecystitis exhibit leukocytosis with a left shift. Some patients may have elevations in aminotransferases, alkaline phosphatase, bilirubin, or amylase caused by choledocholithiasis or cystic duct edema with resulting biliary obstruction. Patients with uncomplicated biliary colic usually have normal biochemical profiles.

Structural Studies
Ultrasound is highly sensitive and specific for diagnosing cholelithiasis. In uncomplicated biliary colic, gallstones may be the only finding. Thickening of the gallbladder wall is a nonspecific finding commonly observed in acute and chronic cholecystitis. Pericholecystic fluid and intramural gas are specific ultrasonographic features of acute cholecystitis. Dilation of the intrahepatic or extrahepatic ducts suggests choledocholithiasis; however, ultrasound is insensitive for imaging common bile duct stones. ^{99m}Tc-labeled iminodiacetic scintigraphy can confirm a diagnosis of acute cholecystitis. The tracer is injected intravenously and excreted in bile. Failure to image the gallbladder within 90 minutes suggests cystic duct obstruction. The gallbladder cannot be visualized in 85% of patients with acalculous cholecystitis. Computed tomography (CT) may be beneficial in evaluating patients with complicated disease (e.g., perforation or gangrene).

Management and Course
Most patients with gallstones remain asymptomatic, but over a 20-year period, 15% to 25% of these asymptomatic patients develop symptoms. Once symptoms occur, there is a high risk of recurrent attacks of pain and complications such as cholecystitis, pancreatitis, and cholangitis.

Although there are many nonsurgical alternatives, cholecystectomy is the definitive treatment for symptomatic cholelithiasis. Laparoscopic cholecystectomy is favored because there are fewer wound-related complications, shorter hospital stays, and more rapid recoveries. The technique results in a 2% to 3% incidence of bile duct injuries, however, a higher incidence than with open cholecystectomy. Open cholecystectomy is preferred if acute cholecystitis is evident, if extensive scarring from prior abdominal surgery exists, if exploration of the common bile duct is planned, or if visualization by laparoscopy is inadequate.

Given the overall benefits of surgical therapy, dissolution therapy with chenodeoxycholic acid or ursodeoxycholic acid should be reserved for patients who are at high risk of surgery. Because of its superior side-effect profile, ursodeoxycholic acid is the preferred agent. Small (<1.5 cm in diameter) noncalcified stones that float on oral cholecystography are suitable for dissolution. Candidate patients should demonstrate adequate gallbladder filling and emptying by oral cholecystography. Dissolution often requires longer than 6 months of therapy. Response rates range from 60% to 70%. There are frequent recurrences after therapy is discontinued. Direct contact dissolution therapy with monooctanoin and methyl-*tert*-butyl ether is often successful in days to weeks, but it has a high rate of complications and thus remains experimental.

Extracorporeal shock wave lithotripsy is 90% successful in achieving stone fragmentation and clearance of solitary, small, radiolucent stones. Most patients also require dissolution therapy. Similar to dissolution therapy, it may take months of extracorporeal shock wave lithotripsy to clear the gallbladder of stones. About 20% of patients experience biliary colic for several weeks after fragmentation.

CHOLEDOCHOLITHIASIS

Incidence and Epidemiology

In the United States, most bile duct stones are cholesterol stones that have migrated from the gallbladder. Ten percent to 15% of patients who undergo cholecystectomy have concomitant bile duct stones, and 1% to 4% exhibit residual postoperative choledocholithiasis, even after the common bile duct is explored. Conversely, more than 80% to 90% of patients with choledocholithiasis have gallbladder stones. The incidence of choledocholithiasis increases with age; one third of octogenarians who undergo cholecystectomy have coexistent bile duct stones. The prevalence of choledocholithiasis and intrahepatic stones is higher in Asian societies. These populations have higher incidences of pigment stones, which usually are formed de novo in the bile ducts.

Etiology and Pathogenesis

Although most bile duct stones originate in the gallbladder, some stones (especially brown pigment stones) form de novo in the bile ducts. The major component of these stones is calcium bilirubinate. Any process that increases the concentration of unconjugated bilirubin in bile or increases bile stasis fosters intraductal brown stone formation. Bacterial β-glucuronidase probably plays a major role in deconjugating bilirubin because most common bile duct stones are culture positive. A diet low in fat and protein may also promote bile duct stone formation; the factors involved are increased deconjugation of excreted bilirubin and sphincter of Oddi (SO) hypertension with associated bile stasis. Other potential risk factors include periampullary diverticula, ampullary stenosis, and foreign material in the bile ducts.

Clinical Features

Unlike with gallbladder stones, most patients with bile duct stones develop symptoms. Some remain asymptomatic for decades, and others present suddenly with potentially life-threatening cholangitis or pancreatitis. Patients with choledocholithiasis often present with biliary colic indistinguishable from the pain of cystic duct obstruction. The pain is steady, lasts for 30 minutes to several hours, and is located in the epigastrium and right upper quadrant.

Cholangitis is the result of superimposed infection in the setting of a biliary obstruction. The Charcot classic triad of right upper quadrant pain, fever, and jaundice may be present in only 50% to 75% of patients with acute cholangitis. Ten percent of episodes are marked by a fulminant course with hemodynamic instability and encephalopathy. *Reynolds pentad* refers to the constellation of the Charcot triad plus hypotension and confusion.

Findings on Diagnostic Testing

Laboratory Studies

Immediately after an attack, levels of serum aminotransferases often are elevated because of hepatocellular injury. Alkaline phosphatase levels are often elevated, mildly in asymptomatic patients, and not more than five times higher than normal in symptomatic patients. Most symptomatic patients have hyperbilirubinemia; the bilirubin level is in the range of 2 to 14 mg/dL. Higher elevations of alkaline phosphatase or bilirubin levels suggest malignant obstruction of the biliary tree.

Structural Studies

In contrast to gallbladder stones, bile duct stones are not readily detected by ultrasound; the sensitivity is less than 20%. The technological advances of helical CT scanning have led to improved accuracy in sensitivity and specificity of 80% to 85% in detecting bile duct stones. Endoscopic retrograde cholangiopancreatography (ERCP) is the procedure of choice for evaluating patients with suspected choledocholithiasis. ERCP has a sensitivity of 90% for diagnosing choledocholithiasis and has the advantage of facilitating therapeutic sphincterotomy and stone extraction. Endoscopic ultrasound can detect 95% or more of common bile duct stones, but current instruments cannot extract stones. Magnetic resonance (MR) cholangiography has a sensitivity similar to ERCP for detecting bile duct stones. It may be used in the initial evaluation of patients for whom the index of suspicion for stones is only low or moderate, to avoid unnecessary exposure to the risks of ERCP.

There is no consensus on the optimal evaluation of choledocholithiasis in patients undergoing elective cholecystectomy for gallstone disease. If open cholecystectomy is planned, intraoperative cholangiography and common bile duct palpation can be used. If stones are found, the common bile duct should be explored and stones should be extracted. Several alternative strategies are available to patients undergoing planned laparoscopic cholecystectomy. One strategy involves minimal preoperative assessment, including ultrasound and CT scanning. An intraoperative cholangiogram is performed during the laparoscopic procedure. Those patients with documented intraductal stones undergo stone extraction laparoscopically or by open cholecystectomy. Alternatively, ERCP with endoscopic sphincterotomy could be performed postoperatively. A second strategy identifies patients preoperatively at high or low risk of coexisting choledocholithiasis on the basis of the biochemical profile and the presence or absence of biliary tract dilation on ultrasound. Patients at high risk undergo preoperative endoscopic ultrasonography or ERCP; those with confirmed biliary stones undergo endoscopic stone xtraction. When the stones are cleared from the bile duct, the patient then roceeds to laparoscopic cholecystectomy. Patients with a low risk of choledoholithiasis undergo laparoscopic cholecystectomy with intraoperative cholangiography, as previously described. Benefits and risks are associated with each strategy; the approach is largely determined by the resources available at individual institutions.

Management and Course

Common bile duct stones, even if asymptomatic, require therapy because of the igh complication rate (e.g., cholangitis and pancreatitis). Secondary biliary cirhosis may develop in cases of persistent biliary obstruction (i.e., >5 years). In uch cases, reversal of portal hypertension and cirrhosis has been reported, suggestng that even late efforts to relieve obstruction are warranted. Definitive therapy nvolves common bile duct exploration and stone extraction, but this procedure ncreases the operative mortality rate of a cholecystectomy from 0.5% to 3% to 4%. The perioperative mortality rate for patients younger than age 60 is 1.5%, whereas ne risk for patients older than 65 is 5% to 10%. On the basis of this high mortality rate, endoscopic sphincterotomy and stone extraction represent a favorable pproach, especially in older patients. The risk of recurrent symptoms is high if atients have intact gallbladders; therefore, cholecystectomy should be performed. n elderly patients with severe comorbid illness, however, the surgical risks may utweigh the risk of recurrent gallstone symptoms. Endoscopic sphincterotomy lone may be an acceptable therapy for these patients. If bile duct stones cannot be xtracted endoscopically, long-term internal stenting is also a therapeutic option or this high-risk group. Young, healthy patients who have minimal operative risk actors may be treated with primary cholecystectomy and common bile duct exploation with stone extraction. The choice of endoscopic versus surgical removal of ile duct stones in this group may be determined by local expertise and resources. t is worth noting that even after surgical common bile duct exploration, 1% to % of patients have retained common bile duct stones.

Patients presenting with cholangitis or pancreatitis are treated initially with conervative measures, including parenteral fluid repletion, bowel rest, and parenteral ntibiotics (for cholangitis). In patients with severe pancreatitis that progresses or ails to improve within 48 hours and in patients with severe cholangitis, emergency ERCP with possible stone extraction reduces morbidity and mortality. Patients who o not pass their stones by ERCP or who have superimposed cholecystitis require mergency surgical intervention.

POSTCHOLECYSTECTOMY SYNDROME

Incidence and Epidemiology

After cholecystectomy, 20% to 40% of patients experience abdominal discomfort, nd 2% to 10% have debilitating pain. Patients who do not have gallstones confirmed n surgical pathological examination are more likely to remain symptomatic after holecystectomy. Most of these patients have functional abdominal pain, but a small ercentage of patients with the postcholecystectomy syndrome have symptoms riginating from the biliary tract. Possible causes include retained common bile duct tones, postoperative bile duct strictures, biliary tumors, and sphincter of Oddi (SO) ysfunction. SO dysfunction is primarily a disease of women who have undergone rior cholecystectomy. The disorder is uncommon and accounts for only 5% to

10% of patients who present with postcholecystectomy pain. SO dysfunction is also the putative cause in 10% to 20% of patients with idiopathic pancreatitis.

Etiology and Pathogenesis

The basic mechanism by which SO dysfunction produces symptoms involves impedance to bile flow at the level of the SO. This can result from an anatomic narrowing, termed *papillary stenosis*, or abnormal motility, termed *sphincter of Oddi dyskinesia*. Stenosis may result from fibrosis or muscle hypertrophy secondary to prior choledocholithiasis. The cause of dyskinesia remains undefined but probably involves dysregulation of neurohormonal influences on the sphincter.

Clinical Features

Patients with SO dysfunction may manifest idiopathic pancreatitis or recurrent abdominal pain after cholecystectomy. The pain is similar to biliary colic; it is localized to the epigastrium and right upper quadrant and often radiates to the scapula.

Findings on Diagnostic Testing

Given the confounding possibility that either small gallbladder stones or sludge is the cause of symptoms, SO dysfunction can be diagnosed reliably only in patients who have undergone prior cholecystectomy. Liver chemistry profiles are obtained during an attack of pain and ultrasound is performed to exclude biliary dilation. ERCP is necessary to exclude alternative diagnoses, such as retained common bile duct stones or postoperative biliary strictures. ERCP can also assess the drainage capability of the biliary tree. The results of laboratory testing, ultrasound, and ERCP can be used to classify patients into groups with distinct probabilities of the presence of physiological SO dysfunction. Type I describes patients with biliary pain, liver chemistry values elevated to at least twice normal on two occasions, dilated common bile ducts, and delayed contrast drainage from the common bile duct during ERCP. Type II is defined by biliary pain with one or two of the above criteria, and type III includes patients with biliary-type pain but none of the other features described. The incidence of manometrically confirmed SO dysfunction is nearly 100% in type I, 50% in type II, and 25% in type III patients.

If ERCP demonstrates biliary dilation and delayed common bile duct contrast drainage (>45 minutes) in a patient with liver chemistry abnormalities during two previous episodes of pain, a presumptive diagnosis of SO dysfunction can be made and the patient can be treated at the time of ERCP with endoscopic sphincterotomy. Papillary stenosis rather than sphincter dyskinesia is the mechanism of dysfunction in most type I patients. SO manometry is indicated to confirm high sphincter pressures in type II and type III patients. It is performed by passing a three-channel, water-perfused catheter into the common bile duct through a duodenoscope. The catheter is slowly withdrawn across the sphincter as basal and phasic pressures are recorded. Although many manometric abnormalities have been observed in patients with SO dysfunction, an elevated basal sphincter pressure (>40 mm Hg) is the only criterion that predicts a therapeutic response to endoscopic sphincterotomy. A basal pressure higher than 40 mm Hg is essential, therefore, to diagnosing SO dysfunction in type II and type III patients.

Management and Course

Pharmacological therapy for SO dysfunction has been disappointing, mostly because of its inefficacy in treating the papillary stenosis variant of the abnormality and the high incidence of side effects. The mainstay of therapy is disruption of the sphincter mechanism. Surgical sphincterotomy has a high success rate, but this approach has been supplanted by endoscopic sphincterotomy, which has become the standard therapy for SO dysfunction. Sphincterotomy alleviates abdominal pain in 90% of patients with manometrically confirmed SO dysfunction. Although results of longer follow-up periods are required, 5% of patients develop restenosis.

Endoscopic sphincterotomy carries a significant complication rate, especially for patients with SO dysfunction. The incidence of post-ERCP pancreatitis in these patients is 10% to 20%. The incidence is higher in patients without common bile duct dilation. A temporary pancreatic duct stent, which is typically left in place for 1 to 5 days following the procedure, may reduce ERCP-related pancreatitis in individuals with SO dysfunction. Hemorrhage and perforation are less common complications.

MISCELLANEOUS COMPLICATIONS OF BILIARY TRACT STONES

Bile Duct Strictures

Trauma and the chronic inflammatory response induced by biliary stones can result in benign strictures of the extrahepatic bile ducts. Other common causes of benign strictures include surgical trauma, chronic pancreatitis, parasitic infection, and sclerosing cholangitis. Patients may present with cholangitis, painless jaundice, or asymptomatic elevations of alkaline phosphatase levels. Diagnosis requires direct bile duct visualization by ERCP or percutaneous transhepatic cholangiography. Given the inadequate long-term efficacy of biliary stenting, surgical decompression is the treatment of choice for benign strictures. Failure to relieve the obstruction predisposes the patient to cholangitis, stone formation, and secondary biliary cirrhosis.

Biliary Fistula

The most common cause of biliary fistula formation is surgical trauma during cholecystectomy. Hepatobiliary scintigraphy can detect bile leaks and fistulae with higher than 90% sensitivity. Most leaks respond to endoscopic therapy using biliary sphincterotomy and/or stenting. Most spontaneous biliary-enteric fistulae are produced by gallstones; alternative causes include malignancy, peptic ulcer disease, and penetrating trauma. Patients with gallstone-induced fistulae can be asymptomatic, or they may present with nonspecific symptoms of anorexia, weight loss, and malabsorption. Gallstone ileus results when a large gallstone (>3 cm) passes into the gut through a cholecystenteric fistula and produces lumenal obstruction in the distal ileum. Biliary fistulae can often be detected on abdominal radiographs or upper gastrointestinal barium radiographs as air or barium in the biliary tree. Treatment requires surgical excision of the fistula, cholecystectomy, and extraction of all bile duct stones.

Hematobilia

Hemorrhage from the biliary tract is a rare complication of gallstones. The more common causes are penetrating trauma or iatrogenic trauma from a liver biopsy. In the United States, hepatobiliary tumors and aneurysms are possible causes, whereas parasitic diseases are possible causes in Asian societies. Diagnosis requires upper gastrointestinal endoscopy to exclude other sources of upper gastrointestinal hemorrhage. Angiography can confirm the site of bleeding. Angiographic embolization is the preferred initial treatment of hepatic causes of hematobilia. Surgical intervention is recommended to treat hemorrhage from the extrahepatic biliary tree.

Oriental Cholangiohepatitis

In selected regions of Southeast Asia, the most common presentation of gallstone disease is a syndrome characterized by intrahepatic bile duct stones, ductal dilation and stricturing, and recurrent cholangitis, known as oriental cholangiohepatitis. It occurs primarily in patients older than 50 and is associated with malnutrition and low socioeconomic status. There are inconsistent associations with infections caused by *Clonorchis sinensis* and *Ascaris lumbricoides,* but the pathogenetic role of these parasites remains unclear.

The stones in this disease are pigmented calcium bilirubinate stones that preferentially involve the left intrahepatic ducts. Patients typically present with relapsing cholangitis and hepatic abscesses. Ultrasound is of limited value because echogenic material often fills the intrahepatic ducts. The diagnosis relies on cholangiography. The primary treatment is surgical and often requires hepatic resection and extensive biliary reconstruction to relieve any obstruction and clear the ductal system of stones. Most patients require reoperation, although long-term prophylactic antibiotics may reduce the frequency of infectious complications.

CHAPTER 58

Abdominal Cavity: Structural Anomalies, Hernias, Intra-Abdominal Abscesses, and Fistulae

EMBRYOLOGY AND ANATOMY OF THE ABDOMINAL CAVITY

The abdominal (peritoneal) cavity appears early in embryonic development as the caudal part of the celomic cavity. It is covered by splanchnic mesoderm. During the migration of the abdominal organs, the mesodermic bands elongate and form the abdominal ligaments, the mesenterium, and the greater and lesser omenta. The dorsal mesogastrium of the foregut develops to a larger extent than its ventral counterpart and folds to the left. The space within the mesogastrial fold becomes the lesser sac. The greater omentum, a structure that hangs free to the pelvis, forms from enlargement of the dorsal mesogastrium and extends from the greater gastric curvature to the transverse colon and mesocolon. The omentum receives arterial blood from the gastroepiploic arteries and becomes laden with fat. In an adult, the remnants of the ventral mesogastrium are the ligaments of the liver—the coronary, falciform, and teres—and the gastrohepatic ligament (lesser omentum). In the developing fetus, the umbilical vein follows the ligamentum teres hepatis and terminates in the portal vein. The mesentery is formed from elongation and folding of the dorsal mesodermic attachment. The mesenteries of the ascending and descending colon fuse with the posterior body wall, and the mesentery of the small intestine extends from the transverse mesocolon to the ileocecal junction.

The abdominal cavity is bounded superiorly by the diaphragm, laterally by the abdominal walls, and inferiorly by the pelvis. The peritoneum is a layer of endoderm that covers the walls and organs of the abdominal cavity. The pancreas, part of the duodenum, the right and left colon, and the rectum are retroperitoneal, whereas the intraperitoneal organs are supported by thickened peritoneal bands (gastrohepatic, gastrosplenic, gastrocolic, splenorenal, splenocolic, falciform, coronary, and teres). The abdominal cavity has three compartments: lesser sac, supramesocolic, and inframesocolic. The lesser sac communicates with the rest of the abdominal cavity through the foramen of Winslow. The supramesocolic compartment (containing the stomach, duodenum, pancreas, liver, and spleen) and the inframesocolic compartment (containing the intestine) are separated by the transverse mesocolon, inserted in the anterior duodenum and pancreas. The area between the colon and the inferior margin of the liver is called the Morison pouch, a potential site for fluid accumulation. The most inferior part of the peritoneum between the rectum and urogenital organs is the pouch of Douglas. The inguinal region is bounded by the arch of the aponeurosis of the transversus abdominis muscle and by the upper ramus of the pubis and the psoas muscle. The inguinal canal contains the vas deferens, spermatic artery and vein, and cremasteric muscle. The omentum and mesentery, rich in lymphatics and blood vessels, provide macrophages and lymphocytes to aid in clearing abdominal foreign bodies and infections.

The parietal peritoneum lines the abdominal cavity, diaphragm, and pelvis, and the visceral peritoneum covers the intraperitoneal organs and forms the mesenteries. The parietal peritoneum is innervated by somatic and visceral afferent nerves and responds to noxious stimuli with a sensation of localized, sharp pain, whereas the visceral peritoneum receives afferent information from the autonomic nervous system and responds to traction and pressure with poorly localized, dull pain. The peritoneum and mesentery are supplied by splanchnic blood vessels and branches of the lower intercostal, lumbar, and iliac arteries.

The retroperitoneum is the space behind the abdominal cavity from the diaphragm to the peritoneal reflection, where it continues as the extraperitoneal pelvic space. The anterior retroperitoneum contains the pancreas, duodenum, and ascending and descending colons. The posterior retroperitoneum contains the kidneys, adrenal glands, vessels, lymphatics, and nervous structures.

DEVELOPMENTAL ABNORMALITIES OF THE ABDOMINAL CAVITY

Omphalocele and Gastroschisis

Etiology and Pathogenesis

The embryonic celomic cavity is too small to accommodate the intestines until the tenth gestational week, when they reenter the abdomen. Omphalocele occurs when the viscera herniate through the umbilical ring and persist outside the body, covered by a membranous sac. At least 50% of infants with omphalocele have associated abnormalities of the skeletal, gastrointestinal, nervous, or genitourinary systems. Gastroschisis is a condition in which the peritoneal sac has ruptured in utero and the viscera are in free contact with the exterior. Associated congenital abnormalities, including incomplete rotation and fixation of the midgut, intestinal atresia, trisomy 13, trisomy 18, vascular disruptions, and renal and gallbladder agenesis, are present in 30% to 50% of cases. Beckwith-Wiedemann syndrome, also known as *EMG syndrome* (exomphalos, macroglossia, gigantism), is characterized by somatic and visceral overgrowth and omphalocele.

Clinical Features, Diagnosis, and Management

The diagnosis of omphalocele or gastroschisis is obvious from examination at birth. It also can be diagnosed prenatally by ultrasound examination. Immediate treatment of these conditions is required to prevent dehydration, visceral desiccation, sepsis, and death. Antiseptic solutions are applied to the sac in infants with omphalocele. With gastroschisis, the viscera are wrapped in a silicone sheet, which is sutured to the abdominal wall until growth of the infant permits reducing the hernia and closing the defect. Amnion inversion is an alternate therapy for high-risk infants. Despite aggressive intervention, the mortality rate for these abnormalities is 40% to 50%. Many of the infants who survive exhibit slow recovery of bowel function.

Diaphragmatic Hernias

Etiology and Pathogenesis

Congenital diaphragmatic hernias are common defects that occur in weak areas of the diaphragm. Anteromedial diaphragmatic hernias through the sternocostal area (i.e., hernia of Morgagni) contain the stomach, colon, or omentum. Posterolateral diaphragmatic hernias through the lumbocostal area (i.e., hernia of Bochdalek) are large and are associated with hypoplasia of the ipsilateral lung (usually on the left) due to displacement of the thoracic contents by the bowel.

Clinical Features, Diagnosis, and Management

Anterior diaphragmatic hernias usually are small and rarely cause significant symptoms. Chest radiographs show an air shadow lateral to the xiphoid. Anterior hernias are corrected surgically with minimal morbidity and mortality. Posterolateral diaphragmatic hernias produce respiratory distress, mediastinal displacement, and nausea and vomiting as a result of intestinal obstruction. Respiratory sounds may be absent on the affected side, heart sounds may be audible in the right side of the chest, and bowel sounds may be audible in the left hemithorax. The abdomen may be scaphoid. Chest radiographs show left thoracic air-fluid levels, mediastinal displacement, and loss of the diaphragmatic line. Upper gastrointestinal radiography using water-soluble contrast may reveal intestinal loops in the thorax. Mortality from congenital diaphragmatic hernias results from respiratory insufficiency, malnutrition, failure to thrive, and intestinal strangulation. Surgery is necessary for posterolateral hernias, but the mortality rate is as high as 50% in the first week of life. Extracorporeal membrane oxygenation may reduce the pulmonary consequences of this condition.

Umbilical Hernias

Etiology and Pathogenesis

Umbilical hernias are caused by congenitally large umbilical rings or by rings that are distended by high intra-abdominal pressures. Predisposing factors include prematurity, Down syndrome, gargoylism, amaurotic family idiocy, cretinism, and Beckwith-Wiedemann syndrome.

Clinical Features, Diagnosis, and Management

Most umbilical hernias reduce and heal spontaneously; strangulation complicates only 5% of cases. Surgery before age 3 is indicated only for large, symptomatic hernias or in the event of incarceration or strangulation. If the hernia does not spontaneously improve by 3 to 4 years of age, elective surgery is performed.

HERNIAS IN ADULTS

Epigastric Hernias

Etiology and Pathogenesis

Epigastric hernias occur in the midline of the abdominal wall between the umbilicus and the xiphoid in a small area of congenital weakness of the linea alba that may contain incarcerated preperitoneal fat. Multiple hernias are reported in 20% of cases.

Clinical Features, Diagnosis, and Management

Although most epigastric hernias are asymptomatic, some produce symptoms ranging from a small, painless nodule to acute obstruction of the small intestine. Pain that is exacerbated by exertion and relieved by reclining is characteristic. Raising the head from the examining table may increase pain. The diagnosis, which may be difficult in obese patients with small hernias, is made by palpation of a tender mass on physical examination. Surgery is indicated for epigastric hernias.

Umbilical Hernias

Etiology and Pathogenesis

Umbilical hernias in adults occur in multiparous women, obese individuals, and up to 40% of cirrhotic patients with ascites. Intestinal or omental incarceration and strangulation complicate 20% to 30% of cases, especially if the umbilical ring is small. Other complications in cirrhotic patients with ascites are hernia ulceration and perforation, which may be further complicated by peritonitis (often caused by *Staphylococcus aureus*) or renal failure.

Clinical Features, Diagnosis, and Management

Large umbilical hernias are obvious from physical examination. If the diagnosis is not self-evident, abdominal radiographs may demonstrate an intestinal loop outside the abdominal wall. Umbilical hernias are treated surgically. In cirrhotic patients, control of ascites with medications or shunting procedures is essential. If perforation occurs, the patient requires hospitalization, antibiotic treatment for gram-positive organisms, and fluid and electrolyte replacement.

Groin Hernias

Etiology and Pathogenesis

Groin hernias represent 85% of all hernias. There are three clinically relevant types: indirect inguinal hernias (through the internal inguinal ring into the inguinal canal), direct inguinal hernias (superior to the inguinal ligament but not through the inguinal canal), and femoral hernias (inferior to the inguinal ligament and medial to the epigastric vessels) (Table 58-1). Most inguinal hernias occur in males, with a male-to-female ratio of about 7:1, whereas there is a female predominance by 2:1 in the incidence of femoral, umbilical, and incisional hernias. Although femoral hernias are more common in women than in men, indirect inguinal hernias are the most common hernias in women. Most groin hernias contain ileum, omentum, colon, or bladder. An indirect inguinal hernia containing a Meckel diverticulum is known as a *Littre hernia*. Inguinal hernias are thought to originate from a patent processus vaginalis in conjunction with conditions associated with increased intra-abdominal pressure such as chronic cough, pregnancy, massive ascites, and extreme athletics.

Clinical Features, Diagnosis, and Management

A patient with a groin hernia presents with an inguinal mass that appears with increased intra-abdominal pressure. Pain usually is mild. Constant pain suggests incarceration; colicky pain indicates strangulation. The diagnosis of hernias of the groin is made on physical examination by inserting the finger through the external inguinal ring into the inguinal canal to the internal ring. Indirect hernias are felt exiting the internal ring at the examiner's fingertip, whereas direct hernias are palpated laterally along the side of the finger. Femoral hernias are felt below the inguinal ligament in the femoral region. Strangulation affects 5% of indirect hernias, and 20% to 30% of femoral hernias strangulate, whereas direct hernias rarely develop this complication. Laparoscopy may visualize the site of herniation and the area of bowel that is trapped. Traditional or laparoscopic surgery is indicated for groin hernias.

TABLE 58-1
Epidemiology of Groin Hernias*

HERNIA TYPE	OCCURRENCE (%)
Inguinal	80
Indirect	(48)
Direct	(24)
Both	(8)
Femoral	5
Inguinal and femoral	2
With a sliding component	12
Sigmoid	(8)
Cecum	(4)
Other	2

*Groin hernias account for 85% of all hernias.

Pelvic Hernias

Etiology and Pathogenesis

Pelvic hernias involve bowel herniation through the obturator foramen, the greater or lesser sciatic foramina, or the perineal muscles. Pelvic hernias are rare; obturator hernias are the most prevalent pelvic hernias. Obturator hernias usually contain ileum and are more common in women.

Clinical Features, Diagnosis, and Management

Patients with obturator hernia often have a history of transient attacks of acute intestinal obstruction. Diagnosis usually is made at laparotomy because the obturator is not easily palpated in the thigh. On rectal or vaginal examination, however, a soft, tender, anterolateral, fluctuating mass may be palpated. The Howship-Romberg sign—medial thigh pain radiating to the knee or hip—is present in 50% of patients. An abnormal gas shadow in the intestine may be detected on radiographs of the obturator foramen. A computed tomographic (CT) scan may be diagnostic if there is hernia incarceration. Pelvic hernias are treated surgically.

Lumbar Hernias

Etiology and Pathogenesis

Lumbar hernias are congenital, or they are acquired through flank or rib trauma, through iliac crest fracture, or by removal of a fragment of the iliac crest for bone grafting. Lumbar herniation in the posterior abdominal wall may be superior (bounded by the twelfth rib, internal oblique, and sacrospinalis) or inferior (bounded by the iliac crest, latissimus dorsi, and external oblique).

Clinical Features, Diagnosis, and Management

Lumbar hernias can be asymptomatic, or they can produce lumbar pain referred to the back or pelvis. Surgery is indicated because these hernias generally increase in size.

Spigelian Hernias

Etiology and Pathogenesis

A spigelian hernia is a small protrusion through the external oblique fascia lateral to the rectus abdominus muscle, below the arcuate line of Douglas. Spigelian hernias are rare and usually occur in elderly persons.

Clinical Features, Diagnosis, and Management

Patients present with discomfort from straining or coughing. Sensation of a mass may be reported. A gas shadow may be seen on radiographs of the abdominal wall, whereas upper gastrointestinal contrast radiography may demonstrate bowel lumen outside the abdominal cavity. Surgery is mandatory.

Traumatic Diaphragmatic Hernias

Etiology and Pathogenesis

Penetrating or blunt trauma may produce diaphragmatic tears. The most common injury is a tear from the esophageal hiatus to the left costal attachment, with herniation of the stomach, spleen, colon, and left hepatic lobe into the thorax.

Clinical Features, Diagnosis, and Management

Diaphragmatic injury produces upper abdominal pain referred to the left shoulder and scapula. Visceral herniation causes nausea and vomiting, central abdominal pain and diaphoresis from traction of the mesentery and blood vessels, and respiratory distress from lung compression and mediastinal deviation. In rare cases, symptoms are mild, and the hernia remains undiagnosed for years. Chest radiographs, upper gastrointestinal contrast radiographs, ultrasound, and CT scans may demonstrate abdominal viscera in the thorax. The disorder requires immediate surgical repair.

Internal Hernias

Etiology and Pathogenesis

An internal hernia is the protrusion of an intraperitoneal viscus into a compartment within the abdomen. Paraduodenal hernias originate from a defect in midgut rotation and may involve bowel herniation into the left fossa of Landzert or the right fossa of Waldeyer. Herniation of the cecum and terminal ileum through the foramen of Winslow into the lesser sac is facilitated by a large foramen and abnormal colonic mobility. The small intestine is involved in 70% of cases and the colon in 25%. Pericecal hernias are characterized by passage of the ileum through the ileocecal fossa into the right paracolic gutter. Loops of the small intestine rarely become incarcerated in the intersigmoid fossa, which is a pocket between the two sigmoid loops. About 5% to 10% of internal hernias in adults occur through defects in the mesentery and omentum. These hernias are the most common type of internal hernias in infants and often are associated with an atretic segment of the intestine.

Clinical Features, Diagnosis, and Management

Internal hernias produce recurrent nausea, vomiting, and pain from intermittent obstruction of the small intestine. The diagnosis relies on abdominal radiography or laparotomy. Arteriography is also useful for diagnosis because it can demonstrate blood vessel displacement or reversal of their course. Radiographs of left paraduodenal hernias show encapsulated small intestine with superior displacement of the stomach and inferomedial displacement of the left colon, whereas right paraduodenal hernias displace the right colon anteriorly. Radiographs of hernias through the foramen of Winslow reveal gas-distended bowel loops in the lesser sac and anterior displacement of the stomach and colon. Intersigmoid hernias produce retrograde ileal filling that can be seen by barium enema radiography. Therapy for internal hernias is surgical.

Iatrogenic Hernias

Etiology and Pathogenesis

Iatrogenic hernias result from surgically created weak areas and abnormal foramina in the abdominal cavity. A retroanastomotic hernia is herniation of the intestine through a mesenteric space left open during construction of an anastomosis (e.g., Billroth II). Incisional hernias are caused by defective abdominal muscle suturing, defects at exteriorized drain sites, vertical laparotomies, multiple incisions (e.g., laparoscopic surgery), infraumbilical incisions, malnutrition, anemia, and wound hematomas or infections.

Clinical Features, Diagnosis, and Management

Retroanastomotic hernias are frequently acute and cause intestinal obstruction. Upper gastrointestinal barium radiography is diagnostic. Immediate surgical treatment is mandatory. Incisional hernias are detected by physical examination. Operative correction is generally required.

ABSCESSES

Etiology and Pathogenesis

Abscesses are fluid collections that contain necrotic debris, leukocytes, and bacteria. The usual causes are operative complications, trauma, visceral perforation, pancreaticobiliary disease, and genitourinary infection. Sources of bacterial contamination include exogenous seeding from penetrating trauma, hematogenous or lymphatic spread from adjacent or distant sites, and local spread from gastrointestinal perforation. Peritoneal inflammation by any mechanism leads to host-protective responses, including transudation of protein-rich fluid, complement production, and leukocyte attraction and activation. These protective responses have both beneficial and undesirable effects. For example, fibrin formation, from activation of tissue thromboplastin, traps bacteria; bacterial proliferation is promoted, lymphatic clearance of bacteria is impaired, and phagocytosis of bacteria by neutrophils is inhibited.

Most intra-abdominal abscesses are contaminated by multiple microbes, including gram-negative facultative organisms (*Escherichia coli* and *Klebsiella*, *Enterobacter*, *Proteus*, and *Pseudomonas* species) and anaerobes (e.g., *Bacteroides fragilis*), although prior antibiotics may influence the bacteriologic spectrum in some cases, leading to fungal infection. Aerobic bacteria promote anaerobe growth by consuming oxygen. Some anaerobes interfere with neutrophil phagocytosis, thereby promoting proliferation of aerobes and anaerobes. Abscesses can develop almost anywhere in the peritoneal cavity. Initially localized inflammatory processes such as appendicitis and diverticulitis may produce localized abscesses in the lower abdomen if perforation occurs after the inflammatory reaction is walled off. If perforation occurs before a localized inflammatory process develops, generalized peritonitis may result. Abscess formation in dependent areas in the recumbent patient, such as the subdiaphragmatic, subhepatic, and pelvic spaces, is associated with generalized peritonitis.

Clinical Features, Diagnosis, and Management

Patients with intra-abdominal abscesses present with intermittent fever (usually >39°C), abdominal pain (localized to the site of inflammation or diffuse), anorexia, and malaise. Subphrenic abscesses may produce shoulder pain, cough, and hiccups. Abscesses adjacent to the bladder or rectum may produce urinary or fecal urgency, respectively. Physical findings are variable, ranging from point tenderness and a focal mass to advanced sepsis with obtundation and hypotension. Bowel sounds may be reduced or absent, and rectovaginal examination may reveal a localized mass or tenderness. Involvement of the psoas muscle may cause pain on flexion of the hip (psoas sign). Even if the physical examination is unrevealing, clinicians must maintain a high degree of suspicion with all patients at risk of abscess formation. After surgery, incisional pain and the effects of analgesics often mask detection of an intra-abdominal abscess. Clinical signs of intra-abdominal abscess typically present 8 days after laparotomy. Factors associated with poor outcome in patients with intra-abdominal abscesses include advanced age, associated organ failure, a recurrent or persistent abscess, and multiple abscesses. Complications of abscesses include sepsis, secondary abscesses caused by direct extension or hematogenous spread, bowel obstruction or fistula formation, and blood vessel erosion with massive hemorrhage.

Blood testing can suggest but not confirm the presence of an abscess. A complete blood count may show mild anemia or leukocytosis. Liver chemistry values may reveal hyperbilirubinemia secondary to the effects of bacteremia. Peripancreatic abscesses can produce hyperamylasemia. Blood cultures may be positive for one or more organisms, usually gram-negative bacilli or anaerobes.

Plain abdominal radiographs, lumenal contrast studies, and radioisotope scans are typically unhelpful for diagnosing intra-abdominal abscesses with accuracy rates that range from 15% to 50%. A CT scan is the imaging test of choice for most patients because it is positive in 90% of cases. Abscesses on CT scans appear as well-defined fluid collections. Ultrasound may be useful in selected regions, including the right upper quadrant, retroperitoneum, and pelvis, but lumenal gas may obscure visualization of other intra-abdominal sites. Endoscopic ultrasound (EUS) is useful for diagnosing pancreatic abscesses and pseudocysts, and it can detect associated varices and direct subsequent therapy. In select cases, EUS-guided aspiration can be used to treat abscesses inaccessible by CT or in patients who are poor candidates for surgery.

The mainstay of treating intra-abdominal abscess is drainage. Percutaneous or EUS-directed drainage may be performed for single abscesses containing thin fluid, whereas operative drainage is usually required for multiple abscesses, loculated abscesses, infected hematomas, or abscesses containing thick viscous fluid. Factors associated with failure of percutaneous drainage include age older than 60 and abscesses that are complex or pancreatic. Patients whose abscesses are drained by any method but who do not respond within 4 days should be restudied with a CT scan or ultrasound, and repeat percutaneous drainage or surgery should be considered. Antibiotics are adjunctive therapy for intra-abdominal abscesses and should be administered prophylactically prior to catheter manipulation. Antibiotic therapy should be broad enough to treat gram-negative and gram-positive aerobes and anaerobes. The duration of antibiotic therapy should be determined by the patient's condition and the results of blood and tissue cultures. Recurrent infection is least likely in those patients who were afebrile and who had normal leukocyte counts.

FISTULAE

Etiology and Pathogenesis

Fistulae are abnormal communications from a hollow organ (gut, biliary tract, pancreatic duct, urinary tract) to another hollow organ or the skin. Fistulae develop in response to surgery, the use of prosthetic mesh to close abdominal wall defects, radiation therapy, inflammatory bowel disease, trauma, and malignancy (Table 58-2). Rarely, fistulae develop when abscesses erode into the adjacent bowel.

Clinical Features, Diagnosis, and Management

The most common presentations of abdominal fistulae include enteric drainage through the skin and signs and symptoms of an intra-abdominal abscess. High-output fistulae (>500 mL per day) that involve the proximal gut produce significant fluid and electrolyte abnormalities; for example, metabolic acidosis from duodenal fistulae, and hypochloremic, hypokalemic metabolic alkalosis from gastric fistulae. Fluid loss may be so severe as to cause dehydration, hypotension, and renal failure. Skin irritation may result from exposure to activated digestive enzymes. Malnutrition may result from protein and nutrient loss from the fistula, decreased oral intake, and the increased energy demands of the underlying illness. Malnutrition

TABLE 58-2
Etiologic Classification of Enteric Fistulae

Congenital
  Tracheoesophageal fistula
  Patent vitelline duct

Postoperative
  Inadvertent injury
  Failure of anastomosis
  Proximity of drain

Posttraumatic
  Direct injury
  Open abdominal wound

Inflammatory
  Crohn's disease
  Adjacent abscess

Postirradiation
  Spontaneous
  Postoperative

Malignant
  Adherence of tumor to adjacent bowel or abdominal wall with subsequent
    tumor necrosis

can significantly increase morbidity and mortality rates associated with fistulae. The presence of multiple, recurrent, or complex fistulae should suggest Crohn's disease. Recurrent urinary tract infection or pneumaturia suggests an enterovesical fistula, whereas diarrhea and malnutrition may be the presenting symptoms of a patient with an enteroenteric fistula that bypasses significant segments of gut. Fistulae are often mistaken for wound infections until fecal contents are identified on the dressings.

Various studies may be needed to diagnose the presence of a fistula accurately. The course of enterocutaneous fistulae can be defined by careful injection of a radiographic contrast medium into the skin opening. Persistently positive urine cultures for enteric organisms may suggest an enterovesical fistula. Upper or lower gastrointestinal contrast radiography may demonstrate disease that leads to fistula formation, but rarely defines the fistula itself. Cystoscopy is the most helpful test for diagnosing enterovesical fistulae. Gastrointestinal contrast radiographs usually demonstrate enteroenteric fistulae, whereas endoscopy is not often helpful. CT scanning and ultrasound may rarely detect fistulae but can be helpful in defining predisposing factors such as intra-abdominal abscess cavities.

The goals of treating an abdominal fistula include correction of fluid and electrolyte abnormalities, drainage of associated abscesses, protection of the skin, nutrient repletion, reduction of fistula drainage, and treatment of the underlying disease. For high-output fistulae, daily adjustments in replacement fluids may require direct measurement of the electrolyte composition in the fistula fluid. Effective drainage of associated abscesses is achieved by placement of sump drains. Skin can be protected with stoma appliances, similar to those used for surgically placed ileostomies or colostomies. The choice of enteral versus parenteral nutrition in patients with gastrointestinal fistulae must be individualized. Enteral feedings may increase fluid output from proximal fistulae of the small intestine, rendering parenteral nutrition more useful. In contrast, patients with fistulae of the distal small intestine or colon may be adequately nourished by enteral feedings without increasing fistulous output. Somatostatin and its analog, octreotide, reduce pancreatic and intestinal secretion and have been proposed for patients with intestinal or pancreatic fistulae. Some studies have shown faster closure of fistulae with these agents; however, further controlled studies are required. Factors that predict an unfavorable response to conservative management of fistulae include malignancy, inflammatory bowel disease, foreign bodies, poorly drained abscesses, distal gut obstruction, disruption of more than 50% of the bowel wall, a fistula tract less than 2.5 cm from the skin or more than 2 cm long, age older than 65, fistula output of more than 500 mL per day, chronicity, and localization to the distal small intestine and colon. Aggressive medical management with parental nutrition, skin care, evacuation of associated abscesses and control of infection results in spontaneous closure in 60% to 75% of cases. Endoscopic obliteration with fibrin sealant has been used with variable success in patients with upper gastrointestinal tract fistulae. Surgery is considered for fistulae that persist after 4 to 6 weeks.

CHAPTER 59

Diseases of the Mesentery, Peritoneum, and Retroperitoneum

DISEASES OF THE MESENTERY

Various diseases processes involve the mesentery and omentum (Table 59-1).

Mesenteric Panniculitis and Retractile Mesenteritis

Etiology and Pathogenesis

Mesenteric panniculitis is a nonspecific inflammation of the adipose tissue of the mesentery. The cause may be trauma, infection, autoimmunity, abdominal malignancy, or ischemia, but it is often unknown. It can be part of the generalized Weber-Christian disease. Pathological features include a thickened mesentery, usually a solid mass, representing excess growth of fat and subsequent degeneration, fat necrosis, xanthogranulomatous inflammation (macrophages, histiocytes, lymphocytes, foreign body giant cells), fibrosis, and calcification. If mesenteric panniculitis

TABLE 59-1
Classification of Mesenteric and Omental Diseases

Mesenteric Diseases
   Primary mesenteric inflammatory diseases
      Mesenteric panniculitis
      Retractile mesenteritis
   Mesenteric cysts
      Embryonic and developmental cysts
      Traumatic or acquired cysts
      Neoplastic cysts
      Infective and degenerative cysts
   Mesenteric tumors
   Benign
      Lipoma
      Hemangioma
      Leiomyoma
      Ganglioneuroma
   Malignant
      Leiomyosarcoma
      Liposarcoma
      Rhabdomyosarcoma
      Metastatic disease
   Mesenteric fibromatosis
   Mesenteric vascular diseases

Omental Diseases
   Mass lesions
      Primary tumors and cysts
      Metastatic disease
   Vascular lesions that compromise blood flow
      Torsion
         Primary
         Secondary (e.g., hernia, adhesion, tumor)
      Infarction
         Primary
         Secondary (e.g., torsion, incarceration in hernia)
   Inflammatory lesions
      Adhesions and inflammation caused by peritonitis

progresses to retractile mesenteritis, the thickened mesentery becomes fibrotic. Fat necrosis may produce mesenteric pseudocysts.

Clinical Features, Diagnosis, and Management

Symptoms of mesenteric panniculitis include abdominal cramps, weight loss, nausea, vomiting, and low-grade fever. Sixty percent of the abdominal masses are palpable, and 40% are discovered at laparotomy. Radiographic findings include displacement and extrinsic compression of bowel, stretching of the vasa recta and vascular encasement on angiography, and an inhomogeneous mass on computed tomographic (CT) scans. Retractile mesenteritis produces similar symptoms, as well as obstruction of the small intestine, mesenteric thrombosis, lymphatic obstruction with ascites, steatorrhea, and protein-losing enteropathy. The prognoses for these conditions depend on the underlying disease. Therapy should rely on surgical bypass; resection usually is not possible. Some patients have reportedly responded to prednisone with azathioprine or cyclophosphamide, but further studies are needed to confirm the effectiveness of this therapy.

Mesenteric Fibromatosis

Etiology and Pathogenesis

Mesenteric fibromatosis (or mesenteric desmoid) is a benign, noninflammatory fibromatous proliferation that arises from the mesentery. The desmoid tumor has an ill-defined margin, lacks encapsulation, and infiltrates into surrounding muscle and fascial planes. The condition may occur spontaneously or in association with the familial polyposis coli syndromes (especially Gardner syndrome). Other cases are associated with trauma, prior surgery, or estrogen use.

Clinical Features, Diagnosis, and Management

Patients with mesenteric fibromatosis may present with an asymptomatic abdominal mass or with intestinal obstruction or perforation from involvement of mesenteric blood vessels. Ultrasound shows a solid mass, and CT scans show a nonenhancing mass with soft tissue density. Wide local excision is the treatment of choice but may be precluded by mesenteric root involvement. Difficult to differentiate from low-grade sarcoma, these lesions can be misdiagnosed during surgery, prompting extensive small bowel resection. Some cases may require palliative intestinal bypass. There are anecdotal reports of successful treatment with prostaglandin synthesis inhibitors and antiestrogens (e.g., tamoxifen) alone or in combination. Cytotoxic chemotherapy and radiation therapy have not proved useful in treating mesenteric fibromatosis. Patients with unresectable disease have relatively good long-term survival.

Mesenteric and Omental Cysts and Solid Tumors

Etiology and Pathogenesis

Lymphangiomas are large cysts of the mesentery of the small intestine, the mesocolon, or the omentum. Lymphangiomas are characteristically found in children. Histologically, these are cystic structures lined with flattened lymphatic endothelium with smooth muscle and abundant lymphoid tissue made up of foam cells containing lipoid material in the cyst wall. Other mesenteric cysts (nonpancreatic pseudocysts, enteric cysts, mesothelial cysts) have cuboidal, columnar, or no epithelial lining. Cystic teratomas, cystic smooth muscle tumors, and cystic mesotheliomas are included in the differential diagnosis of lymphangiomas.

Most mesenteric malignancies arise from other sites and secondarily involve the mesentery through direct spread or metastasis. Primary solid tumors of the mesentery and omentum are rare. These solid tumors may be benign (leiomyoma, hemangiopericytoma, neurofibroma, lipoma, myxoma, xanthogranuloma) or malignant (leiomyosarcoma, fibrosarcoma, liposarcoma, rhabdomyosarcoma, gastrointestinal stromal tumors). Patients present with inflammatory fibrosarcomas at a mean age of 15. These tumors are locally aggressive and possibly metastatic, leading to death.

Clinical Features, Diagnosis, and Management

Lymphangiomas are often large and cause abdominal distention, nausea, and vomiting. Nonlymphangiomatous cysts occur in older persons and may not be symptomatic. Abdominal radiographs demonstrate bowel displacement and proximal bowel dilation. Ultrasound, CT, and magnetic resonance imaging (MRI) studies may show homogeneous or inhomogeneous cysts with unilocular or multilocular characteristics. The definitive management of these lesions is surgical resection. Total excision may require resection of adjacent intestinal segments.

Mesenteric and omental tumors are often detected as palpable abdominal masses. Patients usually present with pain and sometimes with ascites or vomiting. Abdominal radiographs may show bowel loop displacement. The mass can be localized to the mesentery or omentum from CT scans. Angiography may be able to determine if the mass is extrinsic or intrinsic to the mesentery. If possible, primary omental and mesenteric tumors should be surgically excised because 50% of lipomatous, histiocytic, and leiomyomatous mesenteric tumors and 25% of omental tumors are malignant. Metastases to the mesentery produce mesenteric shortening, angulation, and fixation of the bowel, resulting in obstruction or infarction as a result of vascular occlusion. Curative resection usually is not possible in this setting, but surgery may have palliative value for patients with metastatic carcinoid because of the indolent nature of these tumors.

Omental Vascular Accidents

Etiology and Pathogenesis

Primary vascular accidents of the omentum, such as torsion, infarction, and hemorrhage, may occur as complications of hernias or from bifid omentum, obesity, vascular anomalies, embolism from the heart or aorta, thrombosis, abdominal trauma, violent exercise, coughing, straining, and acute changes in body position.

Clinical Features, Diagnosis, and Management

Acute abdominal pain may be generalized or localized to the right abdomen. Other symptoms include nausea, vomiting, anorexia, low-grade fever, and mild leukocytosis. A physical examination may reveal a mobile, tender mass; guarding may or may not be detected. Most patients require surgical resection of the involved omentum.

Mesenteric and Omental Granulomatous Infections

Granulomatous diseases such as tuberculosis or mycoses may be clinically similar to metastatic malignancy, lymphoma, and inflammatory bowel disease. CT scans may show lymphadenopathy, ascites, involvement of the liver, spleen, and adrenals, and nodularity and thickening of the mesentery and omentum. Biopsy specimens stained and cultured for fungi and acid-fast bacillus are necessary for diagnosis.

DISEASES OF THE PERITONEUM

Peritonitis

Peritonitis is a localized or generalized inflammation of the parietal and visceral peritoneum. It may be the primary disease, or it may be secondary to diseases of or injury to the intra-abdominal organs.

Acute Suppurative Peritonitis

Etiology and pathogenesis. Acute suppurative peritonitis results from primary intra-abdominal disease (e.g., perforated ulcer, appendicitis, diverticulitis, and perforated carcinoma), penetrating trauma, or iatrogenic perforation after endoscopy or radiographic procedures.

Clinical features, diagnosis, and management. Patients present with pain that is exacerbated by movement and respirations, anorexia, nausea, vomiting, fever (38°C to 40°C), and signs of hypovolemia (e.g., tachycardia, dry mucous membranes, and hypotension). Abdominal examination may reveal distention, hypoactive or absent bowel sounds, tenderness (point or diffuse), involuntary guarding, and rigidity. Laboratory studies are most remarkable for significant leukocytosis, often with increased bands. Abdominal radiographs may show dilation of the small intestine, colon, and pneumoperitoneum.

Early diagnosis and prompt surgical intervention are essential to reduce morbidity and mortality from multiple organ failure that results from untreated peritonitis. Isotonic crystalloid fluids (e.g., Ringer lactate solution) should be administered to correct hypovolemia and electrolyte imbalances caused by third spacing of fluid. The response to fluid resuscitation requires careful assessment. Central venous pressure monitoring may be necessary and vital signs and urine output should be measured frequently. Nasogastric suction decompresses the stomach, and supplemental oxygen overcomes mild hypoxemia. Broad-spectrum antibiotics to treat aerobic and anaerobic organisms should be started before and continued during and after surgery. The mainstay of therapy for acute suppurative peritonitis is expeditious surgery, including copious irrigation of the peritoneum and repair of the ruptured viscus.

Granulomatous Peritonitis

Etiology and pathogenesis. Granulomatous peritonitis is characterized by peritoneal inflammation with formation of granulomas and development of adhesions. The most common cause is tuberculosis. Tuberculous peritonitis usually is associated with a primary focus of tuberculosis elsewhere, most often the lung, despite normal chest radiographs in about two thirds of cases. The omentum, intestine, liver, spleen, and female genital tract can also be involved. The organism gains entry into the peritoneal cavity transmurally from diseased bowel, from tuberculous salpingitis, or by hematogenous spread from a pulmonary focus. Granulomatous peritonitis may also be caused by infections (e.g., fungal organisms, such as *Candida* and *Histoplasma* species, and parasites, such as amoebas and *Strongyloides*), and iatrogenic sources (e.g., glove talc, and cellulose fibers from gauze, surgical drapes, and gowns).

Clinical features, diagnosis, and management. Generally, the onset of tuberculous peritonitis is insidious. More than 40% of patients have symptoms for at least 4 months before a diagnosis. Symptoms include fever, anorexia, weakness, malaise, weight loss, and abdominal distention from ascites or partial intestinal obstruction. The abdominal examination may reveal tenderness and ascites; the classic doughy abdomen is rare. Laboratory studies usually show no leukocytosis and only mild anemia. Tuberculin skin tests produce positive results in most cases, but results may be negative in anergic persons. Chest radiographs are abnormal in 80% of patients. Abdominal radiographs are rarely useful. CT scans may show thickened bowel and ascites. Ascitic fluid protein levels usually exceed 3.0 g/dL, and glucose levels are less than 30 mg/dL in more than 80% of cases. Ascitic fluid leukocyte counts higher than 250 cells/μL, predominantly lymphocytic, are common. Centrifugation of more than 1 L of ascitic fluid with subsequent acid-fast staining identifies the organism in some cases; ascitic cultures often need 4 to 6 weeks for incubation. Some laboratories use polymerase chain reaction testing, which can detect 10 to 100 mycobacteria in an ascitic fluid sample. Laparoscopy and laparotomy are often diagnostic, revealing characteristic stalactite-like fibrinous masses and granulomatous peritoneal studding. Isoniazid plus two additional drugs for 18 to 24 months is the indicated medical therapy for tuberculous peritonitis. Corticosteroids for 2 to 3 months may prevent development of dense adhesions. There has been a recent emergence of multidrug resistant isolates that fail to respond to isoniazid and rifampin.

Chemical Peritonitis

Etiology and pathogenesis. Peritoneal irritation results from exposure to bile, urine, and chyle, which occurs secondary to injury or surgery. Barium spillage from contrast radiographic procedures produces a severe peritoneal reaction.

Clinical features, diagnosis, and management. Patients present with typical peritoneal findings. Therapy relies on adequate intravenous fluids, broad-spectrum antibiotics, and laparotomy to irrigate the abdomen and control the source of inflammation.

Peritonitis with Chronic Peritoneal Dialysis

Etiology and pathogenesis. Peritonitis, the most common complication of chronic ambulatory peritoneal dialysis (CAPD), occurs 1.4 times per patient-year of treatment. Most CAPD-related peritonitis involves a single organism, which usually is a gram-positive coccus such as *Staphylococcus epidermidis*, *Staphylococcus aureus*, or a *Streptococcus* or *Enterococcus* organism. One fourth of cases results from infection with gram-negative bacteria (e.g., *Escherichia coli*, *Pseudomonas aeruginosa*). Fungal peritonitis is a rare but severe complication of CAPD.

Clinical features, diagnosis, and management. Most patients with CAPD-related peritonitis have less severe symptoms than patients with acute suppurative peritonitis. Some cases may even be asymptomatic and detected only by the presence of a cloudy effluent. Diffuse abdominal pain, fever, hyperhydration, diarrhea, hypotension, and pain over the catheter tunnel are common presenting symptoms. Blood testing usually reveals leukocytosis. The diagnosis relies on the presence of two of three criteria: abdominal pain or tenderness, a turbid dialysate with a neutrophil count that is higher than 100 cells/μL, and a positive peritoneal fluid culture. Most patients are effectively treated by an outpatient course of intraperitoneal antibiotics determined by pathogen susceptibility (e.g., vancomycin, cephalosporins, and aminoglycosides). Heparin is added to the dialysate to prevent postinfection adhesions. CAPD catheters should be removed in cases of persistent peritonitis after 4 to 5 days of treatment, fungal or tuberculous peritonitis, fecal peritonitis, or skin infection at the catheter site.

Peritonitis with AIDS

Peritonitis in patients with AIDS can be caused by perforation of the small intestine or colon secondary to cytomegalovirus enteritis or by infection with *Mycobacterium avium-intracellulare* complex, *Mycobacterium tuberculosis*, *Cryptococcus neoformans*, *Leishmania,* or *Strongyloides.* Most patients present with severe abdominal pain. The principles of management include emergent laparotomy, intravenous fluids, and broad-spectrum antibiotics.

Primary Mesothelioma

Etiology and Pathogenesis

Although most mesotheliomas originate in the pleura, 20% to 40% occur in the peritoneum. The incidence of mesothelioma is linked to exposure to asbestos, exposure to radiation, and use of the angiographic contrast agent Thorotrast.

Clinical Features, Diagnosis, and Management

Patients with peritoneal mesotheliomas present with epigastric or right upper quadrant pain, nausea, vomiting, malaise, fever, weight loss, diarrhea, and anemia. Ascites is present in 90% of patients. Primary mesotheliomas can produce and secrete various hormones such as antidiuretic hormone, growth hormone, and insulin-like factors; all of them can cause paraneoplastic syndromes that manifest as hyponatremia, hypoglycemia, thrombocytosis, and increased production of fibrin-degradation products. Peritoneal mesothelioma is associated with other synchronous neoplasms such as colorectal cancer. Findings on ultrasound and CT scanning can suggest the diagnosis, demonstrate the extent of tumor, and aid in directed biopsy of suggestive lesions. In most cases, the diagnosis is confirmed by laparoscopy or laparotomy. Other neoplasms in the differential diagnosis include benign papillary and fibrous mesotheliomas, adenomatoid tumors, and multicystic peritoneal mesotheliomas. Therapy for mesothelioma rarely prolongs survival. Doxorubicin, alone or in combination with other antineoplastic agents, achieves the best response. Most patients survive less than 1 year after diagnosis.

Pseudomyxoma Peritonei

Etiology and Pathogenesis

Pseudomyxoma peritonei is characterized by the accumulation of large quantities of diffuse, gelatinous material in the peritoneum and omentum that arises from mucinous neoplasms of the appendix or ovary.

Clinical Features, Diagnosis, and Management

Women between the ages of 45 and 55 comprise 75% of cases. Patients most commonly present with increased abdominal girth, secondary to mucinous ascites or intestinal obstruction. Ultrasound shows multiple intraperitoneal multilocular cysts and ascitic septation. A CT scan reveals scalloping of the hepatic and bowel margins from compression by the gelatinous mass. Treatment involves aggressive surgical debulking of the tumor, along with appendectomy and bilateral oophorectomy. Pseudomyxoma peritonei is a low-grade malignancy; the 5-year survival rate is 54%. Recurrence occurs in about 75% of patients and repeat laparotomy is indicated.

DISEASES OF THE RETROPERITONEUM

Retroperitoneal Fluid Collections

Etiology and Pathogenesis

Lymphoceles are cystic masses that contain lymph. They occur in the retroperitoneum after injuries, diseases, or operations (renal or pancreatic transplant) that interrupt the lymph channels traversing the posterior pelvis and abdomen. Duodenal succus results from duodenal injury secondary to endoscopic injury, sphincterotomy, and ulcer or diverticular perforation. Pancreatic duct injury caused by acute and chronic pancreatitis, trauma, or pancreatic surgery can produce localized collections of pancreatic juice. Abdominal trauma and endoscopic or surgical manipulation can injure the distal common bile duct, causing bile leakage. Injury of the collecting system of the kidney can produce perinephric urine extravasation.

Clinical Features, Diagnosis, and Management

CT or ultrasound studies can be used to direct the aspiration of retroperitoneal fluid collections. A lymph collection can be readily distinguished from blood but not urine on CT scans. Duodenal perforations are diagnosed with upper gastrointestinal meglumine (Gastrografin)-enhanced radiography. A CT scan may differentiate a duodenal hematoma from a full-thickness perforation. Preoperative or intraoperative pancreatography can be used to assess pancreatic duct injury. Intravenous pyelography or a CT scan can be used to evaluate the function of an injured renal collecting system.

Surgical intervention is needed to treat many significant retroperitoneal fluid collections. Conservative management may be possible for early duodenal perforation, but retroperitoneal infection mandates operative therapy. Drainage procedures are performed for small pancreatic ductal injuries, but partial pancreatectomy is needed for major duct damage. Isolated bile duct injuries require primary repair or T-tube drainage with secondary repair. Complex injuries that involve the bile ducts, pancreas, and duodenum may need a Whipple procedure. Avulsion of the renal collecting system necessitates nephrectomy, whereas renal pelvis laceration and ureteropelvic junction avulsion can usually be repaired. Ureter injury may be managed by suture repair with or without stenting and nephrostomy.

Retroperitoneal Hemorrhage
Etiology and Pathogenesis

The major cause of retroperitoneal hemorrhage is traumatic vessel injury associated with pelvic or vertebral fracture or avulsion of a renal vascular pedicle. Other causes include anticoagulation therapy, spontaneous hemorrhage into an adrenal gland or retroperitoneal tumor, acute pancreatitis, ruptured aortic aneurysm, and ruptured uteroovarian veins during pregnancy. Massive retroperitoneal hemorrhage has been associated with femoral vein catheterization and liposuction. Most abdominal aortic aneurysms are caused by atherosclerosis; aneurysms secondary to bacterial or fungal infection are less common.

Clinical Features, Diagnosis, and Management

The clinical course of most retroperitoneal hemorrhage depends on the rapidity and volume of bleeding. A rupture of an atherosclerotic abdominal aortic aneurysm manifests as severe back pain and a tender, pulsatile mass on abdominal examination. Inflammatory aneurysms are characterized by discomfort, tenderness, and ureteral obstruction. Ultrasound may confirm the presence of aneurysmal rupture, but this test should not be performed on an unstable patient if doing so would delay surgery. CT scanning and aortography are time-consuming procedures, which precludes their routine use in patients suspected of having aneurysm rupture. Emergency surgery is mandatory for ruptured aortic aneurysms, all cases of massive or persistent retroperitoneal hemorrhage, hemorrhage during pregnancy, and penetrating wounds. Postoperative complications of aortic aneurysm surgery include myocardial infarction, stroke, renal failure, bleeding, and ischemic colitis.

Retroperitoneal Fibrosis

Etiology and Pathogenesis

Retroperitoneal fibrosis is characterized by progressive fibrosis of connective and adipose tissue. It originates in the lower retroperitoneum and spreads bilaterally toward the renal hilus, encircling the vessels and ureters. The fibrosis appears as a white, woody, fibrous plaque with histological features, including lymphocytes, fibroblasts, and collagen bundles, that are typical of chronic inflammation. The most common form of disease is idiopathic; however, fibrosis may result from paraneoplastic phenomena (e.g., carcinoid, Hodgkin disease, and sarcoma), drugs (e.g., methysergide), other fibrotic processes (e.g., mesenteric fibrosis, sclerosing cholangitis, and orbital pseudotumor), radiation therapy, retroperitoneal infection or fluid collections, and inflammatory abdominal aortic aneurysms.

Clinical Features, Diagnosis, and Management

Patients present with abdominal or back pain, anorexia, fatigue, fever, jaundice, edema, protein-losing enteropathy, portal hypertension, peripheral thrombosis, intermittent claudication, hydronephrosis, pyelonephritis, and progressive renal failure with anuria. An abdominal mass is present in 15% of patients. Rarely, the disease involves the duodenum, common bile duct, or colon, resulting in obstruction. Intravenous pyelography shows medial displacement and narrowing of the ureters. A CT scan demonstrates the extent of the fibrous plaque. Disease progression may be slowed by steroid therapy alone or in combination with surgery. Other immunosuppressive drugs such as azathioprine, mycophenolate mofetil, and cyclophosphamide have been used with varying degrees of success. The options for treating renal damage include ureterolysis, renal autotransplantation into the pelvis, ureteral catheter placement, or nephrostomy.

Retroperitoneal Infections

Etiology and Pathogenesis

Retroperitoneal abscesses usually occur in the anterior compartment and result from appendicitis, pancreatitis, a penetrating duodenal ulcer, a perforating colonic carcinoma and diverticulitis, and Crohn's disease. Psoas abscesses may be primary (e.g., *S aureus* in children), or they may be secondary to extension of an intra-abdominal infection (Crohn's disease, appendicitis, diverticulitis, malignancy) or a vertebral infection. One fourth of extrapulmonary tuberculosis infections affect the retroperitoneum, which is seeded at the time of initial dissemination. Renal tuberculosis originates in the cortex and spreads to the medulla, causing papillary necrosis and cavitation. The adrenal glands are susceptible to disseminated histoplasmosis, paracoccidioidomycosis, and blastomycosis. Renal and psoas abscesses may form in the setting of coccidioidomycosis. Opportunistic fungi (e.g., *Candida*, *Aspergillus*, or *Cryptococcus*) may disseminate in the retroperitoneum in patients with altered immune responses. Retroperitoneal actinomycosis may be caused by appendiceal or colonic perforation. It is characterized by chronic abscesses with multiple sinus tracts exuding "sulfur granules." Retroperitoneal infections caused by *Nocardia* usually occur in the kidney and are the result of dissemination from a pulmonary focus. These infections usually affect immunosuppressed patients.

Clinical Features, Diagnosis, and Management

Patients with retroperitoneal abscesses present with fever; malaise; leukocytosis; a retroperitoneal mass; and pain in the flank, back, abdomen, or thigh. A CT scan is most accurate in evaluating retroperitoneal abscesses. It also facilitates needle aspiration of abscess fluid for culture. Operative drainage with broad antibiotic coverage is the treatment of choice. Percutaneous drainage is successful in selected patients with well-defined abscess cavities. The symptoms of retroperitoneal tuberculous infection include dysuria, urinary frequency, hematuria, flank pain, and sterile pyuria. Some symptoms are associated with characteristic findings on intravenous pyelography. Retroperitoneal tuberculous infection is treated with antituberculous chemotherapy. Spinal tuberculosis with a secondary psoas abscess may also require incision and drainage. Involvement of the adrenals in fungal infections may result in life-threatening Addison disease. On CT scans, the findings with retroperitoneal fungal infections include bilateral adrenal enlargement with focal hemorrhage, necrosis, and cavitation. Retroperitoneal fungal infections are treated with amphotericin B; a total 1 to 4 g is administered in the course of the treatment. Actinomycosis is rarely diagnosed without laparotomy. It is treated with incision and drainage, combined with 0.5 to 20 million units of penicillin daily for 4 to 12 weeks. *Nocardia* infections are treated with a combination of trimethoprim and sulfamethoxazole for 3 to 4 months.

Retroperitoneal Neoplasms

Etiology and Pathogenesis

Primary retroperitoneal neoplasms derive from soft tissue, lymphoid tissue, or germ cells. Most are malignant sarcomas: liposarcomas, leiomyosarcomas, and fibrous histiocytomas. Lymphomas (usually non-Hodgkin) result from lymphatic metastases of primary neoplasms. In children, rhabdomyosarcomas, neuroblastomas, ganglioneuroblastomas, and teratomas predominate. Neoplasms of the abdomen, lower extremities, and genitourinary systems can metastasize to the retroperitoneum.

Clinical Features, Diagnosis, and Management

Larger retroperitoneal neoplasms produce fatigue; abdominal pain; radiating pain to the back and posterior thigh; and symptoms of lymphatic, venous, and urinary obstruction. Patients may present with asymptomatic abdominal masses or with nausea, vomiting, and a change in bowel habits from intestinal compression. CT or MRI studies may define the site of origin and the morphology of a retroperitoneal neoplasm; however, angiographic demonstration of invasion of adjacent organs may be necessary to define the malignant nature of the tumor. Percutaneous needle biopsy can determine the histological character of a retroperitoneal neoplasm in 80% of cases. The therapy of choice for retroperitoneal tumors is complete resection of the tumor and involved structures; this is possible in 50% of cases. Debulking may be of value with large, symptomatic sarcomas. Sarcomas respond poorly to adjuvant radiation therapy and chemotherapy. In contrast, lymphomas respond better to these treatments.

CHAPTER 60

Cholestatic Syndromes

Cholestasis is a defect in bile excretion. It can be classified as intrahepatic or extrahepatic based on the anatomic site of the disturbance. Extrahepatic cholestasis is caused by diseases that structurally impair bile secretion and flow in the large bile ducts (see Chapters 56 and 57). Intrahepatic cholestasis is caused by a functional defect in bile formation at the level of the hepatocyte and terminal bile ducts. This chapter reviews the common causes of intrahepatic cholestasis (Table 60-1).

PRIMARY BILIARY CIRRHOSIS

Incidence and Epidemiology

Primary biliary cirrhosis (PBC) is a chronic, progressive, cholestatic disease that affects mainly middle-aged women. Patients may present as early as age 30 or as late as age 90, with a median age between 40 and 55 at presentation. PBC has been observed in all races but is more common in whites. Some of the highest prevalences have been reported in England and Sweden. Worldwide, PBC accounts for 0.6% to 2.0% of deaths from cirrhosis.

Epidemiologic surveys have failed to identify specific environmental risk factors, but developed regions have higher incidences than undeveloped regions. It is not known whether this represents a true difference in disease incidence or a detection bias from health screening.

Etiology and Pathogenesis

Although several disease associations and well-characterized disturbances in immune regulation suggest that PBC is an immune-mediated disease, the etiology remains unknown. Associated immunologic abnormalities include antimitochondrial autoantibodies, increased IgM levels, multiple antinuclear antibodies (~30%), circulating immune complexes, and other associated autoimmune phenomena. Autoimmune diseases associated with PBC include Sjögren syndrome, CREST syndrome, autoimmune thyroiditis, and, possibly, rheumatoid arthritis. PBC has also been linked to the HLA-DR8 antigen, which suggests that the disease may have a genetic component.

Liver injury results from the nonsuppurative destruction of small bile ducts in the lobule. Reduced biliary excretion leads to cholestasis and toxic hepatocyte injury from the accumulation of bile acids and copper. The disease evolves through four histologically described stages. In stage I, the portal tracts are expanded by chronic inflammatory cells and noncaseating granulomas adjacent to the damaged bile ducts, including the classic "florid duct lesion." Stage II is characterized by expansion of the inflammatory infiltrate into the hepatic parenchyma and proliferation of the bile ductules. In stage III, interlobular fibrous septa and ductopenia are present. Stage IV represents cirrhosis.

TABLE 60-1
Differential Diagnosis of Intrahepatic Cholestasis

Primary biliary cirrhosis

Sclerosing cholangitis

Hepatocellular disease
  Viral hepatitis
  Alcoholic hepatitis
  Medications

Intrahepatic cholestasis of pregnancy

Systemic infection

Total parenteral nutrition–associated cholestasis

Postoperative cholestasis

Clinical Features

Forty percent to 50% of persons with PBC are asymptomatic at presentation. The disease is detected in most of these individuals from elevated serum alkaline phosphatase or γ-glutamyltransferase levels. About 50% to 60% of patients have presenting symptoms, usually fatigue and pruritus, and in some, upper right quadrant discomfort. Less than 25% present with jaundice. The pruritus may be relentless and profound, prompting the patient to seek advice from a dermatologist before it is recognized as a complication of cholestasis. The skin may become excoriated and hyperpigmented from incessant scratching. Other physical findings include hepatomegaly, splenomegaly, palmar erythema, spider angiomata, xanthomas, and xanthelasma. The last finding correlates with the hypercholesterolemia (particularly of high-density lipoprotein) which is observed in PBC. The defect in bile acid secretion leads to impaired fat digestion with resultant steatorrhea, weight loss, and fat-soluble vitamin deficiencies. Long-standing cholestasis can also result in bone resorption and osteoporosis, which often lead to vertebral compression fractures and long bone fractures. A rare patient may have hepatic failure or a complication of portal hypertension (e.g., variceal bleeding) as the initial manifestation of PBC.

Most patients with PBC have associated autoimmune diseases. These diseases, of which Sjögren syndrome is by far the most common, usually are mild and survival is dictated by the severity of hepatic dysfunction. Autoimmune thyroiditis with hypothyroidism and CREST syndrome also often occur with PBC and may predate the diagnosis of liver disease. Other diseases associated with PBC include rheumatoid arthritis, gallstones, decreased pulmonary diffusion capacity, psoriasis, Raynaud phenomenon, and distal renal tubular acidosis (Table 60-2). Although the evidence is contradictory, there may be a higher incidence of breast cancer in patients with PBC.

Findings from Diagnostic Testing
Laboratory Studies

All patients with PBC have elevated serum alkaline phosphatase levels. Similar elevations in levels of 5'-nucleotidase and γ-glutamyltransferase help confirm the hepatic origin of the elevated alkaline phosphatase level. Serum bilirubin levels usually are normal at diagnosis. As the disease progresses, more than 50% of patients

TABLE 60-2
Extrahepatic Manifestations of Primary Biliary Cirrhosis

EXTRAHEPATIC DISEASE	PREVALENCE (%)
Sjögren syndrome	30–58
Gallstones	30–50
Decreased pulmonary diffusion capacity	40–50
Renal tubular acidosis	20–33
Osteoporosis	15–40
Bacteriuria	11–35
Arthropathy	4–38
Rheumatoid arthritis	3–26
Hypothyroidism	11–32
Raynaud phenomenon	7–14
CREST* syndrome	3–6
Autoimmune thyroiditis	3–6
Autoimmune anemias	1–2
Psoriasis	1–13
Lichen planus	0.5–6
Ulcerative colitis	0.5–1

*CREST: syndrome of calcinosis, Raynaud phenomenon, esophageal dysmotility, sclerodactyly, and telangiectasias.

develop hyperbilirubinemia, a poor prognostic indicator. As with other cholestatic syndromes, levels of aminotransferases usually are only slightly elevated. Other nonspecific surrogate markers of cholestasis include increased levels of serum bile acids, cholesterol, triglycerides, elevated serum and hepatic copper levels, and decreased levels of fat-soluble vitamins A, D, E, and K.

Serologic Testing
The immunologic abnormalities observed in PBC provide useful diagnostic information. Antimitochondrial antibodies (AMAs) are present in 90% to 95% of patients with PBC. Although other autoantibodies are present in a large number of cholestatic syndromes, elevated titers of AMAs rarely occur in other diseases and therefore are quite specific for PBC. Similarly, the finding of elevated IgM levels on serum protein electrophoresis, often in the absence of hyperglobulinemia, has high predictive value for PBC. Other serologic abnormalities include increased titers of antinuclear antibodies (ANAs) in 25% to 70% of patients and other autoantibodies, but these findings are not specific to PBC and are of limited diagnostic value.

Liver Biopsy
Confirmation of PBC requires percutaneous liver biopsy. The pathognomonic lesion is characterized by patchy destruction of interlobular bile ducts with a mononuclear inflammatory infiltrate. Granulomas may be present in some portal tracts, but their presence is not required to confirm a diagnosis of PBC. The severity of histological damage can be classified into four distinct stages.

Structural Studies
Several imaging procedures may be used to evaluate PBC. These procedures are used primarily to exclude extrahepatic causes of cholestasis. Ultrasound generally

demonstrates bile ducts of normal size. Gallstones are revealed in more than 30% of cases. Computed tomographic scanning also helps to exclude bile duct dilation and may demonstrate portosystemic collaterals that suggest portal hypertension. In patients lacking the serologic markers of PBC, endoscopic retrograde cholangiopancreatography (ERCP) may be necessary. Although the terminal intrahepatic ducts may be irregular, the larger ducts appear to be normal in size and contour on ERCP.

Management and Course

PBC is an invariably progressive disease, but the rate of progression varies. About one half of the patients with PBC are asymptomatic at presentation, but many become symptomatic within 2 to 4 years. As the disease progresses from the asymptomatic to symptomatic stages, serum alkaline phosphatase and α-globulin levels often dramatically increase and subsequently reach a plateau. Once symptoms appear, there is an indolent worsening of fatigue and pruritus, usually over the course of years. Patients eventually develop muscle wasting, progressive jaundice, and hepatic dysfunction. Once jaundice develops, life expectancy declines markedly, with mean survival times of 4 years if bilirubin levels are higher than 2 mg/dL and 2 years if higher than 6 mg/dL. The final stage of PBC is marked by complications of portal hypertension, including ascites, variceal hemorrhage, and encephalopathy.

The chronic inflammatory response and immune dysfunction observed in PBC have prompted clinical trials of several immunosuppressive regimens. Corticosteroids fail to alter the biochemical, histological, and clinical progression observed in PBC. Azathioprine, cyclosporine, colchicine, and D-penicillamine may result in biochemical improvements, but none of these agents alters disease progression or survival. Some clinical trials of weekly regimens of methotrexate have shown improvement in biochemical and histological abnormalities. Given the potential for significant pulmonary toxicity, most experts do not recommend methotrexate until prolonged follow-up shows evidence of improved symptoms and survival.

The synthetic bile acid ursodeoxycholic acid (ursodiol) is the only approved therapy for PBC. Given at a daily dose of 13 to 15 mg/kg, ursodiol may stabilize hepatocyte membranes, decrease the rate of biliary epithelial apoptosis, and decrease the production of more toxic bile acids. Ursodiol also has antioxidant properties, including the ability to inhibit nitric oxide synthase. Several reports describe a decrease in the severity of pruritus in 50% of cases. Most patients experience biochemical improvement, but effects on histological improvement have been inconsistent in short-term trials. Long-term studies of ursodiol treatment have shown improved survival and delay in time to transplantation, but meta-analysis has not confirmed these results, perhaps due to the short duration of the placebo phase before the crossover to ursodiol in several large trials.

The control of pruritus is the goal of symptomatic treatment of PBC. Oral antihistamines are rarely of benefit in cholestasis-associated pruritus. Cholestyramine and colestipol are effective in up to 80% of patients, but they often cause profound constipation and bloating. These ionic resins bind intralumenal bile acids and other pruritogens, thus preventing the absorption of these substances. Cholestyramine and other resins also interfere with the absorption of medications such as digoxin, thyroxine, and penicillins. Steatorrhea and fat-soluble vitamin deficiencies can be exacerbated. Patients intolerant of cholestyramine may respond to phenobarbital or rifampin. Refractory pruritus may respond to naloxone or other opioid antagonists, ondansetron, plasmapheresis, or therapy with ultraviolet B light, but data are limited.

Survival of patients with PBC depends largely on the clinical and histological stage of disease. Patients with asymptomatic PBC have a median survival time of 10 years, which is shorter than that of age-matched controls. The survival times of symptomatic patients are shorter than those of asymptomatic patients. Several models have attempted to predict survival on the basis of clinical variables. The most powerful predictor is the serum bilirubin level. Patients with bilirubin levels higher than 6 mg/dL usually survive less than 2 years. Hypercholesterolemia rarely leads to cardiac disease except in the presence of other cardiac risks or unfavorable lipid profiles. Osteoporosis can be severe; therefore, monitoring the vitamin D level and supplementation of calcium and vitamin D as well as estrogen replacement or bisphosphonate therapy are useful in preventing bone loss.

Prediction of survival is critical in enabling the clinician to select optimal candidates for liver transplantation. Transplantation should be considered for patients with complications of portal hypertension, severe symptomatic osteodystrophy, or a predicted survival of less than 2 years. In properly selected candidates, liver transplantation is highly successful in treating PBC; the 2-year survival rate is higher than 80%.

HEPATOCELLULAR DISEASES

Several liver diseases that characteristically produce hepatocellular injury may demonstrate biochemical and clinical features more consistent with cholestasis. Alcoholic hepatitis may produce profound increases in levels of serum bilirubin and alkaline phosphatase with normal to minimally elevated levels of aminotransferases, a pattern that often correlates with severe hepatocellular injury. Patients with alcoholic hepatitis often have very poor prognoses. Atypical variant forms of acute viral hepatitis A, B, and E include a syndrome of prolonged cholestasis. Although patients with hepatitis C typically manifest acute hepatitis, liver allograft recipients with recurrent infection from hepatitis C virus may rarely develop recurrent cholestatic hepatitis C, which is characterized by pericholangitis and cholestasis with minimal inflammation, rapid graft failure, and poor prognosis.

INTRAHEPATIC CHOLESTASIS
OF PREGNANCY

Pregnancy may be associated with abnormal liver chemistry values attributable to numerous physiological alterations and disease processes. Perhaps the most common finding is a mild increase in the serum alkaline phosphatase level from placental release of this enzyme. Women may also have coincident liver diseases unrelated to their pregnancy, for example, alcohol-, viral-, and immune-mediated liver diseases. The impact of pregnancy on the natural history of these disorders remains unclear. Pregnancy may be complicated by several disorders unique to pregnancy, for example, HELLP syndrome with preeclampsia and the rare but devastating syndrome of acute fatty liver of pregnancy. These two disorders present in the third trimester, often with cholestasis and systemic complications such as disseminated intravascular coagulation and renal and hepatic failure. Acute fatty liver and preeclampsia-related liver injury require prompt delivery of the fetus. Unless diagnosed early, these disorders have high maternal mortality rates.

The most common liver disease unique to pregnancy is intrahepatic cholestasis of pregnancy. It occurs in less than 1% of all pregnancies in the United States and accounts for 30% to 50% of all causes of jaundice in pregnancy. It is distinguished from the other disorders by its benign course. The syndrome is similar to the cholestasis associated with estrogen supplements. Moreover, women with a prior history of intrahepatic cholestasis of pregnancy often manifest cholestasis when challenged with oral contraceptives in the nonpregnant state. The etiology remains unknown, but familial clustering suggests the presence of a genetically acquired sensitivity to the cholestatic effects of estrogens. Patients usually present with pruritus and mild jaundice in the third trimester. Liver chemistry values demonstrate a cholestatic pattern. A biopsy specimen from the liver reveals bland cholestasis with no inflammatory reaction. A biopsy is occasionally needed to differentiate the syndrome from acute fatty liver of pregnancy or other more morbid disorders. Supportive treatment with ursodiol or cholestyramine may relieve the pruritus; cholestasis and pruritus resolve within 24 to 48 hours of delivery.

SYSTEMIC INFECTION

Systemic gram-negative bacterial infections are often accompanied by cholestasis. Endotoxemia decreases bile flow and may result in conjugated hyperbilirubinemia, with bilirubin levels in the range of 5 to 10 mg/dL. Levels of aminotransferases are usually near normal, and the alkaline phosphatase level is variably elevated. Clinical manifestations are dominated by the underlying infection. Cholestasis improves with successful treatment of the responsible microorganisms.

CHOLESTASIS ASSOCIATED WITH TOTAL PARENTERAL NUTRITION

Patients who receive long-term total parenteral nutrition (TPN) may manifest any of several distinct patterns of hepatic dysfunction, including cholestasis. TPN-induced intrahepatic cholestasis is common in premature newborn infants. The mechanism is undefined but probably results from alterations in serum bile acid pools caused by changes in intestinal bacteria. Patients who receive TPN are often subjected to bowel rest; the resulting bile stasis promotes biliary sludge and stone formation. Therefore, extrahepatic cholestasis also should be considered when evaluating patients on long-term TPN.

POSTOPERATIVE CHOLESTASIS

The postoperative state may be complicated by jaundice caused by cholestasis and impaired bile formation or alterations in the production or excretion of bilirubin. Increased bilirubin production, which may exceed the excretory capacity of the liver, can be caused by several factors in a patient undergoing surgery. Hemolysis caused by systemic infections, transfusion reactions, mechanical trauma caused by artificial valves or a circulatory bypass, or preexisting red blood cell defects and hemoglobinopathies increase the production of bilirubin. Similarly, massive transfusions and resorption of large hematomas may overwhelm the liver's ability to excrete bilirubin. Increased bilirubin loads lead to predominantly unconjugated hyperbilirubinemia. Patients with Gilbert syndrome, a common autosomal dominant defect of bilirubin conjugation, often develop unconjugated hyperbilirubinemia from physiological stress and fasting in the perioperative period.

Hepatocellular injury also may cause jaundice in postoperative patients. Hypoxia and hypotension in the perioperative period can produce ischemic hepatitis. Drug-induced hepatotoxicity, especially from anesthetic agents, can cause jaundice. Rarely, viral hepatitis acquired from transfusions results in jaundice, weeks after an operation. All of these insults usually produce a marked increase in levels of aminotransferases in addition to hyperbilirubinemia.

Cholestasis in the postoperative state can be extrahepatic or intrahepatic in origin. Patients undergoing biliary surgery are prone to extrahepatic cholestasis if there are retained bile duct stones and bile duct injuries. Systemic infection, medications, and TPN can produce intrahepatic cholestasis. When all other causes of postoperative jaundice and cholestasis have been excluded, the probable diagnosis is benign postoperative intrahepatic cholestasis. This transient syndrome of unknown etiology usually causes conjugated hyperbilirubinemia and elevated serum alkaline phosphatase levels by the third postoperative day. It gradually resolves over 1 to 2 weeks.

CHAPTER 61

Drug-Induced Hepatic Injury

INCIDENCE AND EPIDEMIOLOGY

Among the many adverse effects of medications, hepatobiliary toxicity is one of the most common. It accounts for 5% of all reported drug reactions. Hepatotoxicity comprises over 50% of all cases of acute liver failure in the United States, and most cases are related to acetaminophen toxicity. The clinical and biochemical patterns of injury can mimic any acute or chronic liver disease (Table 61-1). Medications that predictably produce hepatic injury in a dose-dependent manner are termed *intrinsic hepatotoxins*. Although the exact mechanism of hepatic injury remains poorly defined, intrinsic hepatotoxins or their metabolites (e.g., the acetaminophen metabolite, NAPQI) generally injure hepatocytes by direct structural and functional alterations of vital subcellular elements. Intrinsic hepatotoxins often produce a zonal pattern of injury, which results from metabolic production or accumulation in a particular region of the hepatic lobule. In contrast, idiosyncratic hepatotoxins unpredictably produce hepatic injury in a small percentage of susceptible individuals. However, because an idiosyncratic drug reaction can occur with any agent, these reactions are more common than intrinsic drug reactions. Theories abound to explain idiosyncratic drug reactions. Many reactions appear to be the result of immune-mediated injury caused by a hypersensitive response. Therefore, the onset of idiosyncratic hepatotoxicity typically is delayed several weeks and may be accompanied by fever, rash, eosinophilia, and hepatic granulomas.

TABLE 61-1
Mechanisms of Drug-Induced Hepatic Injury

Hepatocellular: isoniazid, trazodone, diclofenac, nefazodone, venlafaxine, lovastatin
Cholestatic: chlorpromazine, estrogen, erythromycin
Mixed: amoxicillin/clavulanate, carbamazepine, herbs, cyclosporine, methimazole
Immunoallergic: halothane, phenytoin, sulfamethoxazole
Granulomatous: allopurinol, diltiazem, nitrofurantoin, quinidine, sulfa drugs
Steatohepatitis: amiodarone, perhexilline maleate, tamoxifen
Autoimmune: nitrofurantoin, methyldopa, lovastatin
Fibrosis: methotrexate, excess vitamin A
Vascular collapse: nicotinic acid, cocaine, ecstasy
Venoocclusive disease: busulfan, herbal medicines

Etiology and Pathogenesis

One of the principal physiological functions of the liver is the biotransformation of lipophilic substances to polar compounds that are subsequently excreted in bile or urine. Several diverse and overlapping mechanisms have evolved to metabolize and dispose of the ubiquitous xenobiotic and endobiotic chemicals circulating in the human body. Handling these substances requires transcellular transport as well as biotransformation. The enzymes that catalyze the biotransformation reactions are usually found in the endoplasmic reticulum and cytosol of hepatocytes. Many of the substrates for biotransformation are toxic, and in several instances, the products of biotransformation are even more toxic. Because the liver is often the primary site of exposure to these toxins, hepatic injury is a common consequence. Understanding the basic mechanisms of biotransformation is essential to any discussion of drug-induced liver injury.

The biotransformation process is often divided into two phases. In phase 1, the compound undergoes oxidation to a more polar substance, usually using the cytochrome P450 (CYP) superfamily of enzymes. The products are often volatile and may be extremely toxic, as in acetaminophen metabolism. Phase 1 is often referred to as *toxification*. Phase 2 reactions detoxify the metabolites by conjugation with glucuronic acid, glycine, sulfates, and glutathione. Patients with severe liver disease have impaired phase 1 capacity, but phase 2 activities usually are intact, and therefore drug toxicity usually does not occur at higher frequency in patients with preexisting liver disease.

The CYP superfamily is a group of more than 30 different enzymes, found mostly in the endoplasmic reticulum. These enzymes have distinct substrate specificities, but there is often some overlap, that is, two CYPs can contribute to the metabolism of one xenobiotic. CYP3A4, CYP2D6, CYP2E1, and CYP1A1 are among the most important enzymes in the CYP superfamily. The activities of CYP enzymes vary tremendously among individuals. In addition, these enzymes are susceptible to induction and inhibition by numerous specific substrates. These are the primary mechanisms of drug interactions. For example, phenobarbital induces CYP3A4, leading to increased metabolism of cyclosporine. Alternatively, itraconazole inhibits CYP3A4, leading to decreased clearance of cyclosporine and potentially severe systemic drug toxicity. This type of interaction can also increase the risk of drug-induced liver injury. For example, ethanol induces CYP2E1, which increases the conversion of acetaminophen to the toxic intermediate, NAPQI. Because of interindividual variations and the multitude of potential drug interactions, drugs metabolized by the CYP enzymes generally do not have predictable pharmacodynamic profiles.

Uridine diphosphate (UDP)-glucuronosyltransferases are a group of enzymes that catalyze the conjugation of glucuronide to many xenobiotics and endobiotics. As with the CYP enzymes, the substrate specificities of UDP-glucuronosyltransferase isoforms overlap, providing redundant pathways for xenobiotic elimination. The formation of glucuronides is important in the excretion of bilirubin, steroids, and many medications. Glucuronidation is primarily a means of detoxifying substances; however, the glucuronides of several compounds may produce hepatobiliary injury. For example, the glucuronide of estradiol is probably responsible for the cholestasis caused by endogenous and exogenous estrogens. Conjugation with sulfate is an important mechanism in the biotransformation of several drugs to water-soluble compounds. Many of the substrates for UDP-glucuronosyltransferases are also substrates for sulfotransferases.

One of the most important defenses against hepatocellular toxicity is glutathione conjugation by glutathione *S*-transferases. Glutathione is a tripeptide of glutamine, glycine, and cysteine. Glutathione protects cellular enzymes and membranes from oxidative injury by volatile metabolites. The rate-limiting factor for glutathione synthesis is the intracellular concentration of cysteine. In acetaminophen toxicity, an increased concentration of the volatile intermediate NAPQI rapidly exhausts the supply of glutathione. Supplying cysteine, as *N*-acetylcysteine, replenishes glutathione and prevents the accumulation of hepatotoxic levels of NAPQI. Conditions that deplete glutathione levels (e.g., fasting) increase susceptibility to toxicity from substances detoxified by glutathione *S*-transferase.

CLINICAL FEATURES, DIAGNOSIS, AND MANAGEMENT

Cholestasis

Several medications produce biochemical and clinical evidence of cholestasis through multiple structural alterations in hepatocellular membranes and functional alterations in the transport proteins responsible for bile formation (see Table 61-1). Although dozens of drugs have been associated with cholestasis, the most commonly implicated drugs are estrogens, anabolic steroids, sex hormone antagonists, carbamazapine, amoxicillin/clavulanate, trimethoprim/sulfamethoxazole, and erythromycin. Estrogenic and androgenic steroids usually produce bland cholestasis with minimal inflammation, which can be observed in a liver biopsy specimen. Amoxicillin/clavulanate and erythromycin estolate can produce cholangiodestructive cholestasis histologically similar to primary biliary cirrhosis. This inflammatory cholestasis is often accompanied by systemic signs and symptoms of hypersensitivity, including fever, rash, arthralgias, and eosinophilia. In other cases, progressive destruction of the bile ducts may occur, the so-called *vanishing bile duct syndrome*, which can lead to liver failure. Fortunately, drug-induced cholestasis is usually resolved by removing the offending agent, but the cholestasis can persist for months.

Hepatitis

Nonspecific hepatitis is the histological finding in 90% of the cases of drug-induced liver disease. Hepatocellular necrosis is patchy and associated with a variable degree of mononuclear inflammation. Many drugs produce a more severe lesion that is indistinguishable from viral hepatitis. Common culprits include acetaminophen, halothane, isoniazid, and phenytoin. Acute reactions may lead to the development of fulminant or subfulminant hepatic failure. For unclear reasons, the prognosis for patients with drug-induced hepatic failure (except for those cases associated with acetaminophen toxicity) is generally worse than for patients with other causes of fulminant hepatic failure.

Some medications cause a granulomatous hepatitis. Hepatic injuries caused by quinidine, sulfonamides, and allopurinol often are accompanied by noncaseating granulomas. Except for fatal cases of fulminant hepatitis, withdrawing the agent responsible for any variant of hepatitis always results in clinical and histological improvement. Patients with chronic active hepatitis may progress to cirrhosis if the clinician does not recognize the iatrogenic nature of the illness and does not discontinue the drug responsible.

Steatosis and Steatohepatitis

Several drugs disturb the metabolism of fatty acids and triglycerides, leading to triglyceride accumulation in hepatocytes. There are two distinct patterns of bland steatosis. In macrovesicular steatosis, large globules of triglycerides fill the cytoplasm and displace the nucleus peripherally. In microvesicular steatosis, numerous small fat globules uniformly distributed throughout the cytoplasm do not displace the nucleus. Microvesicular steatosis is most commonly associated with valproic acid and intravenous tetracycline. This histological lesion is also seen in Reye syndrome and fatty liver of pregnancy, and similar to the clinical course of these disorders, drug-induced microvesicular steatosis can cause marked elevations in aminotransferase levels, severe hepatic dysfunction, and, eventually, hepatic failure. Macrovesicular steatosis is characteristic of exposure to ethanol, corticosteroids, methotrexate, and amiodarone. The injury from exposure to amiodarone resembles alcoholic hepatitis; both are characterized by the presence of Mallory bodies and an inflammatory infiltrate. Characteristic lysosomal inclusions produced by amiodarone can be observed by electron microscopy, but their presence does not correlate with the magnitude of liver injury. If unrecognized, the steatohepatitis caused by amiodarone can evolve into cirrhosis.

Cirrhosis

Numerous drugs and toxins produce cirrhosis with minimal clinical evidence of antecedent injury. Although high-dose vitamin A, arsenics, and vinyl chloride can be associated with cirrhosis, methotrexate is the agent most often implicated as the cause of cirrhosis. The risk of methotrexate-induced liver injury is poorly defined, but it appears to increase with daily dosing, obesity, ethanol use, and diabetes. Baseline and surveillance biopsies of the liver are often recommended, as liver chemistry values are often normal. The early stages of methotrexate-induced injury are characterized by steatosis with variable degrees of inflammation; drug withdrawal is not necessary. Significant steatohepatitis warrants continued biopsy surveillance. If the patient has progressive fibrosis or established cirrhosis, methotrexate should be discontinued.

Hepatic Tumors

Estrogenic and androgenic steroids have been associated with the development of hepatic adenomas and, rarely, hepatocellular carcinomas. Adenomas can become quite large and may be complicated by hemorrhage and rupture. Cessation of estrogen contraceptives has been associated with regression. Large or hemorrhagic lesions may require surgical intervention. Although focal nodular hyperplasia has been reported with oral contraceptive use, the validity of this association remains in question. The risk of hepatocellular carcinoma appears to be minimal; most reports link the tumor to prolonged use of anabolic steroids. Highly malignant angiosarcomas have been associated with anabolic steroids, and less commonly with vinyl chloride and Thorotrast, a contrast agent no longer used for radiologic procedures.

Portal Hypertension

In addition to drug-induced cirrhosis, portal hypertension may develop secondary to Budd-Chiari syndrome, a disease associated with oral contraceptive use. Underlying myeloproliferative disorders have been noted in many patients with contraceptive-associated Budd-Chiari syndrome. Patients may present with an acute illness characterized by right upper quadrant pain, hepatomegaly, and sudden-onset ascites. Alternatively, portal hypertension may develop insidiously over a period of several months.

Patients who receive high-dose chemotherapy with busulfan, mitomycin C, adriamycin, and 6-thioguanine may present with a clinical illness similar to Budd-Chiari syndrome that is called *venoocclusive disease*, also known as sinusoidal obstruction syndrome. The characteristic histological features of venoocclusive disease are centrilobular necrosis and fibrous obliteration of the central veins. It is most often seen in bone marrow and stem cell transplantations. Patients usually present in the first weeks to months after ablation chemotherapy and radiation therapy. Portal hypertension may be progressive or it may resolve. Rarely, herbal medications have been associated with venoocclusive disease.

Acetaminophen Hepatotoxicity

Acetaminophen is the most common cause of life-threatening hepatic injury. Inadvertent and suicidal ingestions of large doses predictably cause severe acute liver injury and account for up to 20% of liver transplantations performed for fulminant hepatic failure. At therapeutic doses, 90% of acetaminophen is conjugated with glucuronide or sulfate and subsequently excreted in urine. A small percentage of acetaminophen is oxidized by CYP2E1 to the toxic intermediate NAPQI. Under normal physiological conditions, the highly volatile NAPQI is rapidly detoxified by conjugation with glutathione. Any condition that increases the formation of NAPQI or decreases the reserve of glutathione predisposes the patient to acetaminophen hepatotoxicity. The most common scenario is consumption of a supratherapeutic dose of acetaminophen, usually more than 10 to 15 g, which saturates the glucuronidation pathway and increases NAPQI formation. Alternatively, induction of CYP2E1 by chronic ethanol consumption may increase the proportion of acetaminophen metabolized to NAPQI, even at therapeutic doses. In either scenario, the increased NAPQI rapidly overwhelms the reserve of glutathione, and the subsequent accumulation of NAPQI produces hepatocellular injury. Chronic alcoholism and prolonged fasting also deplete glutathione stores, and the small amounts of NAPQI produced with therapeutic doses of acetaminophen cannot be completely detoxified. The residual NAPQI can cause significant hepatocellular injury. These accidental overdoses tend to present later, suffer more severe injury, and have higher mortality rates. Because the centrilobular region is the site of highest CYP2E1 activity and lowest glutathione concentration, acetaminophen toxicity manifests as necrosis in this region in cases secondary either to intentional or accidental overdose.

Acetaminophen is a classic intrinsic hepatotoxin, and ingestion of high doses predictably produces hepatocellular injury. A well-described nomogram, based on serum acetaminophen levels, accurately identifies persons likely to incur hepatotoxicity from a single ingestion of an excessive dose. The first several hours after an overdose, patients may experience nausea and vomiting that resolves rapidly. Over the next 24 to 48 hours, patients may appear deceptively well, with normal aminotransferase levels, but biochemical evidence of acute hepatitis appears within 48 hours of ingestion. By the third to fifth day after ingestion, many patients develop symptoms of acute hepatitis: recurrent nausea, vomiting, jaundice, and abdominal pain. Serum aminotransferase levels usually peak in the thousands. The increase in the bilirubin level and the prolongation of prothrombin time are proportional to the severity of injury. Severe cases may meet the criteria of fulminant hepatic failure, with progression to encephalopathy and other complications of hepatic failure.

All persons suspected of overdosing on acetaminophen should have a toxicology evaluation of serum and urine because many individuals overdose with multiple agents. Gastric lavage and activated charcoal delivered orally or through a nasogastric tube nonspecifically prevent further absorption of residual quantities of intralumenal acetaminophen as well as other medications ingested in an overdose, if performed shortly after ingestion. Their use remains controversial particularly if there is reasonable confidence that acetaminophen was the sole drug ingested. Charcoal therapy may need to be delayed several hours if acetaminophen is the sole medication ingested, to allow administration of the antidote, *N*-acetylcysteine.

Because acetaminophen toxicity results from depletion of hepatic glutathione and the subsequent accumulation of NAPQI, therapy has focused on repletion of glutathione stores. *N*-acetylcysteine delivered orally or intravenously supplies the liver with a source of cysteine, which is the rate-limiting factor in glutathione synthesis. If given within 16 hours of acetaminophen ingestion, there is virtually no risk of developing hepatic failure. Several reports indicate that *N*-acetylcysteine may be beneficial even after the onset of hepatitis, although efficacy clearly declines with increasing delays in therapy.

The nomogram for acetaminophen toxicity predicts that any patient with postingestion serum acetaminophen levels of 150 mg/mL at 4 hours, 70 mg/mL at 8 hours, or 35 mg/mL at 12 hours may suffer severe hepatotoxicity. This nomogram is applicable only to one-time ingestions of large doses by healthy adults. Similarly, the temporal relationship of serum levels to actual ingestion time is often unreliable. Given these limitations and the benign nature of *N*-acetylcysteine therapy, any patient with suspected acute or chronic acetaminophen overdose should receive *N*-acetylcysteine therapy. Further, given the increased susceptibility of alcoholics and fasting patients, any acute liver injury in these settings should prompt clinicians to consider therapy for acetaminophen toxicity.

Most patients with acute hepatic injury secondary to acetaminophen ingestion gradually improve with no long-term sequelae, but the progression to fulminant hepatic failure, which is heralded by the onset of encephalopathy, may be fatal. Any patient with this complication should be referred to a center specializing in liver transplantation. Patients should be monitored in a critical care setting for metabolic complications such as hypoglycemia, acidosis, and renal failure. Reversible causes of encephalopathy should be corrected, and intracranial pressure should be monitored in cases of grade III or IV encephalopathy. Recovery is unlikely if patients have an arterial pH of less than 7.30 or if patients have grade III or IV encephalopathy associated with a prothrombin time international ratio higher than 6.5 and a serum creatinine level higher than 3.5 mg/dL. Patients with these poor prognostic indicators who are otherwise suitable for liver transplantation should be placed at the highest priority for transplantation. Posttransplant survival rates of 80% and higher greatly exceed the chance that patients with these poor prognostic indicators will recover.

CHAPTER 62

Viral Hepatitis

Hepatitis is a nonspecific clinicopathological term that encompasses all disorders characterized by hepatocellular injury accompanied by histological evidence of a necroinflammatory response. Hepatitis is classified into acute hepatitis, which is defined as self-limited liver injury of less than 6 months' duration, and chronic hepatitis, in which the inflammatory response persists after 6 months. These two fundamental forms of hepatitis can be further subdivided on the basis of the underlying disease process or cause. Several diseases, such as drug-induced hepatitis and viral hepatitis B and C, may manifest as both acute and chronic hepatitis. Others, such as viral hepatitis A and E, are strictly acute. Hereditary hemochromatosis, among other diseases, invariably presents as chronic liver injury.

HEPATITIS A

Incidence and Epidemiology

Hepatitis A virus (HAV) causes 200,000 cases of acute hepatitis annually. It is transmitted primarily by fecal-oral routes. Epidemics can be traced to contaminated water or food. HAV is rarely acquired by parenteral exposure. About 30% of the population of the United States has serum IgG antibody to HAV, which suggests prior exposure. Significant racial and ethnic differences in the prevalence of antibody to HAV are likely to reflect both country of origin and socioeconomic status. In developing countries, essentially all children are exposed to the virus, which often produces subclinical illness in this age group. Risk factors for acquiring HAV include male homosexuality, household contact with an infected person, travel to developing countries, and contact with children in day care. Outbreaks have also been associated with the consumption of raw shellfish, frozen strawberries, salads, and raw onions.

Etiology and Pathogenesis

HAV is an RNA virus that produces hepatocellular injury by mechanisms that remain poorly understood. Direct cytopathic or immunologically mediated injury seems probable, but neither has been proven. After exposure, there is a 2- to 6-week incubation period before symptom onset, although the virus may be detectable in the stool 1 week before clinically apparent illness. The immune response to HAV begins early and may contribute to hepatocellular injury. Immunologic clearance of HAV is the rule, and unlike hepatitis viruses B and C, HAV never enters a chronic phase. By the time symptoms are manifest, patients invariably have IgM antibodies to HAV (anti-HAV IgM), which typically persist for 3 to 6 months. IgG antibodies to HAV (anti-HAV IgG) also develop and provide life-long immunity against reinfection.

Clinical Features

Many patients with HAV infection, in particular 80% to 90% of children, are asymptomatic. Only 5% to 10% of patients with serologic evidence of prior HAV infection recall an episode of jaundice. Factors that contribute to subclinical versus clinical infection remain unclear.

The syndrome of acute hepatitis caused by HAV is clinically indistinguishable from other viral causes of acute hepatitis. Patients usually present with a nonspecific prodrome of fatigue, anorexia, nausea, headache, myalgias, and arthralgias. This may be followed by jaundice and right upper quadrant pain. Some patients may experience pruritus, but this rarely requires treatment. Vomiting is common and may become intractable, leading to fluid and electrolyte imbalance. Physical signs include icterus and tender hepatomegaly. The spleen is palpable in a minority of patients. A relapsing variant characterized by recrudescent symptoms 5 to 10 weeks after recovery affects 20% of patients, and the clinical course is rarely protracted, lasting no longer than 12 weeks. Resolution of HAV infection with complete recovery, except in the rare cases of fulminant hepatitis (~1%), is the rule.

Findings on Diagnostic Testing

Elevations in levels of aminotransferases usually occur 1 to 2 weeks before the onset of symptoms and persist for up to 4 to 6 weeks. The alanine aminotransferase (ALT) level usually is higher than the aspartate aminotransferase (AST) level; absolute values often exceed 1000 IU/L. The level of enzyme elevation does not correlate with disease severity. Asymptomatic cases may have serum AST or ALT levels in the thousands. Serum bilirubin levels usually peak 1 to 2 weeks after symptoms appear, but they rarely exceed 15 to 20 mg/dL. HAV infection occasionally produces a cholestatic pattern of liver biochemical abnormalities with a disproportionate elevation in the alkaline phosphatase level. Other laboratory abnormalities include relative lymphocytosis with a normal total leukocyte count.

Diagnosis relies on detecting anti-HAV IgM in the serum. Because this IgM component of the humoral immune response lasts only 3 to 6 months, its presence implies recent or ongoing infection. Liver biopsy is not necessary if the findings from serologic testing are positive and is performed only if the diagnosis is in doubt. Although there are no distinguishing features of any form of viral hepatitis, patchy necrosis and lobular lymphocytic infiltrates are typical findings.

Occasionally, ultrasound scanning may be necessary to exclude biliary obstruction, particularly in patients with the cholestatic variant of HAV infection. This test may confirm hepatomegaly and reveal an inhomogeneous liver parenchyma, but findings usually are nonspecific.

Management and Course

HAV is self-limited, and symptoms resolve in most cases over the course of 2 to 4 weeks. There is no specific treatment, and patients should be encouraged to maintain fluid and nutritional intake. Ten percent of patients require hospitalization for intractable vomiting, worsening coagulopathy, or comorbid illnesses. The overall mortality rate for hospitalized patients is less than 1%. Deaths are mainly the result of the rare case of fulminant hepatitis, which is characterized by signs of hepatic failure, including encephalopathy. These patients should be referred to liver transplant centers for management and potential transplantation.

Infection with HAV can be prevented by either passive or active immunization. Patients exposed to feces of HAV-infected individuals should be given immunoglobulin (0.02 mL/kg) within 2 weeks of exposure. Travelers to endemic areas may be given immunoglobulin, which provides protection for about 3 months, or the formalin-inactivated hepatitis A vaccine, which provides long-term immunity to more than 90% of persons, beginning 1 month after the first dose of the two-dose regimen.

HEPATITIS B

Incidence and Epidemiology

Hepatitis B virus (HBV) is an important cause of acute and chronic hepatitis. In regions of Africa, Asia, and the Mediterranean basin where HBV is endemic, there are high rates of chronic HBV infection. Worldwide, there are 400 million HBV carriers. In the United States during the 1990s, HBV accounted for more than 175,000 cases of acute hepatitis annually, and 5% of these entered a chronic phase. In contrast, perinatal transmission of HBV leads to chronic HBV infection in more than 90% of cases. About 0.3% of the population in the United States suffers chronic infection with HBV.

Although 30% to 50% of infections with HBV have no identifiable source, the main route of transmission is percutaneous. The most common means of transmission are sexual contact with an infected individual, intravenous drug use, and vertical transmission from mother to child. Several epidemiologic surveys have emphasized the importance of contact transmission among individuals in the same household, even in the absence of intimate or sexual contact. The mechanism of this contact-associated transmission remains poorly defined. Blood transfusion is an unlikely source of HBV in Western countries with the use of blood bank screening but poses major risk in developing countries that do not screen blood or blood products for HBV.

Etiology and Pathogenesis

HBV is a DNA virus that has seven genotypes, A through G, based on differences in sequence. One component of HBV is an envelope that contains a protein called *hepatitis B surface antigen* (HBsAg). Inside the envelope is a nucleocapsid that contains the hepatitis B core antigen (HBcAg), which is not detectable in serum. During viral replication, a third antigen termed the *hepatitis B e antigen* (HBeAg) and HBV DNA are detectable in the serum. While in the replicative phase, HBV produces hepatocellular injury primarily by activating the cellular immune system in response to viral antigens on the surface of hepatocytes. The vigor of the immune response determines the severity of acute HBV hepatitis and the probability that the infection will enter a chronic phase. An exuberant response can produce fulminant hepatic failure, whereas a lesser response may fail to clear the virus.

After exposure to HBV, there is an incubation period of several weeks to 6 months before the onset of symptoms. HBsAg appears in the serum, followed shortly by HBeAg late in the incubation period. Detectable levels of HBeAg correlate with active viral replication, as does the quantity of HBV DNA. The first detectable immune response is antibody to HBcAg (anti-HBc), which is usually present by the time symptoms occur. As with HAV, the initial antibody response is primarily IgM, which persists for 4 to 6 months and is followed by a life-long IgG response. Antibodies to HBsAg (anti-HBs) develop in more than 90% of adult ndividuals with acute hepatitis. The appearance of anti-HBs, usually several weeks after the disappearance of HBsAg and resolution of symptoms, signifies recovery. anti-HBs provides life-long immunity to reinfection, although titers may decrease to undetectable levels over the course of years. Antibodies to HBeAg (anti-HBe) appear earlier than anti-HBs and usually signify the clearance of HBeAg and cessation of replication.

In chronic HBV infection, the virus may be in a replicative phase characterized by the presence of HBsAg, HBeAg, and high levels of HBV DNA, along with an immune-mediated chronic inflammatory response. Alternatively, HBV may enter a nonreplicative state, formerly referred to as the carrier state, in which HBV is maintained by insertion into the host genome. In this phase, HBsAg persists, but HBeAg disappears and anti-HBe appears. HBV DNA is present at low levels (fewer than 100,000 copies/mL). The inflammatory response in this nonreplicative state usually is minimal, but due to integrated HBV DNA in the hepatocytes, the risk of hepatocellular carcinoma persists.

Clinical Features

Most acute HBV infections are asymptomatic, especially if acquired at a young age when chronicity is more likely. Thirty percent of infections with HBV in adults result in acute hepatitis, which is indistinguishable from other forms of acute viral hepatitis. The illness usually has a 1-month to 6-month incubation period. Hepatitis may be preceded by a serum sickness syndrome characterized by fever, urticaria, arthralgias, and, rarely, arthritis. This syndrome is probably caused by immune complexes of HBV antigens and antibodies, which may also produce glomerulonephritis and vasculitis (including polyarteritis nodosa) in patients with chronic HBV infection.

Patients with chronic HBV infection may have a history of a distant bout of acute hepatitis, but a history of icterus is unusual. Most patients with chronic HBV infection remain asymptomatic for years. When symptoms develop, they usually are nonspecific, including malaise, fatigue, and anorexia. Some patients exhibit jaundice and complications of portal hypertension, such as ascites, variceal hemorrhage, or encephalopathy. Physical examination in the chronic phase may be normal, although hepatomegaly is common. Some patients may present with stigmata of cirrhosis and portal hypertension, including ascites, dilated abdominal veins, gynecomastia, and spider angiomata.

Findings on Diagnostic Testing

Diagnosis of acute hepatitis B is based on a typical serologic pattern in acute hepatitis. Serum aminotransferase elevations in the thousands and other liver biochemical abnormalities are indistinguishable from alternative causes of acute viral hepatitis. Acute infection is diagnosed by the presence of IgM antibodies to HBcAg (anti-HBc IgM) and evidence of ongoing infection represented by HBsAg, HBeAg, and HBV DNA. In 5% to 10% of patients with acute hepatitis, the latter three markers may be cleared before clinical presentation, leaving anti-HBc IgM as the only indicator of recent infection. It is important to measure the anti-HBc IgM because the isolated presence of IgG antibodies to HBcAg (anti-HBc IgG) is the most common serologic pattern in resolved HBV infection. The timing of HBsAg disappearance is variable, but it is absent in 80% to 90% of cases by 4 months after infection. Persistence of HBsAg beyond 6 months indicates chronic infection. Anti-HBs will appear several weeks after the disappearance of HBsAg. This antibody provides life-long immunity, but titers may drop to undetectable levels over the course of years. As with acute HAV, liver biopsy for acute HBV is needed only if the diagnosis is not substantiated by serologic testing.

Chronic HBV may produce several serologic patterns based on the replicative state of the virus. The presence of HBsAg, HBeAg, and HBV DNA and the absence of anti-HBs and anti-HBe are characteristic of active viral replication. The presence of HBsAg and anti-HBe in the absence of HBeAg, along with low levels of HBV DNA, is representative of the nonreplicative or chronic carrier state. All patients with chronic HBV have anti-HBc IgG. A small number of patients may have low titers of anti-HBc IgM, particularly when the virus is transiting from the replicative phase to the nonreplicative phase. In addition, several mutations exist, including precore mutations that result in negative HBeAg in serum, positive anti-HBe, but significant HBV DNA, as well as pre-S and polymerase mutations. The latter usually arise in response to therapy, such as the YMDD mutation that is associated with lamivudine resistance.

The levels of serum aminotransferases usually are mildly elevated with chronic HBV infection. Biochemical variables and symptoms correlate poorly with the histological severity of liver damage. Liver biopsy provides important prognostic information in patients with chronic hepatitis. Patients with active viral replication demonstrate a variable degree of chronic periportal inflammation. Extension of chronic inflammatory cells into the hepatic lobule is termed *piecemeal necrosis*, whereas inflammation and hepatocellular destruction extending from portal tract to portal tract is termed *bridging necrosis*. Patients in the nonreplicative phase usually have minimal to no inflammation. Variable stages of fibrosis or even cirrhosis can be present in any patient with chronic HBV. Determining the extent of inflammation and fibrosis is often critical in making therapeutic decisions for chronic HBV.

Management and Course

Acute HBV hepatitis usually resolves clinically and biochemically over several weeks to months. As with other forms of acute viral hepatitis, treatment is supportive. One percent of cases follow a fulminant course that results in hepatic failure and encephalopathy. These patients should be referred to transplantation centers.

The risk that HBV infection will become chronic seems to be associated with the patient's age at acquisition. Chronicity rates are 90% for infections acquired perinatally. The rate is lower in older children and is about 5% in adults. The mechanism of this variability in the ability of HBV to enter a chronic phase is probably related to changes in immune tolerance with aging.

Once established, chronic HBV infection is usually life-long. Annually, up to 1% of chronic HBV carriers lose HBsAg and develop anti-HBs, suggesting complete viral eradication. Also each year, the replicative phase of the virus transforms into the nonreplicative phase in 1% to 10% of patients (i.e., HBeAg is lost and anti-HBe is gained). An acute clinical and biochemical flare of the infection often accompanies this seroconversion. The transition to a nonreplicative state does not indicate complete clearance of HBV. Many patients exhibit reactivation of replication with reappearance of HBeAg at some point in the future.

Although cirrhosis may develop at any stage of chronic HBV infection, it usually requires many years of infection. The risk is greatest for patients with bridging necrosis and active viral replication. Because chronic HBV is indolent and produces minimal or no symptoms, complications of cirrhosis, including ascites, variceal hemorrhage, and encephalopathy, may be the initial manifestations of chronic HBV. The lifetime risk of hepatocellular carcinoma is about 20% in persons with chronic HBV infection; therefore, patients with HBV infection that lasts longer than

10 years should be screened every 6 months by serum α-fetoprotein measurements and imaging with ultrasound (or in some cases CT or MRI) to facilitate early detection. The course of acute and chronic HBV infection can also be complicated by superinfection with hepatitis D virus.

Treatment of HBV infection includes antiviral or immunomodulatory therapy with nucleosides, nucleotides and interferon-α. Candidates for interferon therapy should have detectable markers of viral replication (HBeAg and HBV DNA). They should not have histological evidence of cirrhosis or decompensated liver disease. Interferon therapy for HBV requires 15 to 35 million units delivered subcutaneously each week for 4 to 6 months. With this therapy, the virus in 20% to 30% of cases will sustain the transition from the active replicative phase to the nonreplicative phase. Six percent of patients lose circulating HBsAg, which suggests complete viral clearance. Side effects are substantial; there is an almost universal occurrence of an influenza-like illness with myalgia, fever, chills, and headache. Other adverse reactions include depression, bone marrow suppression, alopecia, and autoimmune thyroiditis. Patients should be selected with this side-effect profile in mind, especially if there are preexisting psychiatric conditions and cytopenias. Trials with long-acting pegylated interferons used once weekly are in progress. The Food and Drug Administration has approved two oral therapies, lamivudine and adefovir, for treating HBV infection. Both can be used by individuals who are HBeAg positive or negative, including those with decompensated liver disease. Both drugs are associated with HBeAg seroconversion rates of 20% to 40%, depending on the duration of therapy. Lamivudine has been associated with a high rate of viral resistance (50% to 70% at 3 years), whereas adefovir has been associated with lower rates of resistant virus (<5% at 3 years). Newer antiviral agents, including entecavir and emtricitabine, have a potential for effective combination therapy.

Prevention of HBV has widespread public health implications. A program of universal vaccination of infants with the recombinant hepatitis B vaccine has begun in the United States. This vaccine is also indicated for health care workers, patients on hemodialysis, intravenous drug users, persons who have household contact with HBV carriers, adolescents and individuals who are sexually active with more than one partner, and travelers who reside in an endemic area longer than 6 months. The three-dose regimen is given at time 0, 1 month, and 6 months. It is more than 90% effective in producing protective anti-HBs. Response rates may be lower in immunosuppressed individuals. Although titers may decrease over time, the protective effect is long-lived owing to the amnestic response at the time of exposure.

Postexposure prophylaxis requires the use of hepatitis B immune globulin (HBIG) (0.06 mg/kg) in addition to the recombinant vaccine. Those who have had sexual or parenteral exposure to persons with active HBV infection should receive HBIG within 2 weeks of exposure. Infants born to mothers with HBsAg should receive HBIG at birth and vaccination should be initiated. All exposed persons should receive the vaccine on the usual dosing schedule.

HEPATITIS C

Incidence and Epidemiology

Hepatitis C virus (HCV) is an RNA virus in the *Flaviviridae* family that has been classified into six genotypes, based on sequence variation. Because most infections with HCV assume a chronic phase, preventing transmission is critical. Along with human immunodeficiency virus (HIV), screening of the blood supply for antibodies to HCV has dramatically reduced the incidence of posttransfusion hepatitis to less than 1% of all transfusions. Most HCV infections in the United States result from intravenous drug use.

Given that the main mode of transmission is parenteral, the epidemiology of HCV infection mirrors to some extent that of HBV and HIV infections; however, sexual and perinatal transmission are rare for HCV. In most regions of the world, the prevalence of HCV antibodies ranges from 0.5% to 2%. Higher rates are observed in developing countries and lower socioeconomic groups. Within the United States, there is variation among racial groups with a 7% to 8% HCV positivity rate among inner-city African American and Hispanic populations compared with 0.5% among inner-city whites. In the United States, 70% of HCV infections are caused by genotypes 1a and 1b; the remaining 30% of infections are caused by genotypes and 3.

Although parenteral exposure is the primary means of contracting HCV, 10% of cases still have no identifiable source of infection. Groups at high risk of infection with HCV include intravenous drug users and persons who required transfusions or other blood products prior to 1991 or in countries outside the United States. The risk of sexual transmission is poorly defined but appears to be 3% to 5% in long-standing monogamous relationships. Overall, sexual transmission accounts for up to 20% of the cases of HCV infection. The risk of vertical transmission from mother to fetus is 3% to 5%. The risk is higher (12%–14%) if the mother is seropositive for HIV-1. Intranasal cocaine use, nosocomial infections from contaminated instruments or multidose vials, and needlestick injuries account for a small proportion of HCV infections.

Etiology and Pathogenesis

Based on the observation that HCV infection follows a slightly more aggressive course with immunosuppression secondary to medications or HIV infection, HCV does not appear to solely rely on immune-mediated injury. Dual mechanisms of hepatocellular injury include a direct cytopathic effect of HCV, as well as injury from specific and nonspecific T-cell–mediated immunologic injury. No protective antibodies to HCV have been demonstrated. In addition, the immune response in HCV infection is responsible for the syndrome of mixed cryoglobulinemia observed in a small fraction of chronic HCV infections. In this disorder, HCV antigen associated with monoclonal IgM and polyclonal IgG antibody complexes are deposited in the end organ and activate complement, producing dependent purpura, glomerulonephritis, arthritis, and vasculitis.

The incubation period after exposure is usually 2 to 12 weeks; the average is 6 to 7 weeks. Similar to HBV infection, antibodies develop against several viral proteins and are detected by the enzyme-linked immunosorbent assay (ELISA) and the immunoblot assay (RIBA). Anti-HCVs may not be detectable for up to 2 months after the onset of acute hepatitis; however, HCV RNA is detectable within 1 to 3 weeks after the onset of acute infection. HCV antibodies are neither neutralizing nor protective, and 70% to 85% of HCV infections assume a chronic phase.

Clinical Features

Most patients infected with HCV never develop a clinical syndrome of acute hepatitis. About 15% to 20% of patients develop malaise, fever, fatigue, nausea, vomiting, arthralgia, and right upper quadrant pain. Systemic symptoms may be followed by jaundice. HCV does not appear to be the agent responsible for the large number of cases of fulminant hepatic failure attributed to non-A and non-B hepatitis, and although fulminant HCV has been reported, it is exceedingly rare.

After an acute episode, 75% to 85% of adults and 55% of children with HCV infections enter a chronic phase. Spontaneous clearance of chronic HCV is rare. Many patients remain asymptomatic for years and are detected only during health screening or when donating blood. The most common symptoms of chronic HCV are nonspecific malaise, fatigue, and right upper quadrant abdominal discomfort. Some patients may remain asymptomatic even as the disease progresses to cirrhosis.

Findings on Diagnostic Testing

Patients with acute hepatitis caused by HCV usually have aminotransferase levels lower than 1000 IU/L; less than 10% have levels higher than 2000 IU/L. Serum bilirubin levels rarely exceed 10 to 15 mg/dL. Severe liver dysfunction with abnormal coagulation variables is uncommon.

As with other forms of acute viral hepatitis, the cornerstone of diagnosis is serologic testing. The main obstacle to diagnosing acute infection is the variable delay in the appearance of anti-HCV. Only 65% of patients have anti-HCV within 2 weeks of symptom onset, but 90% are seropositive after 3 months. The remaining 10% usually develops anti-HCV over several months.

Third-generation ELISAs recognize structural (C22, C33, and C100) and nonstructural (NS3, NS4, and NS5) viral proteins with 98.9% sensitivity. The specificity of ELISAs is lower; thus when the pretest probability is low, as in blood donor screening, a confirmatory test is required. One confirmatory test is the third-generation assay RIBA-3, in which antibodies to the individual structural and nonstructural proteins are detected. The presence of antibodies to two or more target proteins is indicative of HCV exposure. In practice, most confirmatory testing is done by testing for the viral RNA using polymerase chain reaction (PCR) or branched DNA (bDNA) amplification methods. Because they are the most sensitive and specific means of detecting active HCV infection, they can be used to detect HCV if serologic assays produce negative results in a patient with a high probability of having disease. Similarly, PCR or bDNA may confirm a positive serologic test result or document clearance of HCV spontaneously or after therapy. Qualitative and quantitative tests for HCV are both available; the qualitative tests are most sensitive (limit of detection ~50 IU/mL or ~10 IU/mL for the HCV transcription-mediated amplification assay [TMA]), whereas the quantitative tests provide more useful data, including the likelihood of response to therapy. Genotype can also be determined using genetic sequence detection techniques. Viral load and genotype do not appear to predict severity of disease but do predict the likelihood of response to antiviral therapy.

Liver biopsy is generally not useful for diagnosing acute HCV infection, but it is important in diagnosing and managing chronic HCV. In chronic HCV, there is a variable degree of periportal chronic inflammation, often with discrete lymphoid aggregates. The severity may vary from a minimal increase in periportal lymphocytes to the confluent destruction of hepatocytes in bridging necrosis. There also is a variable degree of fibrosis, ranging from no fibrosis to cirrhosis. The severity of histological injury correlates poorly with symptoms and elevations in levels of aminotransferases, though newer combinations of tests are being studied as noninvasive predictors of the severity of liver disease. Liver biopsy has been uniformly recommended by the National Institutes of Health and European consensus conferences for individuals being considered for antiviral treatment of HCV infection.

Management and Course

With supportive therapy, most patients with acute HCV experience a gradual resolution of symptoms over weeks to months. The infection is self-limited in 15% to 30% of cases and the virus is cleared, but in the remaining 70% to 85% of cases, the infection becomes chronic.

Chronic HCV infection is an indolent disease. There are often significant fluctuations in levels of serum aminotransferases. Complications generally occur more than 10 years after acquisition. Cirrhosis occurs in 20% to 25% of patients within 20 years of onset. Factors that predict the probability of disease progression are poorly defined, but histological evidence of severe inflammation, male gender, older age at acquisition, alcohol use, coinfection with HBV or HIV are all associated with more rapid progression. Long-term infection with HCV increases the risk of hepatocellular carcinoma, but this risk is limited to patients affected with cirrhosis at a rate of 1% to 5% per year.

The initial approved treatment for HCV, interferon-α, has been replaced by combination therapies of pegylated interferon and ribavirin. Interferon-α (α-2a, α-2b, and α con-1) appears to have both immunomodulatory and antiviral effects in treating HCV infection. Ribavirin has no antiviral activity as a monotherapy, but it is synergistic with interferons through unknown mechanisms. Therapy with pegylated interferon-α-2a or -2b once weekly subcutaneously and ribavirin orally produces an overall rate of long-term clearance of HCV of higher than 50%, as defined by PCR negative testing 6 months after stopping therapy (sustained virologic response). Predictors of a poor response include genotype 1 or 4, high viral load, and histological evidence of cirrhosis. Most individuals who achieve sustained virologic response have a durable remission; few show late relapse. The side effects are similar to those associated with interferon therapy for HBV. Patients with active psychiatric disorders and marked cytopenias generally are not candidates for interferon therapy because of the substantial risk of complications associated with therapy. Sequencing of the entire HCV genome has led to the development of new drugs targeted at specific HCV proteins (e.g., helicase, protease, and polymerase) that offer promise to patients who do not respond to or who cannot tolerate interferon-based therapies.

Liver transplantation should be considered for all patients with symptomatic cirrhosis, complications of portal hypertension (e.g., encephalopathy, refractory ascites, variceal hemorrhage), or small hepatocellular carcinoma limited to the liver. In general, patients with cirrhosis who meet the criteria for Child-Turcotte-Pugh class B or C cirrhosis are best served by transplantation, whereas patients with Child-Turcotte-Pugh class A cirrhosis should be supported by medical therapy. Reinfection of the allograft is the rule, but most transplanted patients will not develop significant disease in the short and medium term. The management of progressive posttransplant HCV infection, which occurs in 15% to 20% of cases, is challenging.

The primary means of preventing HCV infection has been blood donor screening and prevention of parenteral exposure, including universal precautions in hospitals. There is no effective vaccine or passive immune therapy against HCV infection.

HEPATITIS D

The hepatitis D virus (HDV), also termed the *delta agent*, is a defective RNA virus that requires the presence of HBV to replicate. Only patients with acute or chronic HBV infection are susceptible to infection with HDV. HDV is present worldwide, with high incidences in regions of Africa, South America, and the Mediterranean, but a relatively low incidence in the United States. Modes of transmission appear to be both parenteral and sexual.

HDV may increase the severity of acute hepatitis caused by HBV. Diagnosis may be difficult in this setting because there are no clinical or histological features specific to HDV infection and antibody assays may not detect the transient IgM response.

Infection with HDV in chronic HBV carriers may result in an acute phase of hepatitis and clinical decompensation of patients with cirrhosis. Many patients develop chronic HDV infection, which accelerates the progression of chronic HBV hepatitis to cirrhosis. There is no effective therapy for HDV infection, other than suppressing HBV replication. The risk of recurrent HBV infection after liver transplantation is lower in patients coinfected with HDV due to suppression of HBV replication by HDV with very low levels of HBV DNA.

HEPATITIS E

The hepatitis E virus (HEV) is an RNA virus epidemiologically and clinically similar to HAV. It is endemic in developing countries, especially Mexico, Africa, Central Asia, and Southern Asia. Reports in the United States are rare and usually represent infection acquired while traveling in endemic regions. Transmission is mainly by the fecal-oral route. Outbreaks caused by contaminated water or food are common in developing countries.

The incubation period and clinical syndromes of acute hepatitis E are identical to those for HAV. For reasons that remain poorly defined, HEV infection in pregnancy during the third trimester is associated with a fulminant course in 15% to 25% of cases and has a high mortality rate. Diagnosis relies on detecting IgM antibodies to HEV. Detection of IgG antibodies to HEV signifies resolved infection and is associated with immunity. Treatment is supportive, and except for the high rate of fulminant hepatitis in pregnancy, full recovery from HEV infection is the rule.

NON A–E VIRAL HEPATITIS

A small percentage of acute and chronic hepatitis appears to be caused by viruses not detectable by currently available diagnostic assays. Hepatitis G virus (HGV, also called GBV-C), TT virus (TTV), and SEN virus (SENV) have been cloned and appear to be transmitted parenterally. There are no serologic assays, and detection requires PCR of serum to detect viral RNA or DNA. The clinical significance of these viruses remains unclear; only SENV may cause liver disease.

Nonhepatotropic viruses such as cytomegalovirus, Epstein-Barr virus, and varicella-zoster virus may produce acute hepatitis. Herpes simplex virus rarely causes hepatitis, but a few cases of fulminant hepatitis caused by this virus have been reported. Although these viruses cause acute hepatitis, none have been proven to cause chronic hepatitis.

CHAPTER 63

Nonviral Hepatitis

NONALCOHOLIC STEATOHEPATITIS

A form of liver injury histologically indistinguishable from alcoholic hepatitis is often observed in patients who do not have histories of ethanol abuse. This syndrome of steatosis with lobular hepatitis has been termed *nonalcoholic steatohepatitis* (NASH) or *nonalcoholic fatty liver disease type II* (NAFLD). Nonalcoholic steatohepatitis is more common in obese patients and in those with hyperlipidemia, diabetes mellitus, or insulin resistance. Mild elevations in levels of serum aminotransferases are often observed, and nonspecific symptoms of fatigue, anorexia, and abdominal discomfort are present in a minority of patients. There is no specific treatment for nonalcoholic steatohepatitis, but clinicians advise weight loss for obese patients and aggressive treatment of hyperlipidemia and diabetes. Trials of ursodeoxycholic acid (ursodiol) and antioxidants have not provided data to support their use. Insulin-sensitizing agents like metformin have provided the most encouraging data. Although reports suggest that 20% to 40% of cases progress to fibrosis or cirrhosis, further clinical experience will help define the natural history of this disorder.

ISCHEMIC HEPATITIS

An acute form of ischemic liver injury, termed *ischemic hepatitis* or *shock liver*, often complicates the course of critical illness. The portal vein provides about two-thirds of the hepatic blood supply; the residual one-third comes from the hepatic artery. Ischemic injury usually requires reduced flow in both systems. Most patients with ischemic hepatitis have circulatory shock from cardiovascular disease, sepsis, or profound hypovolemia.

In the hours to days after the hemodynamic insult, levels of serum aminotransferases, lactate dehydrogenase, and bilirubin increase to variable degrees. Severe injury is associated with aminotransferase levels in the several thousands and marked prolongation of prothrombin time. The treatment of ischemic hepatitis is largely supportive. Systemic hemodynamics should be optimized, and any coexistent infections should be treated with broad-spectrum antibiotics. Despite apparent severe biochemical dysfunction, most of the laboratory abnormalities improve over 1 to 2 weeks with rapid declines in aminotransferases over the first 24 to 48 hours. If the patient survives, liver function usually returns to normal. The overall prognosis usually is poor because of the underlying critical illness.

WILSON DISEASE

Incidence and Epidemiology

Wilson disease, or hepatolenticular degeneration, is an autosomal recessive disorder caused by mutations in the *ATP7B* gene that lead to excessive accumulation of total body copper. It is a rare disorder with a worldwide incidence of 3 cases per 100,000 of population. Higher incidences may be noted in populations prone to inbreeding. The incidence of heterozygotes is 1 in 90. Abnormal copper metabolism is established from birth. Patients usually are diagnosed in adolescence, although rarely cases manifest after age 50.

Etiology and Pathogenesis

The gene for Wilson disease is a copper-transporting P-type ATPase expressed exclusively in the liver. A defective structure or function of the transporter results in impaired biliary excretion and increased hepatic stores of copper. Free copper is also released into the serum and deposited in end organs. Accumulations in the brain, kidneys, bones, and eyes are responsible for the extrahepatic complications of Wilson disease.

Clinical Features

Patients with Wilson disease almost universally present between ages 5 and 50; the second decade of life is the peak time of onset. Liver disease affects 50% of patients, but the proportion who present with hepatic or neuropsychiatric symptoms varies with age. Potential hepatic manifestations include chronic active hepatitis with associated malaise, fatigue, and anorexia. Alternatively, patients present with complications of cirrhosis or a syndrome of fulminant hepatic failure with marked jaundice, encephalopathy, and hemolytic anemia. The diagnosis might be suggested by asymptomatic elevations of serum aminotransferase levels in an adolescent or young adult, often with a very low alkaline phosphatase level.

Because the primary metabolic defect is localized in the liver, all symptomatic patients with Wilson disease have some degree of liver disease, but 50% of patients present with extrahepatic manifestations. In 40% of patients, neuropsychiatric complications dominate. For unclear reasons, Wilson disease never leads to sensory deficits, but spasticity, choreiform movements, dysarthria, ataxia, and intention tremor result from copper accumulation in the lenticular nuclei. Patients also usually have subtle behavioral or psychiatric changes. The diagnosis should be suspected in adolescents with marked declines in scholastic or social performance. Patients with neuropsychiatric manifestations universally have Kayser-Fleischer rings, which are deposits of copper in the peripheral cornea. Other extrahepatic manifestations include Fanconi syndrome and proximal renal tubular acidosis, osteoporosis with spontaneous fractures, and copper-induced hemolytic anemia.

Findings on Diagnostic Testing

All siblings of Wilson disease patients should undergo diagnostic testing, in addition to young persons with abnormal liver chemistry profiles or clinical symptoms suggestive of Wilson disease. Screening for Wilson disease in a young patient with elevated levels of aminotransferases should include measurement of serum ceruloplasmin, which is decreased in more than 95% of homozygotes. Ceruloplasmin may also be low in 20% of heterozygotes and in patients with malnutrition, protein-losing enteropathy, and other forms of hepatic failure. Therefore, low ceruloplasmin levels should be confirmed by demonstrating 24-hour urinary copper excretion of more than 100 mg. The diagnosis cannot be excluded on the basis of a normal ceruloplasmin level. If Wilson disease is strongly suspected, further diagnostic evaluation with 24-hour urinary copper measurement should be performed with or without penicillamine challenge. Urinary copper also may be elevated in patients with cholestasis from other causes. Detection of Kayser-Fleischer rings may require slit-lamp examination. Although the presence of Kayser-Fleischer rings helps to confirm the diagnosis in the appropriate clinical setting, they may be absent in early Wilson disease. The standard for diagnosis is quantitation of hepatic copper levels in liver biopsy specimens. Histological findings include steatosis, glycogenated nuclei, and variable degrees of periportal mononuclear infiltrates and fibrosis. Genetic testing is not useful because of the large number of mutations described for the *ATP7B* gene.

Management and Course

The critical factor in managing Wilson disease is establishing a definitive diagnosis early in its clinical course. Untreated, the disease is universally fatal. When treated, patients have a normal life expectancy, but because treatment is life-long, the diagnosis should be established with certainty. The cornerstone of treatment has been copper chelation with oral penicillamine (1 g/day). The major obstacle is a 20% incidence of hypersensitivity reactions (e.g., neutropenia, thrombocytopenia, rash, and arthritis). Patients may require dose reduction because of drug-induced nephrotic syndrome. For hypersensitivity reactions other than neutropenia, a 2- to 3-week withdrawal followed by a stepwise increase in the dose may be attempted. Trientine and zinc have fewer side effects and are being used increasingly. Zinc inhibits copper absorption in the gut and cannot be used to treat preexisting copper overload. Although neurological symptoms may not resolve completely, patients with cirrhosis may experience long-term survival if they comply with therapy. Fulminant hepatic failure is not responsive to copper chelation and is universally fatal unless liver transplantation is performed. Transplantation should also be considered in the small fraction of patients with advanced cirrhosis who develop complications of progressive portal hypertension despite therapy.

HEMOCHROMATOSIS

Incidence and Epidemiology

Hemochromatosis is characterized by pathological accumulation of toxic levels of iron in the cells of various organs and tissues, including the liver. Because hepatic inflammation is not a prominent feature of the disease, hemochromatosis technically is not a form of hepatitis, but the iron-induced hepatocellular injury leads to clinical and biochemical features similar to chronic hepatitis. Hemochromatosis may be caused by a genetic disorder of iron homeostasis termed *hereditary hemochromatosis* (HHC), or it may be caused by a secondary disorder, such as transfusional iron overload, sickle cell anemia, or dyserythropoiesis (e.g., thalassemia major). The hepatic manifestations of secondary hemochromatosis are similar to those of HHC, but differentiation is usually apparent from the clinical features of the disorders associated with secondary hemochromatosis. Several hepatic disorders including alcoholic liver disease may be associated with uncomplicated iron overload, and differentiation from HHC may be challenging.

HHC is inherited as an autosomal recessive trait, with the responsible gene, designated *HFE*, localized to chromosome 6. It is one of the most common inborn errors of metabolism; the homozygous frequency is 1 in 300 and the heterozygous frequency is 1 in 9. The disease appears to be more common in persons of Northern European ancestry, but the precise incidence among other racial or ethnic groups is unknown.

Etiology and Pathogenesis

The basic pathophysiological mechanism in HHC is increased intestinal absorption of iron in conditions of normal dietary iron intake. A normal adult absorbs 1 to 2 mg of iron per day, whereas patients with HHC absorb 3 to 4 mg of iron per day. This increased absorption results in an excess accumulation of 700 to 1000 mg total body iron per year. The mechanism of enhanced absorption and intestinal cell transport of iron remains poorly defined.

The clinical features of HHC are produced by intracellular accumulation of toxic levels of iron, which causes hepatocellular destruction and fibrosis in the liver. Although the mechanism of iron toxicity remains poorly understood, damage to cellular and organelle membranes by increased lipid peroxidation has been proposed as an important factor. Iron deposition in the heart, pituitary, pancreas, skin, and gonads is responsible for the extrahepatic manifestations of HHC.

Clinical Features

Liver disease is the most common clinical feature of HHC. Most patients remain asymptomatic until complications of cirrhosis develop, but many cases of precirrhotic HHC are diagnosed after detection of asymptomatic hepatomegaly or mild elevations in levels of serum aminotransferases. Advanced liver disease may present with jaundice, weight loss, fatigue, variceal hemorrhage, ascites, and encephalopathy.

The most common extrahepatic manifestation is diabetes mellitus, which occurs in more than 50% of patients with HHC. An additional 50% of patients develop other endocrinopathies, including hypogonadism from pituitary and primary gonadal iron overload. Most patients with advanced disease have bronze or slate gray discolorations of exposed skin from increased melanin production and iron deposition in the basal layers. Degenerative arthropathy with a characteristic predilection for the second and third metacarpophalangeal joints occurs in 25% of patients.

Findings on Diagnostic Testing

Serum aminotransferase levels rarely exceed 100 IU/L, and they are normal in many cases. Serum measurements of total body iron levels are almost invariably elevated in HHC. The serum ferritin level is usually higher than 500 ng/mL and is often measured in the thousands. However, the serum ferritin level is elevated in any inflammatory disorder or iron overload condition such as alcoholism. Although a transferrin saturation of more than 55% is more specific for HHC, the predictive accuracy is less than 90% and the sensitivity is less than 80%. Therefore, patients with abnormal iron indexes should have their diagnoses confirmed. The standard for diagnosing HHC is liver biopsy with hepatic iron quantification and determination of the hepatic iron index. The hepatic iron index is calculated as micromoles of iron per gram of dry liver divided by the patient's age. An index higher than 2.0 is diagnostic of hemochromatosis, whereas an index less than 2.0 essentially excludes HHC. Patients with alcoholic liver disease and those who are heterozygous for HHC often have markedly abnormal serum iron indexes, but the hepatic iron index is always less than 2.0. Histological evaluation with Prussian blue staining usually shows impressive stores of intracellular iron in more than 50% of hepatocytes, but this finding may also occur in advanced alcoholic liver disease. Noninvasive magnetic resonance imaging may suggest iron overload, but attempts to quantify iron stores with these methods have yet to be validated. Increasingly, diagnosis is made by detecting the C282Y mutation in the *HFE* gene, which detects more than 90% of HHC. A second mutation, H63D, is of less certain clinical import as is the significance of heterozygotes for C282Y and C282Y/H63D compound heterozygotes.

Management and Course

The mainstay of HHC treatment is phlebotomy. The usual regimen removes 1 unit (250 mg of iron) every 1 to 2 weeks. Patients may require a total of 75 to 100 sessions over 2 to 3 years before iron stores return to normal levels. Once the transferrin saturation falls to less than 45% and the serum ferritin level is below 50 ng/mL, patients can be maintained on regimens of phlebotomy every 3 to 4 months. If diagnosed before the onset of cirrhosis or diabetes, patients with HHC compliant with phlebotomy programs can expect normal survival. Although phlebotomy does not reverse cirrhosis, it improves survival and should be considered at all stages of HHC. In patients with dyserythropoiesis or other causes of anemia intolerant of phlebotomy, chelation therapy with desferoxamine is an alternative. Desferoxamine requires parenteral infusion and removes only 50 to 75 mg of iron per dose.

In patients with cirrhosis, the 10-year survival rate is 70%. Most deaths caused by HHC are related to complications of liver disease. Up to 30% of patients with HHC develop hepatocellular carcinoma. Screening patients with established cirrhosis by using biannual α-fetoprotein measurement and ultrasound, computed tomography, or magnetic resonance imaging may result in early detection. Patients with advanced cirrhosis should be considered for liver transplantation, but the posttransplantation survival of patients with HHC is lower than that of patients with other forms of chronic liver disease, possibly because of a higher incidence of diabetes and cardiac disease.

α_1-ANTITRYPSIN DEFICIENCY

Individuals who have inherited the PiZZ phenotype of α_1-antitrypsin may manifest various liver disorders as a result of the accumulation of mutant Z α_1-antitrypsin in the endoplasmic reticulum of hepatocytes. Patients usually present in infancy with cholestatic hepatitis or cirrhosis, but some present in adulthood with chronic hepatitis, cirrhosis, or hepatocellular carcinoma. Only 20% of persons with PiZZ phenotype develop clinical liver disease. The other phenotypes (e.g., PiSS, PiSZ), including those commonly associated with emphysema, are not associated with liver disease. Diagnosis is usually suspected in a patient with liver disease who exhibits decreased levels of the α_1 band in serum protein electrophoresis. Determining the specific phenotype of patients and both parents can provide more direct evidence for the diagnosis. Liver biopsy specimens can confirm the diagnosis by the presence of intracellular periodic acid–Schiff (PAS)-positive globules. There is no specific treatment for α_1-antitrypsin deficiency, and liver transplantation should be considered in patients with complications of cirrhosis. In addition to treating complications of cirrhosis, transplantation cures the underlying metabolic defect.

CHAPTER 64

Autoimmune Liver Disease

INCIDENCE AND EPIDEMIOLOGY

The immune system plays a substantial role in the pathogenesis of a diverse group of liver diseases. The severity and chronicity of many variants of viral hepatitis are influenced by the associated immune response. Similarly, a growing body of evidence suggests that immune mechanisms contribute to liver injury in alcoholic liver disease. Some forms of medication-induced liver disease exhibit histological and clinical characteristics that appear to be autoimmune, including occasional therapeutic response with steroid treatment. Patients with autoimmune hepatitis, a chronic inflammatory liver disorder, have both clinical and serologic features which suggest that it is an immune-mediated condition. Autoimmune hepatitis classically occurs in young women, but it may be seen in children and older adults. In men, the disease often presents later in life. The female-to-male ratio is 4:1.

Autoimmune hepatitis has been classified on the basis of autoantibody markers (Table 64-1). Several variants appear to have divergent epidemiologic features: Type 1 (antiactin), the classic form of autoimmune hepatitis, occurs primarily in young girls and women. Type 1 is associated with antinuclear antibodies (ANAs) and smooth muscle (specifically antiactin) antibodies (SMAs). Type 2 (anti-LKM) autoimmune hepatitis is a disease mainly of young children who present before 15 years of age with liver and kidney microsome (LKM) antibodies, but rarely, ANAs and SMAs. Progression to cirrhosis occurs in 3 years in 82% of patients with type 2 disease, compared to 43% with type 1 disease. Type 3 (anti-SLA) autoimmune hepatitis is rare and follows a clinical and epidemiologic pattern similar to that of type 1, except that serum tests are reliably positive only for antisoluble liver antigen (SLA). ANAs and SMAs may be negative in this third type.

ETIOLOGY AND PATHOGENESIS

The precise etiology of autoimmune hepatitis remains poorly defined, but current evidence suggests that a genetic predisposition to aberrant immunologic responses is the fundamental pathogenic mechanism. Unaffected relatives of patients with autoimmune hepatitis often have autoantibodies. In addition, associations of the antigens HLA-DRB*301 and DRB*401 with type 1 autoimmune hepatitis and DRB1*07, DRB1*15, and DQB1*06 with type 2 autoimmune hepatitis suggest potential genetic components of autoimmune hepatitis relating to immune dysregulation. It is possible that an environmental agent, such as a hepatotropic virus or a medication, triggers an immune response that remains permanently activated in persons with this putative genetic susceptibility, but this hypothesis has not been proven.

The circulating autoantibodies in autoimmune hepatitis are not specific to the liver and do not appear to be pathogenic. They are probably epiphenomena

TABLE 64-1
Comparison of the Clinical and Immunologic Features of Types 1 and 2
Autoimmune Chronic Active Hepatitis

	TYPE 1 (ANTIACTIN)	TYPE 2 (ANTI-LKM)	ANTI-SLA
Age at presentation (y)	10–25 and 45–70	<15	Mean age, 37
Associated disorders	10%	17%	58%
Immunoglobulins			
γ-globulins (g/L)	37 ± 11	23 ± 8	Mean, 32.2; range, 1.8–5.2
IgG	37 ± 16	25 ± 10.4	
IgA	3.7 ± 1.3	1.8 ± 0.9	
IgM	1.7 ± 1.1	2.4 ± 1.5	
Autoantibodies			
anti-SMA (%)	100	0	74
ANA (%)	33	2	29
AMA (%)	2	0	14
Progression to cirrhosis after 3 years (%)	43	82	75

AMA, antimitochondrial antibodies; ANA, antinuclear antibodies; LKM, liver and kidney microsomes; SLA, soluble liver antigen; SMA, smooth muscle antibody.

Data derived from Johnson PJ, McFarlane IG, Eddleston AL. The natural course and heterogeneity of autoimmune-type chronic active hepatitis. *Semin Liver Dis* 1991;11;187.

of a more fundamental immunologic derangement. Abnormal suppressor T-lymphocyte function and associations with many other immunoregulatory disorders are also markers of this poorly defined immunologic defect. Increased immunoglobulins suggest marked B-cell activation. Low complement levels are seen in some patients and may portend a worse outcome. Perhaps the most convincing evidence in favor of the role of immunopathogenic factors in autoimmune hepatitis is the nearly complete resolution of the necroinflammatory response with immunosuppressive therapy. Further understanding of the complex interaction of the immune system with possible environmental triggers may clarify the etiology of autoimmune hepatitis and help identify curative strategies.

CLINICAL FEATURES

Patients with autoimmune hepatitis come to medical attention with a diverse range of presentations from asymptomatic aminotransferase elevations to subfulminant hepatitis. Patients usually present with nonspecific malaise, anorexia, fatigue, arthralgias, and weight loss. Young women often develop amenorrhea. Jaundice occurs in severe cases and is the presenting symptom in more than half of patients. Occasionally, complications of portal hypertension (e.g., ascites, encephalopathy, or variceal hemorrhage) are the initial manifestations of autoimmune hepatitis. Associated autoimmune conditions include thyroiditis, inflammatory bowel disease, and rheumatoid arthritis. In children, 50% present with overlapping features of autoimmune hepatitis and sclerosing cholangitis.

Physical examination findings often are normal in early autoimmune hepatitis, but up to 80% of patients have hepatomegaly. Spider angiomata, jaundice, splenomegaly, and palmar erythema are present in 50% of cases. Advanced disease with portal hypertension can be the presentation of "burned out" disease with ascites (20%), encephalopathy (14%), and variceal bleeding (8%). There is no one clinical feature of autoimmune hepatitis that distinguishes it from other forms of chronic hepatitis or cirrhosis.

FINDINGS ON DIAGNOSTIC TESTING

Laboratory Studies

Before treatment begins, essentially all patients with autoimmune hepatitis have elevated serum aminotransferase levels. Typically, aminotransferase levels are three-fold to tenfold above normal, but occasionally, levels higher than 1000 IU/L are encountered. Patients with advanced disease may present with varying degrees of hyperbilirubinemia or with symptoms of fulminant or subfulminant hepatitis. Similarly, prolongation of prothrombin time, hypoalbuminemia, thrombocytopenia, leukopenia, and anemia may be present in patients with cirrhosis or portal hypertension. Viral testing for hepatitis A, B, and C should be performed to rule out viral infection. Further viral testing (e.g., Epstein-Barr virus) should be performed if infection is considered likely.

Autoantibody Testing

The cornerstone of diagnosing autoimmune hepatitis is documenting the presence of circulating autoantibodies. Three subclassifications of autoimmune hepatitis have been described based on serologic and clinical features (see Table 64-1). Type 1 autoimmune hepatitis, the most commonly encountered, represents the classic form of the disease. Patients have high titers of ANAs or SMAs, or both. Most patients also have polyclonal hypergammaglobulinemia. Type 2 autoimmune hepatitis most often occurs in children and accounts for only 5% of autoimmune hepatitis in adults. It is associated with a high titer of anti-LKM and an extraordinarily high incidence of associated immune disorders. Type 2 autoimmune hepatitis typically lacks ANAs and SMAs, but hypergammaglobulinemia often is pronounced. Patients with type 3 autoimmune hepatitis have anti-SLA, and they may have ANAs and SMAs. Patients with autoimmune hepatitis may have other autoantibodies, including asialoglycoprotein receptor, anti-liver cytosol I, antiactin, antineutrophil cytoplasmic antibodies, and low titers of antimitochondrial antibodies. Conversely, other chronic liver diseases may have low titers of ANAs and SMAs, but titers higher than 1:320 and higher than 1:40, respectively, are unusual. A small group of patients with the typical clinical features of autoimmune hepatitis have no detectable viral serologic features or autoantibodies. Whether this represents infection with an unknown viral agent or a form of autoimmune hepatitis without autoantibodies remains unclear. Some of these patients demonstrate a complete response to corticosteroids; a feature that some consider diagnostic of autoimmune hepatitis.

Liver Biopsy

A liver biopsy is required to establish the diagnosis of autoimmune hepatitis and assess the severity and stage of the necroinflammatory response. Biopsies usually are performed via a percutaneous route, although a transjugular approach may be required if disease is acute and if there is evidence of hepatic decompensation. Autoimmune hepatitis may be histologically indistinguishable from chronic viral hepatitis, with a pattern of periportal mononuclear infiltrate extending into the hepatic lobules, termed *piecemeal necrosis*. Some patients have predominantly plasma cell infiltrates. Severe cases are marked by hepatocellular necrosis extending from the portal tract to the central vein, termed *bridging necrosis*. Although autoimmune hepatitis typically spares the bile ducts, the histological features of autoimmune hepatitis occasionally are indistinguishable from those of primary sclerosing cholangitis or primary biliary cirrhosis. A variable degree of fibrosis may be present. Up to 25% of patients with type 1 disease and 80% of patients with type 2 have cirrhosis at presentation. Patients presenting with jaundice and marked elevations of aminotransferases predictably have bridging or confluent necrosis with variable degrees of fibrosis. The histological picture correlates poorly with the symptoms of patients with mild clinical disease. The autoimmune hepatitis score (Table 64-2) is an assessment of the features of biopsy specimens and the clinical parameters, and may be helpful in evaluating unclear cases or if there appears to be an overlap of autoimmune hepatitis and primary sclerosing cholangitis.

MANAGEMENT AND COURSE

Without immunosuppressive therapy, patients with autoimmune hepatitis usually progress to liver failure, with a mean survival time of 5 years. Fortunately, immunosuppressive therapy is successful in more than 80% of patients. However, because early trials did not include them, it is not known if asymptomatic patients with minimal histological injury benefit from therapy. Most patients with elevated aminotransferase levels and inflammation in biopsy specimens should be treated. Therapy may be divided into an induction phase and a maintenance or withdrawal phase. Therapy is initiated with prednisone alone or in combination with azathioprine. Both regimens are equally effective in inducing remission. Azathioprine alone is not effective for induction. Recommended doses of prednisone have been reduced, with initial doses of 30 to 40 mg/day. The dose is tapered by 10 mg/wk until a dose of 20 mg/day is achieved. The dose is maintained at 20 mg/day until the patient enters remission. Remission is defined as resolution of symptoms, reduction of aminotransferase levels to less than 1.5-fold above normal, lowering of gamma globulin levels to less than 2 g/dL, and improvement to minimal inflammation on liver biopsy. Biochemical remission occurs in 1 to 6 months, but histological improvement may be delayed for 12 to 36 months. The use of azathioprine in doses of 50 to 100 mg/day permits reduction of steroid doses with a concomitant decrease in corticosteroid side effects. Azathioprine should be initiated early because the lag time before therapeutic effect is at least 6 weeks. Azathioprine also has side effects, and patients must be counseled on the risks of bone marrow suppression, immune suppression, and pancreatitis. The increased risk of malignancy with long-term use is controversial, but probably is minimal. Blood counts must be monitored regularly, especially if higher doses are given.

When remission is achieved, corticosteroids should be tapered to the lowest possible maintenance dose or should be discontinued. There is no consensus on the need to repeat the liver biopsy to establish histological improvement. Patients occasionally can be tapered completely off immunosuppressants, but more than 80% of patients will relapse, most in the first few months after stopping therapy. For any patient, the risks of life-long therapy must be weighed against the risk of disease recurrence. Most patients can be maintained with azathioprine (1–2 mg/kg

TABLE 64-2
Summary of Autoimmune Hepatitis Scoring—Revised Sheet

	SCORE
Gender: female	+2
Biochemistry	
(IU ALP: unl ALP): (IU AST: unl AST)	+2, 0, −2
<1.5, 1.5–3, >3	
Total globulin or IgG (fold elevation)	
>2, 1.5−2, 1−1.5, <1	+3, +2, +1, 0
Autoantibodies (ANA, SMA, LKM-1) titer	
>1:80, 1:80, 1:40, <1:40 (IF)	+3, +2, +1, 0
Antimitochondrial antibody	
AMA-positive	−4
Viral hepatitis markers	
Igm HAVAb, HBsAg, IgMHBcAb	positive −3
anti-HCV and HCVRNA ?CMV/EBV	negative +3
Hepatotoxic drug history: (current)	positive −4
	negative +1
Average alcohol intake: (current)	
<25 g/d	+2
>60 g/d	−2
Liver histology	
Interface hepatitis	+3
Mostly lymphoplasmacytic infiltrate	+1
Rosetting of liver cells	+1
None of the above	−5
Biliary changes	−3
Other changes	−3
Other autoimmune diseases in patients or first-degree relatives	+2
OPTIONAL ADDITIONAL PARAMETERS	
Seropositivity of other defined autoantibodies	+2
(pANCA, anti-LC1, anti-SLA, anti-ASGPR, anti-LP, antisulfatide)	+2
HLA DR3 or DR4	+1
Response to therapy	
Complete	+2
Relapse	+3
Nonresponse (cholangiography required)	

ALP, alkaline phosphatase; ANA, antinuclear antibodies; AST, aspartate aminotransferase; CMV, cytomegalovirus; EBV, Epstein-Barr virus; HCV, hepatitis C virus; HLA, human leukocyte antigen; LKM, liver and kidney microsomes; SMA, smooth muscle antibody; unl, upper normal limit.

Data derived from Alvarez F, Berg PA, Bianchi FB, et al. International Autoimmune Hepatitis Group Report: review of criteria for dignosis of autoimmune hepatitis. *J Hepatol* 1999;31:929.

per day) with or without a low dose of prednisone (<10 mg/day). Patients who do not tolerate azathioprine can be maintained on prednisone alone or they may try a newer immunosuppressive agent. Mycophenolate mofetil may be the most preferable because of its favorable side-effect profile and the reports of successful treatment in small series.

At the time of diagnosis, many patients with autoimmune hepatitis will have established cirrhosis. Patients with bridging necrosis progress to cirrhosis in 3 years without therapy. Immunosuppressive regimens have postponed the progression to end-stage liver failure, even in patients with established cirrhosis. Disease progression leads to complications of portal hypertension in a significant number of cases. These patients should be evaluated for liver transplantation. Although recurrent autoimmune hepatitis has been reported in the liver allograft, often requiring higher levels of immunosuppressive therapy, the overall 5-year posttransplant survival rate is higher than 90%. The risk of hepatocellular carcinoma in autoimmune hepatitis–related cirrhosis is much lower than the corresponding risk of cirrhosis caused by chronic viral hepatitis.

CHAPTER 65

Alcoholic Liver Diseases

INCIDENCE AND EPIDEMIOLOGY

Alcohol-related liver diseases are among the most common liver diseases in the United States because more than 14 million persons regularly consume excessive quantities of ethanol. Alcohol-related liver disease is pathologically classified into three forms: fatty liver (steatosis), alcoholic hepatitis, and cirrhosis. There is considerable overlap among these conditions. A liver biopsy specimen may show evidence of all three forms of alcoholic liver disease. Steatosis and hepatitis represent varying degrees of injury that are not required to develop cirrhosis. Steatosis is generally benign, asymptomatic, and reversible with abstinence. Most morbidity and mortality from alcohol-related liver disease are caused by hepatitis and cirrhosis.

Fortunately, lesser degrees of liver injury occur in most alcoholics—only 20% develop severe chronic liver disease. Despite a male-to-female ratio of 10:1 for alcoholism, alcohol-related liver disease is more likely to develop in female alcoholics because they are more susceptible to liver damage from smaller quantities of ethanol. Thus, the male-to-female ratio for clinically significant liver disease is only 3:1, and the peak incidence is between ages 40 to 55 in men and ages 30 to 45 in women, usually after at least 10 years of heavy alcohol consumption. The amount of alcohol required to produce hepatitis or cirrhosis varies among individuals, but as little as 40 g/day (equivalent to four servings of either 12 oz of beer, 4 oz of wine, or 1 oz of 80-proof liquor) for 10 years has been associated with an increased incidence of cirrhosis. There is considerable evidence to suggest that women require less total alcohol consumption (20 g/day) to produce clinically significant liver disease. The incidence of alcoholic liver disease correlates with the national per capita consumption of alcohol. Why only a minority of alcoholics develop cirrhosis remains unknown. Inadequate nutrition, though much discussed, is neither necessary nor sufficient to cause significant alcohol-related liver disease.

ETIOLOGY AND PATHOGENESIS

Metabolism of Ethanol

The mechanisms by which ethanol and its metabolites induce liver injury remain poorly understood, but current evidence suggests several modes of injury. After ingestion, ethanol undergoes partial first-pass metabolism in the stomach and liver and is subsequently distributed throughout the extracellular and intracellular water space. Most ethanol is metabolized by hepatic alcohol dehydrogenase (ADH) to acetaldehyde, which is subsequently converted by acetaldehyde dehydrogenase (ALDH) to acetate. ADH is the rate-limiting enzyme. Its activity is decreased by fasting, protein malnutrition, and chronic liver disease. ADH is not inducible with chronic ethanol ingestion, but several isoforms with disparate rates of ethanol metabolism have been associated with differences in the risk of alcoholism and alcohol-related liver disease among different ethnic groups. There are also several ALDH isoforms with differing metabolic rates. Disulfiram (Antabuse) acts by blocking ALDH; and the accumulation of acetaldehyde leads to the clinical syndrome of flushing, nausea, and vomiting. Isoforms of ALDH with low activities are common among Asian populations and are associated with lower rates of alcoholism. These persons can experience a similar flushing syndrome after consuming ethanol. A smaller portion of ethanol is oxidized by the cytochrome P450IIE1 (CYP2E1). This enzyme is inducible by chronic ethanol ingestion and may contribute to the increased rate of ethanol elimination in alcoholics. More important, because CYP2E1 is responsible for metabolizing other drugs, ethanol can increase or decrease the rate of elimination of some medications (Table 65-1).

The oxidation of ethanol results in increased oxygen consumption and an increased $NADH/NAD^+$ ratio. As a consequence, fatty acid oxidation is inhibited, leading to fat accumulation, which, along with altered protein trafficking and excretion, produces hepatocyte swelling. Increased oxygen demand and compromised sinusoidal blood flow in hepatocyte swelling may produce relative ischemia, particularly in the pericentral zones. Oxygen free radicals formed as a result of cytochrome P450 induction may contribute to lipid peroxidation and to cellular injury. Acetaldehyde may alter membrane and cytoskeletal elements and induce the formation of protein adducts that may serve as antigenic stimuli, leading to an inflammatory response. Finally, alcohol increases gut-derived lipopolysaccharide (endotoxin) in the portal circulation, which leads to Kupffer cell activation. All of these metabolic alterations probably interact with cytokines (e.g., tumor necrosis factor α; transforming growth factor β-1; interleukin 1, 6, 8; and platelet-derived growth factor) to produce cell necrosis, stellate cell activation, collagen deposition, and fibrosis.

Contributing Mechanisms

Excessive ethanol consumption clearly plays a primary role in developing alcoholic liver disease, but other factors are also important. Animal studies and clinical observations of high incidences of malnutrition in alcoholics with liver disease suggest

TABLE 65-1
Interactions Between Chronic Alcohol Abuse and Drug Actions and Metabolism

INCREASED DRUG METABOLISM	INCREASED DRUG/ CHEMICAL TOXICITY	INCREASED DRUG TOLERANCE
Pentobarbital	Acetaminophen	Anesthetics
Meprobamate	Vitamin A	Barbiturates
Warfarin	Isoniazid	Meprobamate
Tolbutamide (and other sulfonylureas)	Phenylbutazone	Benzodiazepines
Phenytoin	Halothane	
Cocaine	Enflurane	
Rifampin	Carbon tetrachloride	
Aminopyrine	Benzene	
Methadone	Nitrosamines	
	Cocaine	

INCREASED PHARMACODYNAMIC EFFECT	ANTABUSE-LIKE REACTIONS
H_1 antihistamines	Tolbutamide
Barbiturates	Metronidazole
Benzodiazepines	Griseofulvin
Chloral hydrate	Quinacrine
Meprobamate	Pargyline
Narcotics	Reserpine
Phenothiazines	Phenylbutazone
Phenytoin	Moxalactam, and several other second- and third-generation cephalosporins

that protein and calorie malnutrition predisposes to alcohol-related liver disease. Moreover, protein and calorie repletion improves the biochemical profile and possibly survival of patients with alcoholic hepatitis. Despite this evidence, the mechanism of enhanced alcohol injury from malnutrition is unclear.

Immunologic, hormonal, and other environmental factors may also modulate individual susceptibility to alcohol-induced liver disease. Sex-related differences in susceptibility to ethanol toxicity suggest that estrogens and androgens may play a role. Alcohol may induce immune-mediated injury through influences on suppressor T-lymphocyte function, and acetaldehyde adducts may promote autoantibody production. Eighteen percent to 50% of alcoholics with liver disease have chronic viral hepatitis C, one third has hepatic iron overload not related to the *HFE* gene mutations that cause hemochromatosis, and cirrhosis is more common in obese alcoholics (who may have increased hepatic steatosis) This suggests that liver injury in some individuals is produced by various causes.

CLINICAL FEATURES

The clinical manifestations of alcoholic liver disease cover a wide spectrum from asymptomatic mild hepatomegaly with fatty liver to hepatic failure caused by severe alcoholic hepatitis or cirrhosis. Although a rare patient may be asymptomatic, patients with alcoholic hepatitis generally experience fever, anorexia, malaise, and abdominal pain. Most have physical examination findings of icterus, tender hepatomegaly, and spider angiomata. Severe alcoholic hepatitis manifests portal hypertension, including splenomegaly, enlarged collateral abdominal veins, ascites in 40% to 70% of cases, encephalopathy in 20%, and upper gastrointestinal bleeding in 30%. Although most patients admitted to hospitals with alcoholic hepatitis have simultaneous cirrhosis by biopsy, portal hypertension may be present in the absence of histological evidence of cirrhosis.

Patients may present with alcoholic cirrhosis without progressing through the stages of steatosis or clinically apparent alcoholic hepatitis. At the time of diagnosis, 10% to 20% of patients with cirrhosis are asymptomatic, but most present with nonspecific complaints of weight loss, malaise, failure to thrive, or complications of portal hypertension (e.g., ascites, spontaneous bacterial peritonitis, variceal hemorrhage, and hepatic encephalopathy). Patients with all forms of alcoholic liver disease, especially alcoholic hepatitis and cirrhosis, often have stigmata of alcoholism, including palmar erythema, Dupuytren contracture, testicular atrophy, gynecomastia, and feminization in male patients.

FINDINGS ON DIAGNOSTIC TESTING

Laboratory Studies

Alcoholic liver disease is characterized by distinctive alterations in serum biochemical profiles. Even in the most severe episodes of alcoholic hepatitis with extensive hepatocyte necrosis and hepatic failure, serum aminotransferase levels are only modestly elevated, typically not above 300 IU/L. Peak levels higher than 500 IU/L should prompt a search for alternative or confounding causes of liver disease, such as viral hepatitis, acetaminophen toxicity, or ischemia. The pattern of elevation is also helpful in distinguishing alcoholic from nonalcoholic steatohepatitis. A ratio of aspartate aminotransferase (AST) to alanine aminotransferase (ALT) higher than 2 is highly predictive of alcoholic liver disease, whereas in nonalcoholic steatohepatitis, the ratio is generally less than 1. However, the AST:ALT ratio is neither highly sensitive nor specific, particularly in patients with cirrhosis. Alkaline phosphatase is elevated in 80% of patients and a small subset of patients with alcoholic hepatitis may demonstrate a predominantly cholestatic biochemical profile, with marked elevations of bilirubin and alkaline phosphatase levels and normal to minimally elevated aminotransferase levels. Although most patients with cirrhosis have abnormal liver chemistry values, patients with well-compensated cirrhosis who abstain from ethanol may have nearly normal laboratory values.

Patients with alcoholic liver disease often have abnormalities of other laboratory profiles that are caused by liver disease or the toxic effects of ethanol. Macrocytosis is common. It usually is caused by the toxic effects of ethanol and occasionally by deficiencies in folate or vitamin B_{12}. Anemia and thrombocytopenia may be manifestations of ethanol toxicity, vitamin deficiency, or sequestration caused by splenomegaly. Prolonged prothrombin time and decreased serum albumin level may indicate severe liver dysfunction with compromised synthetic capacity, but nutritional deficiencies can produce similar abnormalities. Active alcoholics may exhibit ketoacidosis, hypophosphatemia, and hypomagnesemia.

Liver Biopsy

The classification of alcoholic liver disease into fatty liver, alcoholic hepatitis, and cirrhosis is based on clinical and pathological correlations; therefore, confirmation of these abnormalities and exclusion of alternative causes of liver disease require liver biopsy. For patients with coagulopathy, tense ascites, or thrombocytopenia, the risk of biopsy may outweigh the benefit of obtaining pathological confirmation. If there is diagnostic uncertainty, a transjugular liver biopsy should be performed on high-risk patients; this approach is often used when considering urgent transplantation in the case of sudden liver failure. Fatty liver or steatosis is characterized by large intracytoplasmic fat droplets often concentrated in the pericentral zone or zone 3 of Rappaport. By definition, simple steatosis is not accompanied by significant inflammation or necrosis, but pericentral fibrosis, a network of collagen surrounding the central vein, may be observed and is possibly a precursor of cirrhosis. In contrast, inflammation and hepatocellular necrosis are hallmarks of alcoholic hepatitis. The inflammatory infiltrate is primarily neutrophilic, and necrosis may range from ballooning degeneration of isolated hepatocytes to confluent centrilobular necrosis. Alcoholic hyaline (i.e., Mallory bodies) and pericellular and perisinusoidal fibrosis, which has a characteristic "chicken wire" appearance, are common. Cirrhosis, the final stage of alcoholic liver disease, requires documenting the presence of bands of fibrosis extending between the portal tracts and the central veins and the presence of regenerative nodules.

There is no pathognomonic histological feature of alcoholic liver disease. The diagnosis requires synthesizing clinical and pathological information. Mallory bodies are aggregates of perinuclear eosinophilic material once considered diagnostic of alcohol-induced injury. They are present in at least 30% of patients with alcoholic hepatitis or cirrhosis, but they are also present in other liver disorders, including Wilson disease, cholestatic liver disease, nonalcoholic steatohepatitis, drug-induced and total parenteral nutrition–induced liver disease, and hepatitis C. Alcoholic cirrhosis may be confused with primary hemochromatosis because of the high levels of hepatic iron. These two disorders can be distinguished by calculating the iron index: the micromoles of iron per gram of dry liver divided by the patient's age. In hemochromatosis, the iron index is higher than 2, and in alcoholic cirrhosis without hemochromatosis, it is invariably less than 2. Alcoholic cirrhosis may be compounded by the coexistence of other liver disorders, particularly hepatitis C.

Structural Studies

Hepatobiliary imaging is often necessary to exclude biliary obstruction or mass lesions as a cause of cholestasis or hepatomegaly. Ultrasound and computed tomographic scanning may demonstrate diffuse or focal fatty infiltration in steatosis. Alcoholic liver disease often produces nonspecific inhomogeneous ultrasonographic or tomographic patterns, but cirrhosis may exhibit a characteristic nodular pattern. Endoscopic retrograde cholangiopancreatography (ERCP) or percutaneous transhepatic cholangiography (PTC) may be necessary to exclude bile duct obstruction in patients with a cholestatic pattern of liver chemistry values. Magnetic resonance cholangiography may replace diagnostic ERCP and PTC, but it is not useful for patients with ascites. Alcoholic liver disease generally does not produce significant bile duct abnormalities, but gallstones are present in 30% of patients with alcoholic cirrhosis.

MANAGEMENT AND COURSE

The prognosis for alcoholic liver disease is determined mainly by the pathological stage at presentation and the patient's ability to abstain from ethanol consumption. The single most important therapeutic intervention is complete avoidance of ethanol consumption. This often requires a multidisciplinary approach, involving social workers, psychiatrists, primary care physicians, hepatologists, and, most important, social support groups. No therapy for alcoholic liver disease has any proven benefit if heavy drinking continues.

Alcoholic Steatosis

Alcoholic fatty liver is generally benign and resolves completely after 3 to 6 weeks of abstinence. Patients with pericentral fibrosis or alcoholic foamy degeneration may be more likely to develop cirrhosis. The major clinical importance of fatty liver lies in the clinician's ability to recognize significant alcohol-related end-organ damage and to counsel patients to abstain before more severe or irreversible damage ensues.

Alcoholic Hepatitis

In the first 2 weeks after hospitalization for alcoholic hepatitis, hepatic function often declines and serum bilirubin levels increase despite enforced abstinence from ethanol. Early (2 month) mortality rates range from 19% to 78%. Patients with encephalopathy, renal failure, ascites, and variceal bleeding have higher mortalities. Several methods of predicting disease severity and survival have incorporated clinical and laboratory findings, but the most accurate and widely used is the Maddrey discriminant function: serum bilirubin (mg/dL) + [4.6 × (patient's prothrombin time – control prothrombin time)]. A discriminant function of more than 32 identifies patients with severe alcoholic hepatitis who have a 30-day mortality rate higher than 50%.

The management of alcoholic hepatitis centers on abstinence. Eighty percent of patients who continue to drink develop cirrhosis, with a 5-year survival rate of less than 50%. In contrast, 70% of patients abstinent from alcohol have resolution of hepatitis, and only 15% progress to cirrhosis. Patients and clinicians should recognize that clinical improvement occurs gradually over several months to 1 year.

The possible contribution of protein and calorie malnutrition to alcohol toxicity has led to several trials of enteral and parenteral nutritional supplementation for treating patients with alcoholic hepatitis. These supplements result in accelerated biochemical improvement, but only one study demonstrated improved survival. Patients do not have higher incidences of encephalopathy; thus specialized formulas of branched-chain amino acids are not superior to standard formulas and should be given only to patients who have not responded to standard enteral therapy. Patients with alcoholic hepatitis should at least have their calorie intakes monitored and supplemented if deficient. Aggressive enteral supplementation may be warranted if oral intake is inadequate; parenteral nutrition should be used if enteral nutrition cannot be tolerated or if a nasoenteral tube cannot be safely placed or maintained.

Corticosteroids have been used to reduce the inflammatory response of alcoholic hepatitis. Several studies have demonstrated improved survival of patients with a discriminant function of more than 32 or with spontaneous encephalopathy. Studies have used prednisone, prednisolone, or 5-methylprednisolone in doses of 35 to 80 mg/d for 4 to 6 weeks. Treatment should exclude patients with active infection, renal failure, pancreatitis, or gastrointestinal hemorrhage. The mortality rate in this selected group is reduced by 25%.

Anabolic steroids and propylthiouracil have shown some promise in treating alcoholic hepatitis, but these medications are not widely used. Further controlled studies may prove their efficacy. Pentoxifylline in one trial reduced the risk of hepatorenal syndrome by 40% and reduced the mortality rate. Because it can inhibit tumor necrosis factor α and has a low side-effect profile, pentoxifylline is being used to treat moderate alcoholic hepatitis and in conjunction with corticosteroids, to treat severe cases.

Alcoholic Cirrhosis

As with all forms of alcoholic liver disease, long-term survival of patients with alcoholic cirrhosis is directly related to the stage of the disease and the patient's ability to abstain from ethanol consumption. In cirrhotic patients without jaundice, ascites, or gastrointestinal hemorrhage, 5-year survival rates are 85% with abstinence and 60% with continued heavy drinking. In patients with jaundice or ascites, the 5-year survival rates are 50% with abstinence and 30% with continued drinking. Cirrhotic patients with variceal hemorrhage have the worst prognoses: 5-year survival rates of 35% and 20% for nondrinkers and drinkers, respectively. Much of this survival data predates the use of endoscopic variceal banding and transjugular intrahepatic portosystemic shunts, although these therapies have not shown a survival benefit.

Similar to other forms of cirrhosis, treatment is largely supportive. Chronic diuretics are often necessary to correct the total body sodium overload that contributes to ascites and edema. Patients with prior variceal hemorrhage have lower risks of rebleeding with endoscopic obliteration of varices. The β-adrenergic antagonist propranolol reduces the risk of bleeding among patients with varices or portal gastropathy. Encephalopathy is best treated with lactulose, titrated to produce two to three stools per day.

Therapy directed at halting the fibrotic and regenerative processes of cirrhosis has been disappointing. Corticosteroids do not improve survival and have a high incidence of side effects. Limited evidence suggests that colchicine improves outcome in alcoholic cirrhosis. Further tests of colchicine and multicenter trials of lecithin and S-adenosylmethionine (SAM) are ongoing.

Liver transplantation should be considered for patients who have abstained for at least 6 months but continue to suffer from complications of portal hypertension and are in Child class B or C. The period of abstinence selects candidates who will probably have low rates of recidivism. Also, it allows for potential improvement in liver function to a condition that may not warrant transplantation. Patients may be referred to a transplant center before completing this prolonged period of abstinence. The time on the waiting list of potential recipients often serves as the abstinence period. Although guidelines for pretransplant and posttransplant treatment vary from center to center, survival posttransplant has been excellent. With appropriate patient selection, only 10% to 30% of patients return to drinking. Alcohol-related liver disease accounts for about 25% of adult liver transplants in the United States.

CHAPTER 66

Cirrhosis, Portal Hypertension, and End-Stage Liver Disease

The treatment of cirrhosis is largely supportive. Interventions target mainly the complications of portal hypertension, including varices, ascites, and encephalopathy. Treatment may be directed at these complications; for example, beta blockers and endoscopic banding for varices or transjugular intrahepatic portosystemic shunts (TIPS) for decompressing portal hypertension. Orthotopic liver transplantation has become the definitive therapy for advanced liver disease and consequently, the number performed has increased exponentially. Complications of cirrhosis and portal hypertension are the most common indications for orthotopic liver transplantation.

ETIOLOGY AND PATHOGENESIS

Cirrhosis

Cirrhosis represents the final common pathway of many hepatic disorders characterized by chronic cellular destruction. An intervening stage of increased fibrosis is followed by the formation of parenchymal regenerative nodules. The nodular distortion of the lobules and vascular network defines cirrhosis and ultimately plays a critical role in the development of portal hypertension. The cellular and biochemical events leading to this altered growth response and resulting architectural distortion are not well characterized.

Cirrhosis is often classified according to the gross pattern of architectural distortion: micronodular cirrhosis and macronodular cirrhosis. Alcoholic cirrhosis is typically micronodular; uniformly sized parenchymal nodules are separated by thin bands of connective tissue. The cirrhosis that evolves from the bridging necrosis of severe chronic viral hepatitis is often macronodular, characterized by nodules measuring up to several centimeters, separated by thick, asymmetric bands of connective tissue. This classification has limited clinical use because many disease processes present with either variant. Also, micronodular cirrhosis may transform into macronodular cirrhosis. It is not known if there is a difference in the natural history of these pathological variants of cirrhosis.

A more clinically relevant method of classifying cirrhosis is based on the primary disease processes responsible for hepatocellular injury (Table 66-1). In the United States, most cases of cirrhosis are related to alcoholic liver disease and chronic viral hepatitis. Other common causes of cirrhosis include hereditary hemochromatosis, primary and secondary biliary cirrhosis, nonalcoholic fatty liver disease (NAFLD), and autoimmune hepatitis. Several rare disorders that frequently are complicated

TABLE 66-1
Causes of Cirrhosis

Common
  Ethanol
  Chronic hepatitis C
  Chronic hepatitis B, with or without hepatitis D

Infrequent
  Primary biliary cirrhosis
  Primary sclerosing cholangitis
  Secondary biliary cirrhosis
  Autoimmune hepatitis
  Hemochromatosis
  Nonalcoholic fatty liver disease
  Cryptogenic cirrhosis

Rare
  Wilson disease
  α_1-Antitrypsin deficiency
  Small bowel bypass
  Methotrexate
  Amiodarone
  Methyldopa
  Cystic fibrosis
  Sarcoidosis
  Glycogen storage disease
  Hypervitaminosis A

by cirrhosis should always be considered in the differential diagnosis. These include Wilson disease and α_1-antitrypsin deficiency. In certain clinical settings, a metabolic or toxic form of cirrhosis may develop. For example, cirrhosis may occur years after small bowel bypass surgery, possibly secondary to increased serum concentrations of bacterial endotoxins or toxic bile acids from bacterial overgrowth. Medications such as nitrofurantoin, amiodarone, and methotrexate may produce chronic hepatitis and cirrhosis. Cirrhosis in childhood can be caused by congenital anomalies (e.g., biliary atresia), metabolic conditions (e.g., tyrosinemia, galactosemia), α_1-antitrypsin deficiency, cholestatic liver disease (e.g., total parenteral nutrition, progressive familial intrahepatic cholestasis), Wilson disease, glycogen storage disease, cystic fibrosis, and idiopathic neonatal hepatitis. When all other causes of cirrhosis are excluded, the diagnosis is idiopathic (cryptogenic) cirrhosis. This disorder may result from an immunologic or viral disease process that cannot be detected by serologic assays or from "burned out" NAFLD. Cryptogenic cirrhosis may account for 10% to 20% of all cases with cirrhosis; it is clinically indistinguishable from other common causes.

Portal Hypertension

Pressure gradients in portal circulation follow Ohm's law, which states that the pressure gradient is equal to the product of flow and resistance. Portal hypertension occurs if there is increased splanchnic flow or increased resistance in the hepatic

TABLE 66-2
Classification and Differential Diagnosis of Portal Hypertension

Prehepatic causes
  Portal vein thrombosis
  Splenic vein thrombosis
  Arterioportal fistula
  Splenomegaly

Intrahepatic causes
  Cirrhosis
  Fulminant hepatitis
  Venoocclusive disease
  Budd-Chiari syndrome
  Schistosomiasis
  Metastatic malignancy

Posthepatic causes
  Right ventricular failure
  Constrictive pericarditis
  Inferior vena cava web

vasculature. In cirrhosis, both mechanisms contribute to the development of portal hypertension. Nodular regeneration and fibrosis in the space of Disse increase postsinusoidal and sinusoidal resistance, respectively. Cirrhosis is also accompanied by increased splanchnic flow from decreased tone in the splanchnic arterioles. The mechanisms responsible for splanchnic arteriolar vasodilation are poorly understood but may involve nitric oxide. In extrahepatic causes of portal hypertension, such as portal vein thrombosis or massive splenomegaly, either increased resistance or increased flow is the principal mechanism of increased portal pressure. The anatomic site of increased flow or resistance has been used to classify portal hypertension into prehepatic, intrahepatic, and posthepatic portal hypertension (Table 66-2). Intrahepatic causes are often further subdivided into presinusoidal, sinusoidal, and postsinusoidal according to the site of increased resistance. This subclassification has limited value because many forms of cirrhosis may involve more than one site of vascular distortion in relationship to the sinusoids.

CLINICAL FEATURES

Although patients with early cirrhosis may be asymptomatic, the most ubiquitous feature of cirrhosis is a general decline in health with nonspecific complaints of anorexia, weight loss, malaise, fatigue, and weakness. More advanced disease may present with one of the complications of portal hypertension.

Endocrine Manifestations

Patients with cirrhosis may manifest several endocrine disturbances. The prevalence of diabetes mellitus increases in all forms of cirrhosis but particularly in patients with hemochromatosis, alcoholic liver disease, or hepatitis C. Hypogonadism in males and females is also common in hemochromatosis and alcoholic liver disease, primarily because of the direct gonadal toxicities of iron and alcohol, respectively. In addition, androgenic steroids may bypass metabolism in the liver and subsequently undergo conversion in adipose tissue to the estrogenic steroid estrone. Increased plasma estrogen levels may lead to gynecomastia, telangiectasia, and palmar erythema.

Pulmonary Manifestations

End-stage liver disease is often accompanied by pulmonary disorders. Chronic hyperventilation is probably caused by the same central nervous system alterations responsible for hepatic encephalopathy. Patients may have hypoxemia because of mismatches of ventilation and perfusion induced by ascites, which restrict the ventilation of dependent lung spaces. The hepatopulmonary syndrome, a distinct form of right-to-left shunting with impaired gas exchange caused by intrapulmonary vascular dilation, is increasingly recognized. This condition is potentially reversible by transplantation. Portopulmonary hypertension, in contrast, is caused by pulmonary vasoconstriction, which produces markedly elevated pulmonary pressure and is a contraindication to liver transplantation. Patients with or without ascites may develop a transudative pleural effusion, termed *hepatic hydrothorax*, which may impair respiratory function. Hydrothorax probably develops from ascites traversing pores in the diaphragm. The onset of hepatic hydrothorax often signals rapid clinical deterioration.

Renal Manifestations

Numerous disturbances of sodium and water homeostasis are observed in cirrhosis, but the most devastating complication is renal failure caused by the hepatorenal syndrome. In its most severe form, hepatorenal syndrome type I progresses to oliguric renal failure and prerenal physiology despite adequate filling pressure. It is associated with extreme intrarenal vasoconstriction that leads to sodium retention. Potential precipitants include intravascular volume depletion from hemorrhage, diuretics, or paracentesis. Alternative causes of renal failure include acute tubular necrosis caused by hypovolemia, nephrotoxic drugs, nonsteroidal antiinflammatory agents, and radiocontrast agents. These disorders can often be distinguished from hepatorenal syndrome on the basis of a normal or elevated urine sodium concentration. Pulmonary artery catheter placement or central venous pressure monitoring should be considered because they facilitate optimal management of volume status. Hepatorenal syndrome type 1 usually is irreversible without transplantation. A milder form, hepatorenal syndrome type 2, affects many cirrhotics and is characterized by a mildly depressed glomerular filtration rate and marked sodium and water retention refractory to diuretics.

FINDINGS ON DIAGNOSTIC TESTING

Laboratory Studies

Liver chemistry values are obtained in essentially all patients with suspected liver disease or portal hypertension, but the patterns and degrees of abnormality are variable and are determined by the primary disorder. Notably, patients with pathological evidence of cirrhosis may have normal biochemical profiles. Coagulation profiles, complete blood counts, electrolytes, and albumin should all be obtained. Patients with advanced cirrhosis will have a prolonged prothrombin time and a decrease in serum albumin levels because of impaired hepatic synthetic function. Protein malnutrition and vitamin K deficiency, which are particularly common in alcoholics, may also produce these abnormalities. Patients with portal hypertension may have thrombocytopenia, anemia, or leukopenia on the basis of congestive hypersplenism. Thrombocytopenia from splenic sequestration rarely is less than 50,000 per μl; lower levels suggest an alternative diagnosis, such as drug-induced, immune-mediated, or disseminated intravascular coagulation–associated thrombocytopenia. In addition to splenic sequestration, anemia may result from gastrointestinal hemorrhage, nutritional deficiencies (e.g., folate, iron, or vitamin B_{12}), or hemolysis. Hyponatremia, hypokalemia, and renal insufficiency are common complications of the altered renal hemodynamics and sodium and water homeostasis observed in cirrhosis.

An accurate determination of the cause of cirrhosis requires a serologic evaluation, whose extent is largely dictated by the clinical setting. The initial screen should include serum assays for antibody to hepatitis C, antibodies to hepatitis B core antigen and surface antigen, hepatitis B surface antigen, antimitochondrial antibodies, antinuclear antibodies, anti–smooth muscle antibodies, ferritin, transferrin, total iron-binding capacity, and serum protein electrophoresis to measure the α_1 band and gamma globulins. Patients younger than age 50 should be screened for Wilson disease with an assay of serum ceruloplasmin. In the second stage, selected patients may require specialized studies based on the preliminary results above, for example, hepatitis C viral RNA, hepatitis B DNA and e antigen (eAg), α_1-antitrypsin phenotype, or anti–liver and kidney microsomal antibodies.

Structural Studies

Imaging procedures are often helpful in providing evidence of cirrhosis or portal hypertension. Upper gastrointestinal endoscopy permits detecting varices or portal hypertensive gastropathy but does not allow differentiating cirrhosis from other causes of portal hypertension. Ultrasound, computed tomographic (CT), and magnetic resonance imaging (MRI) studies may demonstrate lobular, heterogeneous, hepatic parenchyma or findings attributable to portal hypertension, including ascites, splenomegaly, and portosystemic collaterals. Standard ultrasound and CT scanning are insensitive methods for detecting varices, but Doppler ultrasound may demonstrate portal vein thrombosis or hepatofugal flow. ^{99m}Tc–sulfur colloid scintigraphy is a noninvasive means of assessing liver size and blood flow. A heterogeneous pattern of uptake in the liver and increased uptake in the spleen and bone marrow, which is termed a *colloid shift*, is caused by portal hypertension. Magnetic resonance angiography may help exclude primary vascular causes of portal hypertension, including the hepatic vein thrombosis of Budd-Chiari syndrome and portal vein thrombosis. Patients with suspected secondary biliary cirrhosis caused by primary sclerosing cholangitis should undergo endoscopic retrograde cholangiopancreatography.

Liver Biopsy

Liver biopsy is the only definitive means of diagnosing cirrhosis and often provides clues to the underlying cause. Liver biopsy also can be used to quantify iron and copper if hemochromatosis or Wilson disease is in the differential diagnosis. In coagulopathy, the risk of biopsy-associated hemorrhage often outweighs the benefit of obtaining information from the biopsy specimen. A transjugular biopsy may be performed if histological confirmation is deemed critical. This technique can also provide an estimate of portal pressures.

Portal Venous Pressure Measurement

Although not usually needed in clinical practice, direct and indirect measurements of portal pressure are the definitive means of diagnosing portal hypertension. The more commonly used indirect method involves angiographic positioning of a balloon occlusion catheter in the hepatic vein and, with the balloon inflated, measuring the hepatic vein wedge pressure. Analogous to pulmonary capillary wedge pressure, the hepatic vein wedge pressure measures sinusoidal pressure and is an estimate of portal pressure. It is inaccurate if the causes of portal hypertension are presinusoidal or prehepatic because the major pressure gradient is upstream from the sinusoids. The difference between hepatic vein wedge pressure and free hepatic vein (or right atrial) pressure provides an estimate of the portosystemic gradient, or the pressure drop across the resistance bed of the liver. A portosystemic gradient higher than 5 mm Hg is consistent with portal hypertension, whereas a gradient higher than 12 mm Hg identifies patients at risk for variceal hemorrhage. The pressure in the portal circulation is measured directly by a pressure transducer placed in the portal vein. This can be done through the parenchyma from the hepatic vein, similar to TIPS or transhepatic placement. The risk of bleeding from the transhepatic approach prohibits the routine use of this procedure.

MANAGEMENT AND COURSE

Management of Ascites

The approach to patients with ascites is detailed in Chapter 18.

Management of Variceal Hemorrhage

Any form of portal hypertension can lead to the formation of portosystemic collaterals. The major sites of collateral formation are through the umbilical vein, producing abdominal wall collaterals (the caput medusae); through the superior rectal vein to the middle and inferior rectal vein, producing rectal varices; and through the coronary and left gastric veins to the azygos vein, producing gastroesophageal varices. Collaterals may form in numerous other sites within the abdomen, but hemorrhage from gastroesophageal varices is the primary cause of morbidity from portosystemic collaterals.

The formation of varices is closely related to portal pressure. Varices are not encountered below a threshold portosystemic gradient of 12 mm Hg, but for unclear reasons, many patients with pressures above this level never develop significant varices. Bleeding occurs in 30% of patients with varices, but variables for identifying patients at high risk are less than perfect. Absolute portal pressures above the threshold of 12 mm Hg do not correlate well with the risk of bleeding, but the endoscopic size of varices does seem to indicate the patients at highest risk. Variceal hemorrhage is historically associated with a 50% mortality rate, and without subsequent preventive treatment, the risk of rebleeding is nearly 70%. These high morbidity and rebleeding rates have led to several interventions for treating acute bleeding as well as preventing initial or recurrent variceal hemorrhage.

Primary prevention of acute variceal hemorrhage includes nonselective β-adrenergic antagonists (e.g., propranolol and nadolol). Beta blocker therapy in multiple studies reduced the rate of first bleeds as well as rebleeding. Propranolol should be initiated at 10 to 20 mg, twice daily, and titrated to a 25% decrease in resting heart rate. Contraindications include bradycardia, hypotension, congestive heart failure, reactive airway disease, and peripheral vascular disease. For large varices, endoscopic band ligation reduces the rate of initial variceal bleeding, though this approach remains somewhat controversial because of potential complications. Thus, β-adrenergic antagonists are the most widely recommended therapy for the primary prevention of variceal bleeding.

Acute variceal hemorrhage from esophageal or gastric varices is a medical emergency. Patients should be managed in intensive care; volume resuscitation and optimizing the hemodynamic status are the first priorities. Nonvariceal hemorrhage may account for up to 50% of gastrointestinal bleeding in patients with known cirrhosis. Therefore, early upper gastrointestinal endoscopy is needed to confirm the source of bleeding. Endoscopic band ligation has replaced sclerotherapy as the first-line treatment for both acute and chronic gastroesophageal varices. Band ligation has superior efficacy with fewer side effects. Injection sclerotherapy of varices is occasionally used for acute variceal bleeding that is difficult to control, particularly if extensive bleeding impairs visualization and makes banding difficult. Complications of sclerotherapy include esophageal ulceration, pneumonia, and bacteremia. Combination therapy with banding and sclerotherapy does not have higher rates of efficacy than either technique alone and has more complications. Thus, combination treatment should not be used routinely.

Continuous infusion of the somatostatin analog octreotide ($25-50$ μg/h for 24 to 48 hours) reduces splanchnic blood flow by inhibiting the vasodilating hormones (e.g., glucagon) and lowers portal pressure. It does not cause systemic vasoconstriction and thus is safer than vasopressin. If portal hypertensive bleeding is suspected, therapy should be started immediately and continued for 72 hours. In some studies, octreotide was as effective as endoscopic therapy in controlling acute hemorrhage, but most centers use octreotide and endoscopic therapy together. Continuous infusion of vasopressin (0.1 to 0.4 U/min) may also control acute hemorrhage, but 50% of patients fail to respond, and side effects of systemic vasoconstriction, including myocardial and cerebral ischemia, are common. Vasopressin therapy should be limited to less than 24 to 48 hours. Coadministration of nitrates may reduce systemic vasoconstriction and lead to improved control of hemorrhage.

If bleeding persists despite the above measures, balloon tamponade is sometimes but rarely required. Balloon tamponade is 90% effective in stopping variceal hemorrhage, but it is only a temporizing measure, usually while awaiting TIPS. Adverse effects are common and include esophageal rupture and aspiration. Tamponade should never be continued for longer than 24 to 36 hours and should be limited to inflating the gastric balloon whenever possible. Endotracheal intubation should be performed before balloon insertion to prevent airway compromise.

In refractory or recurrent variceal hemorrhage, portosystemic shunting should be considered by using TIPS or a surgically created shunt. Although both procedures are highly effective in controlling hemorrhage, encephalopathy results in 10% to 20% of patients. The lower morbidity and less invasive nature of TIPS make it the logical choice in this setting.

After acute variceal bleeding has been stopped, secondary prophylactic interventions lower the risk of rebleeding. The preferred therapy is endoscopic band ligation. Complete obliteration of varices is the goal, and several sessions separated by 1 to 2 weeks are often required. Once the varices are obliterated, endoscopic surveillance to detect recurrence is usual, annually or biannually. Pharmacotherapy with the nonselective β-adrenergic antagonists, propranolol or nadolol, also reduces the rate of rebleeding but does not improve survival. Combination therapy with long-acting nitrates may be as effective as endoscopic therapy. Many clinicians use propranolol as an adjuvant means of preventing rebleeding.

Although portosystemic shunt surgery reduces the rate of rebleeding, it has largely been abandoned for secondary prophylaxis because of the high incidence of encephalopathy and the lack of any survival advantage over less invasive therapies. Patients with normal or nearly normal hepatic function may be better served by portal decompression. Due to the long life expectancy of these patients, TIPS may be less desirable than selective shunts like the distal splenorenal (Warren) shunt for those with a well-preserved synthetic function (Child Class A) because of the risk for stenosis of the angiographically placed shunt.

TIPS has added a new dimension to therapies for secondary prophylaxis of variceal bleeding. Although TIPS clearly has a role in patients with hemorrhage refractory to endoscopic therapy, its role in secondary prophylaxis remains to be established. Reports suggest that TIPS improves rebleeding rates compared with endoscopic therapy, but high rates of encephalopathy have generally limited the applicability of TIPS to failure of endoscopic therapy with rebleeding.

Management of Hepatic Encephalopathy

The mechanism for developing encephalopathy in severe liver disease remains ill defined. Possible explanations include decreased clearance of gut-derived neurotoxins, including ammonia; disturbances of central neurotransmission resulting from an accumulation of false neurotransmitters that activate γ-aminobutyric acid receptors or catecholamines; and accumulation of glutamate in astrocytes. None of these explanations is satisfactory. Although serum ammonia is often elevated in hepatic encephalopathy, some patients have normal ammonia levels.

Hepatic encephalopathy is often graded according to the patient's level of consciousness, using the West Haven criteria. Grade I is defined as subtle cognitive deficits with a normal level of arousal or inversion of the sleep–wake cycle. In grade II, asterixis appears, speech is slow, and lethargy is present. Grade III is characterized by an obtunded but arousable patient, and grade IV is represented by a comatose, unarousable patient. Other indexes exist, including the Glasgow coma scale for patients in Stage III to IV and the portosystemic encephalopathy (PSE) index. Minimal hepatic encephalopathy, previously called subclinical, can be measured by Reitan trail testing, other neuropsychiatric testing, electroencephalography, or evoked potentials. Imaging of the brain has little diagnostic yield but may be more important to exclude other causes, such as intracranial hemorrhage in an alcoholic patient with coagulopathy.

New-onset hepatic encephalopathy or acute decompensation of chronic hepatic encephalopathy should always prompt a search for precipitating causes. Common causes include gastrointestinal hemorrhage, psychotropic medications (in particular benzodiazepines), electrolyte and fluid disturbances, infection, new-onset renal insufficiency, constipation, and medical or dietary noncompliance. In addition to providing specific therapy for hepatic encephalopathy, the clinician should always attempt to correct the precipitating factors.

Because many of the responsible neurotoxins appear to be produced by intestinal flora, therapy is directed at altering the colonic microenvironment. Lactulose, titrated to produce two to three soft stools per day, is the first-line therapy. It promotes catharsis and lowers intralumenal pH to decrease ammonia absorption. It can cause flatulence and bloating; higher doses cause diarrhea, with possible fluid and electrolyte disturbances. The antibiotics metronidazole or neomycin decrease urease-producing gut bacteria and may be added to treat refractory hepatic encephalopathy but generally are second-line agents because of side effects, including nephrotoxicity with neomycin and neuropathy with metronidazole. Newer antibiotics are being studied, including rifamaxin, but data are limited. Other agents

TABLE 66-3
Child-Turcotte-Pugh Classification System

PROTHROMBIN TIME	BILIRUBIN	ALBUMIN	ASCITES	ENCEPHALOPATHY	SCORE
0 – 4 seconds above control	0 – 2.0 mg/dL	>3.5 mg/dL	Absent	Absent	1
4 – 6 seconds above control	2.0 – 3.0 mg/dL	2.8 – 3.5 mg/dL	Nontense	Grade I–II	2
>6 seconds above control	>3.0 mg/dL	0 – 2.8 mg/dL	Tense	Grade III–IV	3

Class A = 5 – 6 points; class B = 7 – 9 points; class C = 10 – 15 points.

being studied include benzoate, L-ornithine-L-aspartate, branched-chain amino acids, levodopa, and bromocriptine.

Protein restriction to 1 to 1.5 g/kg per day mostly as vegetables and dairy should be instituted, and any vitamin and mineral deficiencies, particularly zinc, should be supplemented. Given the high incidence of protein malnutrition in cirrhotics, care needs to be used and protein restriction should not be too severe unless portosystemic encephalopathy is difficult to manage.

Orthotopic Liver Transplantation

The decision to perform orthotopic liver transplantation depends mostly on the expected survival of the patient with end-stage liver disease. Several prognostic indicators have been developed, including the Child-Turcotte-Pugh classification (Table 66-3) and the Model for End-Stage Liver Disease (MELD). The 3-year survival rate for patients with Child-Turcotte-Pugh class C disease is 30%, whereas the corresponding survival rate for patients in Child-Turcotte-Pugh class A may exceed 90%. Three-year survival rates for class B patients are intermediate and average 50% to 60%. Because orthotopic liver transplantation has a 1-year mortality rate of 10% to 20%, patients at Child-Turcotte-Pugh stage A are better served with medical therapy. Conversely, the posttransplant 3-year survival rate is higher than 70% to 80% in several centers. Patients in Child-Turcotte-Pugh class B or C clearly benefit from transplantation. The benefit of orthotopic liver transplantation for any person must be weighed against specific clinical indications such as spontaneous bacterial peritonitis, intractable ascites, refractory encephalopathy, recurrent variceal bleeding, or debilitating fatigue. MELD is a mathematical model based on log-transformed serum bilirubin, serum creatinine, and the international normalized ratio (INR) for prothrombin time. It predicts 3-month mortality more accurately than a Child-Turcotte-Pugh score and is now used to prioritize candidates for transplantation.

Pretransplant evaluation should include an assessment for contraindications and an evaluation of factors that may complicate the posttransplant period. Absolute contraindications include active ethanol or substance abuse, extrahepatic or metastatic malignancy, untreated sepsis, and severe cardiopulmonary disease. Relative contraindications include human immunodeficiency virus infection, previous malignancy, and poor social support. Chronologic age is not a contraindication, but patients significantly older than 70 are acceptable candidates for orthotopic liver transplantation only if there are no other comorbidities. The evaluation usually includes ultrasound with Doppler examination, cardiac stress testing, contrast-enhanced (bubble) echocardiography, serologic testing for herpes viruses (e.g., cytomegalovirus, herpes simplex virus, and varicella-zoster virus), serum α-fetoprotein, and tuberculosis skin testing. Women require a Papanicolaou smear. Women older than 40 years should undergo mammography, and all patients older than 50 should have screening colonoscopies. Investigation of a patient's social support system is critical and requires the input of a trained social worker. Psychiatric consultation should be sought for all patients with prior substance or alcohol abuse. Dental evaluation may be necessary in select patients. The complex decision to approve a patient for orthotopic liver transplantation requires the input of several disciplines. This multidisciplinary approach should consider the medical and social implications of transplantation as well as the limited availability of donor organs and the long pretransplant waiting period.

CHAPTER 67

Primary Hepatic Neoplasms

HEPATOCELLULAR CARCINOMA

Incidence and Epidemiology

Hepatocellular carcinoma is the third most common cause of death from cancer worldwide with an estimated 560,000 new cases per year. There is tremendous regional variation in the incidence of hepatocellular carcinoma. Extremely high rates occur in Sub-Saharan Africa, Eastern Asia, Japan, and Korea. Intermediate rates are observed in Singapore, Native Americans, and portions of South America. Hepatocellular carcinoma is uncommon in the United States; the incidence is one tenth the rate of many countries in Southeast Asia. Nonetheless, hepatocellular carcinoma is increasing in the United States and is a major source of morbidity and mortality. Higher rates are seen African Americans and other minority groups. The variation in the incidence of hepatocellular carcinoma is closely related to regional variations in the prevalence of chronic hepatitis B and C infections and circulating hepatitis B surface antigen. All forms of cirrhosis are associated with an increased risk of hepatocellular carcinoma, but the risk is particularly high in patients with cirrhosis secondary to chronic viral infection. Hepatocellular carcinoma can complicate chronic viral hepatitis B infection prior to the development of cirrhosis. Hemochromatosis is associated with a high rate of hepatocellular carcinoma in cirrhotic patients. Of the 90% of patients with hepatocellular carcinoma who have coexistent cirrhosis, there is consistently a male predominance, and in the United States, the male-to-female ratio is higher than 2:1.

Other environmental exposures associated with hepatocellular carcinoma include aflatoxin B1, a toxic metabolite of an *Aspergillus* species that often contaminates grains and nuts and has been demographically linked to hepatocellular carcinoma. At least a portion of the geographic variation in hepatocellular carcinoma rates may be related to differences in levels of aflatoxin B1 in food. Long-term exposure to vinyl chloride or androgenic steroids has also been associated with an increased incidence of hepatocellular carcinoma. The epidemiologic association with anabolic steroids may partially explain the male-to-female ratio in hepatocellular carcinoma.

Etiology and Pathogenesis

Although the precise molecular mechanisms of hepatocellular carcinogenesis are not fully understood, hepatocellular carcinoma probably results from activation of protooncogenes, deactivation of tumor suppressor genes (e.g., *p53* and *pRb*), changes in growth factors or growth factor signaling processes (e.g., insulin-like growth factor [IGF] or transforming growth factors [TGF]), changes in telomeric length and activity, or microsatellite instability. Genetic injury may result from a variety of sources. Perhaps the best described is random integration of the hepatitis B virus (HBV) genome into the host genome, as well as transactivating features of the hepatitis B x protein that can activate protooncogenes such as c-*myc* and c-*fos*. Although hepatitis C virus (HCV) is an RNA virus and does not have the same direct mutagenic capacity as HBV, any chronic inflammatory state can generate free radicals capable of inducing genetic injury. In addition, the HCV core protein appears to be a cell signaling activator. Similarly, the regenerative response in cirrhosis may lead to chromosomal rearrangements that foster unrestrained proliferation. Multiple genetic abnormalities have been identified in hepatocellular carcinoma and in dysplastic nodules. However, it is likely that the process is multifactorial and further genetic studies are needed. For reasons that remain poorly defined, some forms of cirrhosis, such as hemochromatosis and tyrosinemia, have exceptionally high incidences of hepatocellular carcinoma, whereas other diseases, such as Wilson disease and autoimmune hepatitis, have exceptionally low incidences of hepatocellular carcinoma. Further characterization of the cellular and genetic events that lead to hepatocellular carcinoma may clarify these discrepancies.

Clinical Features

Ninety percent of patients with hepatocellular carcinoma have superimposed cirrhosis. The clinical presentations of hepatocellular carcinoma may be subtle; many of the presenting signs and symptoms are often mistakenly attributed to coexisting cirrhosis. Nonspecific symptoms of fatigue, anorexia, weight loss, and jaundice are common. Patients may complain of right upper quadrant pain or increasing abdominal girth. Hepatocellular carcinoma may cause well-compensated cirrhosis to become decompensated, with progressive ascites, encephalopathy, jaundice, or hemorrhage. Invasion of the portal and, less commonly, hepatic veins can greatly worsen portal hypertension that leads to refractory ascites or variceal bleeding. Hepatocellular carcinoma should be suspected in all new cases of portal vein thrombosis. Occasionally, patients with poorly differentiated tumors present with protracted fever and, rarely, with a paraneoplastic syndrome or metastatic disease, usually bony pain or dyspnea from pulmonary tumor emboli or malignant pleural effusion. On physical examination, most patients exhibit hepatomegaly or a discrete mass. Rarely, patients with hepatocellular carcinoma present with an acute abdomen resulting from tumor rupture and hemoperitoneum, which is catastrophic but can be treated with arterial embolization, or hemobilia and jaundice from invasion of the bile ducts. In general, abdominal pain in patients with hepatocellular carcinoma is a poor prognostic sign.

Findings on Diagnostic Testing

Laboratory Studies

Patients presenting with hepatocellular carcinoma as their first manifestation of chronic liver disease should have a complete serologic evaluation to determine the cause of cirrhosis. Aminotransferase levels are often mildly elevated but they can be normal; levels are determined by the underlying liver disease. Alkaline phosphatase levels may be particularly elevated if the tumor assumes an infiltrative pattern. In advanced tumors, serum bilirubin levels may be markedly elevated owing to compromised hepatocellular reserve or, less commonly, extrahepatic bile duct obstruction. Other laboratory abnormalities observed in hepatocellular carcinoma include rare instances of paraneoplastic hypercalcemia and erythrocytosis. Large tumors have been associated with hypoglycemia of uncertain cause.

Tumor Markers

Hepatocellular carcinoma is associated with several serum tumor markers. The marker most often used is serum α-fetoprotein (AFP), the glycosylated protein expressed in proliferating fetal hepatocytes. After the first year of life, AFP levels decrease to less than 10 ng/mL, but several chronic inflammatory states, including viral hepatitis, are associated with AFP elevations to 10 to 100 ng/mL. Although chronic hepatitis in cirrhosis may be associated with levels in the hundreds, levels higher than 400 ng/mL are caused usually by hepatocellular carcinoma. An AFP level higher than 1000 ng/mL associated with a liver mass is diagnostic of hepatocellular carcinoma. Unfortunately, AFP is elevated in only 60% to 70% of patients with hepatocellular carcinoma and may be only mildly elevated only in small tumors, which compromises the measurements of sensitivity of AFP as a screening test for early hepatocellular carcinoma. Other tumors (e.g., testicular, ovarian, gastric) and gallbladder carcinoma are also associated with increased serum levels of AFP. Carcinoembryonic antigen is rarely elevated; marked elevations in the setting of a liver mass suggest metastatic adenocarcinoma.

Structural Studies

Several imaging methods can be used to identify and stage hepatocellular carcinoma. The challenge is to distinguish a small tumor from the regenerative changes associated with cirrhosis. Ultrasound is sensitive for detecting small hepatocellular carcinomas (<2 cm). The hyperechoic pattern in these small tumors differentiates them from hypoechoic metastatic lesions. Ultrasound may be less reliable in distinguishing a small hepatocellular carcinoma from a benign hemangioma, which is also typically hyperechoic. Larger hepatocellular carcinomas are often hypoechoic and may be difficult to differentiate from metastatic lesions, but coexisting cirrhosis or elevated levels of AFP may provide additional diagnostic evidence. A computed tomographic (CT) scan is 80% to 90% sensitive for detecting hepatocellular carcinoma. A spiral CT scan obtains arterial and venous phase contrast images with a single dose of contrast agent. Hepatocellular carcinoma typically is a vascular tumor with marked arterial phase enhancement; the rapid washout of contrast agent leads to the appearance of a hypodense lesion during the venous phase. A hemangioma can be distinguished by a characteristic peripheral-to-central filling pattern and prolonged contrast enhancement. Ultrasound and CT scans demonstrate various patterns of hepatocellular carcinoma growth and extension. One third of hepatocellular carcinomas are infiltrating, with poorly defined borders. Another one third are expanding tumors that are well defined and encapsulated. A small percentage of them manifest as multicentric, space-occupying lesions or large pedunculated masses extending from the liver surface. CT scans are especially useful in defining the tumor capsule and invasion of the portal vein. The accuracy of magnetic resonance imaging (MRI) is similar to that of three-phase spiral CT scanning and avoids the potential adverse effects of intravenous contrast agents. MRI is the procedure of choice for differentiating hemangioma from hepatocellular carcinoma and may be more sensitive for identifying small hypervascular lesions.

A focal area of increased uptake of ^{99m}Tc-sulfur colloid on liver-spleen scanning is virtually diagnostic of the benign lesion, focal nodular hyperplasia, but an unenhanced, or "cold mass," does not differentiate hepatocellular carcinoma from metastatic disease or hepatic adenoma. However, given the ability to diagnose hepatocellular carcinoma reliably without biopsy by using AFP levels and CT or MRI, this test is rarely used. Angiography is used primarily to define the vascular anatomy in patients being considered for resection or for chemoembolization. If there is a high index of suspicion of hepatocellular carcinoma and all other imaging tests fail to localize a mass, CT scans after lipiodol injection may be useful. Lipiodol is an iodinated preparation of poppy seed oil that hepatocellular carcinoma cells preferentially concentrate and retain. Intraarterial injection of lipiodol is followed 2 weeks later by CT scanning. Lipiodol injection can carry some risk of hepatic dysfunction, particularly in patients with portal vein thrombosis. Hepatocellular carcinoma appears as a focal area of enhancement. The most sensitive means of detecting hepatocellular carcinoma is intraoperative ultrasound and laparoscopic biopsy. Given the invasiveness of these last two procedures, repeat CT or MRI scanning after an interval of 2 to 3 months is an alternative means of identifying hepatocellular carcinoma in patients in whom hepatocellular carcinoma is suspected but not detected by initial noninvasive imaging. Screening of patients with cirrhosis and vertical transmission of HBV without cirrhosis by ultrasound and measuring AFP levels every 6 months is recommended, combined with CT or MRI for any unclear lesions or unexplained elevation in AFP.

Histological Studies

When a patient with cirrhosis develops a new hypervascular liver mass associated with elevated serum AFP levels, a biopsy to confirm hepatocellular carcinoma is usually not necessary. The risk of bleeding induced by ultrasound-guided or CT-guided core biopsy of a hepatocellular carcinoma is significant, and there is a small (3% to 5%) risk of needle track spread. Small-gauge needle aspiration often fails to diagnose hepatocellular carcinoma, which often requires architectural features for diagnosis. Histological examination usually reveals cords of undifferentiated hepatocytes, but some tumors are well differentiated and may be difficult to differentiate from a benign hepatic adenoma, particularly on cytology.

Management and Course

Surgical Therapy

The only option for long-term survival from hepatocellular carcinoma is complete surgical excision of the tumor (Fig. 67-1). Unfortunately, resection is limited to unilateral disease in Child A cirrhotic patients; thus, resectability rates range from 5% to 20%. In determining the suitability of a patient for resection, the stage of the tumor and postresection residual hepatic function need to be considered. Any patient with jaundice or significant portal hypertension (wedged hepatic vein pressure gradient >10 mm Hg or varices) will not tolerate further loss of hepatic function. Similarly, any patient with distant metastasis or diffuse hepatic involvement will not benefit from surgery. After successful resection, measurement of serum AFP levels is useful for detecting disease recurrence. The 5-year recurrence rate for patients with resectable tumors is 50% among survivors due to de novo hepatocellular carcinoma or growth of unrecognized intrahepatic metastases. Orthotopic liver transplantation (OLT) for patients with hepatocellular carcinoma offers significant advantages over partial hepatectomy. It can be used for patients with advanced liver disease, and it removes the existing cancer and the diseased liver with its underlying neoplastic potential. Numerous studies have shown that results with liver transplantation are superb in patients with single lesions smaller than 5 cm or up to 3 lesions, each 3 cm or smaller (Stage I–II disease). Patients who meet these "Milan" criteria are now given additional priority for OLT. Other studies have suggested that larger tumors can also be transplanted; such as the University of California, San Francisco (UCSF) criteria that extend to 8 cm hepatocellular carcinoma, suggesting that the current algorithm may be too restrictive. Despite the additional priority given to hepatocellular carcinoma, with the potential for tumor growth and spread while on the waiting list, many centers treat the lesions prior to OLT with ablation and/or chemoembolization therapies (see below). None of these therapies

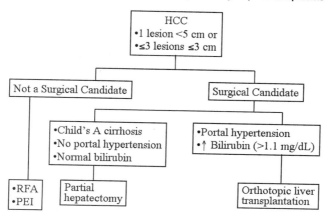

FIGURE 67-1. Management algorithm for curing hepatocellular carcinoma.

has been subjected to randomized controlled trials in combination with OLT and, therefore, the optimal approach remains to be defined. Living donor liver transplantation has also been used to shorten waiting time and may be an optimal use of the reduced-sized graft because of the usually reasonably preserved hepatic function in patients with hepatocellular carcinoma. The impact of regeneration on the risk of hepatocellular carcinoma recurrence after living donor liver transplantation remains controversial.

Locoregional forms of treatment are reasonable for patients who are not candidates for surgical approaches. These options include percutaneous alcohol injection, radiofrequency ablation, and transcatheter arterial chemoembolization.

Percutaneous Alcohol Injection

Percutaneous alcohol injection (PEI) has become a widely accepted form of therapy for small, localized hepatocellular carcinomas. The advantage of PEI over other local ablative minimally invasive therapies is the relatively simple technique and low cost. PEI can be safely performed on patients who are not candidates for resection or OLT, even in the presence of advanced cirrhosis. Hepatocellular carcinomas less than 3 cm in size and fewer than three nodules are suitable for PEI. It is likely that absolute alcohol kills cells by a combination of cellular dehydration, coagulative necrosis, and vascular thrombosis.

PEI has a complication rate of 1.7% and a mortality rate of 0.1%. Patients may experience abdominal pain and low-grade fever. Contraindications to PEI include massive ascites, coagulopathy, and obstructive jaundice. The survival rates of PEI in most studies are equivalent to surgical resection and relate to the severity of the underlying liver disease.

Radiofrequency Ablation

Radiofrequency ablation (RFA) uses thermal energy generated by an alternating electric current generator in the radiofrequency range (200 to 1200 kHz) to create focal coagulative necrosis. RFA is usually performed by a percutaneous approach but can be done laparoscopically or during open surgery for difficult to reach lesions. Ultrasound guidance is used to place the probe in the outpatient department. Lesions 5 cm or larger can be treated, but lesions near large blood vessels are poorly treated because blood acts as a heat sink. Spiral contrast-enhanced CT scanning is usually used to assess tumor necrosis after RFA because lesions rarely shrink and the degree of enhancement with contrast provides an estimate of viable tumor.

The results of RFA appear comparable to other ablative techniques though there is increased concern about needle track seeding because of the larger caliber probe used in RFA.

Transcatheter Arterial Chemoembolization

Transcatheter arterial chemoembolization (TACE) uses angiographic emboliza-tion of the arterial supply with lipiodol, gel foam, or microspheres, in combina-tion with local delivery of high levels of chemotherapeutic agents (e.g., doxoru-bicin, mitomycin C, cisplatin) to create ischemic and cytotoxic damage to the hepatocellular carcinoma. The technique spares healthy liver because it receives only 20% to 30% of its blood flow from the hepatic artery. In contrast, a he-patocellular carcinoma obtains 80% to 100% of its blood flow from the hepatic artery.

The risks of TACE include contrast allergy, renal insufficiency, increased liver function tests, and bleeding. Fever and right upper quadrant pain are common and many centers routinely use postprocedure antibiotics. Hepatic abscesses are rare, however, as is ischemic cholecystitis. Advanced cirrhosis with hyperbiliru-binemia (usually >3 to 5 mg/dL or INR >1.7) is a relative contraindication for TACE because of the risk of liver failure. Other contraindications include hepatic encephalopathy, biliary obstruction, portal vein occlusion, portosystemic shunt, a transjugular intrahepatic portosystemic shunt (TIPS) device, or creatinine higher than 1.8.

The efficacy of TACE is determined by the size of the lesion. Because TACE also avoids the risk of needle track seeding, transplant centers often use chemoem-bolization as a bridge to transplantation for patients with hepatocellular carcinoma. TACE prevents progression of the lesions and potential micrometastases while the patient waits for a donor organ. The role of chemoembolization as a palliative pro-cedure remains controversial; however, recent data suggest a survival advantage of TACE but not embolization without chemotherapy.

Cytotoxic Chemotherapy

Hepatocellular carcinoma is unfortunately refractory to most available cytotoxic therapies. Moreover, the presence of cirrhosis with impaired clearance of drugs me-tabolized by the liver increases drug toxicity. Leucopenia and thrombocytopenia from splenic sequestration can exacerbate bone marrow toxicity. The overall re-sponse rate is less than 20% for systemic chemotherapy. Intraarterial therapy with a pump has been tried but does not affect survival. Newer trials with a blockade of neoangiogenesis and other agents are awaited.

Hormonal and Other Therapy

The presence of androgen receptors in tumors and the male predominance of he-patocellular carcinoma have led to the use of antiandrogen therapy for this cancer. Similarly, estrogen receptors in the liver also led to using tamoxifen (an anti-estrogen) to treat this disease. Thalidomide with and without TACE is also being studied. Though current data have not supported a survival benefit from any of these therapies, the lower toxicity and lack of efficacy of systemic cytotoxic ther-apies have led to their use for patients with advanced or disseminated disease in some centers.

FIBROLAMELLAR HEPATOCELLULAR CARCINOMA

Fibrolamellar hepatocellular carcinoma is clinically and pathologically distinct from the hepatocellular carcinoma that complicates cirrhosis. Fibrolamellar hepatocellular carcinoma is not typically associated with cirrhosis. It often occurs in young adults and there is no sex predominance. Patients usually present with abdominal pain, weight loss, hepatomegaly, and an abdominal mass. Serum AFP levels are characteristically normal, and imaging procedures often demonstrate intralesional calcification or, rarely, a central scar. Prognosis is favorable relative to the more common variant of hepatocellular carcinoma. Fifty percent to 75% of patients have resectable tumors, and long-term survival is common. Transplantation should be considered in this group given the decreased propensity of fibrolamellar hepatocellular carcinoma to metastasize and the younger age of the patient population.

HEPATOBLASTOMA

Less than 1% of primary liver tumors, termed *hepatoblastomas*, derive from fetal hepatocytes. Most cases occur in young children, but adults may be affected. Patients present with abdominal pain, weight loss, and a palpable right upper quadrant mass. Unlike fibrolamellar tumors, serum AFP levels usually are elevated, but similar to fibrolamellar tumors, calcification is often evident on ultrasound or CT images. At presentation, a hepatoblastoma often is massive in size. Complete surgical excision is the optimal treatment, but chemotherapy may be beneficial for unresectable tumors. Long-term survival rates average 25%.

MESENCHYMAL TUMORS

Mesenchymal tumors account for less than 1% of primary malignant liver neoplasms. Angiosarcoma is associated with exposure to anabolic steroids, arsenic, and vinyl chloride. Other histological variants include rhabdomyosarcoma, leiomyosarcoma, and liposarcoma. Patients often present later in life with advanced disease and survival is limited.

BENIGN LIVER MASSES

Hepatic Adenomas

The incidence of benign hepatic adenomas has increased with the use of oral contraceptives. Isolated adenomas occur mainly in women who are of reproductive age. These lesions are usually found incidentally by abdominal imaging performed for other reasons. However, they can grow to large sizes before symptoms occur; most symptomatic patients present with abdominal pain or palpable abdominal masses. Intratumor hemorrhage and rupture are frequent complications, especially if the adenoma is associated with contraceptive use. Patients rarely present with hepatic adenomatosis, characterized by multiple adenomas throughout the liver. These patients frequently have glycogen storage disorders, and malignant degeneration is a well-described complication. Hepatic adenomas are at risk of malignant degeneration though this risk is small for isolated lesions. In addition, well-differentiated hepatocellular carcinoma may be difficult to distinguish from adenomas, and histological misclassification of hepatocellular carcinoma as adenoma may later be interpreted as malignant transformation. Adenomas typically appear as hypodense areas on CT scans and as "cold lesions" on ^{99m}Tc–sulfur colloid images. MRI will show the absence of a central scar seen in focal nodular hyperplasia. Discontinuing oral contraceptives may resolve the condition, but if the lesion persists or hepatocellular carcinoma is suspected, surgical excision is recommended.

Focal Nodular Hyperplasia

Focal nodular hyperplasia is a space-occupying lesion composed of all the normal cell populations usually found in the liver, including reticuloendothelial cells. The etiology is unknown. Lesions usually are detected incidentally during imaging procedures performed for unrelated symptoms. Twenty-five percent are multicentric and most are less than 5 cm in diameter. Diagnosis is often possible based on a classic appearance in imaging procedures. CT or MRI scans may demonstrate a central stellate scar that is often calcified. ^{99m}Tc–sulfur colloid imaging often but not invariably demonstrates a focal area of increased signal from the presence of reticuloendothelial cells. Characteristically photopenic adenomas, hepatocellular carcinomas, and metastatic tumors appear as "cold spots" on ^{99m}Tc–sulfur colloid images. Biopsy is often required to differentiate focal nodular hyperplasia from adenoma in women at risk of both lesions. Focal nodular hyperplasia is benign and no treatment is necessary.

Hemangioma

Cavernous hemangiomas are focal collections of dilated vascular channels and are the most common benign space-occupying lesions of the liver, with an estimated prevalence of 5% to 10%. Most are asymptomatic and are detected incidentally, but large hemangiomas can produce symptoms such as abdominal pain. The main clinical importance of this lesion lies in differentiating it from more serious disorders. Radiologic procedures play a primary role in diagnosing hemangioma. Hemangiomas are typically hyperechoic on ultrasound and retain contrast for prolonged periods on CT scanning. MRI is the most sensitive and specific means of diagnosing hemangioma. Percutaneous biopsy, which carries some risk of hemorrhage, is rarely required. Surgical excision is necessary only for large, symptomatic lesions.

CHAPTER 68

Gastrointestinal Complications of the Acquired Immunodeficiency Syndrome

EPIDEMIOLOGY AND ETIOLOGY

It was estimated that by the year 2002, 40 million people worldwide had been infected with human immunodeficiency virus type 1 (HIV-1), the causative agent of the acquired immunodeficiency syndrome (AIDS), and 20 million had died from complications of this disease. Although progress has been made in developing medications to prevent or treat the complications of AIDS, an effective vaccine is not available and therapy is expensive; thus, there will be a continued need for clinicians to care for patients with AIDS.

The most common gastrointestinal manifestations of AIDS are diarrhea and esophageal disease (dysphagia and odynophagia); however, patients may also present with hepatobiliary disorders, abdominal pain with or without pancreatitis, hemorrhage, and neoplasia.

ESOPHAGEAL DISORDERS

Etiology and Pathogenesis

Primary infection of the esophagus in immunocompetent people is rare, but it occurs in as many as 30% of patients with AIDS. The most common cause is infection with *Candida albicans*, which is characterized by superficial esophageal erosions and thick, white plaques of exudate that coat the esophageal mucosa. Other causes include herpes simplex virus (usually HSV type 1), cytomegalovirus (CMV), and idiopathic ulceration associated with AIDS. HSV generally produces multiple, small, discrete ulcerations that may coalesce to form deep linear ulcerations. CMV esophagitis generally presents with shallow ulcers but may also coalesce to form large ulcers with raised edges. CMV is typically a disseminated disease, and by the time esophagitis is diagnosed, patients often have CMV infection at other sites. Severely immunocompromised patients may develop large, deep ulcers, termed *idiopathic* or *aphthous ulcers*, that are not associated with a diagnosable pathogen. HIV itself has been isolated from these ulcers and may be the causative agent.

Mass lesions of the esophagus are uncommon in AIDS, but Kaposi sarcoma and lymphoma can metastasize to the esophagus and produce dysphagia. Dysphagia can also result from mediastinal adenopathy, inflammation-induced dysmotility, or a stricture complicating a large esophageal ulcer. It is important to differentiate oropharyngeal dysphagia from esophageal dysphagia. Patients with AIDS are susceptible to a number of central nervous system diseases that can manifest as choking or aspiration caused by an uncoordinated oropharyngeal phase of swallowing.

Clinical Features and Diagnosis

The most common presenting symptoms of esophageal disease associated with AIDS are dysphagia and odynophagia. Although the presence of oral candidiasis supports the diagnosis of esophageal candidiasis, the absence of thrush does not rule out this infection. Upper gastrointestinal endoscopy with brushing and biopsy of mucosal abnormalities is the standard for evaluating AIDS patients with symptoms referable to the esophagus. *Candida* esophagitis has a typical endoscopic appearance of thick, white plaques coating the esophagus that may coalesce to form pseudomembranes. Brush cytology and biopsy specimens will confirm the presence of fungal pseudohyphae. HSV may be identified by Cowdry type A intranuclear inclusions in infected squamous cells, but occasionally viral culture of the biopsy material is necessary to confirm HSV infection. CMV can be identified histopathologically based on the presence of multinucleated cells with characteristic intracytoplasmic inclusions or "owl's-eye" intranuclear inclusions. Idiopathic ulcers are large, excavating lesions that may have a cobblestone appearance by endoscopy. Biopsy specimens of idiopathic ulcers, by definition, lack identification of opportunistic organisms other than HIV and demonstrate intense inflammation with necrosis and granulation.

Management

Esophageal candidiasis accounts for approximately half of the esophageal infectious complications of AIDS, so it is acceptable to observe the response to empirical therapy before extensive diagnostic evaluation. Therapy with an oral imidazole, such as ketoconazole (200 to 400 mg/d), fluconazole (100 mg/d), or itraconazole (200 mg/d) may be initiated. Symptom response is expected in 80% of patients with *Candida* infection, and the duration of therapy should be 7 to 14 days. The side effects of these medications include nausea, hepatotoxicity, and adrenal insufficiency. Failure to achieve a complete response within 1 week should prompt evaluation by upper endoscopy. Nonresponders in whom *Candida* infection is confirmed may require higher doses or low-dose parenteral amphotericin B. Long-term prophylactic antifungal therapy usually is required once a patient responds.

HSV esophagitis responds to high-dose oral (400 mg, five times per day) or parenteral acyclovir. The side effects of this drug include rash and irritation of veins if administered parenterally. Valacyclovir (a prodrug of acyclovir) is administered three times per day (1 g orally) and may be equipotent to acyclovir. Rare drug resistance requires changing therapy to the viral DNA polymerase inhibitor foscarnet (90 mg/kg, twice daily, intravenous). As with other opportunistic infections, long-term secondary prophylaxis is needed to prevent relapses.

First-line therapy for CMV esophagitis consists of parenteral ganciclovir (5 mg/kg, twice daily). Clinical and endoscopic improvement is expected in 77% of patients after 2 to 4 weeks of therapy. The main side effect is myelosuppression, which is often compounded by the use of other components of highly active antiretroviral therapy (HAART). Low-dose maintenance therapy provided through a long-term central venous catheter is required to prevent relapses. Refractory esophagitis and infections caused by resistant strains of CMV can be treated with foscarnet. Foscarnet also requires parenteral access and is associated with renal insufficiency, congestive heart failure, electrolyte disturbances, and anemia. A newer systemic antiviral, cidofovir, has efficacy and can be administered weekly (5 mg/kg, intravenous).

AIDS-associated idiopathic esophageal ulcers may respond to intralesional or systemic corticosteroid treatment. Studies have shown that prednisone (40 mg/d, orally) administered for 4 weeks or more is effective in more than 90% of cases. Thalidomide (200 to 300 mg/d, orally) has also been effective in inducing symptomatic and endoscopic remission.

In rare cases, patients with refractory esophageal disease require parenteral nutrition. Volume deficits and electrolyte disorders should be corrected. A topical anesthetic agent (e.g., viscous lidocaine) may palliate odynophagia. Patients with CMV and idiopathic ulcers can develop esophageal strictures that require endoscopic dilation. Other more rare complications of AIDS-associated esophageal ulcers include hemorrhage or fistula formation. Patients with CMV esophagitis often have poor prognoses with median survival time of 6 to 8 months; patients with esophagitis caused by other agents have a longer median survival time.

DIARRHEA

Etiology and Pathogenesis

Diarrhea complicates the course of disease in more than one half of patients infected with HIV. Depending on the etiologic agent, the clinical presentation may vary widely. Patients with colorectal infections generally present with frequent, low-volume, watery stools, often accompanied by occult or frank blood. Systemic signs of fever and anorexia are common. In addition to opportunistic infections, patients infected with HIV have a higher incidence of infection with bacteria, such as *Salmonella* species, *Shigella flexneri*, and *Campylobacter jejuni*, which affect immunocompetent patients as well. These bacteria are more likely to produce bacteremia and prolonged or relapsing infections in patients with AIDS. In addition, because antibiotics are frequently needed to treat complications associated with AIDS, *Clostridium difficile* and antibiotics should be considered causes of AIDS-associated diarrhea.

Mycobacterium avium-intracellulare complex (MAC) is the most common cause of systemic bacterial infection among patients with AIDS in the United States. Patients often present with diarrhea, profound wasting, and fever. Abdominal adenopathy may be associated with abdominal pain. Infiltration of the small intestine with infected macrophages results in obstruction of lymphatic flow and malabsorption.

In addition to mycobacteria, other organisms responsible for small bowel–type diarrhea include protozoa. *Cryptosporidium* causes self-limited diarrhea in immunocompetent hosts; however, in patients with AIDS, *Cryptosporidium* infection is associated with severe chronic diarrhea and wasting. The organism usually affects the small intestine, producing histological findings similar to celiac sprue, but may also involve the biliary tract and colon. The two Microsporidia species, *Enterocytozoon bieneusi* and *Septata intestinalis*, are associated with a clinical syndrome indistinguishable from cryptosporidiosis and may be responsible for up to one third of AIDS-associated diarrhea. *Isospora belli* and *Cyclospora* are protozoans related to *Cryptosporidium* and have been associated with chronic diarrhea and malabsorption in AIDS, especially in undeveloped countries. *Entamoeba histolytica* and *Giardia lamblia* can also cause symptomatic disease among patients with AIDS.

Viral infection with CMV and HSV can present with colitis in AIDS patients. CMV can involve any portion of the gastrointestinal tract and is the most common cause of hematochezia in AIDS. The endoscopic appearance of CMV ranges from focal erythema to diffuse colitis with deep ulcerations. HSV may also produce diarrhea, but infection is generally limited to the rectum. Patients with HSV proctitis usually suffer from rectal pain and tenesmus, rather than diarrhea. Adenovirus can be isolated from inflamed colonic mucosa in AIDS patients; however, a causal relationship between infection and diarrhea has not been established.

Some patients with AIDS-associated diarrhea and wasting have extensive histological changes in the small intestine, including villous atrophy and focal crypt necrosis. However, an identifiable pathogen other than HIV cannot be identified. This syndrome has been termed *AIDS-associated enteropathy*, but as with other idiopathic gastrointestinal disorders in AIDS, the pathogenic role of HIV remains unclear.

Clinical Features and Diagnosis

The management of diarrhea in patients with AIDS is complicated by the fact that although a thorough evaluation including endoscopy and biopsy can identify pathogens in 44% to 85% of cases, many pathogens are unresponsive to currently available antimicrobial agents. In addition, 25% of patients are infected with more than one organism; therefore, identifying and treating a single pathogen may not yield a clinical response. Conversely, some infections are responsive to therapy, but because of toxicity from medications, a definitive diagnosis should be obtained before initiating therapy. In any diagnostic approach to diarrhea in patients with AIDS, the overall prognosis of the patient along with the potential risks and benefits of identifying the responsible pathogens should be considered.

After a thorough history and physical examination, including a detailed drug history, the initial noninvasive evaluation should include an examination of a stool sample for *Salmonella*, *Shigella*, and *Campylobacter* species and a stool assay for *C difficile* toxin. Examination for parasites requires processing three separate stool samples with a modified acid-fast stain (*Cryptosporidium*, *Isospora*, *Cyclospora*, MAC), a modified trichrome stain (Microsporidia), and a standard saline wet mount (*G lamblia*). When fever, weight loss, and other systemic symptoms suggest a diagnosis of MAC infection, blood should be cultured with a special transport medium (e.g., Du Pont isolator). Stool examination identifies an enteric pathogen in 48% to 55% of HIV-1 patients with diarrhea.

If no pathogen is identified or treatment of identified pathogens fails to result in clinical improvement, endoscopic evaluation and biopsy may be required to identify additional pathogens. Esophagogastroduodenoscopy (EGD) alone yields a diagnosis in 26% of AIDS patients with diarrhea and negative stool studies, compared to a 44% to 50% yield using EGD plus colonoscopy. Histopathological examination may demonstrate the viral inclusions of CMV or any of the pathogenic protozoa. Special stains identify Microsporidia. Biopsy specimens should be cultured for viruses and mycobacteria in addition to histological preparation with acid-fast stains to increase the yield for MAC and CMV. Electron microscopy is rarely necessary to identify Microsporidia.

Therapy

In addition to supportive therapy for symptoms and specific therapy targeting identified pathogens (Table 68-1), treatment of diarrhea in AIDS has been advanced by the development of HAART. HAART combines reverse transcriptase inhibitors

TABLE 68-1
Therapy for Intestinal Infections in HIV-1–Infected Adults

PATHOGEN	TREATMENT	ALTERNATIVE TREATMENT
Protozoal		
Cryptosporidium parvum	Paromomycin, 25 – 35 mg/kg in 3 or 4 doses	Paromomycin, 1 g bid + azithromycin
Microsporidium species	Albendazole, 400 mg bid × 4 wk (*Septata intestinalis*)	600 mg qd × 4 wk
	Fumagillin, 20 mg tid × 2 wk (*Enterocytozoon bieneusi*)	
*Isospora belli**	Trimethoprim-sulfamethoxazole, 1 DS[†] qid × 10 day	
	then bid × 3 wk	
Giardia lamblia	Metronidazole, 250 mg tid × 5 day	Tinidazole, 2 g single dose
		Furazolidone, 100 mg qid × 7 – 10 day
Cyclospora cayetanensis	Trimethoprim-sulfamethoxazole, 1 DS qid × 10 day	
Viral		
Cytomegalovirus*[†§]	Ganciclovir, 5 mg/kg IV q12h × 2 – 3 wk	Foscarnet, 60 mg/kg IV q8h or 90 mg IV
		q12h × 2 – 3 wk
Herpes simplex*[†§]	Acyclovir, 200 – 800 mg 5/d × 7 – 14 day	Foscarnet, 40 mg/kg IV q8h × 3 wk
Adenovirus	NA[∥]	
Rotavirus[#]	NA	
Astrovirus	NA	
Picobirnavirus	NA	
Bacterial		
Salmonella species*[§]	Ceftriaxone, 1 – 2 g qd × 7 day	Amoxicillin, 1g tid × 7 – 14 day
	Ciprofloxacin, 500 mg bid × 7 day	Trimethoprim-sulfamethoxazole, 1 DS
		bid × 10 – 14 day
		(Continued)

TABLE 68-1 (Continued)

Shigella flexneri[*][#]	Ciprofloxacin, 500 mg bid × 7 day	Trimethoprim-sulfamethoxazole, 1 DS bid × 10 – 14 day
Campylobacter jejuni[*][#]	Ampicillin, 500 mg qid × 5d Erythromycin, 500 mg qid × 7 day Ciprofloxacin, 500 mg bid × 7 day	Ceftriazone, 1 – 2 g qid × 7day Tetracycline, 500 mg qid × 7 day
Mycobacterium avium complex[*][§]	Clarithromycin, 500–1000 mg bid Rifabutin, 300 mg pd and ethambutol, 15 – 25 mg/kg qd	Azithromycin, 500 mg qd
Prophylaxis:	Clarithromycin, 500 mg qd or azithromycin, 500 mg qd	Rifabutin, 300 mg qd
Clostridium difficile	Metronidazole, 500 mg tid × 7 – 10 day	Vancomycin, 15 mg qid × 7 – 10 day
Bacteriosis[#]	Ciprofloxacin, 500 mg bid × 4 wk	
Fungal		
Histoplasma capsulatum suppression[*]	Amphotericin B, 0.5 – 1.0 mg/kg IV qd × 7 day then qod to total 10 – 15 mg/kg Itraconazole, 200 mg qd	Itraconazole, 200 mg bid × 4 – 8 wk[**]

[*] Chronic suppression at reduced dosage may be necessary.
[†] Double-strength tablet.
[‡] Reduce dosage for decreased creatinine clearance.
[§] Resistance may develop; susceptibility testing necessary.
[‖] Not available.
[#] Pathogenicity in HIV-1 infection under investigation.
[**] Also maintenance regimen.

HIV-1, human immunodeficiency virus type 1.

552

with protease inhibitors. It has reduced the mortality of patients infected with HIV-1, in addition to decreasing the frequency of opportunistic infections and the severity of symptoms. The gastrointestinal side effects of HAART include nausea, vomiting, abdominal pain, and diarrhea. Hepatic toxicity may complicate long-term therapy, and other specific organs may be adversely affected, such as with dideoxyinosine-induced pancreatitis.

Note that in contrast to cases of immunocompetent patients presenting with uncomplicated bacterial colitis, antibiotics are indicated for patients with AIDS infected by *Salmonella*, *Shigella*, or *Campylobacter* species. MAC is treated with combination regimens that include a macrolide azole agent, rifabutin, and ethambutol. Symptomatic improvement has been observed among patients with *Cryptosporidium* infection treated with paromomycin with or without azithromycin. Microsporidia are usually not responsive to antimicrobial agents, but albendazole has decreased symptoms including weight loss in patients with *S intestinalis*, whereas fumagillin is the preferred drug for *E bieneusi*.

Because antimicrobial agents often fail to resolve infection, symptom-based therapy is often implemented. Opiates (e.g., diphenoxylate, codeine, paregoric, tincture of opium) may help reduce stool volume. In patients with refractory AIDS-associated diarrhea, the somatostatin analog octreotide can also reduce stool frequency and volume. Implementation of a low-fat, low-lactose, high-protein, high-calorie diet can minimize symptoms of malabsorption and help maintain the patient's nutritional status. Occasionally, elemental supplements or even total parenteral nutrition (TPN) are necessary. The decision to use invasive therapy such as TPN or enteral feedings through a gastrostomy tube should be based on the disease prognosis and on the potential for controlling the acute illness.

HEPATOBILIARY DISEASES

Etiology, Pathogenesis, and Clinical Features

Evidence of hepatobiliary injury is a common manifestation among patients with AIDS and may be induced by medication, infection, and structural disease. Many of the drugs used to treat HIV-1 and AIDS produce cholestasis (e.g., sulfonamides, rifampin) or hepatitis (e.g., isoniazid, imidazoles). Chronic infection with hepatitis B virus (HBV) or hepatitis C virus (HCV) is common among HIV-infected patients owing to shared routes of exposure. Granulomatosis hepatitis may be caused by infection with MAC, fungus, or miliary tuberculosis. AIDS cholangiopathy, which may present in the form of papillary stenosis or sclerosing cholangitis, has been linked to infections with *Cryptosporidium* species, Microsporidia, *I belli*, and CMV. Patients present with pruritus, abdominal pain, and progressive cholestasis. Infiltrative liver disease secondary to Kaposi sarcoma and lymphoma may also produce cholangiopathy. Bacillary angiomatosis is a form of sinusoidal dilation, also termed *peliosis hepatis*, which has been associated with the bacillus *Bartonella henselae*. Patients usually present with abdominal pain, elevated liver chemistry values, and a disproportionate increase in serum alkaline phosphatase levels.

Diagnosis and Management

The initial evaluation for abnormal liver chemistries consists of serologic analysis for HBV and HCV and blood cultures for MAC. Further diagnostic evaluation is generally reserved for patients with significant symptoms or a progressive rise in liver chemistry profiles. Ultrasound may reveal biliary dilation in patients with AIDS cholangiopathy; endoscopic retrograde cholangiopancreatography (ERCP) is required to confirm this diagnosis. Computed tomographic scans may demonstrate the dilated sinusoids characteristic of bacillary angiomatosis and may also provide ancillary evidence of infiltrative diseases of the hepatic parenchyma, such as adenopathy associated with MAC or lymphoma. Exclusion of granulomatous hepatitis requires liver biopsy, and in addition to histological examination with special stains, care must be taken to culture the biopsy specimen for mycobacteria and fungi.

Based on the lack of specific therapy for most hepatobiliary disorders associated with AIDS, treatment is largely supportive. Implementation of disease-specific therapy, however, requires definitive diagnosis with liver biopsy or ERCP. The role of interferon therapy for chronic HCV is expanding as HAART prolongs the life expectancy of the AIDS population. Granulomatous hepatitis caused by mycobacterial or fungal infection and peliosis hepatis caused by *B henselae* require long-term antimicrobial therapy. Patients with the papillary stenosis form of AIDS cholangiopathy often experience relief of abdominal pain with endoscopic sphincterotomy, despite biochemical evidence of the progression of cholestasis. Kaposi sarcoma and lymphoma require systemic chemotherapy and radiation therapy.

GASTROINTESTINAL HEMORRHAGE

Severe gastrointestinal bleeding is uncommon in HIV-1–infected patients. The most common AIDS-associated etiologies include viral esophagitis, gastroduodenal lymphoma, and MAC disease of the small intestine. Upper gastrointestinal bleeding is more often caused by HSV ulceration, whereas lower tract bleeding is more frequently caused by CMV colitis. Other etiologies of gastrointestinal hemorrhage include ulcers associated with non-Hodgkin lymphoma, idiopathic ulcerations, and extensive mucosal Kaposi sarcoma.

ACUTE ABDOMINAL PAIN

Abdominal pain is less common than diarrhea in HIV-1 infected patients. Patients with HIV infection may present with acute abdominal pain caused by diseases prevalent among immunocompetent patients, such as calculous cholecystitis and appendicitis, in addition to diseases specific to AIDS. The most common etiologies of abdominal pain associated with AIDS are non-Hodgkin lymphoma of the gastrointestinal tract, CMV disease of the small or large intestine, and pancreatitis. Although peptic ulcer disease is uncommon in AIDS, CMV ulcers or ulcers associated with lymphoma throughout the gastrointestinal tract may perforate and produce peritonitis. MAC may present with necrotic bulky adenopathy that mimics peritonitis, with guarding and rebound tenderness. Tuberculosis and fungal peritonitis are potential causes of acute abdomen in patients with AIDS. Pancreatitis may be caused by other opportunistic infections, such as those produced by CMV, *Cryptococcus neoformans*, and *Toxoplasma gondii*, in addition to certain medications (e.g., pentamidine, dideoxyinosine, sulfonamides). Kaposi sarcoma and lymphoma may present with mass lesions causing intussusception or bowel obstruction, with subsequent development of strangulation and perforation. Previously, the high operative mortality rate associated with surgery for AIDS-related complications diminished enthusiasm for surgical interventions. However, improvement in managing AIDS complications and extending life expectancy with HAART has reversed this trend. Currently, laparotomy should be considered for AIDS patients with an acute abdomen.

CHAPTER 69

Parasitic Diseases: Protozoa and Helminths

PROTOZOA

Entamoeba histolytica

Etiology and Pathogenesis

Amebiasis is caused by the protozoan *Entamoeba histolytica*. The life cycle of *E histolytica* includes a host infective stage (cyst) and a tissue invasive stage (trophozoite). Fecal-oral transmission of cysts occurs from ingesting contaminated food or water or sexual contact. Excystation occurs in the small intestine or colon, after which motile trophozoites colonize the colon, produce cysts, and invade the colonic epithelium. Clinical disease is attributed to direct invasion of the intestinal epithelium, in addition to production of proteases, collagenases, and extracellular enterotoxin that disrupt mucosal barriers and induce inflammation. Infection of the liver may occur by migration of amebas from the colon through the portal vein.

Amebiasis is most prevalent in Central and South America, Indonesia, India, and the tropical regions of Africa. In developed countries, populations at risk of infection include immigrants from, or long-term visitors to endemic areas, patients with acquired immunodeficiency syndrome (AIDS), and institutionalized persons. Malnourished individuals, very young and old persons, pregnant women, and patients on corticosteroids are also at risk of severe infection.

Clinical Features, Diagnosis, and Management

The clinical features of amebiasis include intestinal and extraintestinal disease (see Table 69-1). The severity of intestinal disease may range from asymptomatic infection to dysentery and fulminant colitis. The latter is characterized by severe bloody diarrhea, fever, and abdominal pain with tenderness. Toxic megacolon is a complication that is often fatal and is associated with administration of corticosteroids. Alternatively, the disease course may be chronic and confused with inflammatory bowel disease. The development of a localized colonic infection that forms a mass of granulation tissue is a rare complication. These masses, or amebomas, are located in the cecum, ascending colon, rectosigmoid, transverse colon, and descending colon, in decreasing order of frequency. Amebic strictures also form in the anus, rectum, and sigmoid colon.

Diagnosis of intestinal amebiasis depends on the microscopic demonstration of cysts or trophozoites in the stool or on biopsy specimens obtained during lower gastrointestinal endoscopy. Because parasites are excreted intermittently, at least three stool specimens from different days should be evaluated, using a wet preparation to look for motile trophozoites containing erythrocytes and formalin–ethyl acetate to identify cysts. Fecal antigen tests are available that can differentiate

TABLE 69-1
Clinical Manifestations of Infection with *Entamoeba histolytica*

Intestinal disease
   Noninvasive intestinal colonization
   Diarrhea in patients with acquired immunodeficiency syndrome
   Acute amebic proctocolitis
   Chronic nondysenteric intestinal amebiasis
   Ameboma
   Toxic megacolon
   Amebic peritonitis secondary to perforation
   Amebic strictures

Extraintestinal disease
   Liver abscess, rarely with extension to thorax, pericardium, or peritoneum
   Brain abscess
   Cutaneous amebiasis
   Venereal infection

between *E histolytica* and nonpathogenic *Entamoeba dispar*. Colonoscopy or sigmoidoscopy with biopsy may be useful for patients with dysentery to differentiate infection from inflammatory bowel disease. The endoscopic appearance of amebiasis consists of discrete shallow ulcers covered with yellow or white exudates on a background of mucosal edema and erythema.

Amebic liver abscesses develop in 10% of patients who have had invasive amebiasis. The primary symptoms of amebic liver abscess are fever and right upper quadrant abdominal pain. Note that only a third of patients with amebic abscess have symptoms of active colonic disease. Physical findings may include hepatomegaly and tenderness of the right upper abdominal quadrant. Laboratory tests reveal leukocytosis and an elevated alkaline phosphatase level, whereas hyperbilirubinemia is uncommon. Ultrasound or CT may be used to locate the abscess. The lesion should be aspirated in febrile patients with right upper quadrant pain to exclude a pyogenic process after excluding echinococcal cyst, which may induce anaphylaxis if subjected to needle aspiration. Complications of amebic hepatic abscess include pulmonary involvement from direct extension of a liver abscess, peritonitis from rupture of the abscess, pericarditis, cutaneous amebiasis, brain abscess, and amebic penile or cervical ulceration.

Metronidazole is the drug of choice for both invasive colonic disease and liver abscess (750 mg orally, three times daily; or 500 mg intravenously every 6 hours, for 5 to 10 days). A second antimicrobial such as dehydroemetine (1 to 1.5 mg/kg per day, intramuscular injection for 5 days) may be added for critically ill patients. After completing therapy for invasive intestinal amebiasis or hepatic amebiasis, a second phase of treatment is necessary to eradicate the intestinal carriage. Poorly absorbed drugs, such as diloxanide furoate, iodoquinol, and paromomycin, are recommended because of their intralumenal activity and lower incidence of systemic side effects. These agents are also used to treat asymptomatic persons with intestinal disease to prevent complications and the spread of infection to others. Colonic surgery is generally not necessary, except in cases involving toxic megacolon or perforation. Surgical drainage of hepatic amebic abscesses may be required in complicated cases.

Giardia lamblia

Etiology and Pathogenesis

Giardia lamblia, a flagellated protozoan, is the most commonly identified intestinal parasite in the United States. Waterborne outbreaks have occurred in the Northeast, Northwest, and Rocky Mountain regions of the United States and Canada. Person-to-person transmission is the second most common mode of acquisition. Food has been documented as a vehicle for *G lamblia* transmission in commercial food establishments. *G lamblia* can infect sheep, beavers, cattle, dogs, and cats, but it is unknown if these reservoirs are implicated in human disease. Patients at risk of acquiring giardiasis include those with common variable immunodeficiency, X-linked agammaglobulinemia, previous gastric surgery, achlorhydria, and, possibly, AIDS.

The life cycle of *G lamblia* consists of a trophozoite stage and a cyst stage. Infection may result from inocula of as few as 10 to 25 cysts. The organism adheres to enterocytes, after which diarrhea is produced by a calcium-dependent secretory process, as well as by malabsorption from local zinc depletion and decreases in brush-border enzymes and surface area. An immune response develops that contributes to organism clearance by producing secretory antibodies and provides partial immunity against reinfection.

Clinical Features, Diagnosis, and Management

The presentation of *G lamblia* infection varies from asymptomatic cyst passage to acute, self-limited diarrhea or chronic diarrhea with malabsorption and weight loss (Table 69-2). There is a 1- to 2-week incubation period prior to development of acute symptoms of diarrhea, abdominal pain, bloating, flatulence, eructation, malaise, nausea, and anorexia. Stools may initially be watery but later are described as greasy, foul-smelling, and may float. Weight loss of more than 4.5 kg occurs in most cases. Prolonged or recurrent diarrhea may persist for months and may be associated with lactose intolerance and malabsorption of fat, protein, D-xylose, and vitamins A and B_{12}. Nodular lymphoid hyperplasia is associated with *Giardia* infection.

Giardiasis is traditionally diagnosed by examining stool for cysts or trophozoites. The diagnostic sensitivity may reach 90% from collecting three stool samples. Antigen detection assays for stool using enzyme-linked immunosorbent assay (ELISA) or direct fluorescent antibody tests may also be used to diagnose infection. Stool tests may be negative because the organism resides mainly in the small intestine; thus, duodenal aspiration, biopsy, or brush cytology may be required to confirm the diagnosis. Histopathology of the small intestine may reveal spruelike changes. The serum may be positive for anti-*Giardia* IgM antibodies indicating active infection, whereas the level of IgG antibodies may remain elevated for years.

Metronidazole (250 mg, three times daily for 5 to 7 days) is the most commonly used therapy in the United States. Side effects include a metallic taste, nausea, dizziness, headache, neuropathy, a disulfiram-like effect if taken with alcohol, and, rarely, neutropenia. Tinidazole, which is not available in the United States, is also effective. Furazolidone (pediatric dose: 2 mg/kg, three times daily for 7 to 10 days) is advocated as an alternative for treating giardiasis in children. Albendazole has also been efficacious. Oral paromomycin may be considered for treating pregnant women. Recurrent symptoms from either persistent infection or reinfection are common and may be treated with combination therapy, including metronidazole and furazolidone. The role of treatment for asymptomatic cyst passers is controversial. Prevention of giardiasis includes water purification and good personal hygiene.

TABLE 69-2
Symptoms of Infection with *Giardia lamblia*

SYMPTOM	PERCENTAGE OF PATIENTS (RANGE)
Diarrhea	90 (64 – 100)
Malaise	86 (72 – 97)
Flatulence	75 (35 – 97)
Foul-smelling, greasy stools	75 (57 – 87)
Abdominal cramps	71 (44 – 85)
Bloating	71 (42 – 97)
Nausea	69 (59 – 79)
Anorexia	66 (41 – 82)
Weight loss	66 (56 – 76)
Vomiting	23 (11 – 36)
Fever	15 (0 – 24)
Constipation	13 (0 – 26)
Urticaria	10 (5 – 14)

Adapted with permission from Hill DR. Giardiasis. In Mandell GR, Douglas RG, Bennett J, eds, *Principles of Infectious Diseases*. New York: Churchill-Livingstone; 1990;2113.

Cryptosporidium Species

Etiology and Pathogenesis

Although *Cryptosporidium* species have been most commonly associated with diarrhea in patients with AIDS, disease may also be produced in immunocompetent hosts. *Cryptosporidium* species have caused diarrhea in malnourished children in developing areas, children in day-care centers, travelers, and veterinary and health care workers. Several notorious waterborne outbreaks of *Cryptosporidium parvum* in the United States involved failure of treatment and purification of drinking water. *C parvum* is the primary mammalian pathogen infecting humans, calves, piglets, foals, mice, and goats. Infection can be transmitted person-to-person, via contaminated food and water, and by contact with infected animals. Transmission is initiated by ingesting oocysts that are excreted in the feces of infected humans or animals, which excyst in the small intestine after exposure to gastric acid, bile, and digestive enzymes. The sporozoites infect the mucosal epithelium, causing villous atrophy, crypt elongation, and lamina propria inflammation, especially in immunocompromised individuals. *Cryptosporidium* infections cause malabsorption or secretory diarrhea by unknown mechanisms.

Clinical Features, Diagnosis, and Management

In immunocompetent hosts, intestinal cryptosporidiosis manifests as self-limited diarrhea (usually for 10 to 14 days) and may be associated with symptoms of abdominal cramping, anorexia, malaise, myalgias, weight loss, and fever ($<39°C$) after a mean incubation period of 9 days (range: 5 to 22 days). In immunocompromised patients, the organism causes severe diarrhea that may be in excess of 17 L per day and may contribute to malnutrition or death. The most widely used method for diagnosis is acid-fast staining of stool specimens to detect oocysts visually. Direct immunofluorescence staining may add sensitivity by detecting smaller numbers of oocysts. Elevated serum IgM or IgG antibody titers are detected in 95% to 100% of patients within 2 weeks of symptom onset; increased IgG titers may persist for long periods. Intestinal biopsy specimens are positive in some cases, but usually biopsy is not necessary if stool samples have been collected properly.

No antimicrobial or antiparasitic agent consistently eradicates *Cryptosporidium* infection. The disease is self-limited in immunocompetent hosts, and therapy is conservative, concentrating on fluid resuscitation. One study of AIDS patients with intestinal cryptosporidiosis illustrated the potential benefit of azithromycin (600 mg daily) and paromomycin (1 g, twice daily); however, the response was not universal. Spiramycin, hyperimmune bovine colostrum, and immunoglobulin concentrate have shown promise in other clinical studies. Prevention of infection involves careful hand washing, avoidance of contaminated water, and avoidance of infected persons for 1 to 2 weeks after their symptoms resolve.

Other Enteric Protozoa

Cyclospora Species

Cyclospora can induce prolonged, nonbloody diarrhea with anorexia, fatigue, and weight loss. Transmission occurs from ingestng fruit or water contaminated with oocytes. A large outbreak in the United States was associated with contaminated raspberries. The organism targets the proximal small intestine, and after a 7- to 10-day incubation period, symptoms may persist for a mean of 14 days, although diarrhea has reportedly lasted as long as 60 days. Acid-fast stains of stool samples or duodenal aspirates can diagnose the organism. Treatment with trimethoprim-sulfamethoxazole (160 mg TMP/800 mg SMX, twice daily for 7 to 10 days for immunocompetent hosts, or four times daily for 10 days for immunocompromised patients) has been effective.

Isospora belli

Isospora belli is a coccidian protozoan that causes a prolonged diarrheal illness in AIDS patients and other immunocompromised individuals and also causes disease in immunocompetent travelers. Sporulated oocysts excyst after ingestion and invade the intestinal epithelium. After an incubation period of 2 to 3 days, the organism produces severe nonbloody diarrhea, cramping, nausea, and weight loss. Diagnosis is by identifying oocysts in stool samples or in biopsy specimens of the small intestine. Trimethoprim-sulfamethoxazole (160 mg/800 mg, four times daily for 7 days, followed by 10 days of twice daily administration) is effective. Patients with AIDS may require prolonged therapy and should be given prophylactic therapy to decrease the incidence of relapse (trimethoprim-sulfamethoxazole 160 mg/800 mg, three times weekly, or sulfadoxine-pyrimethamine 500 mg/25 mg, once weekly).

Blastocystis hominis

Blastocystis hominis is a protozoan commonly detected in the stool of patients with diarrhea. Its pathogenic role is controversial. The organism is frequently detected in asymptomatic individuals. In symptomatic individuals, eradication does not always result in symptom improvement. Symptoms attributed to *B hominis* infection include diarrhea, abdominal pain, anorexia, weight loss, and flatulence. The parasite is detected by stool examination. Treatment with metronidazole, iodoquinol and furazolidone has had variable success.

Trypanosoma cruzi

Chagas disease is caused by *Trypanosoma cruzi*, which is acquired from the bite of an infected reduviid bug. Acute infection is usually asymptomatic, but some patients exhibit unilateral periorbital edema (Romaña sign), fever, adenopathy, hepatosplenomegaly, myocarditis, and constitutional symptoms. Chronic disease is characterized by cardiac or gastrointestinal manifestations including a progressive loss of visceral innervation, especially in the esophagus and colon, that results in dysphagia, regurgitation, and constipation. Chagas disease is diagnosed by detecting parasites in Giemsa-stained blood, cultivating organisms in specialized media, performing xenodiagnosis with reduviid bugs, or using serologic tests. Currently, there are no effective treatments for chronic disease.

Miscellaneous

Microsporidian protozoa, predominantly *Enterocytozoon bieneusi* and *Septata intestinalis*, most frequently cause diarrhea in AIDS patients. Diagnosis requires intestinal biopsy with electron microscopic examination of the specimens. *Balantidium coli* is a ciliate protozoan that causes rectosigmoid colon ulcerations with dysentery or secondary bacteremia.

HELMINTHS

Nematodes

Trichuris trichiura (Whipworm)

Etiology and pathogenesis.   Humans are infected with *Trichuris trichiura* through a fecal-oral route. After excystation, larvae penetrate the intestinal mucosa, molt, mature, and reattach to the colonic wall as adults. Mature female worms deposit 2000 to 6000 eggs daily into the stool. Infection is most frequent in areas without latrines and in communities where human feces are used as fertilizer.

Clinical features, diagnosis, and management.   The diagnosis is confirmed by finding ova in the stool or adult worms in the colonic mucosa. Mebendazole is the recommended therapy, and albendazole has also been effective.

Enterobius vermicularis (Pinworm)

Etiology and pathogenesis.   *Enterobius vermicularis* is frequently found in school-age children living in areas of high population density in both temperate and tropical climates. Ingested ova hatch in the small intestine, producing larvae that mature during their migration to the ileum. Adult females exit the anus to lay eggs on the perianal or perineal skin. Poor personal hygiene and exposure to infected peers contribute to infection in children aged 5 through 10 years.

Clinical features, diagnosis, and management.   Symptoms of infection with *E vermicularis* include perianal pruritus, local skin trauma, secondary bacterial dermatitis, vulvovaginitis, urinary tract infection, and secondary enuresis. Complications of infection include intestinal perforation secondary to appendicitis, diverticulitis, or malignancy. Applying transparent adhesive tape to the perianal skin early in the morning and transferring the contents to a microscope slide to detect the ova most efficiently provides the diagnosis. Three specimens provide a diagnostic sensitivity of 90%, whereas traditional stool examination for ova and parasites detects only 10% to 15% of cases. Treatment consists of pyrantel pamoate, mebendazole, or albendazole. Prevention of infection is enhanced by handwashing, laundering contaminated clothing, and possibly treating the entire household to interrupt transmission.

Capillaria philippinensis

Etiology and pathogenesis. *Capillaria philippinensis* infection is acquired after ingesting infected, raw, freshwater fish. Endemic regions include the Philippines, Thailand, Indonesia, Japan, Taiwan, Egypt, and Iran. Adult organisms invade the mucosa of the small intestine and cause inflammation of the lamina propria. Ova are released into the intestinal lumen; some ova are passed in the stool, and others excyst in the intestine and can result in autoinfection.

Clinical features, diagnosis, and management. The clinical presentation of *C philippinensis* infection includes chronic diarrhea, abdominal pain, borborygmi, constitutional symptoms, malabsorption, weight loss, and, in rare cases, death. It is diagnosed by detecting ova, larvae, or adult worms in multiple stool examinations. Therapy consists of mebendazole, albendazole, or flubendazole, in addition to fluid and electrolyte replacement.

Trichostrongylus Species

Etiology and pathogenesis. *Trichostrongylus* species are parasites of herbivorous animals that infect humans in the Middle East and Asia. Ingesting food or water contaminated by feces from infected animals is usually the cause of infection, although larvae may also directly invade through the skin. Adult worms live in the proximal small intestine.

Clinical features, diagnosis, and management. The clinical presentation is variable; the majority of patients complain of mild epigastric pain, diarrhea, and flatulence. Associated signs include anemia, eosinophilia, and emaciation. Diagnosis is made by identifying ova in the stool. Therapy consists of pyrantel pamoate, mebendazole, or albendazole.

Ascaris lumbricoides

Etiology and pathogenesis. *Ascaris lumbricoides* is the most prevalent intestinal nematode; it infects 1.2 billion people worldwide in tropical and temperate areas. After ingestion of contaminated food or water, eggs hatch in the duodenum where the larvae penetrate the intestinal wall, enter the venous circulation, and migrate to the lungs. The organisms then exit the circulatory system into the pulmonary tree, travel to the trachea and pharynx, are reswallowed, and complete their development in the small intestine. Female ascarids produce 200,000 eggs per day, 10 to 12 weeks after the ingestion of ova.

Clinical features, diagnosis, and management. Patients present with pulmonary manifestations (bronchospasm, mucus hypersecretion, bronchiolar inflammation), with production of sputum that contains Charcot-Leyden crystals and larvae, urticaria, and gastrointestinal findings, which may include abdominal pain, nausea, anorexia, diarrhea, and, possibly, growth retardation in children. Serious complications of *A lumbricoides* infection include partial or complete intestinal obstruction, an abdominal mass, intussusception, volvulus, perforation, and localized abscesses. Biliary complications result from migration of adult *A lumbricoides* into the common bile duct and include cholecystitis, ascending bacterial cholangitis, secondary liver abscess, bile peritonitis, biliary calculi, and acute pancreatitis. Diagnostic evaluation may include chest radiographs that show pulmonary infiltrates or abdomen radiographs that reveal adult worms in the gastrointestinal tract or bile duct. Eosinophilia may be present. It is usually diagnosed by identifying ova in feces. Treatment of *A lumbricoides* consists of mebendazole pyrantel pamoate, or albendazole. Intestinal obstruction may require surgery. Biliary obstruction may need surgical or endoscopic extraction of dead worms after anthelmintic chemotherapy.

Trichinella spiralis

Etiology and pathogenesis. *Trichinella spiralis* infection typically occurs after ingestion of incompletely cooked meat containing larvae. The reservoir for *T spiralis* includes pigs, wild boars, bears, walrus, and horses. Ingested larvae excyst in the small intestine and molt to become adults. After mating, females remain embedded in the mucosa and release larvae, which invade the mucosa, enter the lymphatics or bloodstream, and encyst in skeletal muscle cells.

Clinical features, diagnosis, and management. Trichinosis presents initially with an intestinal phase characterized by nausea, vomiting, pain, and diarrhea. A systemic phase begins 1 to 3 weeks later and manifests as fever, myalgia, facial or periorbital edema, headache, conjunctivitis, and a rash. Lethal complications include cardiac involvement and meningoencephalitis. Laboratory abnormalities include eosinophilia and elevated serum levels of creatine phosphokinase. It is diagnosed by serologic testing using indirect immunofluorescence or ELISA; however, muscle biopsies are required to detect cysts in rare cases. Mebendazole is the recommended treatment. NSAIDs and corticosteroids may control symptoms. Trichinosis can be prevented by thoroughly cooking meat (to at least $76.6°C$).

Hookworms

Etiology and pathogenesis. Ova of *Ancylostoma duodenale, Ancylostoma ceylanicum,* and *Necator americanus* are excreted in the feces and excyst in soil, becoming filariform larvae that can invade the human host through cutaneous fissures or hair follicles in the feet or hands. The larvae migrate to the lungs, ascend the trachea to the pharynx, and are swallowed. Hookworms are widely distributed worldwide but are rare in the United States. Poor sanitation is a risk factor for infection, as is the practice of not wearing protective footwear.

Clinical features, diagnosis, and management. The cutaneous phase of infection induced by larvae causes an edematous, pruritic, papulovesicular eruption; the pulmonary phase of infection manifests with coughing, wheezing, pulmonary infiltrates, and eosinophilia (Löffler syndrome). Intestinal symptoms include epigastric pain, tenderness, flatulence, and, rarely, acute hemorrhage. Chronic disease characteristically causes iron deficiency anemia and hypoalbuminemia. Pediatric manifestations include growth retardation and impaired intellectual development. It is diagnosed by detecting ova in stool samples. Pharmacological therapy includes mebendazole, pyrantel pamoate, or albendazole in addition to iron supplementation.

Strongyloides stercoralis

Etiology and pathogenesis. *Strongyloides stercoralis* is acquired cutaneously from soil contaminated with feces that contain larvae. After entering through the skin, larvae migrate first to the lungs, then to the small intestine. Adults reside in the mucosa and release ova into the lumen. The ova hatch quickly, releasing larvae that may either pass through the feces or autoinfect the host by penetrating the intestinal mucosa or perianal skin. Because of the latter, *S stercoralis* infection may persist for decades. The organism is endemic in tropical Africa, Asia, and Latin America, and is also found in Eastern Europe and southern United States.

Clinical features, diagnosis, and management. The cutaneous phase produces a maculopapular rash or linear urticaria (larva currens). The respiratory phase may not cause symptoms, or it may be associated with coughing, shortness of breath, wheezing, fever, pulmonary infiltrates, and eosinophilia. Intestinal infection leads to symptoms and signs, including abdominal pain, diarrhea, vomiting, malabsorption, steatorrhea, weight loss, and obstruction. Bacterial superinfection may be life-threatening if present in immunocompromised patients; this manifests with sepsis, meningitis, peritonitis, or endocarditis. *Strongyloides* is diagnosed by identifying larvae in stool samples, duodenal aspirates, or biopsy specimens of the small intestine. Serologic tests provide presumptive evidence of infection. Thiabendazole is the treatment of choice; ivermectin and albendazole are alternatives.

Cutaneous Larva Migrans

Etiology and pathogenesis. Dog and cat hookworms (*Ancylostoma braziliense*, *Ancylostoma caninum*) are present in the Caribbean, Africa, South America, and the Gulf and southern Atlantic coasts of North America. These organisms also enter the host by cutaneous penetration.

Clinical features, diagnosis, and management. The name of the disease syndrome is derived from the generation of creeping eruption, a dermatitis characterized by serpiginous, papulovesicular, erythematous, pruritic lesions. Topical thiabendazole is the treatment of choice, and oral albendazole is an effective alternative.

Visceral Larva Migrans

Etiology and pathogenesis. Infection is caused by fecal-oral transmission of larvae of dog and cat ascarids (*Toxocara canis*, *Toxocara cati*). Larvae are released in the intestine but cannot complete their life cycle in humans.

Clinical features, diagnosis, and management. Patients may be asymptomatic or may have symptoms of fever, cough, abdominal pain, urticaria, hepatomegaly, dermatitis, ocular involvement, eosinophilia, or hypergammaglobulinemia. Diagnosis is best confirmed using an ELISA to detect anti-*Toxocara* antibodies. Treatment consists of thiabendazole or diethylcarbamazine.

Anisakiasis

Etiology and pathogenesis. Anisakiasis results from ingesting raw or incompletely cooked infected seafood (e.g., squid, cod, herring, salmon, mackerel, Pacific pollock, and Pacific red snapper). In human hosts, larvae attempt to penetrate the stomach, small intestine, or colon, producing local inflammation but usually no eosinophilia.

Clinical features, diagnosis, and management. Acute gastric anisakiasis presents with abdominal pain, nausea, vomiting, and occasionally hemorrhage 12 to 24 hours after ingestion of contaminated fish. Abdominal radiographs may demonstrate thumbprinting of the bowel wall, lumenal narrowing, or a mass lesion. It can be diagnosed by upper gastrointestinal endoscopic extraction of worms from the stomach or duodenum. Surgery may be necessary to relieve obstruction or to repair perforation.

Angiostrongylus costaricensis

Etiology and pathogenesis. *Angiostrongylus costaricensis* typically resides in mesenteric arteries. From this point, larvae migrate through the intestinal wall, are passed in the feces, and invade slugs. Human infection results from ingesting slug-infested vegetation.

Clinical features, diagnosis, and management. Adult worms and ova elicit a granulomatous arteritis in the ileocecal region, which can produce arteritis, thrombosis, infarction, and perforation. Clinical features include nausea, vomiting, right lower quadrant pain, a palpable abdominal mass, fever, eosinophilia, and leukocytosis. Surgery is often necessary, and it is diagnosed by identifying organisms in surgical specimens. Thiabendazole has been used effectively in case series.

Cestodes (Tapeworms)

Taenia saginata

Etiology and pathogenesis. Human infection results from ingesting beef or meat from camels or other herbivores that contains cysticerci, the larval form of *Taenia saginata.* After digestion of the infected meat, the cysticercus breaks down, and a scolex is released that attaches in the jejunum. The tapeworm may grow to several feet in length, depositing proglottids and ova in the stool. Cattle ingest ova from human feces, after which larvae migrate to the muscle, thus completing the life cycle.

Clinical features, diagnosis, and management. Most infections do not cause symptoms; however, the clinical presentation may include abdominal discomfort, anxiety, vertigo, nausea, vomiting, diarrhea, and weight loss. Finding ova or proglottids in the stool confirms the diagnosis of *T saginata* infection. Treatment consists of niclosamide.

Taenia solium

Etiology and pathogenesis. *Taenia solium* infects humans who ingest infected pork. Infection is common in Latin America.

Clinical features, diagnosis, and management. *Taenia solium* infection manifests with cysticercosis, a disease caused by encystment of cysticercus larvae in the brain (which can be fatal), subcutaneous tissue, skeletal muscle, eyes, or other organs. Intestinal infection is diagnosed by detecting ova or proglottids in the stool. CT or magnetic resonance imaging (MRI) studies may demonstrate cysticerci in involved areas. Antibodies in the serum or cerebrospinal fluid are detected in some cases. Niclosamide or praziquantel are effective in treating intestinal infection; however, praziquantel and albendazole are required to treat neurological involvement. Corticosteroids may prevent cerebral edema.

Diphyllobothrium latum

Etiology and Pathogenesis. The fish tapeworm, *Diphyllobothrium latum,* infects humans after ingestion of raw or incompletely cooked fish that contains the tapeworm in its procercoid stage. *D latum* is found in pike, salmon, trout, whitefish, and turbot in northern regions of Europe, Asia, and North America and in temperate regions of South America. Humans excrete tapeworms in the coracidia stage, thereby infecting crustaceans inhabiting freshwater that is contaminated by human feces. Finally, freshwater fish eventually consume infected crustaceans.

Clinical features, diagnosis, and management. The classic presentation of vitamin B_{12} deficiency caused by tapeworm competition for the vitamin is not always present. It is diagnosed by identifying ova or proglottids in stool samples. Niclosamide is recommended for treatment.

Hymenolepis nana

Etiology and pathogenesis. Infection with the dwarf tapeworm, *Hymenolepis nana*, follows ingestion of ova. Transmission is hand-to-mouth or by ingestion of fecally contaminated food or water. An oncosphere is liberated that penetrates the intestinal mucosa and forms a cercocystis. The cercocystis releases a scolex at maturity, which anchors in the small intestine and releases ova.

Clinical features, diagnosis, and management. Patients may present with anorexia, abdominal pain, diarrhea, flatulence, or weight loss. Infection with *H nana* is diagnosed by identifying eggs in the feces. Praziquantel is the treatment of choice.

Echinococcus Species

Etiology and pathogenesis. Humans are infected with ova of *Echinococcus granulosus* after ingesting fecally contaminated food or water. After excystment, larvae invade the intestinal mucosa and disseminate through the lymphatics and blood circulation to form cysts in the liver, lungs, bones, brain, muscles, eyes, heart, and other organs. Infection is endemic in areas of poor sanitation in Australia, New Zealand, North Africa, the Middle East, and South America. The typical echinococcal or hydatid cyst contains an external hyaline cuticula, an inner germinal membrane with brood capsules, protoscoleces, and daughter cysts. Infection from another organism, *Echinococcus multilocularis*, is acquired by ingesting plants contaminated with canine feces.

Clinical features, diagnosis, and management. Hydatid cysts generally grow slowly. Complications may occur from rupture into the biliary system (which can cause obstructive jaundice or ascending cholangitis), peritoneum (producing anaphylaxis or peritoneal seeding), or lung. The diagnosis is based on identifying a hydatid cyst by CT, MRI, or ultrasound studies. Serologic tests are available, but results are not always positive in affected patients. Surgical excision is a common approach to therapy, although some case reports claim successful percutaneous aspiration and drainage of liver cysts that avoided the classic risk of anaphylaxis. Administration of mebendazole or albendazole has been advocated before surgery. A scolicide (20% sodium chloride) should be injected into the cyst at the time of surgery or drainage. High-dose albendazole is recommended as suppressive therapy for patients for whom surgery is contraindicated.

E multilocularis produces an alveolar hepatic cyst with a jelly-like matrix. The clinical presentation includes hepatomegaly, abdominal pain, and obstructive jaundice. It is diagnosed from typical findings in imaging studies. The presence of antibodies against *Echinococcus*-specific antigen 5 has high specificity for *E multilocularis* infection. Surgery is the only reliable treatment for *E multilocularis*. Mebendazole or albendazole is used to treat inoperable disease.

Trematodes

Schistosomiasis

Etiology and pathogenesis. Adult *Schistosoma* worms live as pairs within venules in their human host. The ova produce lytic enzymes that allow invasion through the intestinal wall and ova excretion in the stool. Miracidia, released from hatching ova, infect snails. After maturation into cercariae, the organisms penetrate human skin during water-related exposures and make their way to the portal circulation. After 3 weeks, the organism migrates to the superior mesenteric veins or inferior mesenteric veins. *Schistosoma mansoni* is endemic in Africa, Latin America, and the Middle East. *Schistosoma japonicum* is found in China,

Japan, the Philippines, and Indochina. *Schistosoma intercalatum* occurs in Western and Central Africa, and *Schistosoma mekongi* is found along the Mekong River in Indochina.

Clinical features, diagnosis, and management.   The cutaneous phase of infection may produce mild, pruritic dermatitis. The systemic phase of acute schistosomiasis (Katayama fever) occurs 3 to 8 weeks after invasion and consists of fever, malaise, urticaria, abdominal discomfort, diarrhea, weight loss, cough, hepatosplenomegaly, adenopathy, and eosinophilia that may last for months. Chronic intestinal disease is characterized by mucosal congestion, hypertrophy, and ulceration of the mucosa. Patients may complain of abdominal pain, bloody diarrhea, intestinal polyps, and strictures. Liver disease manifests as periportal fibrosis, which may progress to Symmers clay pipestem (portal) fibrosis with presinusoidal portal hypertension. The pathological picture in the liver is predominantly mesenchymal; the parenchyma and liver function are preserved until late in the disease. Esophageal variceal hemorrhage and ascites may complicate liver involvement. Pulmonary manifestations of schistosomiasis include obliterative arteritis, pulmonary hypertension, and cor pulmonale. Other sites of involvement include the gallbladder (cholecystitis, cholelithiasis), spinal cord, brain, and kidneys (glomerulonephritis, nephrotic syndrome).

    The diagnosis of schistosomiasis is confirmed by identifying ova in stool or in biopsy specimens. Colonoscopic findings include hyperemia, friability, and polyps. Praziquantel is recommended for treating all *Schistosoma* species. Oxamniquine is a therapeutic alternative. Portal hypertension and bleeding esophageal varices may require endoscopic band ligation or radiographic portosystemic shunts.

Liver Flukes

Etiology and pathogenesis.   The liver flukes, *Clonorchis sinensis* and *Opisthorchis viverrini* are indigenous to the Far East and cause human disease as a result of the consumption of infected raw fish. Adult flukes can live in the biliary tract for up to 30 years, releasing eggs into the bile and eventually into the stool. Humans may become infected with *Fasciola hepatica* after ingesting watercress contaminated with encysted metacercariae. The larvae excyst, penetrate the gut wall, migrate through the peritoneum, and invade the liver before penetrating the bile ducts, where they spend their adult lives.

Clinical features, diagnosis, and management.   Symptoms of infections with *C sinensis* and *O viverrini* may include hepatomegaly and liver tenderness, dyspepsia, anorexia, icterus, edema, and diarrhea. Long-term complications include pyogenic cholangitis, cholelithiasis, chronic cholecystitis, pancreatitis, and cholangiocarcinoma. The diagnosis is confirmed by demonstrating ova in the stool or bile. Ultrasound may show liver enlargement; sludge, dilation, and thickening of the wall of the gallbladder; and bile duct dilation or cholangiocarcinoma. Endoscopic retrograde cholangiopancreatography may show biliary dilation and filling defects, tortuosity and irregular dilation of the intrahepatic ducts, and blunting of the terminal branches of the biliary tree. Praziquantel is the only drug that is active against liver flukes.

    Patients with *F hepatica* develop fever, hepatomegaly, right upper quadrant pain, weight loss, anemia, eosinophilia, and diarrhea more than 6 weeks after infection. The diagnosis is suggested by serologic testing and confirmed by demonstrating ova in the stool, duodenal aspirates, or bile. Bithionol is the recommended treatment.

Intestinal Flukes

Etiology and Pathogenesis. The intestinal fluke, *Fasciolopsis buski*, is acquired by ingesting cercariae on water plants (e.g., water caltrop, water hyacinth, water chestnut, water bamboo). After ingestion, adult organisms attach to the mucosa of the upper small intestine and release ova into the feces. Heterophyidae are trematodes that infect human hosts who ingest infected, raw, or incompletely cooked fish in the Middle East or Asia. *Nanophyetus salmincola* is found in the Pacific Northwest and Siberia and is acquired by ingesting incompletely cooked salmon. Infection with *Echinostoma* species occurs after ingesting contaminated raw snails, fish, and amphibians.

Clinical features, diagnosis, and management. Infection with *F buski* is associated with intestinal inflammation and ulceration. Patients may present with epigastric pain, nausea, and diarrhea. Heterophyidae infections produce colicky abdominal pain, tenderness, diarrhea, and eosinophilia. Abdominal pain, diarrhea, nausea, vomiting, and eosinophilia characterize *N salmincola* infections. Praziquantel is the drug of choice for treating these infections.

CHAPTER 70

Gastrointestinal Manifestations of Systemic Diseases

CARDIOVASCULAR DISEASES

Fifteen percent to 41% of patients with gastrointestinal angiodysplasias also have aortic stenosis. Most bleeding angiodysplasias in patients with aortic stenoses occur in the right colon. The association between the two conditions remains controversial. Aortic valve replacement may result in cessation of bleeding, but the angiodysplasias usually persist. A possible mechanism is that aortic stenosis is complicated by a deficiency in large multimers of the von Willebrand factor and impaired shear-induced platelet aggregation.

Heart failure promotes congestion of the splanchnic bed, which may cause anorexia, nausea, abdominal pain, distention, ischemic injury, diarrhea, malabsorption, or protein-losing enteropathy. Hepatic congestion may produce jaundice, right upper quadrant pain, low protein ascites, abnormal liver chemistry values, prolonged prothrombin time, and rarely, cirrhosis (if congestion is prolonged). Medications for heart failure produce gut toxicity, including anorexia, nausea, vomiting, and intestinal ischemia (with digoxin); nausea, anorexia, and diarrhea (with antiarrhythmics); electrolyte disturbances and constipation (with diuretics); mucosal damage (with potassium); and pancreatitis (with diuretics).

Cardiac disease has other gastrointestinal consequences. Dysphagia may result from left atrial enlargement. Intestinal infarction may be caused by embolism from cardiac thrombi or myxomas and endocarditis. Gastroesophageal reflux disease occurs with cardiac medications that relax the lower esophageal sphincter. Aspirin given for cardiac prophylaxis is a common cause of ulcer bleeding. Complications of cardiac surgery include acalculous cholecystitis, pancreatitis, intestinal infarction, and hepatic necrosis.

CHROMOSOMAL AND GENETIC ABNORMALITIES

Abetalipoproteinemia is an autosomal recessive disorder that causes hypolipidemia, diarrhea, malabsorption, growth failure, retinitis pigmentosa, acanthosis, and cerebellar ataxia. The condition results from mutations of the microsomal triglyceride transfer protein.

Anderson-Fabry disease, an X-linked glycosphingolipidosis, is caused by mutations in the gene that encodes the lysosomal exoglycosidase, α-galactosidase A, which causes deposition of ceramide trihexose in endothelial, neural, and smooth muscle cells. Patients present with episodic constipation, diarrhea, nausea and vomiting, abdominal pain, intestinal ischemia, and perforation, as well as renal failure, peripheral paresthesias, and cerebrovascular events.

Down syndrome (trisomy 21) is associated with duodenal stenosis and atresia, malrotation, annular pancreas, tracheoesophageal fistula, esophageal stenosis, hiatal hernia, esophageal reflux, celiac disease, imperforate anus, and Hirschsprung disease. Acquired hepatitis A and B infections are more common in institutionalized persons.

Familial Mediterranean fever, an autosomal recessive disorder, results from mutations in the MEFV gene. The target organs are blood vessels. Symptoms, including fever, synovitis, peritonitis, and pleurisy, begin in childhood. The disease is complicated by amyloidosis, joint degeneration, renal vein thrombosis, and narcotic addiction.

Gaucher disease is an autosomal recessive condition with deposition of glucocerebroside in lysosomes of macrophages in the reticuloendothelial system, including the liver and spleen. Patients present with hepatosplenomegaly, hepatic fibrosis, or cirrhosis (with ascites and esophageal varices).

Acute intermittent porphyria, hereditary coproporphyria, variegate porphyria, and δ-aminolevulinic acid deficiency are characterized by recurrent abdominal pain, nausea, vomiting, constipation, hypertension, neuropathy, and neuropsychiatric disturbances (Table 70-1). Variegate porphyria and coproporphyria also may cause photosensitivity. Multiple mutations underlie each type. Drugs, surgery, and pregnancy are common precipitating causes. Porphyria cutanea tarda may present with photodermal and mechanical dermal sensitivity without abdominal pain and is associated with selected chronic liver diseases.

Hereditary angioedema is an autosomal dominant deficiency of activated C1 inhibitor that presents with recurrent nonpitting swelling of the orofacial region, extremities, and gut. The swelling may be provoked by stress or trauma. Abdominal manifestations include pain, tenderness, bloating, nausea, and vomiting. "Thumbprinting" and other signs of mucosal edema are evident on barium radiography. Synthetic androgens (e.g., danazol, methyltestosterone) may ameliorate attacks. Analgesics and epinephrine are used to treat acute abdominal symptoms.

TABLE 70-1
Characteristics of Hepatic Porphyrias

DISORDER	ABDOMINAL PAIN	SKIN LESIONS	BIOCHEMICAL MARKERS
Acute intermittent porphyria	Yes	No	High PBG, ALA
Variegate porphyria	Yes	Yes	High PBG, ALA, and coproporphyrin
Hereditary coproporphyria	Yes	Yes	High PBG, ALA, and coproporphyrin
ALA dehydratase deficiency	Yes	No	High ALA, normal PBG
Porphyria cutanea tarda	No	Yes	High uroporphyrin

ALA, δ-aminolevulinic acid; PBG, porphobilinogen.

Hyperlipidemia type I (hyperchylomicronemia) and type V (hyperlipoproteinemia) are associated with recurrent pancreatitis. An increased incidence of gallstone formation occurs in type IV. The use of statins (3-hydroxy-3-methylglutaric acid [HMG-CoA] reductase inhibitors) is associated with increases in hepatic aminotransferases.

Niemann-Pick disease is an inherited disorder of sphingomyelinase activity that occurs mostly in people of Jewish ancestry. Patients manifest hepatosplenomegaly and hepatic failure in infancy from an accumulation of sphingomyelin.

Tangier disease is an autosomal recessive deficiency of α-lipoprotein characterized by cholesterol deposition in the reticuloendothelial system; it leads to hepatosplenomegaly, enlarged tonsils, adenopathy, peripheral neuropathy, and yellow-orange patches in the colonic mucosa. The defect is localized to chromosome 9q31.

Turner syndrome (X chromosome monosomy) is associated with gastrointestinal hemorrhage caused by intestinal vascular malformations, an increased incidence of inflammatory bowel disease, and greater development of anorexia nervosa.

Von Hippel–Lindau disease is an autosomal dominant inherited disorder with retinal and central nervous system retinoblastomas, renal cell carcinoma, pheochromocytoma, and endolymphatic sac tumors. Patients also present with cysts, serous cystadenomas, and neuroendocrine tumors of the pancreas.

CONNECTIVE TISSUE DISEASES

Ehlers-Danlos syndrome is a group of inherited diseases of collagen formation. Gastrointestinal bleeding occurs in type I (gravis) Ehlers-Danlos, whereas type IV disease presents with intra-abdominal bleeding secondary to ruptured aneurysms of the splanchnic system and spontaneous bowel perforation.

Pseudoxanthoma elasticum, an inherited disorder of connective tissue synthesis, is complicated by gastrointestinal bleeding caused by ineffective vasoconstriction and vessel retraction after injury from elastic fiber degeneration in visceral blood vessels.

Most patients with progressive systemic sclerosis or scleroderma have gastrointestinal complications, including tightening of the perioral skin, gingival inflammation, impaired taste, diminished esophageal body contractions and reduced lower esophageal sphincter pressure, delayed gastric emptying, acid hypersecretion, intestinal hypomotility and dilation, small bowel and colonic pseudodiverticula, bacterial overgrowth, and telangiectasias. Chronic iron deficiency anemia may result from telangiectasias or gastric antral vascular ectasia.

Polymyositis and dermatomyositis are characterized by inflammation of striated muscle and, to a lesser degree, smooth muscle. The gastrointestinal tract may be involved along its entire length, but the proximal esophagus is most commonly affected and produces dysphagia, regurgitation, and aspiration. Other gut manifestations include esophageal reflux, small bowel and colonic dysmotility, colonic pseudodiverticula, and pneumatosis intestinalis. An association of dermatomyositis with gastric and colonic malignancy has been observed.

Gastrointestinal manifestations of rheumatoid arthritis include temporomandibular joint arthritis with impairing chewing, sicca syndrome, stomatitis, gingivitis, esophageal dysmotility, secondary amyloidosis, mesenteric vasculitis, cholecystitis, appendicitis, perisplenitis, splenic infarction, pancreatitis, and hepatic arteritis. Patients with Felty syndrome are prone to intra-abdominal sepsis. Chronic NSAID use may produce gastrointestinal mucosal damage. Therapy with methotrexate can cause hepatic fibrosis and cirrhosis. Gold preparations can cause colitis.

Systemic lupus erythematosus affects the gastrointestinal tract in several ways. Serosal inflammation produces lupus peritonitis and ascites. Mesenteric vasculitis elicits intestinal ischemia or perforation. Pancreatitis, enteritis, intussusception, gut dysmotility, and pneumatosis intestinalis may be seen. Terminal ileitis from lupus may mimic Crohn's disease. Hepatomegaly and elevated aminotransferases may be observed.

Sjögren syndrome is associated with reduced saliva production, impaired esophageal motility, esophageal webs, celiac disease, pancreatic insufficiency, primary biliary cirrhosis, and chronic active hepatitis.

The seronegative spondyloarthropathies include ankylosing spondylitis, psoriatic arthritis, reactive arthritides (e.g., Reiter syndrome), arthritis associated with inflammatory bowel disease, and Whipple disease. Most patients are positive for human leukocyte antigen B27.

DERMATOLOGIC DISEASES

Ataxia-telangiectasia is an autosomal recessive condition with ataxia, telangiectasia on sun-exposed areas, sinopulmonary infection, immunodeficiency, hepatic venoocclusive disease, and increased risk of malignancy.

Blue rubber bleb nevus syndrome is associated with hemorrhage, iron deficiency anemia, and intussusception secondary to rubbery visceral angiomas.

Cowden syndrome is an autosomal dominant disease with ectodermal, mesodermal, and endodermal hamartomas. Multiple hamartomatous polyps from the esophagus to the colon cause blood loss and intestinal obstruction. Other manifestations include mucocutaneous papular lesions, esophageal glycogen acanthosis, and strong propensities for goiter, thyroid cancer, and breast cancer.

Epidermolysis bullosa is a group of diseases in which minor trauma disrupts the cohesion of the epidermis and dermis. Epidermolysis bullosa lethalis is a fatal autosomal recessive disease of infancy with oral, anal, and esophageal blistering and pyloric atresia. Epidermolysis bullosa dystrophica is characterized by thin-walled esophageal bullae, which progress to erosions, ulcers, pseudodiverticula, webs, strictures, and obstruction.

Pemphigus is a group of diseases characterized by acantholysis resulting in bullae formation, occasionally involving the esophagus. The medication D-penicillamine causes pemphigus.

Hereditary hemorrhagic telangiectasia is an autosomal dominant disorder with formation of telangiectasias, aneurysms, and arteriovenous malformations throughout the body. Gastrointestinal hemorrhage develops in 10% to 40% of patients. Large vascular ectasias occasionally form mass lesions. Hepatic vascular malformations lead to hepatomegaly, hemobilia, portal hypertension, esophageal varices, hepatic encephalopathy, and high-output heart failure. Bile duct lesions similar to Caroli disease have been described.

Neurofibromatosis is an autosomal dominant disease that presents with hemorrhage, obstruction, and development of leiomyomas, sarcomas, and neurogenic neoplasms. Rarely, neurofibromas may involve the gallbladder and liver.

Stevens-Johnson syndrome is a severe hypersensitivity reaction with fever, mucositis, and a diffuse rash that may progress to an exfoliative dermatitis. The oropharyngeal mucosa may exhibit erosions and sloughing. The entire gut may be affected in severe cases. Mucosal injury produces dysphagia, odynophagia, esophageal strictures, and gastrointestinal hemorrhage.

Sweet syndrome is characterized by acute eruption of tender, erythematous, nonulcerating plaques that may mimic erythema nodosum. The condition is associated with ulcerative colitis and Crohn's disease.

Tylosis is an autosomal dominant disorder characterized by thickening of the skin on the palms and soles. Papillomas form in the esophageal mucosa. The disease has a 95% probability for the development of esophageal carcinoma. The responsible locus on chromosome 17q25.1 has been termed the tylosis esophageal cancer gene.

Patients with chronic urticaria develop abdominal pain, gastroduodenitis, peptic ulcer, and mucosal edema. Urticarial vasculitis presents with persistent urticaria with residual bruising and may accompany collagen vascular disease, familial complement deficiency, or infection.

ENDOCRINOLOGIC DISORDERS

Acromegaly promotes enlargement of the tongue and visceral organs from increased secretion of growth hormone. Patients may have a proclivity for developing colonic adenomas and cancer.

Addison disease produces steatorrhea, anorexia, nausea, vomiting, weight loss, and abdominal pain. The disorder is associated with atrophic gastritis, antibodies against the gastric proton pump and intrinsic factor, and, rarely, achlorhydria and pernicious anemia. Cushing syndrome causes increases in hepatic aminotransferases secondary to fatty infiltration.

Diabetes has profound gastrointestinal consequences. Nausea, vomiting, anorexia, and abdominal pain are manifestations of diabetic ketoacidosis. Long-standing disease produces esophageal dilation, delayed esophageal emptying, esophageal reflux, and weak esophageal peristalsis with nonperistaltic contractions. *Candida* esophagitis may cause odynophagia in some diabetics. Gastroparesis is a symptomatic disorder associated with delayed gastric emptying, which produces early satiety, bloating, heartburn, nausea, vomiting, and bezoars and contributes to poor glycemic control. Diarrhea with or without steatorrhea results from bacterial overgrowth, increased secretion, dysmotility, anal neuropathy, bile acid malabsorption, associated celiac disease, and pancreatic insufficiency. Constipation is a consequence of colonic motor dysfunction, whereas fecal incontinence results from neuropathic damage to the anal sphincter. Thoracic radiculopathy produces severe abdominal pain. Intestinal angina, malabsorption, diarrhea, and hemorrhage may result from mesenteric atherosclerosis or microvascular disease. Impaired gallbladder contractility predisposes to gallstone formation. Hepatomegaly, steatosis, and, rarely, hepatitis may develop secondary to poor control of blood sugar.

Hyperparathyroidism leads to anorexia, nausea, vomiting, constipation, and abdominal pain as a consequence of hypercalcemia. Hypercalcemia also predisposes to pancreatitis and peptic ulcer formation. Gastrointestinal manifestations of hypocalcemia from hypoparathyroidism include abdominal pain, intestinal tetany, diarrhea, steatorrhea, and intestinal pseudoobstruction, as well as esophageal candidiasis from associated immune dysfunction.

Gastrointestinal symptoms of hyperthyroidism include anorexia, nausea, vomiting, increased stool frequency, and mild steatorrhea. Moderate to severe hyperthyroidism causes heart failure and subsequent passive congestion of the liver. Primary biliary cirrhosis, atrophic gastritis, and chronic active hepatitis are associated with autoimmune thyroid disease. Goiters may produce esophageal displacement and dysphagia in the absence of hyperthyroidism. The consequences of hypothyroidism include dysphagia from delayed esophageal emptying, constipation, distention, diarrhea from bacterial overgrowth, intestinal pseudoobstruction, megacolon, and poor gallbladder contractility. Other manifestations include impaired salivary, gastric, intestinal, and pancreatic secretion; ascites; and central congestive fibrosis of the liver.

Common gastrointestinal symptoms in pregnancy include altered appetite, pica, ptyalism, gingivitis, nausea, vomiting, heartburn, constipation, and hemorrhoids. Gastroesophageal reflux is worse in the third trimester, whereas nausea is most severe in the first trimester. Constipation results from mechanical compression of the colon, motor inhibitory effects of circulating hormones, and lack of exercise. The incidence of cholecystitis is slightly increased, perhaps secondary to delayed gallbladder emptying. Benign intrahepatic cholestasis is the most common cause of jaundice in pregnancy. Toxemia may produce indirect hyperbilirubinemia secondary to hemolysis. The HELLP (hemolysis, elevated liver enzyme levels, low platelet levels) syndrome is a catastrophic variant of toxemia that produces features suggestive of a thrombotic microangiopathic process. Acute fatty liver of pregnancy occurs in young primigravidas in the third trimester and causes vomiting, jaundice, encephalopathy, and acute renal failure. Splenic artery rupture is a life-threatening complication that presents as acute abdominal pain and shock.

GRANULOMATOUS DISEASES

Many infectious and noninfectious diseases are associated with granuloma formation in the liver and intestine (Table 70-2). Hepatic sarcoidosis presents with fever, hepatomegaly, and elevations in alkaline phosphatase. In rare cases, portal hypertension and hepatic dysfunction develop. Granulomatous cholangiopathy may mimic primary biliary cirrhosis. In the stomach, sarcoidosis produces thickened folds, ulcers, or nodules, whereas the disease may mimic ileal Crohn's disease when it involves the small intestine.

Tuberculosis may involve any portion of the gastrointestinal tract and causes abdominal pain, fever, and weight loss. Peritoneal disease with ascites is common in countries where tuberculosis is endemic.

TABLE 70-2
Causes of Hepatic Granulomas

Infections
  Tuberculosis
  Atypical mycobacteria
  Brucellosis
  Cat scratch disease
  Tularemia
  Lymphogranuloma venereum
  Blastomycosis
  Coccidiomycosis
  Histoplasmosis
  Nocardiosis
  Candidiasis
  Enterobiasis
  Strongyloidiasis
  Toxocariasis
  Toxoplasmosis
  Leishmaniasis
  Q fever
  Secondary syphilis
  Cytomegalovirus
  Mononucleosis

Medications
  Allopurinol
  Amoxicillin-clavulanate
  Diphenylhydantoin
  Halothane
  Hydralazine
  Methyldopa
  Nitrofurantoin
  Procainamide
  Quinidine
  Quinine
  Sulfasalazine
  Sulfonamides
  Sulfonylureas

Lymphoma

Metals
  Beryllium
  Copper

Vasculitis
  Giant cell arteritis
  Systemic lupus erythematosus
  Polyarteritis nodosa
  Polymyalgia rheumatica
  Rheumatoid arthritis
  Wegener granulomatosus

Miscellaneous
  Bacille Calmette-Guérin immunotherapy
  Crohn's disease
  Idiopathic granulomatous hepatitis
  Immunodeficiency
  Jejunoileal bypass surgery
  Mineral oil
  Primary biliary cirrhosis
  Sarcoidosis
  Silica
  Whipple disease

HEAVY METAL TOXICITY

Lead poisoning results from ingesting or removing lead-based paints, battery or jewelry manufacture, welding, automobile radiator repair, or eating from painted dishes acquired abroad. It presents with recurrent, severe abdominal pain, oral ulcers, constipation, paresthesias, psychiatric symptoms, a metallic taste in the mouth, a gingival lead line, anemia, renal dysfunction, mild hepatitis, and secondary porphyria.

Arsenic poisoning occurs in persons who are involved in wood preservation and glass and metal manufacturing and in those who are victims of intentional poisoning. Doses of 100 to 300 mg may be fatal. Acute poisoning produces abdominal pain, vomiting, diarrhea, garlicky breath, dysphagia, hepatomegaly, jaundice, and circulatory collapse from the blockade of cellular oxidative processes. Chronic arsenic toxicity produces insidious weakness, nausea, diarrhea, constipation, macular skin pigmentation, leukoderma, palmar and plantar keratoses, pancytopenia, edema, peripheral vascular disease, neuropathy, cirrhosis, and portal hypertension. An association with cutaneous, hematologic, respiratory, and hepatic angiosarcoma has been observed.

Gold-induced enterocolitis affects both the small intestine and colon and produces severe ulcers in the small intestine and colon. Reversible cholestatic hepatitis has also been reported.

HEMATOLOGIC DISORDERS

Hemolytic uremic syndrome is characterized by hemolysis, thrombocytopenia, and acute renal failure. Thrombotic thrombocytopenic purpura is likely the same illness manifesting with fever and central nervous system sequelae. Enteric infection with *Salmonella*, *Shigella*, *Campylobacter* species, or *Escherichia coli* (especially O157:H7) is frequently causative. Thrombotic thrombocytopenic purpura also is reported in solid organ transplant recipients taking cyclosporine or tacrolimus. Gastrointestinal consequences include diarrhea, segmental colitis, ischemia, fulminant colitis with toxic megacolon, and perforation.

Hypercoagulability produces mesenteric vein thrombosis with intestinal ischemia and infarction. Hepatic vein occlusion produces ascites and the Budd-Chiari syndrome. Causes of hypercoagulability include oral contraceptives, pregnancy, inflammation, and surgery. Antithrombin III deficiency, protein C deficiency, and factor V Leiden mutations are inherited hypercoagulable disorders. Gastrointestinal hemorrhage may occur in patients with coagulation factor deficits, whether the condition is inherited (e.g., factor VIII deficiency in hemophilia A, factor IX deficiency in hemophilia B, factor XI deficiency), acquired (e.g., in the presence of lupus anticoagulant, vitamin K deficiency, liver disease), or iatrogenic (e.g., warfarin therapy). Gastrointestinal bleeding also occurs with platelet defects secondary to inherited diseases (von Willebrand disease, Bernard-Soulier syndrome, and Glanzmann thrombasthenia) and medications such as aspirin and nonsteroidal antiinflammatory drugs.

Acute sickle cell crisis produces abdominal pain, ileus, mucosal ulcers, and gastrointestinal hemorrhage, as well as jaundice, hepatomegaly, cholelithiasis, cholecystitis, and transfusion-related hemosiderosis or chronic hepatitis C infection. Splenomegaly is prevalent in early disease, but recurrent splenic infarctions lead to autosplenectomy and hyposplenism. Hemoglobin C disease has manifestations similar to those of sickle cell anemia, but attacks are milder and splenomegaly persists into adulthood. Transfusions also produce iron overload and chronic hepatitis C in patients with β-thalassemia. Hereditary spherocytosis is an autosomal dominant disorder with fragile erythrocytes that presents with indirect hyperbilirubinemia (as a result of hemolysis), jaundice, pigment gallstones, splenomegaly, and relapsing pancreatitis.

Plummer-Vinson (Paterson-Kelly) syndrome produces dysphagia (from hypopharyngeal or esophageal webs), iron deficiency anemia, glossitis, cheilosis, dyspepsia, diarrhea, flatulence, hoarseness, paresthesias, pyorrhea, koilonychia, atrophic gastritis, splenomegaly, and an increased risk of developing hypopharyngeal and esophageal malignancies. The role of iron deficiency anemia in the pathogenesis of the syndrome is not understood.

METABOLIC DISEASES

The systemic amyloidoses are a group of diseases with extracellular deposition of insoluble fibrillar proteins. Gastrointestinal manifestations include macroglossia, disrupted esophageal contractions, reduced lower esophageal sphincter pressure, prominent gastric and intestinal folds, gastric outlet obstruction, gastric ulcer, gastrointestinal hemorrhage, mesenteric retraction, intestinal obstruction, pseudoobstruction, bacterial overgrowth, intestinal ischemia, hepatosplenomegaly, and pancreatic exocrine insufficiency.

Gastrointestinal consequences of the capillary leak syndrome, an episodic illness characterized by increased small vessel permeability and fluid shifts, include nausea, vomiting, and diarrhea secondary to impaired gut fluid absorption.

NEOPLASTIC DISORDERS

Cancer cachexia is characterized by marasmus with anorexia, early satiety, weight loss, anemia, and edema secondary to increased catabolism of muscle and adipose tissue. Possible pathogenic factors include circulating substances with hormone-like effects as well as proinflammatory cytokines. Cancer chemotherapy produces a range of gastrointestinal side effects, including constipation, nausea, vomiting, diarrhea, hemorrhage, abdominal pain, and perforation. Necrotizing enterocolitis (also called typhlitis) complicates chemotherapy-induced neutropenia.

Gastrointestinal involvement with leukemia is common. Visceral leukemic infiltration causes oral pain and bleeding, dysphagia, obstruction, hemorrhage, and enterocolitis. Hepatosplenomegaly, portal hypertension, subcapsular splenic hemorrhage, and splenic rupture may also result from leukemic infiltration. Immunosuppressed leukemics are at risk for opportunistic infections caused by *Candida* organisms, herpesvirus, or cytomegalovirus. Up to 10% of patients with non-Hodgkin lymphoma exhibit gastrointestinal tract involvement that produces obstruction, hemorrhage, abdominal masses, and perforation. Hepatic and splenic invasion is frequent. In Hodgkin disease, presinusoidal portal hypertension is a consequence of increased intrahepatic blood flow from splenomegaly or intrahepatic infiltration with malignant cells. Rarely, enlarged mesenteric lymph nodes manifest as an abdominal mass or cause obstruction.

Plasmacytomas occurring during multiple myeloma produce abdominal pain, gastrointestinal ulceration, hemorrhage, and obstruction. Hyperviscosity may cause intestinal ischemia and mesenteric thrombosis. Amyloidosis is a recognized complication of multiple myeloma. Waldenström macroglobulinemia, an IgM-secreting variant of myeloma, produces hepatosplenomegaly and malabsorption from plasma cell infiltration of the liver, intestine, and lymph nodes. α-Heavy-chain disease causes infiltration of the intestine and abdominal lymph nodes with malignant B lymphocytes and α-chains. Symptoms and complications include abdominal pain, palpable masses, vomiting, weight loss, malabsorption, hypocalcemia, obstruction, intussusception, and perforation.

Polycythemia vera may cause Budd-Chiari syndrome from hepatic vein thrombosis, as well as abdominal fullness from hepatosplenomegaly due to extramedullary hematopoiesis). Essential or primary thrombocytosis predisposes to gastrointestinal bleeding, mesenteric thrombosis, and hepatosplenomegaly from extramedullary hematopoiesis or Budd-Chiari syndrome. Myelofibrosis with myeloid metaplasia presents with splenomegaly, portal hypertension, ascites, and variceal hemorrhage. Paroxysmal nocturnal hemoglobinuria is a myeloproliferative disorder characterized by intravascular hemolysis and severe venous thrombosis.

Nonhematologic malignancies also produce significant gastrointestinal complications. Malignant melanoma metastasizes to the stomach, small intestine, colon, liver, pancreas, and gallbladder. Symptomatic manifestations include abdominal pain, anorexia, hemorrhage, obstruction, intussusception, perforation, jaundice, and cholecystitis. Malignancies derived from breast, thyroid, and lung also can metastasize to the gut. Ovarian cancer can encase the abdominal viscera, producing intestinal obstruction. Renal cell carcinoma directly invades or metastasizes to the gut. Nonmetastatic hepatic dysfunction also complicates renal cell carcinoma. Gastrointestinal symptoms of mastocytosis include abdominal pain, nausea, diarrhea, fecal urgency, and malabsorption. Multiple endocrine neoplasias produce a variety of clinical syndromes that depend on the hormones secreted by tumors in different organ systems.

The main gastrointestinal manifestations of paraneoplastic syndromes are anorexia, dysphagia, nausea, vomiting, bloating, constipation, and diarrhea. Impaired gastrointestinal motor function results from paraneoplastic visceral neuropathy and from tumor-induced hypercalcemia.

NEUROMUSCULAR DISORDERS

Autonomic nervous system dysfunction in Parkinson disease, pandysautonomia, and paraneoplastic syndromes presents with vomiting, small intestinal bacterial overgrowth, intestinal pseudoobstruction, fecal incontinence, and constipation. In some patients, ingesting a meal may produce postprandial hypotension.

Dementia and chronic brain injuries are associated with oropharyngeal dysfunction, which increases the risk of aspiration pneumonia, progressive inanition, and malnutrition. Other consequences include fecal impaction and fecal incontinence. Acute brain injury secondary to stroke, trauma, tumor, or surgery produces gastric erosions, ulcerations (Cushing ulcer), and hemorrhage.

Gastrointestinal diseases associated with hiccups include gastroesophageal reflux, gastric obstruction, and stomach and esophageal tumors. Nongastrointestinal causes include foreign bodies in the ear canal; cervical tumors or adenopathy; central nervous system disease; metabolic disease; alcoholism; and disease of the mediastinum, pericardium, pleura, or diaphragm.

Gastrointestinal manifestations of migraine headaches include nausea, vomiting, abdominal pain, and diarrhea. Abdominal migraines are characterized by recurrent identical attacks of abdominal pain, no abdominal symptoms between attacks, a family history of migraine headache, and response to migraine therapy. Cyclic vomiting syndrome, a disorder primarily of children, presents with discrete episodes of relentless emesis and is associated with an increased tendency to develop migraine headaches later in life.

Multiple sclerosis causes anorectal dysfunction, gastroparesis, abnormal colonic motor activity, and oropharyngeal motor disturbances. Patients present with incontinence, nausea, vomiting, constipation, megacolon, and dysphagia.

Duchenne muscular dystrophy may cause nausea, vomiting, abdominal distention, constipation, acute gastric dilation, and pseudoobstruction as a consequence of impaired smooth muscle function. Myotonic dystrophy produces prominent gastrointestinal symptoms, including oropharyngeal dysphagia, aspiration, nausea, abdominal distention and pain, ileus, diarrhea, constipation, and symptomatic cholelithiasis. Mild aminotransferase elevations also may develop. Oculopharyngeal muscular dystrophy is associated with oropharyngeal dysphagia and pharyngo-oral and pharyngonasal regurgitation.

Gastrointestinal manifestations of Parkinson disease include oropharyngeal dysphagia, esophageal hypomotility, gastroparesis, constipation, megacolon, and pseudoobstruction. Many of these consequences of Parkinson disease are further exacerbated by medications given to treat the disorder.

Acute spinal cord injury causes ileus and predisposes to gastrointestinal bleeding. Constipation and fecal incontinence are chronic consequences of spinal injury. High spinal cord damage can impair gastric and small intestinal motor function, which causes gastric distention, gastroesophageal reflux, and ileus.

Amyotrophic lateral sclerosis commonly produces dysphagia due to loss of pharyngeal and upper esophageal control and rarely is associated with gastroparesis. Oropharyngeal dysfunction also occurs with myasthenia gravis and Kearns-Sayre syndrome. Stiff man syndrome may lead to dysphagia as a result of cricopharyngeal and upper esophageal spasm.

NUTRITIONAL DISTURBANCES

Kwashiorkor-marasmus syndromes are caused by protein-calorie undernutrition. Vitamin and mineral deficiencies, diarrhea (resulting from intestinal and pancreatic atrophy), and infectious complications (resulting from malnutrition-induced immunodeficiency) accompany this type of illness. Hepatomegaly, fatty liver, and chronic calcific pancreatitis may develop. Rapid refeeding with carbohydrate-rich solutions produces hypophosphatemia, hypokalemia, hypomagnesemia, and death in some cases.

Obesity predisposes to cholelithiasis, esophageal reflux, and fatty liver. Gastric surgery for obesity may lead to cholecystitis and deficiencies of vitamin B_{12}, folate, and iron, whereas jejunoileal bypass is associated with significant intestinal and hepatic complications.

ORGAN TRANSPLANT COMPLICATIONS

Gastrointestinal complications of bone marrow transplantation result from induction regimens (lethal doses of chemotherapy and radiation therapy), immunosuppression, graft-versus-host disease, and venoocclusive disease. Induction regimens cause oropharyngeal pain, nausea, vomiting, abdominal pain, diarrhea, and hemorrhage. Immune system dysfunction predisposes to bacterial and fungal (usually *Candida albicans*) infections in the initial 30 days after transplant and viral and parasitic infections thereafter. *Clostridium difficile* can cause severe and prolonged diarrhea without pseudomembrane production in neutropenic patients. Graft-versus-host disease may be acute (onset <100 days posttransplant) or chronic (onset >100 days posttransplant). Early manifestations include watery diarrhea, anorexia, nausea, vomiting, abdominal pain, hemorrhage, gastrointestinal perforation, and jaundice. Rarely, graft-versus-host disease occurs when blood is transfused from a first-degree relative to an immunocompromised recipient. Venoocclusive disease presents as hyperbilirubinemia, hepatomegaly, right upper quadrant pain, or sudden weight gain within 20 days of bone marrow transplantation.

Renal transplant recipients have increased risks of intestinal ischemia, diverticulitis, cytomegalovirus-induced colitis, intestinal tuberculosis, intra-abdominal abscess, and chronic hepatitis B and C infection. Complications of cardiac transplantation include gastrointestinal hemorrhage, pancreatitis, cholecystitis, and bowel perforation. Lung transplantation is associated with postoperative colonic perforation and an increased risk of vagal injury that causes dysphagia and gastric stasis. In addition to liver rejection and postoperative common bile duct ischemia, liver transplant patients can present with cytomegalovirus colitis or enterocolitis, pancreatitis, and gastrointestinal bleeding. Consequences of immunosuppressive therapy after solid organ transplant include opportunistic infections, medication-induced pancreatitis, and lymphatic malignancies.

PSYCHOLOGICAL DISORDERS

Emotional factors may cause or contribute to globus symptoms, noncardiac chest pain, functional dyspepsia, and irritable bowel syndrome. The complications of anorexia nervosa are mostly those of starvation, although gastroparesis that resolves with weight gain has been reported. Bulimia produces acute gastric dilation with rupture, dental enamel erosion, esophagitis, Mallory-Weiss tears, esophageal rupture, salivary type hyperamylasemia, and pancreatitis. Rumination syndrome may cause weight loss. Psychogenic vomiting, constipation, and other gastrointestinal complaints are manifestations of major depression or conversion disorder. Schizophrenics may present after ingesting a foreign body. Antipsychotic medications have significant anticholinergic activity that may cause gastric retention, megacolon, and constipation. Patients with Munchausen syndrome often feign gastrointestinal illnesses, including abdominal emergencies, hematemesis, and inflammatory bowel diseases.

PULMONARY DISEASES

Chronic cough and nocturnal asthma are atypical manifestations of gastroesophageal reflux disease. Life-threatening respiratory distress or pneumonia can result from aspiration of gastroenteric contents. Respiratory failure and mechanical ventilation may be complicated by gastrointestinal hemorrhage from erosive gastritis and ulcer disease. Chronic respiratory failure may also predispose to development of pneumatosis intestinalis. Acute exacerbation of chronic respiratory failure may lead to ischemic hepatitis secondary to arterial hypoxemia and elevated central venous pressure. The ZZ phenotype of α_1-antitrypsin deficiency is associated with the development of hepatic cirrhosis. Infants with cystic fibrosis may present with meconium ileus, intussusception, intestinal atresia, volvulus, and perforation. Chronic constipation, small intestinal obstruction, and rectal prolapse may develop in older children. Gastroesophageal reflux results from reduced saliva production, gastrointestinal hypomotility, chronic coughing, and postural drainage of pulmonary secretions. Pancreatic insufficiency leads to malabsorption of fat and nonfat nutrients. High doses of pancreatic enzyme supplements can lead to a fibrosing colopathy that presents with bloody diarrhea. Osteomalacia is a common sequela of chronic steatorrhea. Children with cystic fibrosis can develop biliary cirrhosis and progressive portal hypertension with secondary variceal hemorrhage.

RENAL FAILURE

Uremia produces dysgeusia, oral inflammation, parotitis, sicca syndrome, abdominal pain, anorexia, nausea, vomiting, diarrhea, constipation, pseudoobstruction, and intussusception. Gastrointestinal hemorrhage results most commonly from hemorrhagic gastritis or angiodysplasia. The incidence of pancreatitis in chronic renal failure is unknown. Mild hyperamylasemia is common, secondary to impaired renal clearance. Duodenal pseudomelanosis, pigmentation of the proximal duodenum with iron sulfide or hemosiderin, occurs with renal failure. Metastatic calcifications may be deposited in the mesenteric vessels, resulting in ischemia, hemorrhage, or infarction. Uremic patients develop hepatic friction rubs. Elevations in alkaline phosphatase are common, as are chronic hepatitis B and C infections. Chronic ambulatory peritoneal dialysis may predispose to bacterial peritonitis. Polycystic kidney disease is associated with hepatic cysts that may become infected.

SUBSTANCE ABUSE

Ethanol consumption can produce chest pain and esophagitis. Binge drinking may result in gastric erosions and hemorrhage. Diarrhea and malabsorption occur as consequences of enhanced small intestinal transit, reduced brush border enzyme activity, impaired absorption, pancreatic insufficiency, liver disease, and malnutrition. Other complications include pancreatitis, hepatic steatosis, hepatitis, cirrhosis, and carcinoma of the larynx, nasopharynx, esophagus, and liver. Hepatotoxicity is common with amphetamines and results from both immune mechanisms and hyperthermic liver injury. Anorexia and diarrhea are common with cocaine use, whereas intestinal ischemia, hepatocellular necrosis, and retroperitoneal fibrosis are rare complications. The practice of smuggling cocaine in swallowed condoms can produce intestinal obstruction or death if a condom ruptures internally. Gastrointestinal symptoms of opiate abuse include anorexia, nausea, vomiting, abdominal pain, and constipation. Intravenous use may lead to viral hepatitis, cirrhosis, hepatic abscess, or talc granulomas. Complications of tobacco smoking include carcinoma of the oropharynx, esophagus, and pancreas. Smokers are also at increased risk for exacerbations of ulcer disease and Crohn's disease.

VASCULITIDES

Gastrointestinal manifestations of Behçet disease include oral lesions resembling aphthous ulcers, esophageal ulcers (which may bleed, perforate, or lead to stricture), intestinal involvement resembling Crohn's disease (which may result in bleeding or perforation), and rare cases of Budd-Chiari syndrome. Disseminated fibrinoid necrosis of smaller arteries that occurs in giant cell arteritis can produce intestinal ischemia, abdominal pain, nausea, anorexia, weight loss, hemorrhage, and perforation. Henoch-Schönlein purpura causes abdominal pain, diarrhea, vomiting, obstruction, and intussusception, which may precede the onset of the characteristic purpuric rash. The bowel may exhibit edema, submucosal or subserosal hemorrhage, and thickened folds on radiographic or endoscopic evaluation. Polyarteritis nodosa is a systemic necrotizing vasculitis of small to medium-sized arteries, often caused by hepatitis B infection; it presents with epigastric pain, nausea, anorexia, mucosal ulceration, bleeding, diarrhea, appendicitis, cholecystitis, pancreatitis, obstruction, hepatic infarction, pseudomembranous colitis, pneumatosis intestinalis, peritonitis, and intra-abdominal abscess formation. Churg-Strauss syndrome is a systemic vasculitis that may lead to nausea, vomiting, hemorrhage, perforation, and cholecystitis. Vasculitis associated with Wegener granulomatosis can result in odynophagia secondary to esophageal ulcers, granulomatous inflammation of the stomach, intestinal or colonic ischemia, hemorrhage, and perforation. Circulating immune complexes in cryoglobulinemia may initiate vasculitis that involves the gut and produces cramping, enterocolitis, and, rarely, ischemia of the small intestine or colon.

CHAPTER 71

Gastrointestinal Manifestations of Immunologic Disorders

IMMUNODEFICIENCY DISEASES OF THE GUT

B-Lymphocyte (Antibody) Defects

X-Linked (Congenital or Bruton) Hypogammaglobulinemia

Etiology and Pathogenesis: X-linked (congenital or Bruton) hypogammaglobulinemia occurs predominantly in males and is characterized by low serum levels of all immunoglobulins (<100 mg/dL). The genetic defect results from mutations in the cytoplasmic signal transduction molecule, Bruton tyrosine kinase. An intrinsic B-lymphocyte defect with a maturation block in B-cell differentiation is present. Pre–B cells are present in bone marrow, but circulating B cells are absent.

Clinical features, diagnosis, and management: Patients present in infancy or early childhood (after loss of maternal IgG) with recurrent pyogenic infections that affect the gastrointestinal tract in 30% of cases. Diarrhea caused by *Campylobacter* species is the most common infectious condition. Perirectal abscesses, small intestinal bacterial overgrowth, and viral infections (hepatitis, enterovirus) also occur. Giardiasis is surprisingly uncommon. An increased incidence of lymphomas and leukemias has been reported. Rectal biopsies show a neutrophilic lamina propria infiltrate, crypt abscesses, and an absence of plasma cells. Treatment is with parenteral immunoglobulin replacement.

Selective Immunoglobulin A Deficiency

Etiology and pathogenesis: Selective IgA deficiency is the most prevalent primary immune deficiency. It usually occurs sporadically, although familial cases are reported and drugs (e.g., phenytoin, penicillamine, sulfasalazine) can produce reversible deficiency. Most patients lack serum and secretory IgA1 and IgA2. IgA deficiency is associated with celiac disease, pernicious anemia, Crohn's disease, and food allergies (Table 71-1).

Clinical features, diagnosis, and management: Most IgA-deficient persons are asymptomatic, but some people develop recurrent bacterial and viral sinopulmonary infections. Giardiasis occurs at the same rate in IgA-deficient patients as in the general population. Jejunal biopsies appear normal, but immunofluorescence reveals few or no IgA-producing cells and increased numbers of IgM-secreting cells. There is no specific treatment for IgA deficiency.

580

TABLE 71-1
Disorders that May Occur in Association with Immunoglobulin A Deficiency

Gastrointestinal associations
  Celiac disease
  Pernicious anemia
  Vitamin B_{12} deficiency secondary to bacterial overgrowth
  Intrinsic factor deficiency
  Nodular lymphoid hyperplasia
  Food allergy
  Crohn's disease
  Disaccharidase deficiencies (unproven)

Extraintestinal associations
  Collagen vascular diseases
  Atopy
  Malignancy (lymphoma, carcinoma [?])

Common Variable Hypogammaglobulinemia

Etiology and pathogenesis: Common variable hypogammaglobulinemia is a heterogeneous group of disorders that usually are sporadic but can be familial. It is characterized by an intrinsic defect in terminal B-cell differentiation and variable alterations in T-cell function. One third of patients exhibit atrophic gastritis and pernicious anemia, which confer an increased risk of gastric cancer. In contrast to classical pernicious anemia, common variable hypogammaglobulinemia exhibits an absence of mucosal plasma cells, a lack of autoantibodies, involvement of the entire gastric mucosa, and normal gastrin levels with defective gastrin release in response to meal or bombesin stimulation. Nodular lymphoid hyperplasia may involve most of the gut. The nodules consist of lymphoid follicles with germinal centers within the lamina propria with reduced or absent plasma cells. Lymphoid hyperplasia is thought to reflect B lymphocytes that cannot fully differentiate and is not a premalignant condition.

Clinical features, diagnosis, and management: Common variable hypogammaglobulinemia presents at a later age (second or third decade of life) with less severe infections than those of X-linked hypogammaglobulinemia. Recurrent respiratory infections or diarrhea (60% of cases) and steatorrhea are prevalent. Giardiasis is common and may cause extensive mucosal damage with malabsorption. Cryptosporidiosis, strongyloidiasis, and bacterial overgrowth with anaerobic species also occur but are less common. Infections caused by *Campylobacter* species may mimic ulcerative colitis. Intestinal biopsy specimens often show villous atrophy, but the lesion differs from celiac sprue in that there is a paucity of lamina propria plasma cells and the condition rarely responds to dietary gluten exclusion. Chronic liver disease occurs in 10% to 15% of patients, in many cases secondary to viral hepatitis acquired from intravenous immunoglobulin preparations; other causes include cholelithiasis, autoimmune hepatitis, sclerosing cholangitis, and biliary cryptosporidiosis. Nearly all patients require parenteral immunoglobulin replacement therapy.

Secretory Component Deficiency

The secretory component is essential for transepithelial delivery of IgA and IgM from the lamina propria to the lumen. Secretory component deficiency reduces lumenal IgA and IgM and is associated with intestinal candidiasis and diarrhea.

T-Lymphocyte Defects

Congenital Thymic Hypoplasia

Etiology and pathogenesis: Congenital thymic hypoplasia (DiGeorge syndrome) results from defective embryonic formation of the third and fourth pharyngeal pouches. It is characterized by absent T-lymphocyte function, hypoparathyroidism, and cardiovascular abnormalities. The syndrome is due to deletions in the short arm of chromosome 22.

Clinical features, diagnosis, and management: Neonates present with tetany or seizures and other congenital anomalies. Gastrointestinal manifestations include esophageal atresia, candidiasis, chronic diarrhea, and malabsorption.

Chronic Mucocutaneous Candidiasis

Etiology and pathogenesis: Chronic mucocutaneous candidiasis is a spectrum of syndromes characterized by increased susceptibility to *Candida* infections. The disease has variable association with Addison disease, diabetes, hypothyroidism, and hypoparathyroidism. One subset comprises the autoimmune polyglandular syndrome type I, a recessive disorder due to mutations in the AIRE gene.

Clinical features, diagnosis, and management: Patients present with recurrent oropharyngeal or esophageal candidiasis, which may be complicated by stricture formation and nutritional deficits. Therapy is with systemic antifungal agents.

Combined B-Lymphocyte and T-Lymphocyte Defects

Severe Combined Immunodeficiency Syndromes

Etiology and pathogenesis: Severe combined immunodeficiency syndromes are a group of disorders with defective B-lymphocyte and T-lymphocyte function and sometimes natural killer cells. The X-linked variant is caused by a mutation of the common cytokine receptor γ-chain, a component of receptors for several interleukins. Autosomal recessive types usually result from deficiencies of purine degradation enzymes. The variant syndrome of reticular dysgenesis has a coexisting granulocyte deficiency.

Clinical features, diagnosis, and management: Infants present with life threatening infection (cytomegalovirus, rotavirus), diarrhea, malabsorption, and failure to thrive. Graft-versus-host disease may develop because of exposure to maternal lymphocytes during delivery. Intestinal biopsies show absent plasma cells, partial villous atrophy, and macrophages in the lamina propria that stain positive to periodic acid–Schiff stain. Bone marrow transplantation is needed to prevent a fatal outcome. For associated adenosine deaminase deficiency, enzyme replacement with irradiated erythrocytes or enzyme conjugated to polyethylene glycol is possible.

Wiskott-Aldrich Syndrome

Etiology and pathogenesis: Wiskott-Aldrich syndrome is an X-linked recessive condition caused by defective T-lymphocyte function and poor antibody response to polysaccharide antigens. The defective gene encodes for a member of a family of proteins responsible for signal transduction from the cell membrane to the actin cytoskeleton in hematopoietic cells.

Clinical features, diagnosis, and management: Patients present with eczema, thrombocytopenia, recurrent infections, and development of lymphoma, as well as gastrointestinal manifestations (i.e., hemorrhage, diarrhea, malabsorption, colitis). Stem cell transplantation is curative.

Ataxia–Telangiectasia

Etiology and pathogenesis: Ataxia-telangiectasia is an autosomal recessive disorder of defective DNA repair mechanisms, with frequent chromosomal abnormalities and increased sensitivity to radiation. The responsible gene encodes a product similar to phosphatidylinositol-3-kinases, which are involved in signal transduction and cell cycle control. IgA deficiency is common.

Clinical features, diagnosis, and management: Manifestations include ataxia, oculocutaneous telangiectasia, recurrent sinopulmonary infections, and high incidences of lymphoreticular malignancies and adenocarcinoma. Mild abnormalities of liver function may be noted, and levels of α-fetoprotein are elevated.

Phagocytic Cell Defects

Chronic Granulomatous Disease

Etiology and Pathogenesis: Chronic granulomatous disease represents a group of disorders of defective phagocytic cell oxidative metabolism. The X-linked type is caused by mutation of the gene that encodes the β-subunit of cytochrome $\beta558$ that generates superoxide in phagocytes. Autosomal recessive types are caused by mutations in the α-subunit of $\beta558$ or in cytosolic proteins needed to activate NADPH. Microbicidal activity is defective because toxic oxygen metabolites (e.g., hydroxyl radical, hydrogen peroxide) are not generated. Susceptibility to pyogenic (*Staphylococcus* species, *Serratia marcescens*, *Salmonella* species, gram-negative enterococci) and fungal (*Candida* and *Aspergillus* species) infections increases, especially if organisms are catalase-positive.

Clinical features, diagnosis, and management: Patients usually present in infancy with infection, granuloma formation throughout the body, and pigmented, lipid-bearing tissue histiocytes. Hepatomegaly is common. Liver abscesses form in one third of cases and often require surgery. Gastrointestinal manifestations include gingivitis, stomatitis, antral strictures, perianal abscesses, *Salmonella* gastroenteritis, diarrhea, and malabsorption. Aggressive antimicrobial therapy is indicated.

Complement Deficiency

Hereditary Angioedema

Etiology and pathogenesis: The most common complement deficiency syndrome is hereditary angioedema, a disorder with decreased levels (85% of cases) or impaired function (15% of cases) of C1 esterase inhibitor. Most cases are inhibited in autosomal dominant fashion. The condition is believed to result from increased vascular permeability that is mediated by kinins, the production of which is inhibited by

C1 esterase inhibitor. Lymphoproliferative disorders, collagen vascular diseases, and certain drugs produce acquired deficiencies of C1 esterase inhibitor. Defective C5α inhibitor protein in serosal fluid occurs in familial Mediterranean fever.

Clinical features, diagnosis, and management: Patients present with painless, nonpruritic, nonpitting, subepithelial edema of the skin and mucous membranes. Attacks develop over the course of hours and may be precipitated by trauma, infections, or surgery. Gastrointestinal manifestations include abdominal pain, vomiting, diarrhea, tenderness, intussusception, fever, hypotension, and increased bowel sounds. Barium radiographs may show mucosal edema, whereas biopsy specimens show an absence of inflammatory infiltrates. The diagnosis is confirmed by measuring C1 esterase inhibitor. C4 levels may also be reduced. Anabolic steroids (e.g., danazol, stanozolol) can prevent attacks. C1 esterase inhibitor concentrate may be given for acute attacks.

SECONDARY IMMUNODEFICIENCIES

Immunodeficiency due to protein loss may complicate protein-losing enteropathy secondary to Ménétrier disease and Crohn's disease, as well as primary or secondary lymphatic obstruction. Protein-calorie malnutrition depresses the cell-mediated immune function. Corticosteroids increase the risk of infectious illness, including candidiasis. Systemic immune deficiency has been associated with increasing age.

FOOD HYPERSENSITIVITY

Etiology and Pathogenesis

Food hypersensitivity or allergy refers to reactions that are mediated by the immune system, whereas food intolerance describes non–immune-mediated adverse reactions. Reactions to food additives may be as important as allergy to natural food components. True food hypersensitivity is rare (0.3% to 7.5% in children), declines with age, and is more prevalent in atopic individuals. Conversely, food intolerance is reported by 20% of adults. Uptake of ingested antigens and presentation to the mucosal immune system occurs by three routes: M cells overlying lymphoid follicles, intestinal enterocytes that absorb antigens and stimulate suppressor T cells, and antigen sampling across the epithelium by dendritic cells. Local IgA secretion follows ingestion of dietary antigens, but a systemic immune response rarely develops because of immune tolerance. Food hypersensitivity from a breakdown in oral tolerance usually results from ingesting milk, eggs, nuts, fish, shellfish, soybeans, and wheat. Food hypersensitivity may be immediate (IgE-mediated, type I) or delayed (late-phase IgE-mediated, immune complex–mediated, and cell-mediated). Plasma histamine levels rise in patients who have gastrointestinal symptoms elicited by food challenge, which indicates a central role for mast cell degranulation in food hypersensitivity. Eosinophils may partially mediate in the late phase of food allergy and may contribute to allergy-related dysmotility.

Clinical Features, Diagnosis, and Management

Patients present with eczema, urticaria, rhinitis, asthma, abdominal symptoms, and even anaphylaxis within minutes to hours of ingesting food. Chronic diarrhea and malabsorption may arise from non–IgE-mediated delayed hypersensitivity. Th diagnosis of food hypersensitivity relies on demonstrating that ingesting the implicated food reproducibly induces symptoms and on showing that immune mechanisms are involved. Because food challenges and skin testing may trigger anaphylaxis, diagnostic testing should be performed in facilities that can manage serious allergic reactions. Direct skin testing using the prick technique with food extracts is a simple and sensitive method for detecting mast-cell–bound IgE antibodies. A positive test result (i.e., a wheal >3 mm larger than a control solution wheal) indicates the presence of sensitizing antibodies but does not confirm food hypersensitivity. Skin testing should not be performed on patients with known anaphylaxis. Rather, in vitro assays for allergen-specific IgE antibodies may be used. Systematic elimination of different foods may identify foods that induce allergic reactions. The most restrictive elimination diet is an elemental diet, which can provide useful information if patients report allergies to multiple foods or cannot identify specific foods to which they are allergic. Double-blinded, placebo-controlled food challenges are the most reliable method of confirming food hypersensitivity but should be avoided in patients with prior anaphylaxis. Direct challenge of the intestinal mucosa with food antigen extracts using colonoscopy has been used in some instances.

The only acceptable treatment of food hypersensitivity is avoiding the offending food. Antihistamines and corticosteroids may play secondary roles in symptom control. Oral or parenteral immunization (hyposensitization) has not been shown to reduce food allergy, but breast feeding until the age of 6 months may have a protective effect against its development.

EOSINOPHILIC GASTROENTERITIS

Etiology and Pathogenesis

Eosinophilic gastroenteritis is probably not a single condition but rather a heterogeneous group of disorders with similar features, including eosinophilic infiltration of the gut wall. Allergic phenomena have been proposed as one cause for eosinophilic gastroenteritis; however, some patients have no atopic symptoms, the response to dietary elimination is usually disappointing, and many patients have no family history of allergy.

Clinical Features, Diagnosis, and Management

With mucosal involvement, patients present with diarrhea, cramping, nausea, vomiting, abdominal pain, malabsorption, weight loss, protein-losing enteropathy, occult fecal bleeding, anemia, growth retardation in children, and, rarely, perforation. Charcot-Leyden crystals secondary to lumenal eosinophil extrusion may be seen on stool inspection. Barium radiographs show diffuse mucosal nodularity, lumenal narrowing, widening of small bowel segments, and antral cobblestoning. Intestinal biopsies exhibit diffuse eosinophilic infiltration of the mucosa. When eosinophilic gastroenteritis involves the muscular layers of the gut, patients report nausea, vomiting, pain, and distention. Barium studies demonstrate irregular antral or intestinal narrowing, but mucosal biopsies may not be helpful. Eosinophilic infiltration of the serosa produces eosinophilic ascites or pleural effusions. Some cases of gastroesophageal reflux represent a localized form of eosinophilic infiltration, eosinophilic esophagitis, that may reflect food allergy or a hypersensitivity phenomenon.

A trial of an elemental diet can eliminate a role for food hypersensitivity. Prednisone is effective therapy for most patients with eosinophilic gastroenteritis, although repeat courses or prolonged administration is often necessary. The long-term prognosis is favorable, although the disease follows a waxing and waning course. Some patients require total parenteral nutrition.

GASTROINTESTINAL COMPLICATIONS OF ORGAN TRANSPLANTATION

Intestinal Disease Secondary to Induction

The combination of chemotherapy and radiation therapy before bone marrow transplantation produces immediate intestinal necrosis. Regeneration of the mucosa can take up to 3 weeks (Table 71-2). Anorexia, cramping, abdominal pain, and diarrhea result from damage to the small intestine and colon. Stool cultures are obtained to exclude infection. Rectal biopsies show no evidence of graft-versus-host disease or opportunistic infection. Treatment includes supportive measures and total parenteral nutrition.

Acute Graft-Versus-Host Disease

Etiology and Pathogenesis

Acute graft-versus-host disease (GVHD), which may occur 3 or more weeks after bone marrow transplantation, consists of dermatitis, mucositis, enteritis, and hepatic dysfunction. Acute GVHD is characterized by epithelial cell death. The induction phase involves primarily CD4 lymphocytes transferred with the donor graft that recognize disparities with recipient major histocompatibility complex antigens as foreign. Activation of donor T cells within tissues is followed by clonal expansion and subsequent cytokine and chemokine release to recruit additional inflammatory cells.

Clinical Features, Diagnosis, and Management

The typical presentation of acute GVHD is profuse, watery diarrhea (up to 10 L per day). The severity of gastrointestinal symptoms usually parallels the severity of skin (erythematous, maculopapular rash on the palms, soles, and trunk) and liver involvement. Other symptoms include anorexia, vomiting, buccal mucositis, abdominal pain, hemorrhage (esophagitis, gastric erosions), and protein loss. Barium radiography exhibits bowel wall edema, pneumatosis cystoides intestinalis, and mucosal ulcerations that may normalize or, in some cases, take on a chronic, segmental ribbon-like appearance. Endoscopy shows erythema or mucosal sloughing, which is most prominent in the ileum, cecum, and ascending colon. The earliest histological change is apoptosis of individual intestinal crypt cells, which is diagnostic if observed in normal-appearing tissue 20 days after transplantation. Later changes, including total denudation of the mucosa, are not as specific. Cholestasis and mild hepatocellular necrosis are common with acute GVHD. Management consists of nutritional support, fluid and electrolyte resuscitation, administration of steroids and immunosuppressants (cyclosporine, antithymocyte globulin, anti–T-cell monoclonal antibodies), and vigilance for secondary infections. Octreotide may reduce high-output diarrhea.

TABLE 71.2

Gastrointestinal Complications of Bone Marrow Transplantation

VARIABLE	SECONDARY TO INDUCTION	ACUTE GVHD	CHRONIC GVHD
Onset after transplant	0 – 20 days	20 – 80 days	>80 days
Clinical features	Anorexia, abdominal pain, diarrhea	Large-volume diarrhea, pain, ± rash, ± liver disease	Dysphagia, oral ulcers, diarrhea
Radiography	Not helpful	Mucosal edema, mucosal ulcers, pneumatosis	Esophageal strictures and webs
Endoscopy and manometry	Nonspecific	Normal, erythema, sloughing	Esophageal bands, webs
Histology	Cell atypia, crypt cell regeneration	Apoptosis (early) mucosal disintegration (late)	Neutrophil infiltration, basal cell necrosis
Stool findings	Negative	Negative for pathogens, cellular debris, increased protein	Negative

GVHD, graft-versus-host disease.

Chronic Graft-Versus-Host Disease
Etiology and Pathogenesis
Chronic GVHD occurs 80 to 400 days after bone marrow transplantation, most often in patients who have had prior acute GVHD. It predominantly involves the skin, liver, and gastrointestinal tract and is characterized by fibrosis and atrophy rather than inflammation.

Clinical Features, Diagnosis, and Management
Gastrointestinal involvement affects the mouth (mucositis), esophagus (dysphagia, gastroesophageal reflux), and small intestine (patchy fibrosis of the lamina propria and submucosa and bacterial overgrowth secondary to dysmotility). Esophageal disease is often associated with skin involvement (hyperpigmentation and scleroderma-like changes). Endoscopic findings range from generalized desquamation of the upper and middle esophagus to web-like fibrous bands. Esophageal manometry and pH testing may reveal nonspecific motor abnormalities and prolonged acid exposure. Histological changes in the esophagus include infiltration with neutrophils and lymphocytes, necrosis of individual cells of the basal mucosa, and submucosal fibrosis. The liver in chronic GVHD exhibits abnormal interlobular bile ducts followed by destruction of small bile ducts and proliferation of ductules. Prednisone alone or in combination with azathioprine is often effective. Antireflux therapy should be initiated, but esophageal dilation may be needed to treat progressive web and stricture development.

Small Intestinal Transplantation

Small intestinal transplantation has high morbidity and mortality because of rejection, sepsis, and posttransplant lymphoproliferative disorder. Rejection predisposes to sepsis because of loss of the mucosal barrier function. Crypt cell apoptosis characterizes acute rejection, whereas chronic rejection exhibits fibrosis, focal ulcers, and obliterative arteriopathy. Lymphoproliferative disorder is likely to be related to infection with Epstein-Barr virus. Graft-versus-host disease is not a major obstacle to intestinal transplantation.

CHAPTER 72

Skin Lesions Associated with Gastrointestinal and Liver Diseases

CUTANEOUS MANIFESTATIONS OF INFLAMMATORY BOWEL DISEASE

Patients with inflammatory bowel disease (IBD) may present with several immunologically mediated cutaneous disorders (Table 72-1). Reactive inflammatory vascular dermatoses manifest as generalized, localized, or annular erythema. These may be associated with drug or transfusion reactions, occult carcinoma, infections, or the underlying inflammatory condition. Urticaria is dermal edema and erythema that resolve within 24 hours; angioedema is a similar lesion that occurs in deep dermal or subcutaneous regions. In patients with IBD, urticaria usually results from medications or from causes independent of the underlying gastrointestinal illness. Therapy for urticaria relies on removing the offending agent and using antihistamines.

Erythema multiforme is an acute, self-limited mucocutaneous syndrome with target-like skin lesions that may be accompanied by serum sickness symptoms (e.g., fever and arthralgias), which may result from IBD or the drugs used to treat it. The minor form of erythema multiforme is limited to the skin, whereas the major form is more severe with significant mucosal involvement, a condition known as the Stevens-Johnson syndrome. Toxic epidermal necrolysis, which overlaps the Stevens-Johnson syndrome, manifests as a burn-like appearance, is usually drug-induced, and has a 30% mortality rate. Gastrointestinal complications of toxic epidermal necrolysis include esophagitis and esophageal stricture. Therapy generally consists of corticosteroids; ophthalmologic consultation is recommended for eye involvement.

Tender, nonulcerated, subcutaneous nodules that are found usually on the lower extremities characterize erythema nodosum. Associated symptoms include fever, malaise, arthralgias, and arthritis. The incidence of erythema nodosum is 7% with ulcerative colitis but is lower with Crohn's disease. The lesion is thought to be caused by immune complex deposition in vessels within subcutaneous fat. Erythema nodosum generally resolves with control of the underlying disease, although NSAIDs or acetaminophen may be used to reduce systemic symptoms.

Palpable purpura is caused by leukocytoclastic vasculitis, which affects postcapillary venules and is characterized by endothelial swelling, leukocytoclasis, extravasation of erythrocytes, neutrophilic invasion, and fibrinoid necrosis of blood vessel walls. Similar vascular lesions may occur in the central and peripheral nervous system, synovium, pleura, pericardium, gastrointestinal tract, and kidneys. The mainstay of treatment consists of controlling the underlying disease. Severe cases may require corticosteroids, immunosuppressives, or plasmapheresis.

TABLE 72-1
Cutaneous Conditions Associated with Inflammatory Bowel Disease

Erythemas (including annular erythemas)

Urticaria

Erythema nodosum

Necrotizing vasculitis

Larger vessel necrotizing vasculitis

Pustular vasculitis

Pyoderma gangrenosum

Oral lesions
    Specific granulomas (Crohn's disease only)
    Aphthosis
    Angular cheilitis
    Pyostomatitis vegetans

Metastatic Crohn's disease

Finger clubbing

Acquired acrodermatitis enteropathica (zinc deficiency)

Striae

Epidermolysis bullosa acquisita

Psoriasis

Exfoliative erythroderma

Vitiligo

Lichen nitidus

Lichen planus

IBD, celiac disease, rheumatoid arthritis, diabetes mellitus, dermatitis herpetiformis, and select chronic infections are associated with erythema elevatum diutinum. This lesion is a chronic fibrosing dermatosis that is caused by immune complexes. Firm, tender, red to yellow-brown papules and plaques appear on the extensor surfaces of extremities. Histologically, there is a leukocytoclastic vasculitis, subepidermal fibrin deposition, and dermal papillary edema. Oral dapsone is the treatment of choice.

Pyoderma gangrenosum appears as a cutaneous ulcer with a purple undermined border that worsens with local trauma and may heal with cribriform scarring. Underlying IBD should be excluded for any patient with pyoderma gangrenosum, although chronic hepatitis, rheumatoid arthritis, and myeloproliferative disorders may produce similar cutaneous findings. Pyoderma gangrenosum is treated aggressively with corticosteroids, immunosuppressives, or sulfones because of the risk of local infection or sepsis. Anti–tumor necrosis factor (TNF) antibody therapy may prove beneficial.

A lesion similar to pyoderma gangrenosum, Sweet syndrome, or acute febrile neutrophilic dermatosis, appears as tender cutaneous erythematous papules and plaques located on the upper extremities, head, and neck. The lesions may ulcerate and become purulent and may be accompanied by fever and peripheral blood neutrophilia. The etiology is thought to be a hypersensitivity reaction, and the histological appearance includes a vascular reaction with dermal inflammatory neutrophilic infiltrates and leukocytoclasia. Therapy consists of dapsone, prednisone, or other immunosuppressive agents.

Oral lesions are common in IBD. Aphthous ulcers or angular stomatitis are seen in 30% of patients with ulcerative colitis. Crohn's disease is associated with granulomas of the lips and mouth, which may be nodular or present in a cobblestone pattern. Patients with numerous oral aphthous ulcers should be evaluated to exclude ulcerative colitis, Crohn's disease, and Behçet disease. Pyostomatitis vegetans is an oral papular eruption with a cobblestone appearance and is associated with IBD.

Other cutaneous manifestations of IBD include "metastatic" Crohn's disease (i.e., noncaseating cutaneous granulomas), pustular vasculitis, and other skin disorders that relate to specific nutritional deficiencies.

CUTANEOUS MANIFESTATIONS OF RHEUMATOLOGIC DISEASES

Dermatomyositis is an inflammatory condition affecting skin and muscle, which may manifest gastrointestinal symptoms such as dysphagia because striated muscles of the pharynx and esophagus are involved. Cutaneous lesions include periungual telangiectasia, cuticular dystrophy, and violaceous poikiloderma (hypopigmentation or hyperpigmentation, telangiectasia, epidermal atrophy), which may present over the eyes (heliotrope rash), knuckles (Gottron sign), and extensor surfaces. Dermatomyositis may develop as a paraneoplastic phenomenon.

Scleroderma may present as one of several forms: a localized cutaneous form (morphea); a relatively mild systemic CREST variant (calcinosis, Raynaud phenomenon, esophageal dysmotility, sclerodactyly, telangiectasia); or more severe, progressive systemic sclerosis. Sclerosis occurs acrally, periorally, and on the trunk. A salt-and-pepper pigment change may be noted over sclerotic areas in darker skinned patients. Telangiectases are boxlike or matlike on the face, hands, oral mucosa, and other sites. Esophageal disease leads to acid reflux; therefore acid suppression should be administered to reduce esophageal fibrosis.

Behçet disease is defined by the presence of oral aphthous ulcers in the absence of IBD or collagen vascular disease plus two or more of the following symptoms: genital aphthous ulcers, synovitis, posterior uveitis, cutaneous pustular vasculitis, and meningoencephalitis. Aphthous ulcers may occur at any gastrointestinal site with Behçet disease. The oral aphthous ulcers of Behçet disease can be differentiated clinically from the psoriasiform oral lesions of Reiter disease. Recurrent herpes simplex must be excluded as a cause of the oral and genital lesions. Histological examination of cutaneous pustular vasculitis reveals either leukocytoclastic vasculitis or a neutrophilic vascular reaction. The synovitis produces an asymmetric, migratory, nonerosive oligoarthritis.

A bowel-associated dermatosis-arthritis syndrome develops in 20% of patients after jejunoileal bypass for morbid obesity. Pustular vasculitic lesions, arthritis, and a serum sickness–like illness with fever, myalgias, and arthralgias characterizes this syndrome. A similar syndrome may occur with IBD or after creating a blind loop during ulcer surgery (e.g., Billroth II). The skin lesions appear in crops that last 1 to 2 weeks and occur at intervals from one to several months. The syndrome may resolve with systemic antibiotics (e.g., metronidazole, tetracycline, or erythromycin), systemic corticosteroids, oral dapsone, or by the restoration of normal intestinal anatomy.

Amyloidosis is characterized by the deposition of an abnormal protein with characteristic staining properties and electron microscopic features in the extracellular space. Primary amyloidosis is associated with gastrointestinal, cardiac, and renal disease. Other features may include macroglossia and cutaneous lesions such as papules, plaques, and nodules with pinch purpura; however, patients with secondary amyloidosis do not manifest cutaneous disease.

SKIN DISEASE AND GASTROINTESTINAL HEMORRHAGE

A variety of disorders exhibit cutaneous lesions and present with gastrointestinal hemorrhage. Hereditary hemorrhagic telangiectasia, or Osler-Weber-Rendu disease, is an autosomal dominant disorder that is associated with numerous 1-mm to 3-mm telangiectasias on the lips, tongue, face, hands, chest, and feet. Aneurysms and arteriovenous malformations may affect mucocutaneous and internal organs.

Blue rubber bleb nevus syndrome is an autosomal dominant disorder characterized by cutaneous, blue-colored, rubbery, compressible, and sometimes painful nodular vascular malformations up to 10 cm in diameter. Bleeding or intussusception may result from involvement of the small or large intestine, oropharynx, nasopharynx, esophagus, stomach, peritoneal cavity, mesentery, liver, lung, penis, eye, and central nervous system.

Kaposi sarcoma, which occurs in the acquired immunodeficiency syndrome (AIDS) and in an endemic form in elderly persons of Mediterranean descent, is a tumor derived from proliferating endothelial cells. The cutaneous lesions range from reddish-purple macules to large vascular tumors. The lesions typically begin on the lower extremities, extending proximally in association with peripheral edema. Gastrointestinal involvement includes the small intestine, stomach, esophagus, and colon, in decreasing order of frequency, and may result in hemorrhage and partial bowel obstruction.

Malignant atrophic papulosis (Degos disease) is an idiopathic disease that affects the skin, gastrointestinal tract, and central nervous system. The cutaneous lesions are discrete, painless papules with umbilicated porcelain-white centers surrounded by telangiectatic rims. Patients who have gastrointestinal involvement with this condition may present with fatal gastrointestinal hemorrhage.

In addition to the aforementioned vascular diseases, gastrointestinal bleeding may complicate the course of many connective tissue diseases. Pseudoxanthoma elasticum is a genetic disorder characterized by elastic fiber alterations that produce cutaneous, visceral, ocular, and cardiovascular lesions. Cutaneous findings include yellow papules and plaques that affect the buccal mucosa, neck, axilla, and other flexures. Intestinal lesions consist of yellow, cobblestone-appearing mucosa that is associated with upper and lower tract hemorrhage. Ehlers-Danlos syndrome, a heterogeneous group of genetic disorders with defective collagen production, produces hyperextensible and fragile skin with impaired wound healing, purpura from easy bruising, cigarette burn–like scars, "fish-mouth" scars, and pseudotumors over joints. Visceral involvement leads to hemorrhage and perforation. Cutis laxa, a group of autosomal and X-linked disorders characterized by abnormalities of elastic fibers, leads to the appearance that the skin is too large for the patient's body, with areas of sagging and wrinkling. Gastrointestinal involvement includes diverticula and hernias. Neurofibromatosis (von Recklinghausen disease) is an autosomal dominant disorder with cutaneous lesions consisting of café au lait macules axillary freckles, and cutaneous neurofibromas. Gastrointestinal ulceration, bleeding, volvulus, obstruction, perforation, and intussusception may occur as a result of neurofibroma formation in the tongue, gallbladder, stomach, and jejunum, or less commonly, in the esophagus and colon. Therapy for symptomatic disease is surgical.

CUTANEOUS FINDINGS IN GASTROINTESTINAL POLYPOSIS SYNDROMES

A variety of cutaneous features suggest the presence of hereditary or sporadic gastrointestinal polyposis syndromes. Gardner syndrome is a form of familial adenomatous polyposis that presents in adolescence with osteomas and epidermoid cysts of the scalp, face, and extremities. Patients with Gardner syndrome also develop desmoid tumors, which are locally aggressive but nonmetastatic fibrous tumors that affect the mesentery and abdominal wall. Peutz-Jeghers syndrome, like Gardner syndrome, is an autosomal dominant disease. Patients present in childhood with multiple gastrointestinal hamartomatous polyps and melanotic macules involving the lips, palms, soles, digits, periorbital skin, anus, and buccal mucosa. Cronkhite-Canada syndrome is a sporadic disorder defined by alopecia, onychodystrophy, intestinal polyps, and cutaneous hyperpigmented macules that coalesce to form plaques primarily on the upper extremities, occasionally with the development of vitiligo. Multiple hamartoma syndrome, or Cowden disease, is an autosomal dominant disorder whose cutaneous lesions include facial and oral mucosal papules (trichilemmomas), oral cobblestoning, acral keratoses, lipomas, hemangiomas, neuromas, café au lait macules, and a scrotal appearance of the tongue. Muir-Torre syndrome is an autosomal dominant condition with multiple visceral carcinomas in association with cutaneous sebaceous neoplasms (i.e., hyperplasia, adenoma, epithelioma, and carcinoma), basal cell carcinomas, and keratoacanthomas. Adenomatous polyps are not present in all patients with Muir-Torre syndrome, but colonic adenocarcinoma may develop in addition to urogenital, hematologic, and breast cancers.

CUTANEOUS SIGNS OF GASTROINTESTINAL MALIGNANCY

Certain characteristic skin lesions should raise concern for gastrointestinal malignancy. Metastatic nodules derived from gastrointestinal adenocarcinoma appear as firm, pink, dermal to subcutaneous masses in the abdomen or pelvis. The Sister Mary Joseph nodule is an indurated nodule of the umbilicus that suggests gastric or colonic adenocarcinoma. Carcinoma erysipeloides, an erythematous plaque that mimics cellulitis, results from direct involvement of the lymphatics by tumor. Extramammary Paget disease is a cutaneous adenocarcinoma that appears as an erythematous scaling or lichenified patch with surface erosion and crusting. If it is located in a perianal site, it suggests rectal or cloacogenic carcinoma. Therapy includes surgery or radiation therapy, but recurrence is common. Acanthosis nigricans is a condition characterized by smooth, thickened, hyperpigmented skin in body fold areas such as the axilla and neck. It is associated with gastric adenocarcinoma and other tumors. Interestingly, acanthosis nigricans precedes the diagnosable tumor by several years in up to 20% of patients; alternatively, it may indicate metastatic disease in patients with known malignancy. Remission of acanthosis nigricans parallels the cure of the underlying neoplasm. Tylosis is a diffuse or punctate yellow hyperkeratosis of the palmar or plantar surfaces that may be present in patients with gastrointestinal malignancy, especially esophageal squamous cell carcinoma. The Howel-Evans syndrome is an autosomal disorder in which 95% of those affected develop esophageal carcinoma and tylosis by age 65. Generalized erythroderma is observed in some patients with gastrointestinal lymphoma, esophageal, or occult carcinoma, although it may also be seen with primary skin disease or drug reactions. Hypertrichosis lanuginosa acquisita is the rapid appearance of fine, downy hair on the trunk and face that is associated with pulmonary and gastrointestinal malignancy, including colon, gallbladder and pancreatic cancer. Patients with Plummer-Vinson (Paterson-Kelly) syndrome have koilonychia (brittle, spoon-shaped nails), atrophic tongue, and angular stomatitis in association with iron deficiency anemia and dysphagia.

The carcinoid syndrome is characterized by flushing (a bright-red color on the face, chest, trunk, and extremities lasting 10 to 30 minutes), rosacea-like telangiectasia, and edema. It may be exacerbated by alcohol, certain foods, and stress. Therapy consists of octreotide, the synthetic octapeptide of somatostatin. Necrolytic migratory erythema is associated with glucagonoma, an islet cell tumor of the pancreas. The lesion consists of erythema, erosions, superficial necrosis, and scale involving the perioral, abdominal, and perineal regions. Angular cheilitis and a red, swollen tongue may also be present. Intravenous amino acid supplementation or octreotide may be useful therapy.

BULLOUS SKIN DISEASES THAT AFFECT THE GASTROINTESTINAL TRACT

Epidermolysis bullosa is a spectrum of diseases, inherited either dominantly or recessively, in which blisters occur spontaneously, often at sites of friction. The major gastrointestinal sites of involvement are the mouth, esophagus and anus. Esophageal lesions present with dysphagia, often caused by bullae or web-like scar ring near the cricopharyngeal area. Anal involvement may produce constipation. Pyloric atresia is rarely the presenting manifestation in infants. Epidermolysis bullosa acquisita, an acquired form, is a late-onset disorder that is associated with IBD.

Pemphigus vulgaris presents with oral erosions and cutaneous lesions that are characterized by acantholytic blistering and by the presence of IgG in the intraepidermal space on biopsy. Lower gastrointestinal involvement may produce hemorrhage.

Bullous pemphigoid occurs in older patients and consists of tense cutaneous bullae, with oral involvement in one third of cases and less often in the esophagus or anus. Bullous pemphigoid has been associated with gastrointestinal malignancy, especially colonic carcinoma. Biopsies of the cutaneous lesion reveal subepidermal blistering with linear IgG deposition in the basement membrane zone.

SKIN CONDITIONS ASSOCIATED WITH ABDOMINAL PAIN

Patients with variegate porphyria present with episodic abdominal pain and blisters and erosions in sun-exposed areas, which may progress to milia formation, hyperpigmentation, facial hypertrichosis, and sclerosis. The skin findings in the lysosomal storage condition, Fabry disease, consist of punctate, small (1 mm), nonblanching red-blue angiokeratomas from the abdomen to the knees. Reduced sweat production may occur with this disease. Mastocytosis is a disorder of mast cell proliferation with pruritic red-brown macules (urticaria pigmentosa) that develop wheals or vesicles when stroked (Darier sign). Varicella-zoster virus reactivation in the T7 through L1 dermatomes may produce abdominal pain in association with clustered vesicles. Angioedema, characterized by edema in a deep dermal or subcutaneous location, may present as part of a hereditary or acquired C1 esterase deficiency syndrome or after ingesting certain medications. The condition may result in gastrointestinal mucosal edema and abdominal pain.

Pancreatic disease is associated with certain cutaneous findings. Periumbilical purpura (Cullen sign) and left flank purpura (Grey-Turner sign) represent the retroperitoneal dissection of blood along fascial planes from acute hemorrhagic pancreatitis. Pancreatitis may also be associated with panniculitis that appears as tender, red, subcutaneous nodules, most commonly in the pretibial region. Pancreatic carcinoma or pancreatitis may induce fat necrosis, which produces regions of fluctuance in the skin. The eruption of yellow-red papules over extensor surfaces and the buttocks in a patient with pancreatitis suggests eruptive xanthomatosis secondary to hypertriglyceridemia or type IV or V hyperlipoproteinemia.

CUTANEOUS LESIONS ASSOCIATED WITH LIVER DISEASE

Jaundice is the yellow discoloration of skin, mucous membranes, and sclera from the accumulation of bilirubin and its metabolites. It is generally recognizable when blood levels of bilirubin exceed 2.5 mg/dL. Pruritus may be a symptom of patients with cholestasis, cirrhosis, chronic hepatitis C, primary sclerosing cholangitis, and the cholestasis of pregnancy. The last may be successfully treated with ursodeoxycholic acid (ursodiol); other forms of pruritus may respond to corticosteroids, photochemotherapy, antihistamines, opiate antagonists (naloxone, nalmefene, naltrexone), bile acid sequestering agents (cholestyramine, colestipol), rifampin, and serotonin antagonists (ondansetron).

Polyarteritis nodosa is characterized by tender, palpable purpuric nodules and livedo. It is associated with fever, arthralgias, malaise, and fibrinoid necrotizing arteritis. Its presence is linked to hepatitis B, hepatitis C, parvovirus B19, and human immunodeficiency virus infection. Treatment consists of corticosteroids. Cryoglobulins are immune complexes that deposit in blood vessels, creating a clinical syndrome similar to polyarteritis nodosa. Symptoms are worsened by exposure to cold weather. Hepatitis C, hepatitis B, and persistent hepatitis A are viral infections associated with cryoglobulinemia.

A variety of other skin lesions are associated with liver disease. Gianotti-Crosti syndrome, or papular acrodermatitis of childhood, presents as erythematous papules on the extremities and face that resolve after 2 to 4 weeks and is associated with hepatitis B or Epstein-Barr virus infection. Hepatitis C, primary biliary cirrhosis, and other liver diseases are associated with lichen planus, a mucocutaneous condition consisting of pruritic, purple, polygonal papules with Wickham striae and white mucosal plaques. Therapy includes corticosteroids, dapsone, photochemotherapy, methotrexate, and thalidomide. Chronic hepatitis C can be documented in 90% of patients presenting with porphyria cutanea tarda (PCT). Clinically, PCT appears as subepidermal bullae, milia, and scarring that usually affect the back of the hands, along with photosensitivity, hypertrichosis and hyperpigmentation of the face, and iron overload. Therapy includes phlebotomy, antimalarials, deferoxamine, and thalidomide. The melanin content of the skin may be increased in chronic liver disease, manifesting as diffuse or patchy grayish mucocutaneous pigmentation. Vascular changes, such as spider angiomata and palmar erythema, are thought to occur secondary to altered estrogen metabolism. Nails may take on an opaque whitish and pink discoloration (Terry nails) in cirrhosis or a blue discoloration of the distal nail (azure lunula) among patients with Wilson disease. Urticaria, urticarial vasculitis, erythema multiforme, erythema nodosum, and pyoderma gangrenosum can occur in liver disease.

SKIN CONDITIONS FROM MALNUTRITION AND MALABSORPTION

Certain cutaneous lesions may suggest specific malabsorptive disorders. Dermatitis herpetiformis is strongly associated with celiac sprue. This skin condition is characterized by intense pruritus and multiple, grouped vesicles distributed symmetrically, especially on the scalp and extensor surfaces of the extremities. Histologically, there is subepidermal blistering with neutrophilic infiltration of the dermal papillae and IgA deposition at the dermal-epidermal junction or within the dermal papillae. Even in the absence of gastrointestinal symptoms, patients with dermatitis herpetiformis generally display villous atrophy of the small intestine with an inflammatory infiltration that is gluten sensitive. The skin lesions respond to dietary gluten restriction, dapsone, or sulfapyridine.

There is considerable overlap in the cutaneous manifestations of the specific nutrient deficiency syndromes. Marasmus (total starvation) is characterized by dry, loose skin, loss of subcutaneous fat, and thinning of hair. In kwashiorkor (carbohydrate excess with protein deficiency), there are hypopigmented or hyperpigmented scaling patches and purpura with epidermal peeling over joints or flexural areas (flaky paint sign). In contrast to marasmus, edema is present. Hair pigment may show alternating dark and light bands (flag sign). Cutaneous lesions in essential fatty acid deficiency, especially linoleic acid, include diffuse, erythematous scaling, alopecia, and traumatic purpura.

Vitamin A deficiency is characterized by multiple keratotic papules on the extremities (phrynoderma) with mucosal keratinizing metaplasia. Conversely, vitamin A excess causes alopecia, a sunburned appearance, cheilitis, skin fragility, and brittle nails. Deficiencies in B vitamins (riboflavin, pyridoxine, niacin) produce seborrheic dermatitis of the face, perioral and groin regions, and a smooth tongue. Niacin deficiency (pellagra) causes painful, eroded, pigmented, scaling patches in sun-exposed sites. Appearance of this lesion on the upper chest is known as a *Casal necklace*. Cutaneous manifestations of vitamin B_{12} deficiency include generalized hyperpigmentation of the palms, soles, and nails, whereas white hair, alopecia areata, or vitiligo may occur in pernicious anemia. Folate deficiency may cause a lemon-yellow skin discoloration. Purpura, petechiae, perifollicular hemorrhages, corkscrew hairs, and gingival erosions are manifestations of vitamin C deficiency. Zinc deficiency (acrodermatitis enteropathica) is associated with erythematous, scaling, vesiculopustular or eroded plaques that are acrally distributed. Alopecia, impaired wound healing, stomatitis, and secondary candidal infections are common.

PERINEAL SKIN LESIONS

A variety of distinct cutaneous findings may occur in the perianal or perineal area (Table 72-2). Crohn's disease causes perianal erosions and ulcers. Vesicles or erosions on an erythematous base suggest possible herpes simplex, whereas infection

TABLE 72-2
Perineal Skin Lesions

Erythema with scale or maceration
  Contact dermatitis
  Seborrheic dermatitis
  Psoriasis
  Candidiasis
  Dermatophytosis
  Secondary syphilis
  Extramammary Paget disease
  Nutritional deficiencies
  Bowen disease

Vesicles, erosions, ulcers
  Herpes simplex
  Varicella-zoster virus
  Impetigo (streptococcal, staphylococcal)
  Syphilis (primary or secondary)
  Chancroid
  Deep, fungal, acid-fast bacilli, or protozoal infections
  Bullous pemphigoid
  Pemphigus
  Ecthyma

Nodules, tumors, ulceration
  Condyloma acuminata
  Hidradenitis suppurativa
  Squamous or basal cell carcinoma
  Crohn's disease
  Carcinoma
  Kaposi sarcoma
  Granulomatous herpes simplex

with varicella-zoster virus produces dermatomal clustering of vesicles. Other infections such as amebiasis, primary and secondary syphilis, and nontreponemal venereal disease also cause ulcers and erosions in this region. Condyloma acuminata (venereal warts) appear as flesh-colored, pedunculated papules. Erythema with scaling or maceration in the gluteal fold suggests candidal infection, psoriasis, seborrheic dermatitis, contact dermatitis from fecal soiling, or bacterial impetigo. The clinical presentation, skin scrapings prepared with potassium hydroxide, and culturing may be used to determine the etiology. Biopsy is indicated to exclude extramammary Paget disease if lesions do not respond to treatment. Idiopathic pruritus ani presents commonly in middle-aged men with superimposed psychological factors and responds to removal of any triggering factors, careful cleaning techniques, topical or locally injected corticosteroids, or cryosurgery.

CHAPTER 73

Vascular Lesions: Ectasias, Tumors, and Malformations

A variety of vascular lesions manifest in the gastrointestinal tract. They can be broadly categorized as ectasia, vascular neoplasia, and other vascular lesions (Table 73-1).

DIEULAFOY LESION

Incidence and Epidemiology

The Dieulafoy lesion is an arterial malformation associated with massive gastrointestinal hemorrhage; it accounts for 1.5% of acute upper gastrointestinal bleeding episodes. In addition to lesions in the stomach and duodenum, Dieulafoy lesions have also been reported in the jejunum, ileum, colon, and rectum. The mean age at presentation is 55, although the range is wide. Men are affected twice as often as women.

Etiology and Pathogenesis

The Dieulafoy lesion is a caliber-persistent arteriole; an abnormally large submucosal vessel. It is not known whether the lesion is congential or acquired. Relatively minor trauma may injure the vessel and initiate hemorrhage. In 75% of patients with upper gastrointestinal Dieulafoy, the lesion is located in the proximal stomach. It rarely forms in the esophagus but can affect the distal stomach (13%) and duodenum (12%). It is not associated with the use of alcohol, nonsteroidal antiinflammatory agents, tobacco, or *Helicobacter pylori* infection.

Clinical Features

Upper gastrointestinal Dieulafoy lesions usually present with massive upper gastrointestinal bleeding and an absence of associated gastrointestinal symptoms. Hypotension, orthostasis, tachycardia, and prerenal azotemia are common. Lower gastrointestinal lesions manifest as hematochezia with hemodynamic instability.

Findings on Diagnostic Testing

Upper gastrointestinal endoscopy is the principal means of diagnosing an upper tract Dieulafoy lesion. There may be a pigmented protuberance, identifying the vessel stump, and an adherent clot with little surrounding edema. No ulceration is present; if one is seen, the visualized lesion is a visible vessel in an ulcer, not a Dieulafoy lesion. Lesions of the colon are similar in appearance to upper tract

TABLE 73-1
Vascular Lesions of the Gastrointestinal Tract

Vascular ectasia disorders
Angiodysplasia
Gastric antral vascular ectasia ("watermelon stomach")
Telangiectasia associated with multisystem disease (e.g., hereditary hemorrhagic
telangiectasia, CREST syndrome, Turner syndrome)

Vascular tumors
Hemangiomas
Multiple-hemangioma syndromes (e.g., intestinal hemangiomatosis, universal
hemangiomatosis, blue rubber bleb nevus syndrome, Klippel-Trénaunay-Weber
syndrome)
Malignant vascular tumors (e.g., angiosarcoma, hemangiopericytoma, Kaposi
sarcoma)

Other vascular lesions
Dieulafoy lesion
Miscellaneous (e.g., multiple phlebectasia, pseudoxanthoma elasticum,
Ehlers-Danlos syndrome)

CREST syndrome = calcinosis, Raynaud phenomenon, esophageal dysmotility, sclerodactyly, and
telangiectasia.

lesions. Active bleeding may obscure endoscopic visualization, in which case angiography may be used to identify the bleeding vessel.

Management and Course

Initial management consists of fluid resuscitation and replacement of blood loss. Acid suppression is of no benefit. Endoscopic therapy is used to treat the Dieulafoy lesion: injection therapy with epinephrine or polidocanol, bipolar electrocoagulation, thermal coagulation, laser photocoagulation, band ligation, and hemoclips. Up to 85% of patients achieve long-term hemostasis with this approach. Angiography with selective left gastric artery embolization has been used with limited success to treat gastric Dieulafoy lesions. If nonsurgical attempts to control bleeding fail, surgical vessel ligation, wedge resection, or proximal partial gastrectomy may be necessary. Colonic lesions unresponsive to endoscopic therapy should be managed surgically. Mortality averaged 25% in the past, but diagnostic and therapeutic advances have dramatically improved the survival of patients with this condition.

ANGIODYSPLASIA

Incidence and Epidemiology

Angiodysplasia consists of dilated, tortuous, thin-walled blood vessels lined by endothelium with little or no smooth muscle. Vascular ectasias that occur in association with lesions of the skin or other organs are termed *telangiectasias*. Angiodysplasia and telangiectasia are endoscopically and histologically identical; the terminology only separates the clinical syndromes.

About 2% to 5% of upper and 3% to 6% of lower gastrointestinal hemorrhage is attributed to angiodysplasia. Precise estimates are difficult, in part because angiodysplasia is commonly found in asymptomatic people; about 1% of healthy subjects who undergo colonoscopy have colonic angiodysplasia. Patients who bleed from colonic angiodysplasia are generally older than 60 years, but cases have been reported in infants and children. Race and gender do not influence the prevalence of these lesions. Angiodysplasia is not familial, although hereditary hemorrhagic telangiectasia is. Although the majority of angiodysplasias occur in the right colon and cecum, 40% are found distal to the hepatic flexure.

Etiology and Pathogenesis

The increased prevalence of angiodysplasia in the elderly has led to the theory that it results from aging-associated degeneration of vascular integrity. Chronic obstruction of venous outflow at the level of the muscularis appears to be the initial pathophysiological defect, leading to dilation of submucosal veins and capillaries. It is possible that neurovascular or hormonal mechanisms may induce angiodysplasia in response to local hypoperfusion.

Angiodysplasia has been associated with several diseases. The prevalence of angiodysplasia reportedly increased with aortic stenosis; however, more recent studies fail to confirm this association. Angiodysplasia is cited as the most common cause of gastrointestinal bleeding in patients with renal failure (19% to 32%), but the pathophysiological link between angiodysplasia and chronic renal failure is controversial. Increased prevalence of angiodysplasia with scleroderma or CREST syndrome, Turner syndrome, and portal hypertension has also been reported.

Clinical Features

Angiodysplasia clinically manifests with painless gastrointestinal hemorrhage. Most colonic lesions are located in the right colon and are associated with low-grade chronic bleeding or iron deficiency anemia, but 10% to 15% of patients present with acute massive hemorrhage. Up to 60% of patients have multiple angiodysplasias within the same portion of the intestinal tract. Although the percentage of angiodysplastic lesions that bleed is unknown, autopsy series suggest that most do not produce clinically evident bleeding.

Findings on Diagnostic Testing

Endoscopy is the procedure of choice for diagnosing angiodysplasia. Upper gastrointestinal endoscopy, small bowel enteroscopy, capsule endoscopy, and colonoscopy are the primary methods for identifying angiodysplasia in the gastrointestinal tract. The lesions range in diameter from 0.2 to 1.0 cm and typically are discrete and bright red, composed of a dense reticular network of vessels. Angiography may identify colonic angiodysplasia overlooked on colonoscopy or angiodysplasia lesions in the small intestine not visualized by enteroscopy plus capsule endoscopy. The characteristic angiographic findings include a vascular tuft during the arterial phase of the study, rapid filling of the dilated vein, and slowly emptying veins. Because angiodysplasias bleed only intermittently, angiography demonstrates active bleeding in only 10% to 20% of patients. ^{99m}Tc-labeled erythrocyte scintigraphy is more sensitive in detecting acute hemorrhage, but it can identify only the general region of bleeding. Patients with acute lower tract bleeding should undergo emergency colonoscopy or erythrocyte scintigraphy as the initial imaging procedure. Positive erythrocyte scans should be followed by angiography or colonoscopy.

Management and Course

Many angiodysplasias are asymptomatic and are incidentally noted by endoscopy for nonbleeding indications. About one quarter of patients who bleed from angiodysplasia experience recurrent hemorrhage within 1 year, and one half rebleed over a 3-year period. Any therapeutic intervention for these patients must consider this natural history of angiodysplasia. Patients with mild, chronic blood loss who do not require transfusion are best managed conservatively with oral iron supplements. Several reports have suggested a benefit from estrogen alone or in combination with progesterone, especially for patients with renal failure or hereditary hemorrhagic telangiectasia. Other series have failed to demonstrate decreased transfusion requirements. Although the efficacy of hormonal therapy for sporadic angiodysplasias remains in question, an empirical trial of oral contraceptives containing low-dose estrogen is often worthwhile for selected patients. Gynecomastia in males and recurrent menstruation in postmenopausal females may limit compliance. Hormonal therapy should be avoided for patients with histories of thromboembolism, atherosclerotic disease, or hormone-sensitive neoplasms.

Patients with acute bleeding or chronic bleeding who require transfusion should undergo more invasive therapy. Successful outcomes have been reported using multiple endoscopic methods, including heater probe thermocoagulation, electrocoagulation with multipolar or argon plasma coagulation, photocoagulation using Nd:YAG lasers, and injection therapy with alcohol or epinephrine. Local expertise and availability dictate the preference for instruments to control hemorrhage. In all series evaluating endoscopic therapy, multiple sessions are often necessary, and 50% of patients experience persistent or recurrent bleeding (presumably from angiodysplasia at other sites).

Angiography may be used to provide selective intraarterial infusion of vasopressin to control acute bleeding, which is successful in 50% to 90% of cases. One third of patients rebleed after infusion; thus angiographic embolization is often required to prevent recurrent hemorrhage. Complications of embolization include abdominal pain, fever, and occasionally bowel infarction, which necessitates emergency colectomy.

If medical and endoscopic therapies fail to control bleeding, surgical resection should be considered. Preoperative angiography can often define the extent of angiodysplasia in the small intestine and the colon. Recurrent hemorrhage after surgery occurs in one quarter to one third of patients and is generally from unresected lesions in the remaining intestine.

GASTRIC ANTRAL VASCULAR ECTASIA

Incidence and Epidemiology

Gastric antral vascular ectasia (GAVE), also known as "watermelon stomach," is a distinctive syndrome of vascular ectasias localized in the gastric antrum. The mean age at presentation is 70 (range: 50 to 90), with a female-to-male ratio of 5:1. Although endoscopic surveys have been limited, the disorder is rare and is observed in less than 0.03% of upper endoscopic examinations.

Etiology and Pathogenesis

The etiology of GAVE remains unknown, although a trophic mechanism is suggested by elevated tissue concentrations of gastrin, prostaglandin-E2, and 5-hydroxytryptamine. Alternatively, repeated mucosal trauma secondary to pyloric prolapse is suggested based on the location of similar lesions elsewhere in the body. GAVE is associated with hypochlorhydria, cirrhosis, bone marrow transplantation, and scleroderma, which may also provide insight into its pathogenesis.

Clinical Features and Diagnosis

GAVE generally presents with iron deficiency anemia from chronic occult gastrointestinal bleeding. Acute upper gastrointestinal hemorrhage is uncommon, and the lesion is painless.

Upper gastrointestinal endoscopy is the only definitive means of diagnosing GAVE. There is a characteristic appearance of erythematous longitudinal antral folds that converge toward the pylorus in a pattern reminiscent of a watermelon. Distinguishing GAVE from other gastropathies is based on the endoscopic pattern of dilated vessels or by demonstrating that the lesions blanch when compressed with biopsy forceps. Biopsy specimens reveal hypertrophied mucosa, dilated and tortuous mucosal capillaries occluded by fibrin thrombi, and dilated or tortuous submucosal veins. Angiography and barium radiography are generally of limited diagnostic value for this condition.

Management and Course

Patients may require iron supplementation and blood transfusion. Endoscopic therapy with multipolar or argon plasma electocoagulation, heater probe coagulation, or laser therapy successfully controls bleeding, but multiple sessions may be required. Endoscopic therapy is generally well tolerated but is associated with complications, including perforation, stenosis, ulceration, and recurrent hemorrhage. Estrogen-progesterone therapy and other medical therapies have been largely anecdotal and are of uncertain clinical benefit. A transjugular intrahepatic portosystemic shunt (TIPS) is not effective in controlling hemorrhage. If patients do not respond to endoscopic therapy, antrectomy is essentially curative.

SYSTEMIC TELANGIECTASIA SYNDROMES

When vascular ectasias occur in conjunction with vascular lesions of the skin or other organs, they are termed *telangiectasias*. Hereditary hemorrhagic telangiectasia, also known as *Osler-Weber-Rendu syndrome*, is an autosomal dominant disorder associated with vascular ectasia of the skin, mucous membranes, and internal organs. The disease prevalence is about 10 per 100,000 population, with equal gender distribution. Patients usually present in childhood with recurrent and severe epistaxis. Gastrointestinal hemorrhage occurs in 25% of cases. Bleeding from a source in the upper intestinal tract, characterized by melena and hematemesis, is more common than lower tract bleeding. Bleeding from a posterior nasal or pharyngeal source presents similarly and should be considered in the differential diagnosis. The diagnosis of hereditary hemorrhagic telangiectasia should be considered in individuals with telangiectasia, recurrent epistaxis, and compatible family histories. Gastrointestinal lesions are identified by endoscopic examination, and most are located in the stomach and duodenum. Endoscopic thermocoagulation, electrocoagulation, and photocoagulation are effective in controlling bleeding. Estrogen-progesterone therapy improves epistaxis and may reduce the rate of gastrointestinal bleeding. The role of surgery is limited because of the diffuse nature of the disorder.

Bleeding gastrointestinal telangiectasias also occur in the CREST (calcinosis, Raynaud phenomenon, esophageal dysmotility, sclerodactyly, and telangiectasia) variant of progressive systemic sclerosis. These patients have vascular lesions on the hands, lips, face, and tongue, as well as other signs of systemic sclerosis. Gastrointestinal hemorrhage is not a dominant feature of this disorder but has been reported from telangiectasias in the colon, stomach, and small intestine. The therapeutic approach is similar to that for sporadic angiodysplasia.

HEMANGIOMAS

Incidence and Epidemiology

The prevalence of hemangiomas is about 1 per 15,000 population. Hemangiomas are benign vascular growths that usually are detectable at birth or shortly after birth but often do not produce symptoms until young adulthood (often in the third decade of life). They are a rare etiology of gastrointestinal hemorrhage, although the precise incidence is unknown.

Etiology and Pathogenesis

Hemangiomas are hamartomas that result from abnormal vascular development in the intestinal wall. There are three types: capillary, cavernous, and mixed. Capillary hemangiomas are usually located in the small intestine and are composed of discrete clusters of thin-walled, tiny vessels, the caliber of normal capillaries. Cavernous hemangiomas are found mainly in the rectum and distal colon and can be polypoid (circumscribed) or expansive (diffuse). Cavernous lesions are clusters of dilated, thin-walled vascular channels separated by scant stromal tissue. Mixed lesions exhibit both capillary and cavernous features. Growth characteristics, especially of cavernous hemangiomas, suggest that hemangiomas are benign neoplasms rather than congenital hamartomas.

Clinical Features

Many hemangiomas are asymptomatic, but the most common clinical presentation is gastrointestinal hemorrhage. Capillary hemangiomas tend to cause low-grade chronic bleeding with iron-deficiency anemia, but cavernous lesions may produce massive bleeding. Most cavernous lesions are located in the rectosigmoid region, so painless hematochezia is a common presenting symptom. Polypoid and expansive lesions may cause nausea, vomiting, and abdominal pain as a result of obstruction or intussusception. Multiple hemangiomas throughout the digestive tract, a condition termed *intestinal hemangiomatosis*, affect 10% of patients. In the rare neonatal syndrome of universal hemangiomatosis, cavernous lesions are disseminated to other organs, including the brain and skin. Two other rare disorders associated with diffuse cutaneous and gastrointestinal hemangiomas are the blue rubber bleb nevus syndrome and Klippel-Trénaunay-Weber syndrome. In the former, cutaneous lesions affect the limbs, trunk, and face. Their blue color and rubbery consistency are the source of the syndrome's descriptive name. Lesions also occur throughout the gastrointestinal tract and may produce occult bleeding. In the latter syndrome, patients have distinctive soft tissue and bony hypertrophy of one limb. Gastrointestinal lesions are cavernous and are usually located in the rectum.

Findings on Diagnostic Testing

Upper and lower gastrointestinal endoscopy can diagnose hemangiomas in the stomach, proximal duodenum, and colon. Capillary lesions appear as punctate red nodules, whereas cavernous lesions are violet-blue, sessile, polypoid lesions. The color, submucosal location, and compressibility distinguish the latter from colonic adenomas. On barium radiography, larger lesions can be mistaken for adenomatous polyps or carcinoma. Angiography and capsule endoscopy are useful for detecting hemangiomas in the small intestine. The characteristic pooling of contrast in the venous phase is a typical finding in angiographic images of large cavernous lesions but may be absent in images of small lesions.

Management and Course

Small capillary hemangiomas may be amenable to endoscopic obliteration by coagulation, band ligation, or polypectomy, but large cavernous lesions have high rates of massive hemorrhage or perforation using this therapy. Symptomatic sporadic hemangiomas are best managed by surgical resection. In disorders with multiple gastrointestinal hemangiomas, conservative therapy with iron supplementation is recommended initially. Persistent hemorrhage or obstruction at a defined site requires surgical resection.

MISCELLANEOUS VASCULAR LESIONS

Angiosarcomas, epithelioid hemangioendotheliomas, and hemangiopericytomas are malignant neoplasms that originate from the cellular components of blood vessels. All may be complicated by gastrointestinal hemorrhage or obstruction. Kaposi sarcoma is another vascular neoplasm that frequently disseminates to the gastrointestinal tract. This represents one of the most common causes of gastrointestinal bleeding in patients with acquired immunodeficiency syndrome. Gastrointestinal bleeding also occurs in patients with pseudoxanthoma elasticum, as a result of an abnormal vascular structure. This disorder of elastin synthesis typically presents with bleeding from arterioles in the gastric fundus. Gastrectomy is the definitive therapy.

Ehlers-Danlos syndrome is a heterogeneous group of genetic disorders of collagen metabolism. Patients characteristically have skin hyperextensibility, bruise easily, and have hypermobile joints. Diagnosis is by clinical presentation, family pedigree analysis, and identifying genetic or biochemical defects. Patients with type IV Ehlers-Danlos syndrome can present with gastrointestinal hemorrhage from spontaneous arterial rupture due to vascular and perivascular connective tissue fragility. There is an increased risk of intramural intestinal hematomas, colonic diverticular hemorrhage, and intestinal perforation.

CHAPTER 74

Mesenteric Vascular Insufficiency

ISCHEMIA OF THE SMALL INTESTINE

Incidence and Epidemiology

Intestinal ischemia accounts for about 1 in 1000 hospital admissions. Both acute and chronic forms of mesenteric ischemia exist. Embolization to the superior mesenteric artery accounts for about one half of all cases of acute mesenteric ischemia; arterial thrombosis (15%), venous thrombosis (5% to 10%), and nonocclusive ischemia (20% to 30%) comprise the remainder of cases (Table 74-1). A common source of an embolus is the heart of a patient who is in atrial fibrillation or who has an akinetic ventricular wall. Thrombotic occlusion usually occurs in mesenteric vessels that are atherosclerotic. Acute mesenteric venous thrombosis can be the consequence of an intra-abdominal inflammatory process such as appendicitis, inflammatory bowel disease, or diverticulitis. Although many cases are idiopathic, a large proportion of these patients have underlying hypercoagulable conditions. Conditions associated with low-flow states such as congestive heart failure also predispose to venous thrombosis. Nonocclusive mesenteric ischemia almost invariably occurs in profound hypotension caused by hemorrhagic or cardiogenic shock. Chronic mesenteric ischemia, otherwise known as intestinal angina, is characterized by transient, recurrent episodes of inadequate intestinal blood flow to meet metabolic requirements. This form of ischemia generally affects middle-aged and elderly people, with a female-to-male ratio of 3:2. Atherosclerosis is the most common cause of chronic mesenteric insufficiency, thus this syndrome is associated with diabetes, hyperlipidemia, and tobacco use. Mesenteric ischemia affects young persons less commonly, in which case the disorder is secondary to penetrating trauma, strangulation obstruction of the small intestine, vasculitis, and celiac artery compression syndrome.

Etiology and Pathogenesis

Mesenteric ischemia occurs when splanchnic blood flow is insufficient to maintain adequate nutrient delivery to the small intestine. The microvascular network of the splanchnic circulation embodies several anatomic and physiological adaptive mechanisms to maintain oxygen delivery. An acute reduction in the arterial perfusion pressure of the intestinal tract results in a compensatory dilation of the resistance arterioles. This autoregulation maintains adequate tissue perfusion in acute mesenteric artery occlusion. In systemic hypotension, however, the more efficient autoregulatory mechanisms in other organs and activation of the autonomic nervous system and the renin-angiotensin axis result in disproportionate decreases in splanchnic blood flow. This systemic response also increases the tone of venous

---

TABLE 74-1
Factors That Predispose to Mesenteric Ischemia

Arterial embolism
Atrial fibrillation (recent cardioversion)
Prior embolic event
Prosthetic valve
Recent myocardial infarction or myocardial dyskinesia
Recent vascular instrumentation
   Cardiac catheterization
   Angioplasty
   Angiography

Arterial thrombosis
Aortic dissection or aneurysm
Atherosclerosis
Diabetes
Hypercholesterolemia
Hypertension
Trauma
Vasculitis

Venous thrombosis
Cardiopulmonary bypass
Congestive heart failure
Hypercoagulable states
Inflammatory conditions (appendicitis, inflammatory bowel disease)
Pericardial tamponade
Venous obstruction

Nonocclusive mesenteric ischemia
Aortic insufficiency
Cardiogenic or hypovolemic shock
Congestive heart failure
Dialysis
Pulmonary edema
Major cardiac or abdominal surgery
Vasoconstrictive drugs

---

capacitance vessels, augmenting systemic venous return to the heart to maintain cardiac output. The net result is a redistribution of blood flow from the gastrointestinal tract to the brain, heart, kidney, and skeletal muscles. Angiotensin-mediated vasoconstriction of the splanchnic resistance arterioles results in nonocclusive mesenteric ischemia and most cases of ischemic colitis.

Injury to the bowel occurs from both the initial decrease in blood flow and the restoration of flow, known as reperfusion injury. Several mechanisms have been implicated in the pattern of injury, including initiation of an inflammatory response, production of reactive oxidants, and an imbalance between proinflammatory and protective mechanisms. The rolling phenomenon refers to a transient adhesive interaction mediated by the selectin family of adhesion molecules that regulates leukocyte infiltration, which is a key component of the inflammatory response in low-flow states. Xanthine oxidase is an important enzyme for producing superoxide and hydrogen peroxide and is abundant in intestinal epithelial cells. Finally, reperfusion injury may result from decreases in nitric oxide production coupled with increases in the production of reactive oxygen species that occur in the reperfusion period. Loss of the gut barrier permits entry of enteric bacteria. Bacterial endotoxins and exotoxins may play an important role in the systemic and hemodynamic complications of mesenteric ischemia.

An extensive network of collaterals between the systemic and splanchnic circulation and between the three major splanchnic vascular beds provides additional protection from ischemia caused by segmental occlusion. The celiac axis communicates with the superior mesenteric vessels through the pancreaticoduodenal cascade, and the superior mesenteric vessels connect with the inferior mesenteric vessels by way of marginal vessels connecting the middle colic and left colic arteries. In chronic ischemia, these collaterals can become quite large; therefore, the clinical syndrome of intestinal angina does not occur unless at least two of the three major mesenteric arteries are diseased. A small number of patients with chronic mesenteric ischemia may have obstruction of the celiac axis from extrinsic compression by the median arcuate ligament of the diaphragm. It is important to understand that collateral flow is established by vasodilation of resistance arterioles in the ischemic segment. Therefore, vasodilating agents used to treat intestinal ischemia caused by nonocclusive vasospasm may preferentially dilate other vascular beds, compromising collateral flow in the spastic segment.

Risk factors for small intestinal ischemia include hypercholesterolemia, diabetes, and hypertension. Both hypercholesterolemia and diabetes appear to be associated with increased production of radical oxygen species and enhanced recruitment of leukocytes in hypoperfused tissue. Hypertension may alter the inflammatory response to ischemia.

Clinical Features

Acute Mesenteric Ischemia

Abdominal pain out of proportion to physical findings is the hallmark of acute mesenteric ischemia. The character of the pain may be either localized or diffuse; it is generally colicky but may become constant with the progression of ischemia. The onset of pain caused by thrombus formation may be more gradual than the onset of pain related to embolic occlusion. The clinical severity of the syndrome usually depends on the presence or absence of collateral flow from the celiac axis and inferior mesenteric circulation. If collaterals are well developed, thrombotic occlusion may not produce significant morbidity. Pain may not be present in up to 20% of patients with nonocclusive mesenteric ischemia and may be difficult to elicit in confused or critically ill patients. Other presenting signs and symptoms include abdominal distension, gastrointestinal bleeding, fever, diarrhea, nausea, vomiting, and diminished bowel sounds. The presence of abdominal tenderness, rebound, rigidity, decreased urine output, or hyperventilation due to acidosis is indicative of transmural bowel infarction.

Chronic Mesenteric Ischemia

Chronic mesenteric ischemia, also called intestinal angina, is characterized by the classic triad of postprandial abdominal pain, chronic weight loss, and sitophobia (fear of eating). The abdominal pain is analogous to angina pectoris and lower extremity claudication. Pain typically develops 30 to 90 minutes postprandially and may last several hours. Physical examination usually reveals evidence of peripheral vascular disease. Abdominal findings are nonspecific, although many patients have abdominal vascular bruits. Despite the diffuse reduction in splanchnic arterial flow, acute mesenteric infarction rarely complicates the course of intestinal angina.

Findings on Diagnostic Testing

Laboratory Studies

Patients with acute intestinal ischemia may not have laboratory abnormalities. Only with intestinal infarction will patients develop leukocytosis, lactic acidosis, and hyperamylasemia. Other nonspecific abnormalities include elevations of serum alkaline phosphatase and creatine phosphokinase levels. However, these abnormalities are nonspecific and simply reflect the systemic inflammatory response or tissue necrosis. Elevations in the hematocrit are indicative of fluid sequestration, which is particularly severe in mesenteric venous thrombosis.

Structural Studies

Abdominal radiographs should be obtained to exclude obstruction of the small intestine. Occasionally, edematous or hemorrhagic mucosa will appear as a "thumbprinting" pattern on the bowel wall. As intestinal infarction occurs, air may dissect the bowel wall, producing pneumatosis cystoides intestinalis. Twenty-five percent of abdominal radiographs of mesenteric ischemia will be normal. Although free intraperitoneal air indicates perforation, this finding is not always present. Ultrasound with Doppler evaluation of the splanchnic vessels is especially useful in documenting large vessel stenosis in chronic intestinal angina. Dynamic contrast-enhanced computed tomographic scans are a sensitive means (90% to 100%) for diagnosing mesenteric venous thrombosis; however, it is an insensitive method for detecting arterial occlusion or nonocclusive mesenteric ischemia. In contrast to ischemic colitis, endoscopy is not useful in evaluating patients with suspected mesenteric ischemia.

Magnetic Resonance Angiography

Magnetic resonance angiography (MRA) is more sensitive than computed tomography for diagnosing severe stenoses or occlusion of the origins of the celiac axis and superior mesenteric artery. It is also highly sensitive and specific for venous thrombosis. MRA cannot assess more peripheral arterial occlusions, nor is it helpful in diagnosing nonocclusive mesenteric ischemia.

Angiography

The cornerstone for evaluating patients with mesenteric ischemia is angiography. In addition to its diagnostic and therapeutic capacity, angiography is often critical in planning operative reconstruction. In arterial embolic occlusion, there is usually an abrupt obstruction within the initial 3 to 10 cm of the superior mesenteric artery. A lack of associated collaterals provides ancillary evidence that the obstruction is acute. It may be difficult to distinguish arterial thrombosis from embolic occlusion, but with thrombosis, atherosclerotic narrowing of the superior mesenteric artery usually is prominent and collaterals are often well developed. The venous phase of angiography can identify the presence and site of mesenteric thrombosis. In nonocclusive mesenteric ischemia, arteriography usually reveals multiple areas of narrowing and irregularity in the main vessels, with an absence of small to medium sized arterial branches. In most cases, there is evidence of vasospasm and absence of the typical arterial blush in the bowel wall. Chronic mesenteric ischemia invariably presents with high-grade stenosis of at least two vessels. Because most patients with mesenteric ischemic syndromes have associated cardiovascular and atherosclerotic disease, many patients have coexisting atherosclerotic stenosis of the splanchnic arteries. Distinguishing clinically significant lesions from incidental atherosclerosis requires synthesizing historical, physical, and radiologic information.

Surgery for Diagnosis

Diagnostic laparoscopy or laparotomy is indicated for patients with suspected intestinal infarction or suspected obstruction and strangulation of the small intestine, for both diagnosis and definitive surgical therapy.

Management and Course

The initial goal of therapy for patients with acute mesenteric ischemia is fluid resuscitation and restoration of hemodynamic stability. Hypovolemia is multifactorial, caused by sequestration of fluids due to ischemic injury of the bowel, angiotensin-mediated splanchnic vasoconstriction, or hemorrhage. Central venous and pulmonary artery pressures should be monitored to ensure that the volume status is optimized. The onset of intestinal infarction is heralded by lactic acidosis, which may require bicarbonate replacement or mechanical ventilation. Broad-spectrum antibiotics should be administered in anticipation of bacteremia from breakdown of the mucosal defense barrier. The prognosis of acute mesenteric ischemia depends largely on the extent of intestinal injury at the time of diagnosis. Unfortunately, in most patients, acute mesenteric ischemia is recognized after infarction has occurred, and the comorbid conditions often present in these syndromes contribute to mortality rates as high as 50% to 90%.

Superior mesenteric artery emboli may be treated by surgical revascularization, intraarterial perfusion of thrombolytic agents or vasodilators, or systemic anticoagulation. Emergent laparotomy is indicated for peritoneal signs, at which time the infarcted bowel is resected and embolectomy performed. In the absence of intestinal infarction, embolism has been treated using intraarterial infusion of heparin and thrombolytic agents (e.g., urokinase, streptokinase, recombinant tissue plasminogen activator). Thrombolytic therapy is more likely to be successful if administered within 12 hours of the onset of symptoms. Intraarterial infusion of papaverine to treat vasoconstriction may be useful as an adjunctive measure.

Emergent surgical intervention is indicated for diagnosing acute superior mesenteric artery thrombosis. At the time of surgery, necrotic tissue is resected and the vascular obstruction is relieved. Intravascular injection of fluorescein dye is helpful in defining bowel viability. The extent of necrotic tissue is highly variable and depends largely on the anatomic site of vascular compromise. Sudden occlusion of the only remaining patent vessel may lead to infarction of the entire small intestine and colon, whereas occlusion of a superior mesenteric artery tributary usually causes segmental necrosis. After the initial resection, a second-look operation often is performed to assess bowel viability further. Reestablishing flow after arterial thrombosis is difficult and usually requires a bypass with a synthetic graft or a saphenous venous segment.

Patients in the early phase of mesenteric venous thrombosis can be treated with anticoagulation therapy. In studies of patients with superior mesenteric vein thrombosis, intravenous heparin has decreased thrombus propagation and recurrence and has improved survival. Thrombolytic therapy is rarely indicated for superior mesenteric vein thrombosis. Signs of peritonitis warrant surgical exploration.

In patients with nonocclusive mesenteric ischemia, vasodilators can be administered by angiographic catheterization. If repeat contrast injection demonstrates a response, a continuous infusion of papaverine (30 to 60 mg/h) can be administered through the angiographic catheter for 24 hours. This often results in clinical improvement, but surgical intervention may be required if peritoneal signs or other indications of transmural necrosis develop.

The goals of therapy for chronic intestinal angina are relief from symptoms, improvement of nutritional status, and prevention of mesenteric infarction. The primary mode of treatment is surgical, using either revascularization with anterograde or retrograde bypass grafting, transaortic mesenteric endarterectomy, or reimplantation of the diseased vessels to the aorta. Most patients who undergo successful revascularization have long-term relief from symptoms. Percutaneous transluminal angioplasty has been increasingly used for definitive therapy but has a higher rate of recurrence than surgery.

ISCHEMIC COLITIS

Incidence and Epidemiology

Ischemic colitis, the most common form of intestinal ischemia, occurs primarily among middle-aged and elderly persons. The overall incidence is unknown because many cases resolve spontaneously and are unrecognized.

Etiology and Pathogenesis

Tributaries of the superior mesenteric artery serve the cecum, right colon, and transverse colon, whereas the left colon receives blood from the inferior mesentery artery. A watershed region susceptible to ischemic insult is present between the superior and inferior mesenteric arteries, located anatomically at the splenic flexure. The rectum is well protected by an overlapping vascular supply from the inferior mesenteric artery and the internal iliac artery. Most cases of ischemic colitis are associated with systemic hypoperfusion or surgical disruption of blood flow in the inferior mesenteric artery after aortic surgery. Systemic hypoperfusion is often accompanied by angiotensin-mediated vasoconstriction, similar to the pathophysiological events of nonocclusive mesenteric ischemia. In contrast to acute mesenteric ischemia, spontaneous occlusion of the inferior mesenteric artery is an uncommon cause of ischemic colitis.

Clinical Features

Ischemic colitis commonly presents with symptoms of crampy lower abdominal pain, nausea, vomiting, and bloody diarrhea several hours to days after an episode of hemodynamic instability. The low-flow state is transient and may not be recognized in many patients. The physical findings of acute ischemic colitis are nonspecific and include fever, abdominal distention and tenderness, and occult or overt rectal blood. A minority of patients with chronic colonic ischemia present with obstructive symptoms caused by a segmental ischemic stricture.

Findings on Diagnostic Testing

Laboratory abnormalities are usually mild and nonspecific in patients with ischemic colitis, unless infarction is present. Plain abdominal films may demonstrate thickening of the bowel wall or "thumbprinting" of the mucosa. In contradistinction to mesenteric ischemia, angiography is rarely informative in ischemic colitis because most spontaneous episodes are the result of systemic low-flow states rather than acute occlusion of the inferior mesenteric artery. Colonoscopy can confirm the diagnosis based on characteristic features and is preferred to sigmoidoscopy because half of the lesions are proximal to the sigmoid colon. There is usually rectal sparing because the systemic and splanchnic vascular supplies overlap in this region, and thus abnormal mucosa may be first encountered in the rectosigmoid region. The mucosa is generally edematous and friable in the early stages of ischemic colitis and progresses to frank ulceration in the late stages. Endoscopic biopsy reveals nonspecific inflammation, submucosal hemorrhage, interstitial edema, vascular congestion, and intravascular platelet thrombi. A characteristic pattern of hemosiderin deposition with transmural fibrosis and mucosal atrophy is pathognomonic of chronic ischemia.

Management and Course

Most patients with ischemic colitis improve with conservative measures that optimize cardiovascular function. Vasodilators have not been useful in treating ischemic colitis, unlike nonocclusive mesenteric ischemia. Vasoconstricting agents and volume depletion should be avoided. Emergent surgical exploration is required for evidence of frank peritonitis, during which time all necrotic segments should be resected. Patients with symptomatic colonic strictures should undergo elective resection. Revascularization is not indicated for ischemic colitis. Although a small percentage of patients succumb to complications of ischemic colitis, survival is most often limited by the comorbid illness that precipitated the compromised colonic perfusion.

CHAPTER 75

Radiation Injury

ETIOLOGY AND PATHOGENESIS

During gamma irradiation therapy, photons collide with outer orbital electrons that are then ejected from the atom. This process leads to secondary ionization of other atoms or generation of reactive elements such as free radicals. These interactions damage DNA, proteins, and lipids, resulting in genetic damage and cell death. Ionizing radiation is delivered in units; the accepted SI (Système International d'Unités) unit of dose is the gray (Gy), which is equivalent to 100 rad or 1 joule of energy distributed over 1 kg of tissue. Most modern radiation therapy regimens use megavoltage photons that disperse high-energy electrons in targeted tissues.

The cytotoxicity of a given dose of radiation therapy depends on the amount of radiation and also on the form of radiation delivered. In general, alpha particles are more damaging than gamma rays, and beta particles produce an intermediate degree of injury. The deeper penetration and more widespread use of gamma irradiation make this procedure the most commonly associated with visceral injury. The toxicity of a given dose can be amplified by coadministering chemotherapy such as 5-fluorouracil, doxorubicin, bleomycin, and actinomycin D.

Gastrointestinal injury from radiation therapy can be separated into acute and chronic presentations. In acute injury, radiation-induced cellular toxicity destroys epithelial cells and interferes with proliferation. Small doses of radiation can cause villous blunting and minor alterations in mucosal function, but larger doses can denude extensive regions of mucosa. This can result in massive fluid and electrolyte losses and also bacteremia from disruption of the mucosal barrier. Simultaneous damage to vascular endothelial cells increases vascular permeability and edema. Most injuries caused by smaller doses are self-limited; however, larger cumulative doses can lead to persistent or progressive disease.

Chronic radiation injury will present months or years after exposure. This disorder is from small vessel ischemic injury, mediated by endothelial inflammation that is coupled with smooth muscle and fibroblast proliferation that compromise blood flow in small vessels. Histologically, chronic radiation injury is characterized by the presence of excessive fibrosis and atypical fibroblasts. Progressive ischemic injury and fibrosis may lead to stricturing, ulceration, fistulization, and perforation.

CLINICAL FEATURES, DIAGNOSIS, AND MANAGEMENT

Radiation Injury to the Esophagus

Radiation esophagitis is a frequent complication of therapy directed at hematologic, pharyngeal, or thoracic tumors. Acute injury occurs from doses of 6000 cGy or larger. Odynophagia and chest pain are the most common symptoms, and usually they develop after the second week of treatment. The chest pain is usually substernal, constant, and exacerbated by swallowing. Dysphagia in this early phase may be present as a result of esophagitis, which interferes with esophageal motility.

The diagnosis of acute radiation esophagitis is usually apparent from the clinical setting and generally does not require confirmation by upper gastrointestinal endoscopy. Supportive care and adjustment of the radiation dose or modification of the radiation field usually facilitates healing. Viscous lidocaine, antacids, antisecretory agents, and antihistamines often alleviate odynophagia and dysphagia. The nutritional status of the patient should be monitored closely, and patients with prolonged and severe episodes may require enteral feeding by a nasoenteric or gastrostomy tube.

Chronic radiation injury to the esophagus usually presents 6 months or more (sometimes >5 years) after completing therapy. The principal symptom is dysphagia, caused by fibrotic strictures, the risk of which correlates with the radiation dose. One percent to 5% of patients who receive 6000 cGy and 50% of patients who receive 7500 cGy develop radiation-induced esophageal injury. Fistulae formation is also a form of chronic radiation injury that causes recurrent aspiration pneumonia in the case of a tracheoesophageal fistula or, rarely, massive hemorrhage resulting from an aortoesophageal fistula. Fistulae are usually caused by tumor necrosis of primary esophageal or lung neoplasms or may result from vasculitis induced by chronic radiation injury. Barium swallow radiography is helpful in diagnosing a stricture or fistula. Upper gastrointestinal endoscopy with brushing and biopsy of strictures is necessary to exclude malignancy. This is especially important if the patient presents with dysphagia more than 10 years after radiation exposure, given the increased risk of secondary squamous cell carcinoma. If a stricture is short and straight, endoscopic balloon dilation may alleviate dysphagia. Endoscopic placement of self-expanding metal stents (SEMS) has decreased the need for surgical intervention for many patients. Coated stents may be used to manage tracheoesophageal fistulae; however, some of these patients may also require enteral feeding to reduce the complications of aspiration. Complications of SEMS include intractable chest pain, hemorrhage, migration, and perforation.

Radiation Injury to the Stomach

The stomach is relatively resistant to radiation damage. Ulceration and stenosis generally require doses larger than 4500 cGy, but transient hypochlorhydria is commonly seen with smaller doses. Stricture formation is more common in the antrum and in the cardia than in other regions of the stomach. Endoscopic or radiographic methods are used to identify the lesion. Therapy for gastric radiation injury is usually supportive; obstruction, hemorrhage, and perforation are extremely rare.

Radiation Injury to the Small Intestine

The small intestine is the most radiosensitive organ in the gastrointestinal tract. The high turnover rate of the mucosa of the small intestine makes it particularly susceptible to radiation injury. Radiation enteritis occurs most commonly after radiation therapy for gynecologic, urologic, rectal, or retroperitoneal malignancies. Because their positions within the abdominal cavity are fixed, the duodenum, distal ileum and cecum are particularly vulnerable to injury. Additionally, patients with a thin body habitus or chronic mesenteric vascular insufficiency, or those receiving radiosensitizing chemotherapy are at increased risk of developing radiation enteritis. There is a dose-response relationship in which clinically significant acute toxicity occurs in 20% of patients who receive 1000 cGy, in 40% of patients who receive 1000 to 3000 cGy, and in 90% of patients who receive more than 3000 cGy. Methods to prevent radiation injury include placing mesh material to displace or protect the small intestine during therapy or maintaining a full bladder, when the dose is delivered, to displace the small intestine from the radiation field. The former is useful when radiation is delivered as adjuvant therapy after a primary surgical resection.

Both acute and chronic injury may manifest from radiation therapy. Acute injury is characterized by loss of regenerative epithelium, malabsorption, diarrhea, and abdominal pain. Perforation rarely complicates the course of acute enteritis. Supportive therapy consists of antispasmodics, bulk-forming agents, and antidiarrheals, carefully administered, because these patients are also at risk of bowel obstruction. Data concerning the efficacy of aminosalicylates are conflicting. Most cases of radiation injury are self-limited, but with large doses, the injury may be severe and persistent.

Chronic injury occurs in 5% of treated patients and typically presents 1 to 2 years after the exposure, but lag times of up to 20 years have been reported. Vascular damage leads to ischemia-mediated fibrosis, ulceration, and fistulization. Strictures may cause signs or symptoms of obstruction; additionally, resulting stasis in the small intestine may promote bacterial overgrowth. Patients frequently present with diarrhea, which may be caused by bile salt malabsorption, bacterial overgrowth, impaired mucosal absorptive capacity, or an enteric fistula. Fistulae may also communicate with the genitourinary system. In rare cases, patients present with acute gastrointestinal hemorrhage or peritonitis from ulceration or infarction.

Treatment of diarrheal symptoms usually is supportive. Dietary manipulation, including avoidance of fats and lactose, may improve malabsorptive symptoms. Loperamide and diphenoxylate are advocated. A peripheral opiate antagonist, loperamide-*N*-oxide, has provided benefit in small cohort studies. Cholestyramine and antibiotics are often given empirically for bile salt malabsorption and bacterial overgrowth, respectively. Nutritional status should be monitored closely. Patients with severe disease may require enterally administered elemental diets or even parenteral nutrition. If severe symptoms persist or the course is complicated by obstruction or bleeding, surgical resection may be necessary; however, surgery should be limited to truly refractory cases because of the high rate of anastomotic failures and adhesions that can further complicate the clinical course. Unless there is extensive fistulization, resection of the diseased segment is preferred to a bypass.

Radiation Injury to the Colon and Rectum

Radiation injury of the colon and rectum is a common complication of treatments targeting the cervix, uterus, prostate, bladder, and testes. Radiation therapy for testicular cancer often involves an extensive field that may include the transverse colon. The majority of cases of radiation colitis develop in the rectosigmoid colon after pelvic irradiation. The use of radiation implants and external beam irradiation increases the risk of colitis.

Acute injury occurs in the first 6 weeks after exposure and manifests as diarrhea and tenesmus. Lower gastrointestinal endoscopy usually demonstrates minimal nonspecific mucosal injury. Treatment is primarily supportive, and symptoms resolve within 2 to 6 months.

The most common symptoms of chronic radiation colitis are rectal bleeding and diarrhea. Patients may also develop rectovaginal or rectovesical fistulae and present with symptoms related to the genitourinary tract. Endoscopically, radiation colitis has a characteristic appearance of scattered telangiectasias on a background of pale, friable mucosa. Biopsy is not necessary for the diagnosis unless there is a coexisting stricture, in which case recurrent malignancy must be excluded. Barium enema radiography is often necessary to define the extent of complicating strictures or fistulae.

Multiple forms of medical therapy have been studied; however, none stands out as superior. Sucralfate delivered either orally or by enema (2 g in 20 mL water) is effective. Short-chain fatty acids have had encouraging results, as has antioxidant therapy with vitamin E (400 IU, three times daily) and vitamin C (500 mg, three times daily). Local application of formalin (50 mL of 4% solution) to obliterate telangiectatic vessels has decreased bleeding in open label trials, although complications of severe pain or acute colitis have been reported. Most trials evaluating 5-aminosalicylates and steroid enemas have demonstrated no response. Chronic rectal bleeding is best managed initially with endoscopic argon plasma coagulation, laser photocoagulation, or electrocautery. Although several sessions are necessary, ablation of mucosal telangiectasias reduces transfusion requirements and hospitalization rates. Endoscopic dilation is also effective in relieving symptoms caused by short, discrete, colonic strictures. Surgical resection is reserved for patients with long, tortuous strictures or refractory bleeding.

Radiation Injury to the Hepatobiliary System

Hepatic injury induced by radiation typically occurs 4 to 8 weeks after therapy. Symptoms include malaise, fatigue, weight gain, ascites, right upper quadrant abdominal pain. Radiation liver damage can manifest as Budd-Chiari syndrome, with progressive weight gain, ascites, and jaundice. Alkaline phosphatase levels are elevated more so than bilirubin or aminotransferase levels. Primary parenchymal injury results in focal necrosis and, eventually, bridging fibrosis. CT findings include low-attenuation areas adjacent to the tumor mass and atrophy in the treated segment or lobe with hypertrophy of the untreated liver. The differential diagnosis of these findings includes metastatic disease and drug toxicity.

Venoocclusive disease can be a complication of radiation therapy in addition to certain chemotherapeutic agents, and occurs more frequently when used concomitantly for bone marrow ablation. The disease results from thrombotic and fibrotic obliteration of small central veins, leading to centrilobular congestion. The clinical syndrome occurs 1 to 4 weeks after exposure and presents with jaundice, weight gain, ascites, right upper quadrant pain, and, occasionally, encephalopathy. Treatment is usually supportive with fluid restriction and diuretics. The mortality rate is 30% to 50%.

Radiotherapy-induced hepatotoxicity has been reduced through the use of three-dimensional multiplanar delivery techniques. There is no specific therapy other than correction of fluid and electrolyte disorders. Patients with jaundice have poor prognoses. The overall mortality rate is 10% to 20%.

CHAPTER 76

Endoscopy

PRINCIPLES OF ENDOSCOPIC EVALUATION OF THE GASTROINTESTINAL TRACT

Utility of Endoscopy

Gastrointestinal endoscopy has transformed all aspects of diagnosing and treating patients with diseases of the gastrointestinal tract. Each endoscopic procedure has a specific set of indications and contraindications. In general, an endoscopic procedure is indicated only when the results are expected to influence the course of patient management. In some cases, however, the attendant risks of endoscopy may outweigh the benefits. Before proceeding with endoscopic intervention, a patient should give a complete history and have a complete physical examination to establish the indication for the study and exclude the presence of any contraindications. Many procedures require bowel cleansing or prolonged fasting; therefore, the clinician must be aware of comorbid conditions, such as diabetes, heart failure, or renal dysfunction, which may require adjusting the instructions for patient preparation. All patients should be counseled on the risks and benefits of endoscopy; written and verbal informed consent is mandatory.

Principles of Conscious Sedation

Most endoscopic procedures require conscious sedation to permit a safe and complete examination. The optimal agents and dosages vary, but all carry the risk of cardiopulmonary complications. All patients should be monitored for changes in blood pressure, heart rate, and respiratory rate throughout the course of sedation. Many centers use pulse oximetry and electrocardiographic monitoring, but it is uncertain if routine use of these more expensive monitoring procedures improves treatment outcomes. No electronic monitoring can replace clinical judgment. Therefore, if significant cardiopulmonary signs or symptoms arise, the procedure should be aborted. The benzodiazepine antagonist flumazenil and the opiate antagonist naloxone can be used to reverse the effects of benzodiazepines and narcotics, respectively, in patients with complications of oversedation, but they should not be used routinely to reverse sedation. Slow titration of the initial dose of the sedative agent is the best way to avoid oversedation.

Antibiotic Prophylaxis

The role of preprocedure antibiotics to prevent endocarditis or bacteremia in patients with vascular or other prostheses is undefined. Based on the documented risks of bacteremia with given procedures and the risks of establishing an infection in certain preexisting conditions, the American Society of Gastrointestinal Endoscopy promotes guidelines for antibiotic prophylaxis before endoscopic procedures (Table 76-1). In many circumstances, no definitive recommendations can be made and the decision is made at the clinician's discretion. Antibiotics can be costly, and many have a substantial risk of allergic reactions. These issues must be considered when contemplating the use of prophylactic antibiotics. The standard regimen includes parenteral ampicillin (1 to 2 g) and gentamicin (1.5 mg/kg, up to 80 mg) 30 minutes before the procedure, followed by oral amoxicillin (1.5 g) 6 hours after the procedure. Amoxicillin may be replaced by a repeat dose of the parenteral regimen 8 hours after the procedure. Intravenous vancomycin (1 g) is substituted for ampicillin in patients with penicillin allergies.

Coagulation Disorders

Although coagulation abnormalities are not absolute contraindications to endoscopy, the use of endoscopic biopsy can be associated with an increased risk of bleeding. Before any therapeutic intervention, including percutaneous gastrostomy tube placement and electrocoagulation for polypectomy or hemostasis, attempts should be made to correct coagulation disorders. Prolongation of prothrombin time unrelated to the administration of warfarin may require parenteral vitamin K therapy. If there is no response to vitamin K or if emergency therapy is necessary, coagulation factors should be supplemented with fresh, frozen plasma. Antiplatelet agents (e.g., aspirin) should ideally be withheld for 7 to 10 days before and after these therapeutic measures, although there is no evidence that routine endoscopy including polypectomy is associated with an increased risk of bleeding complications in patients using daily aspirin. Depending on the underlying medical condition, warfarin can often be withheld for 5 to 7 days before the procedure and reinstituted 1 to 2 days after therapy. If medical conditions prohibit discontinuation, one of two potential management pathways can be used. In the first, the patient is hospitalized, warfarin is discontinued, and heparin is initiated. When the prothrombin time normalizes, the patient is prepared for the procedure, and heparin is discontinued 4 hours before the intervention. Heparin can be restarted 4 hours after the procedure, and warfarin can be reinstituted 12 to 24 hours after heparin if no procedure-related hemorrhage occurs. Alternatively, warfarin may be stopped 5 days prior to the procedure and subcutaneous low molecular weight heparin (e.g., dalteparin) initiated, once or twice daily, according to the patient's

TABLE 76-1
Recommendations for Antibiotic Prophylaxis

RISK GROUP	PROCEDURE	ANTIBIOTIC PROPHYLAXIS
High risk of endocarditis (prosthetic valve, prior endocarditis, systemic pulmonary shunt, or synthetic vascular graft <1 y old)	Stricture dilation, sclerotherapy	Recommended
	Esophagogastroduodenoscopy or colonoscopy	Insufficient data (endoscopist's discretion)
Moderate risk of endocarditis (rheumatic valvular disease, mitral valve prolapse with insufficiency, hypertrophic cardiomyopathy, and most congenital malformations)	Stricture dilation, sclerotherapy	Insufficient data (endoscopist's discretion)
	Esophagogastroduodenoscopy or colonoscopy	Not recommended
Low risk of endocarditis (coronary bypass surgery, pacemakers, and implantable defibrillators)	All endoscopic procedures	Not recommended
Prosthetic joints	All endoscopic procedures	Not recommended
Obstructed biliary system or pancreatic pseudocyst	Endoscopic retrograde cholangiopancreatography	Recommended
Cirrhosis and ascites	Stricture dilation, sclerotherapy	Insufficient data (endoscopist's discretion)
	Esophagogastroduodenoscopy or colonoscopy	Not recommended
All patients	Percutaneous gastrostomy	Recommended

weight. The last low molecular weight heparin dose is given the night before the procedure and then restarted the evening of the procedure and continued for 5 days, whereas warfarin is restarted the evening of the procedure and continued as previously taken. This second approach avoids hospitalization because the subcutaneous low molecular weight heparin is self-administered in an outpatient setting.

UPPER GASTROINTESTINAL ENDOSCOPY

Indications and Contraindications

Many symptoms attributable to diseases of the esophagus, stomach, and duodenum are best assessed by esophagogastroduodenoscopy (EGD) or upper gastrointestinal endoscopy. The American Society of Gastrointestinal Endoscopy has established consensus guidelines for the appropriate use of EGD (Table 76-2). Therapeutic endoscopy is often indicated for control of variceal and nonvariceal bleeding, dilation of strictures, removal of some foreign bodies, palliation of advanced malignancies with stents or tumor ablation, and placement of a percutaneous gastrostomy tube. The advent of longer endoscopes has expanded the capability of upper gastrointestinal endoscopy in diagnosing and potentially treating diseases of the small intestine. Enteroscopy is indicated when investigating chronic bleeding presumed secondary to a source in the small intestine or if visualization or sampling the small intestine is warranted by radiologic abnormalities.

The major contraindications to upper gastrointestinal endoscopy include perforation, hemodynamic instability, cardiopulmonary distress, and inadequate patient cooperation. Coagulation disorders are relative contraindications to therapeutic intervention. Percutaneous gastrostomy tube placement is contraindicated if the stomach is inaccessible because of a prior gastrectomy or interposed bowel, liver, or spleen.

Patient Preparation and Monitoring

Patients should not ingest solid food for 6 to 8 hours or liquids for 4 hours before elective upper gastrointestinal endoscopy. If delayed gastric emptying is suspected, a liquid diet can be instituted 24 hours before the procedure and the fasting interval increased to 8 to 12 hours. For complete gastric outlet obstruction, evacuation of the stomach with a nasogastric tube is usually necessary. If an emergency endoscopic procedure is required for gastrointestinal bleeding, measures should be taken to avoid aspiration. Evacuation of the stomach with an orogastric tube before the procedure, attentiveness to oral suction during the procedure, and prophylactic endotracheal intubation in an obtunded patient protect the patient's airway.

Immediately before the procedure is begun, the posterior pharynx is anesthetized with a topical spray or a gargle anesthetic. The clinical benefit of these agents has been called into question; their use should be avoided in patients with acute hemorrhage or delayed gastric emptying, given the increased risk of aspiration. A short-acting benzodiazepine (e.g., midazolam) usually provides a sufficient level of conscious sedation for diagnostic upper gastrointestinal endoscopy. Some endoscopists add intravenous opiates, although the synergistic cardiopulmonary depressant effects of this combination may increase the rate of complications. Longer therapeutic procedures, including percutaneous gastrostomy tube placement, require administering opiates for patient comfort. Throughout the

TABLE 76-2
Indications for Upper Gastrointestinal Endoscopy

Diagnostic

Upper abdominal distress despite an appropriate trial of therapy

Upper abdominal distress associated with signs or symptoms of organic disease (weight loss, anorexia)

Refractory vomiting of unknown cause

Dysphagia or odynophagia

Esophageal reflux symptoms unresponsive to therapy

Upper gastrointestinal bleeding

When sampling of duodenal or jejunal tissue or fluid is indicated

To obtain a histological diagnosis for radiographically demonstrated gastric or esophageal ulcers, upper intestinal tract strictures, or suspected neoplasms

To screen for varices so that patients with cirrhosis can be identified as possible candidates for prophylactic medical or endoscopic therapy

To assess acute injury after caustic ingestion

When management of other disease processes is affected by the presence of upper gastrointestinal pathological conditions (e.g., use of anticoagulants)

Therapeutic

Treatment of variceal and nonvariceal upper gastrointestinal bleeding

Removal of foreign bodies

Removal of selected polypoid lesions

Dilation of symptomatic strictures

Palliative treatment of stenosing neoplasms

Placement of percutaneous feeding gastrostomy tube

Surveillance

Follow-up of selected gastric, esophageal, or stomal ulcers to document healing

Barrett esophagus

Familial adenomatous polyposis

Adenomatous gastric polyps

Follow-up of varices eradicated by endoscopic therapy

procedure, a trained assistant should work together with the endoscopist to monitor the oral secretions as well as the overall clinical condition of the patient.

Performance of the Procedure

The endoscope is introduced blindly or under direct visualization by passing the instrument into the posterior pharynx and instructing the patient to swallow. Direct visualization is preferred because it is less traumatic and provides a view of the larynx. A standard EGD involves a complete inspection of the esophagus, stomach, and the first two portions of the duodenum. A pediatric colonoscope or push enteroscope can be advanced into the proximal jejunum. Enteroscopy can also be performed with the sonde enteroscope, which relies on peristaltic movement to propel the instrument into the distal jejunum or ileum, but this instrument does not provide biopsy or therapeutic capabilities.

Endoscopic biopsy or brush cytology studies may provide a pathological diagnosis. For some disease processes (e.g., infections caused by *Helicobacter pylori* and causes of malabsorption in the small intestine), random biopsies of normally appearing mucosa may be indicated. Upper gastrointestinal endoscopy also provides the capability of therapeutic intervention. Dysphagia from esophageal strictures or achalasia can be relieved with endoscopic dilation using pneumatic balloon or sequential bougienage techniques. The safest means of bougienage dilation involves passage of the dilator over a guidewire that is placed endoscopically into the distal stomach. Although fluoroscopy reduces the complication rate of dilation, radiation exposure and resource limitations have precluded its routine use in many centers. Acute or chronic nonvariceal hemorrhage can be controlled with electrocoagulation, heater probe application, injection therapy, or laser photocoagulation. Large or bleeding esophageal varices may be treated with injection sclerotherapy or band ligation. Mucosal polyps can be excised with electrocoagulation using hot biopsy forceps or with snare polypectomy. Deep tissue sampling and excision of mucosal lesions may be accomplished with submucosal injection and endoscopic mucosal resection (EMR). Large stenosing esophageal or gastric malignancies can be ablated with laser photocoagulation or electrocoagulation. Esophageal malignancies can also be palliated by deploying metallic expandable stents.

Complications

Diagnostic upper gastrointestinal endoscopy is usually very safe, and rates of serious complications are low. Most complications are related to oversedation, emphasizing the need for preprocedural patient assessment and vigilant patient monitoring throughout the period of sedation. The high rate of wound infections associated with gastrostomy tube placement can be substantially reduced by prophylactic antibiotics. The benefit of prophylactic antibiotics for other indications remains unproven.

VIDEO CAPSULE ENDOSCOPY

Indications and Contraindications

Wireless capsule endoscopy or video capsule endoscopy (VCE) uses a wireless, short focal length lens to capture two images per second as the capsule traverses the gastrointestinal tract. The video images are transmitted by radiotelemetry to an array of aerials attached to the body via a recording belt. The primary indication for VCE is for evaluating obscure gastrointestinal bleeding. However, indications continue to evolve, and it has been used for evaluating small bowel tumors and small intestinal Crohn's disease. Contraindications to VCE include esophageal stricture and intermittent or partial small bowel obstruction. Relative contraindications include dementia, gastroparesis, and the presence of a pacemaker because of potential interference as the capsule traverses the chest. No cases of complications in patients with pacemakers who have undergone VCE have been reported.

Performance of the Procedure

The procedure is generally performed in ambulatory patients after an overnight fast with or without a polyethylene glycol preparation. An eight-lead sensor array is fastened to the abdomen in a designated pattern that allows image capture and continuous triangulation of the capsule location in the abdomen. The images are stored on a small portable recorder carried on the belt and are subsequently downloaded for interpretation. Patients may proceed with normal activities and can consume clear liquids 2 hours after capsule ingestion and food 4 hours after capsule ingestion. The capsule itself is disposable and is passed by normal excretion.

Complications

The primary risk of VCE is capsule retention, which occurs in up to 25% of patients but requires surgical intervention in less than 1%. Retained capsules rarely cause obstructive symptoms, and most cases can be observed for extended periods during which most capsules will pass spontaneously, thereby avoiding surgery.

LOWER GASTROINTESTINAL ENDOSCOPY

Indications and Contraindications

Diseases or symptoms referable to the colon and rectum are best evaluated by colonoscopy or flexible sigmoidoscopy. The American Gastroenterology Association, the American Cancer Society, and the American Medical Association have deemed colonoscopy superior to flexible sigmoidoscopy for detecting colonic lesions (even within the limited area seen on sigmoidoscopy) but recognize sigmoidoscopy with or without barium enema as an acceptable alternative to colonoscopy (in average risk individuals) when patient preference or local expertise limits the use of full colonoscopy. Patients with increased risk because of personal or family history of previous colon cancer or colon polyps or with a genetic syndrome predisposing to colon cancer should undergo full colonoscopy for colon cancer screening. Sigmoidoscopy is used to complete the examination of the colon in conjunction with barium enema radiography and to investigate rectosigmoid symptoms in young persons who are at extremely low risk of colorectal neoplasia. All patients older than 40 years with symptoms referable to any portion of the colon are best evaluated by total colonoscopy. The American Society of Gastrointestinal Endoscopy has established recommendations for using colonoscopy (Table 76-3) that are intended as guidelines. They should not replace the clinical judgment of the clinician.

As with any endoscopic procedure, colonoscopy is contraindicated if a perforation is suspected or if the patient is uncooperative. Lower gastrointestinal endoscopy specifically is contraindicated in fulminant colitis and the suppurative phase of acute diverticulitis. Recent myocardial infarction is a relative contraindication to colonoscopy and should delay elective procedures for several weeks.

Patient Preparation and Monitoring

Most lower gastrointestinal endoscopic procedures require cleansing the colon. Limited preparation of the left colon is usually sufficient for flexible sigmoidoscopy and can be achieved with two tap water or small volume sodium phosphate enemas administered 1 hour before the examination. This limited preparation precludes the use of electrocautery because of the hazard of residual explosive gases. Colonoscopy or any lower gastrointestinal endoscopic procedure using electrocautery requires full preparation of the colon. The two most commonly used agents are sodium phosphate and balanced electrolyte solutions containing polyethylene glycol (PEG). Sodium phosphate is given orally in 45-mL aliquots the evening before and 3 hours before colonoscopy, whereas PEG solutions are administered in 1-gallon to 2-gallon volumes over a period of 4 to 6 hours the evening before colonoscopy. Mannitol and other carbohydrate purgatives should be avoided if electrocoagulation is anticipated because bacterial fermentation produces explosive

TABLE 76-3
Indications for Colonoscopy

Diagnostic
Fecal occult blood
Hematochezia in the absence of a convincing anorectal source
Melena, if an upper intestinal source is excluded
Unexplained iron deficiency
Abnormality on barium enema that is probably significant (filling defect, stricture)
To exclude the presence of synchronous cancer or polyps in a patient with confirmed
    colorectal neoplasia
Chronic, unexplained diarrhea
Selected patients with altered bowel habits at risk of colonic neoplasia
Inflammatory bowel disease, if establishing a diagnosis or determining the extent of
    disease will alter management decisions

Therapeutic
Excision of polyps
Bleeding from vascular ectasias, neoplasia, polypectomy site, or ulceration
Foreign body removal
Decompression of acute colonic pseudoobstruction or volvulus
Balloon dilation of stenotic lesions
Palliative treatment of inoperable stenosing or bleeding neoplasms

Surveillance
Prior history of colorectal cancer or adenomatous polyps
Family history of hereditary nonpolyposis colon cancer
Family history of colorectal cancer in a first-degree relative (< age 55) or in several
    family members
Long-standing (>7–10 y) chronic ulcerative pancolitis with biopsies to detect dysplasia;
    colitis limited to the left side may require less intensive surveillance

hydrogen gas. Both sodium phosphate and PEG solutions yield adequate bowel cleansing, but patients often prefer the small-volume sodium phosphate solution to the unpleasant tasting, large-volume PEG solutions. However, sodium phosphate may lead to dangerous fluid and electrolyte shifts in patients with heart failure or renal insufficiency; PEG solutions are preferred for patients with these conditions.

Sedation and monitoring are similar to the practices used for upper gastrointestinal endoscopy. Colonoscopy, however, almost invariably requires adding opiates to standard benzodiazepine sedation to minimize the visceral pain from colonic distention and stretching. This combination of a benzodiazepine and an opiate has a synergistic depressant effect on the cardiopulmonary system, emphasizing the need for standard cardiopulmonary monitoring. Unlike colonoscopy, flexible sigmoidoscopy to the splenic flexure is often accomplished without sedation. A skilled endoscopist can often perform this procedure with minimal discomfort to the patient.

Performance of the Procedure

Flexible sigmoidoscopy involves introducing the instrument into the descending colon or splenic flexure, whereas total colonoscopy involves passing the instrument to the cecum. Although experienced endoscopists may reach the cecum in 90% to 98% of examinations, a significant number of patients have colonic anatomies that preclude safe completion of the procedure. Therefore, the well-trained endoscopist should be willing to abandon a colonoscopic study that appears unreasonably traumatic.

As with upper gastrointestinal endoscopy, colonoscopy provides the capability of obtaining biopsy specimens to establish the diagnosis of endoscopic abnormalities and to sample normally appearing mucosa if occult conditions (e.g., microscopic colitis) are suspected. Therapeutic colonoscopic techniques include polypectomy with hot biopsy forceps or with snare polypectomy using electrocoagulation to promote hemostasis. Acute and chronic bleeding from angiodysplasias can be treated with electrocoagulation, heater probe application, and laser photocoagulation. Less common procedures include through-the-scope pneumatic balloon dilation of discrete benign strictures, decompressive colonoscopy with tube placement for acute pseudoobstruction, and palliative laser ablation of inoperable neoplasms.

Complications

The overall risk of serious complications, including perforation and uncontrolled hemorrhage, is approximately 1 in 500 for diagnostic colonoscopy. Therapeutic maneuvers increase the risk of complications, although there are wide variations in reported rates. Hemorrhage after polypectomy is common. It may occur in up to 1% to 2% of patients and often occurs up to 7 to 10 days after the procedure when residual necrotic tissue and scar tissue are sloughed. The risk of perforation is also increased in therapeutic maneuvers. The transmural burn syndrome represents a localized, contained perforation that may be associated with localized pain, fever, and leukocytosis 6 to 24 hours after polypectomy or after any therapy that uses electrocoagulation. Many patients can be treated conservatively with parenteral broad-spectrum antibiotics, but any patient with signs of frank perforation should undergo surgical exploration.

ENDOSCOPIC RETROGRADE CHOLANGIOPANCREATOGRAPHY

Indications and Contraindications

Endoscopic retrograde cholangiopancreatography (ERCP) is indicated for evaluating patients with suspected biliary or pancreatic disorders when noninvasive imaging with ultrasonography or computed tomographic (CT) scanning is equivocal and when therapeutic intervention is necessary (Table 76-4). Various abdominal symptoms can be attributed to the pancreaticobiliary system, and the decision to proceed with ERCP should be made by a clinician experienced in caring for patients with these disorders. ERCP has a role in the preoperative evaluation of selected patients undergoing laparoscopic cholecystectomy, pancreatic resection, or surgical pseudocyst drainage. Many of the available therapeutic options, including endoscopic sphincterotomy, stone extraction, endoscopic cystgastrostomy, and biliary or pancreatic stent placement, also require the availability of surgical support. Thus, the treatment of patients undergoing ERCP often requires the combined expertise of the endoscopist and a surgeon.

In addition to the standard contraindications for all endoscopic procedures, ERCP is relatively contraindicated in the presence of an obstructed biliary system or a documented pancreatic pseudocyst, unless immediate endoscopic or surgical

TABLE 76-4
Indications for Endoscopic Retrograde Cholangiopancreatography

Suspected Biliary Disorders
Unexplained jaundice or cholestasis
Postcholecystectomy complaints
Postbiliary surgery complaints
Acute cholangitis
Acute gallstone pancreatitis
Evaluation of bile duct abnormalities in other imaging studies
Sphincter of Oddi manometry

Suspected Pancreatic Disorders
Chronic upper abdominal pain consistent with pancreatic origin
Unexplained weight loss
Steatorrhea
Unexplained recurrent pancreatitis
Evaluation of pancreatic abnormalities in other imaging studies
To obtain pancreatic duct brushings or pure pancreatic juice

Before Therapeutic Intervention
Endoscopic sphincterotomy
Endoscopic biliary drainage
Endoscopic pancreatic drainage
Endoscopic cystgastrostomy
Balloon dilation of pancreaticobiliary strictures
Preoperative mapping for pancreatic or biliary resections

drainage is planned. Any procedure performed under these conditions should be accompanied by administration of prophylactic antibiotics (see Table 76-1). Therapeutic interventions, particularly endoscopic sphincterotomy, are contraindicated in patients with severe coagulopathy.

Patient Preparation and Monitoring

All patients undergoing ERCP should be prepared in the same manner as patients undergoing EGD. Attention should be given to several factors specific to ERCP. First, because the endoscope used for ERCP is equipped with side-viewing rather than with forward-viewing optics, special attention should be given to patients with dysphagia. Passing the instrument through the esophagus is done blindly, increasing the risk of perforation if there is a Zenker diverticulum or esophageal stricture. The ductal injection of contrast material can result in significant systemic absorption, as demonstrated occasionally by the appearance of a postinjection nephrogram. Although anaphylactic reactions have not been reported, erythema and rash can occur, and some clinicians choose to pretreat patients who have histories of reactions to contrast agents with antihistamines and corticosteroids 12 and 2 hours before the procedure. Because ERCP involves radiographic imaging of the upper abdomen, any residual gastrointestinal contrast agent should be evacuated with purgatives. Immediately before sedating the patient, abdominal radiographs should be obtained to ensure that all contrast material is gone and to establish the location of soft tissue shadows and calcifications.

The sedation of patients undergoing ERCP is similar to the procedure used for patients undergoing upper gastrointestinal endoscopy. Because biliary manipulation and injection are often associated with visceral pain, opiates are frequently added. Patient movement should be minimized to obtain optimal imaging. Because the patient is in the prone position on the fluoroscopic table rather than in the left decubitus position used for upper gastrointestinal endoscopy, special attention should be given to removing oral secretions.

Performance of the Procedure

ERCP involves passing a side-viewing endoscope into the second portion of the duodenum and visualizing the ampulla of Vater. Both the pancreatic and biliary system can be cannulated with specialized catheters that are advanced through the duodenoscope. After selective cannulation of the pancreatic or biliary system, radiologic contrast dye is injected under fluoroscopic guidance until the entire ductal system is visualized. Care should be taken to avoid injecting air because bubbles may be mistaken for biliary or pancreatic stones. Overinjection of dye into the pancreas leads to staining of the parenchyma, a pattern termed *acinarization*, which is associated with an increased risk of ERCP-induced pancreatitis. Abdominal radiographs are obtained during the injection and periodically as the contrast dye drains from the duct. After one ductal system is examined, the alternate system is cannulated and injected. For some disorders, only cholangiography or pancreatography is necessary. Biliary manometry can be performed in specialized centers as part of the ERCP examination with a specialized water-perfused manometry catheter positioned across the sphincter of Oddi. The ampulla of Vater may not be easily accessible in patients whose anatomy has been altered by a Billroth II or Roux-en-Y gastrojejunostomy.

ERCP is a nonoperative method of treating many pancreaticobiliary disorders. Endoscopic sphincterotomy is often performed to facilitate biliary stone extraction. The procedure involves cannulation of the common bile duct with a papillotome, a specialized catheter with an exposed wire that extends across the most distal portion of the catheter. Positioning the wire across the papilla and applying electrical current produces a cut through the papilla. After sphincterotomy, stones may pass spontaneously, but extraction with balloon catheters or baskets placed through the endoscope and into the bile duct is often necessary. If endoscopic stone extraction fails, a nasobiliary tube or endoscopic stent can be placed while the patient awaits definitive surgical therapy. Sphincterotomy also relieves obstruction caused by sphincter of Oddi dyskinesia or papillary stenosis. Specialized centers may perform sphincterotomy of the minor papilla to treat pancreas divisum.

Biliary or pancreatic strictures can also be treated with ERCP. Inoperable, malignant obstruction of the extrahepatic bile ducts is best relieved by endoscopic placement of a plastic or metallic stent, in many cases after sphincterotomy. Occasionally, patients with primary sclerosing cholangitis will have dominant strictures of the extrahepatic bile ducts, which are amenable to pneumatic balloon dilation followed by stent placement. For most benign biliary strictures, however, surgical therapy is preferred because of superior long-term patency. Transpapillary placement of a pancreatic stent has been used to treat symptomatic pancreatic ductal strictures and pseudocysts in patients with chronic pancreatitis.

Complications

Acute pancreatitis is the most common complication of ERCP. Sixty percent to 80% of patients undergoing ERCP develop asymptomatic elevations in serum amylase and lipase levels, but clinically overt pancreatitis is much less common. Retrospective series report an incidence of 1% to 2%, but prospective series suggest that symptomatic acute pancreatitis occurs in 4% to 7% of patients undergoing ERCP. The risk is increased by acinarization of the pancreas, repeated attempts at cannulation, and sphincter of Oddi manometry. Conservative management leads to resolution for most patients, but severe necrotizing pancreatitis occurs in a small subset of patients. Placement of a temporary pancreatic duct stent following free-cut sphincterotomy or sphincterotomy for sphincter of Oddi dysfunction reduces the risk of ERCP-induced pancreatitis.

Endoscopic sphincterotomy has an overall complication rate of 5% to 8%, equally divided among bleeding, perforation, cholangitis, and pancreatitis. One percent to 2% of patients undergoing sphincterotomy require surgical intervention for related complications; the mortality rate for sphincterotomy is 0.5% to 1%. Attempted biliary drainage with endoprosthesis placement has an 8% risk of cholangitis, but most of these episodes occur when drainage is unsuccessful or incomplete. Stent occlusion and cholangitis are delayed complications that occur in 40% of patients in a mean of 5 to 6 months after endoprosthetic insertion.

ENDOSCOPIC ULTRASOUND

Indications and Contraindications

Endoscopic ultrasound (EUS) provides the capability of obtaining high-resolution ultrasound images within the upper and lower gastrointestinal tracts. Specialized endoscopes with ultrasound probes at the tips and oblique-viewing optics can generate acoustic images of gastrointestinal wall layers and surrounding strictures. The increased availability of the instruments and clinical experience with the technique has expanded the list of clinical indications for EUS (Table 76-5). Focal intramural and extramural mass lesions and wall thickening are easily identified by EUS. Localization to a specific wall layer (i.e., mucosa, submucosa, muscularis, serosa, extralumenal) often helps to identify the histological origin of the lesion. EUS is useful in detecting anal sphincter defects in patients with incontinence and has been used to localize enterocutaneous fistulae in Crohn's disease. EUS is also of value in identifying and staging several tumors, including esophageal carcinoma, gastric carcinoma, gastric lymphoma, ampullary carcinoma, distal bile duct carcinoma, pancreatic carcinoma, and rectal carcinoma. EUS is both sensitive and specific in determining the local extent of the tumor (T stage) and the presence of regional lymph nodes (N stage), but it is not a reliable means of establishing distant metastatic disease (M stage). EUS is superior to CT and magnetic resonance imaging studies and to transabdominal ultrasound for pancreatic imaging, and it is the most accurate means for defining vascular invasion by tumors in the peripancreatic bed. Similarly, EUS can localize pancreatic islet cell tumors not detected by conventional imaging studies. Evidence suggests that the sensitivity of EUS is equivalent to that of ERCP for detecting common bile duct stones and chronic pancreatitis.

The introduction of instruments to obtain ultrasound-directed fine-needle aspiration has further expanded the role of EUS. Sampling of pancreatic mass lesions has proved useful, particularly in patients with unresectable disease who are candidates for palliative radiation therapy or chemotherapy. EUS-directed transesophageal aspiration of mediastinal lymph nodes has proved superior to other nonsurgical methods of staging non–small-cell lung cancer and often provides information critical to the decision to pursue surgical or nonsurgical therapy in these

TABLE 76-5
Indications for Endoscopic Ultrasound

Tumor staging (esophageal, gastric, pancreatic, ampullary, distal bile duct, rectal, non–small-cell lung)
Neuroendocrine tumor localization
Evaluation of submucosal mass lesions
Suspected chronic pancreatitis
Detection of distal bile duct stones
Fine-needle aspiration of adjacent lymph nodes or mass lesions
Evaluation of anal sphincters
Suspected enterocutaneous fistula
Direct endoscopic cystgastrostomy for pancreatic pseudocysts

patients. The same instrumentation used in tissue sampling has launched EUS into therapeutics. EUS-guided needle injection of the celiac ganglia has been used to control chronic pain caused by chronic pancreatitis or pancreatic cancer. Endoscopic ultrasound can direct needle placement and detect pericystic blood vessels in patients undergoing endoscopic cystgastrostomy, thereby improving the safety profile of the procedure. Future refinements in endosonographic image quality and performance will probably expand the diagnostic and therapeutic capabilities of EUS.

Because EUS is a specialized form of upper and lower gastrointestinal endoscopy, contraindications are identical to those for diagnostic endoscopy in their respective locations in the gastrointestinal tract.

Patient Preparation and Monitoring

Preparation of the patient for EUS of the upper gastrointestinal tract is identical to that for EGD. Similarly, EUS of the rectum or colon requires bowel cleansing in accordance with the techniques used for flexible sigmoidoscopy or colonoscopy, respectively. The principles of sedation and monitoring are also based on the standard practices for upper and lower gastrointestinal endoscopy.

Performance of the Procedure

There are two principal types of echoendoscopes. The linear or curved array instruments provide 100-degree sector images parallel to the longitudinal axis of the endoscope, whereas radial scanning instruments provide 360-degree images perpendicular to the longitudinal axis of the endoscope. Although upper echoendoscopes usually have oblique-viewing optics, echocolonoscopes are available with forward-viewing optics. The ultrasound frequency can be altered on most of the available instruments. Higher frequency imaging (12 to 20 MHz) provides increased resolution, and lower frequency imaging (5.0 to 7.5 MHz) provides increased depth of penetration. Because images from linear or curved array instruments are oriented along the axis of the endoscope, specialized needles can be advanced through the working channel and directed under real-time ultrasound guidance into a lesion for tissue aspiration.

EUS provides high-resolution images of the bowel wall and, in most structures, identifies five echolayers that correlate with the mucosa, muscularis mucosae, submucosa, muscularis propria, and serosa or adventitia. Directing the instrument to a focal submucosal mass or to an area of wall thickening can identify the layer from which the abnormality originates. The pancreas can be visualized from the duodenum or posterior wall of the stomach, whereas the bile duct and gallbladder can be identified from the duodenum. The major vascular structures of the splanchnic circulation can also be identified from the duodenum or stomach. Flow within these structures can be assessed by the color flow and pulse Doppler modes that are available on curved array instruments.

Complications

EUS has a safety profile similar to that of diagnostic upper and lower gastrointestinal endoscopy. The larger diameter of the echoendoscope makes traversing lumenal strictures more hazardous, which is problematic for esophageal tumors. Patients with significant dysphagia should undergo preliminary forward-viewing endoscopy or barium swallow radiography, so that the severity of lumenal narrowing can be assessed. Although pancreatitis following EUS fine-needle aspiration has been reported, EUS-directed biopsy is relatively safe, with a complication rate of 1% to 2%.

CHAPTER 77

Imaging Procedures

Imaging of the abdomen and gastrointestinal tract is an essential element of the diagnostic evaluation of many patients who exhibit signs and symptoms suggestive of digestive disorders. In some instances, these procedures also provide a means for obtaining histological diagnoses by using image-guided biopsies or needle aspiration. Moreover, radiologic testing plays an important role in facilitating many therapeutic interventions.

CONTRAST RADIOLOGY

Pharynx

Pharyngoesophagography provides structural and functional assessments of patients with swallowing disorders. A cine or video recording of the swallowing of a bolus of liquid or solid barium provides a detailed examination of the activation and coordination of the muscles involved in deglutition. Periodic radiographs are obtained to identify morphologic abnormalities. Single-contrast and double-contrast barium esophagrams are an integral part of this examination and help exclude associated motility or structural abnormalities of the esophagus.

Barium examination of the pharynx and esophagus is the procedure of choice in evaluating patients with oropharyngeal dysphagia or recurrent aspiration.

Swallowing dysfunction is particularly common in patients with cerebrovascular disease, neuromuscular disorders, head and neck tumors, and previous head and neck surgery or radiation therapy. Barium swallow radiography is a sensitive means for detecting laryngeal penetration and aspiration. *Penetration* refers to the entry of barium into the larynx because of abnormal coordination during the swallowing process; *aspiration* refers to the entry of barium into the larynx because of poor pharyngeal clearance during normal breathing. Pharyngograms are more sensitive than upper gastrointestinal endoscopy in identifying diverticula and are more than 95% sensitive in detecting mucosal neoplasms.

Upper Gastrointestinal Tract

Contrast radiography of the upper gastrointestinal tract can provide diagnostic information on patients who exhibit various signs and symptoms referable to the esophagus, stomach, or duodenum. Patients should fast for 6 to 8 hours before the study. A complete examination involves both single-contrast and double-contrast studies. For a double-contrast study, the patient swallows barium and an effervescent agent, and the gaseous distention in conjunction with a series of changes in the patient's position makes it possible to obtain detailed images of the mucosa. The single-contrast study is particularly useful for defining gross lumenal abnormalities (e.g., strictures).

In most settings, upper gastrointestinal barium radiography is less sensitive and specific than upper gastrointestinal endoscopy for detecting mucosal disease, although studies by a radiologist who specializes in double-contrast examinations may have an accuracy approaching that of upper gastrointestinal endoscopy. The sensitivity of barium swallow radiography for detecting reflux esophagitis can be as high as 90%, but it is an unreliable means for detecting Barrett mucosa. Similarly, although double-contrast examinations can detect ulcers and strictures of the esophagus, endoscopic biopsy is necessary to confirm the histological diagnosis. Double-contrast studies are also sensitive for detecting gastric erosions and ulcers. There are radiographic features that suggest a benign gastric ulcer, including prepyloric location and symmetric radiating folds, but some clinicians advocate endoscopic biopsy of all gastric ulcers. Contrast examination of the duodenum may identify duodenal ulcer disease, and it is superior to endoscopy in defining lumenal strictures. Occasionally, it is difficult to distinguish active from healed gastroduodenal ulcers in barium radiographic studies. Upper gastrointestinal endoscopy is the procedure of choice when examining patients with acute gastrointestinal hemorrhage.

Although there are no absolute contraindications to contrast radiography of the upper gastrointestinal tract, the use of barium is contraindicated in patients with suspected perforation. In these cases, a water-soluble agent (e.g., meglumine [Gastrografin]) should be substituted. Because Gastrografin may trigger an intense inflammatory response if aspirated, however, barium is the agent of choice if a tracheoesophageal fistula or a swallowing disorder is suspected. A thorough examination requires extensive maneuvering of the patient, which means that studies of immobile or uncooperative patients are often of limited diagnostic value.

Small Intestine

The small intestine may be examined by dedicated barium radiography or by small bowel enema (enteroclysis), which provides more detail. In dedicated barium radiographic studies of the small intestine, the patient is often given metoclopramide 20 minutes before ingesting 500 mL barium. The upper gastrointestinal tract is examined briefly, and the barium is followed through the small intestine with periodic fluoroscopy and abdominal radiography. Enteroclysis requires a skilled and dedicated radiologist. The duodenum is intubated with a balloon occlusion catheter; the injection of barium is followed by the infusion of 1500 to 2000 mL of a 0.5% solution of methylcellulose, which distends the loops of the small intestine and provides a detailed, double-contrast examination of the mucosa. Enteroclysis is more sensitive than dedicated barium radiography of the small intestine in defining small tumors or subtle mucosal abnormalities, but enteroclysis is more time-consuming and labor-intensive and is more uncomfortable for the patient because of the duodenal intubation and distention. As a result, dedicated barium radiography of the small intestine is often used initially, and if there is a high suspicion of a pathological condition in the small intestine and the standard examination findings are normal, enteroclysis can be performed.

Contrast studies are the procedures of choice in evaluating patients with symptoms of partial or incomplete obstruction of the small intestine. In addition to defining the level of obstruction, the study may identify the cause of obstruction. Barium radiography of the small intestine is particularly useful for diagnosing and defining the extent of Crohn's disease. Disease complications (e.g., strictures and fistulae) are best identified by barium studies. Benign and malignant tumors of the small intestine can be detected, but the clinician must remember that small tumors can be overlooked on dedicated barium radiography of the small intestine. Enteroclysis is the best test for detecting subtle mucosal abnormalities. Enteroclysis is also the preferred test if a mucosal malabsorptive process or Meckel diverticulum is suspected. Although barium studies are often used for patients with unexplained gastrointestinal bleeding, the diagnostic yield is extremely low, primarily because barium studies cannot identify vascular ectasias.

Colon

To achieve an adequate examination of the mucosa of the colon, the patient must undergo colonic cleansing before barium enema radiography. Preparative regimens vary, but a common procedure involves a diet of clear liquids for 24 hours followed by ingestion of 300 mL magnesium citrate and 10 mg bisacodyl the evening before the study and a repeat dose of bisacodyl the morning of the procedure. Patients with renal failure should not be given purgatives that contain magnesium. Single-contrast barium enema radiography involves filling the entire colon with low-density barium, whereas double-contrast evaluation uses a small amount of high-density barium followed by insufflation of air, which produces a thin coating of barium over the entire colonic mucosa.

Single-contrast agents provide only limited views of mucosal structures and are primarily indicated if a colonic stricture or diverticular disease is suspected. Double-contrast studies are superior to single-contrast examinations for defining mucosal disease including colorectal polyps. Areas of the rectum and sigmoid colon are often difficult to visualize by barium radiography, and no examination of the colon should be considered complete without flexible sigmoidoscopy. Conversely, the cecum cannot be visualized in up to 10% of patients undergoing colonoscopy, and barium enema radiography is often necessary in these circumstances for a complete examination of the colon.

Although colonoscopy is superior to barium enema radiography in detecting small colorectal polyps and subtle mucosal disease, barium enema radiography is 95% sensitive in detecting colorectal cancer. Double-contrast barium radiography can reliably define polyps larger than 1 cm in diameter and can detect ulcerations in advanced inflammatory bowel disease. However, the superior sensitivity and specificity of endoscopy as well as the capability of obtaining biopsy specimens and performing a polypectomy have established colonoscopy as the procedure of choice for these disorders.

Barium enema radiography is less expensive and safer than colonoscopy, but it requires adequate patient mobility. Barium enema radiography is contraindicated in the setting of toxic megacolon, ischemic colitis, or confirmed perforation. If a perforation is suspected, water-soluble contrast agents should be used. Colonic perforation is a rare complication of barium enema radiography.

ULTRASOUND

Diagnostic ultrasound relies on differences in acoustic impedance between distinct tissues. Acoustic impedance determines the speed of sound in a given tissue, and when a sound wave encounters an interface of tissues with different densities, a portion of the sound wave is reflected. As sound travels through acoustically homogeneous substances (e.g., fluid), echoes are minimal or absent. When sound encounters the border between substances with dramatically different acoustic densities (e.g., an air-tissue interface), however, all of the acoustic energy is reflected, producing an intense echo signal. Ultrasound images are generated by transformation of returning echoes into electrical signals with a magnitude proportional to the intensity of the sound wave amplitude.

Currently available ultrasound units provide real-time images with a resolution that is based on the frequency of the transducer. Higher frequency probes increase the resolution but diminish the depth of penetration. Pulse and color-flow Doppler units can qualitatively and quantitatively assess the flow in vascular strictures. Despite improvements in instrument standardization, the overall accuracy of ultrasound continues to depend on the skill of the technician and the interpreting radiologist.

Liver

Ultrasound is a noninvasive method for diagnosing several hepatic disorders. The normal hepatic parenchyma appears homogeneous and relatively hypoechoic, but in cirrhosis, the liver usually appears small, lobular, heterogeneous, and relatively hyperechoic. Other diffuse hepatocellular disorders are inconsistently associated with nonspecific changes in parenchymal echo texture. Documenting the dimensions of the hepatic lobes is helpful in establishing the small size. Collateral vessels or ascites caused by portal hypertension can also be identified. Furthermore, Doppler assessment can establish the presence and direction of flow (hepatofugal versus hepatopetal) in the portal vein. Doppler ultrasound should be the initial procedure for patients with suspected occlusion of the portal or hepatic vein.

Ultrasound is also instrumental in examining hepatic mass lesions; several series have documented sensitivity equivalent to that of CT scanning. The lack of intravenous contrast and radiation exposure has prompted recommendations that ultrasound be the initial imaging method for detecting liver masses. Ultrasound is particularly accurate in defining cystic lesions of the liver. Moreover, ultrasound has a sensitivity of 90% and a specificity of 93% in detecting hepatocellular carcinoma and is more sensitive than CT scanning in detecting tumors less than 3 cm in diameter. Conversely, contrast-enhanced CT scanning is more sensitive than ultrasound in defining liver metastases. Similarly, hemangiomas characteristically appear as peripheral hyperechoic lesions, but confirmation of the diagnosis usually requires contrast-enhanced CT or magnetic resonance imaging (MRI) studies or tagged erythrocyte nuclear scintigraphy. Because ultrasound provides real-time images, it is often the procedure of choice for obtaining image-guided biopsy specimens of hepatic mass lesions.

Biliary Tract

Ultrasound is the noninvasive procedure of choice for examining patients with suspected biliary disorders. The sensitivity and specificity for detecting gallstones are 98% and 95%, respectively. Stones typically appear as focal hyperechoic densities with acoustic shadowing distal to the stone because of nearly complete reflection of the sound wave. Ultrasound also is a sensitive means for detecting gallbladder sludge, which appears as an amorphous hyperechoic collection, without shadowing, in the dependent portion of the gallbladder. Ultrasound is far less accurate in detecting common bile duct stones, with sensitivities ranging from 15% to 60%; however, the associated biliary dilation is usually evident. CT scanning is superior to ultrasound in identifying distal bile duct stones and other causes of extrahepatic bile duct obstruction.

Ultrasound is often used as the primary diagnostic test for acute cholecystitis. Ultrasound criteria include the presence of increased gallbladder wall thickness, a sonographic Murphy sign, a distended gallbladder, pericholecystic fluid, and stones or sludge. The sonographic Murphy sign is defined as maximal tenderness with the ultrasound transducer positioned over the gallbladder. This finding has a sensitivity of 65%, but it is often absent in gangrenous cholecystitis. Based on the above criteria, ultrasound has an overall accuracy of 90% in diagnosing acute cholecystitis. In many centers, radionuclide imaging is used as a complementary test if the results of ultrasound are equivocal.

Pancreas

Ultrasound of the pancreas often is limited by the organ's retroperitoneal location and ultrasound's inability to image through overlying bowel gas. As a result, a CT scan is the noninvasive procedure of choice for excluding pancreatic disease. Ultrasound still has a substantial role in evaluating patients with pancreatic disorders, however. Ultrasound should be the initial imaging procedure for patients with acute pancreatitis, primarily because it can detect gallstones. In addition, when the pancreas is visualized, complications of acute and chronic pancreatitis, including fluid collections, abscesses, and pseudocysts, may be identified. Ultrasound often is preferable to CT scanning for following a pseudocyst over time because of the lower cost and lack of radiation exposure.

Ultrasound may detect up to 80% to 90% of pancreatic adenocarcinomas and 50% of pancreatic endocrine tumors. Contrast-enhanced CT scanning has superior sensitivity and provides added staging information, making it the noninvasive procedure of choice for evaluating pancreatic neoplasms. If a mass lesion is identified by ultrasound, however, an image-guided biopsy can establish the diagnosis for up to 90% of tumors.

Miscellaneous Abdominal Structures

Ultrasound is the best imaging technique for establishing the presence of ascites. As little as 30 mL of fluid can be detected in the hepatorenal recess. Acute appendicitis usually is a clinical diagnosis, but ultrasound can provide corroborative evidence for the diagnosis. In acute appendicitis, the appendix is visualized as a thick-walled, noncompressible target lesion. The finding of a complex fluid collection distinct from the ovaries suggests an associated abscess. Ultrasound is also helpful in identifying other intra-abdominal inflammatory processes, including diverticulitis and abdominal abscesses, but CT scanning is a more sensitive method for diagnosing these disorders.

COMPUTED TOMOGRAPHY

CT produces cross-sectional images of the body by reconstructing radiographic images obtained using a thin, fan-shaped collimated x-ray beam that penetrates the body at varying angles and is detected by an opposing array of detectors. Tissues are represented on a gray-scale continuum measured in Hounsfield units. Imaging of abdominal structures requires orally administered contrast agents to identify lumenal structures and intravenous contrast agents to identify vascular structures and focal abnormalities in specific organs. Axial images can be obtained every 1 to 10 mm. The introduction of helical CT scanning significantly shortened scan times such that large areas (such as the entire abdomen) can be scanned in a single breath-hold, resulting in less motion artifact and improved image quality. Arterial phase and venous phase scans can be obtained with a single injection of contrast. As with ultrasound, CT can guide needle biopsies and catheter drainage of collected fluid.

In preparation for abdominal CT scanning, the patient should drink water-soluble contrast material 12 and 2 hours before the procedure. If the contrast agent is given intravenously, the patient should fast or ingest only clear liquids for the 6 hours preceding the test. Anaphylactic reactions are rare, but milder reactions (e.g., rash, urticaria, and vomiting) are more common. The risk of contrast-induced renal failure is increased significantly in patients with diabetes and preexisting renal dysfunction or if the contrast agent is administered with other nephrotoxins (e.g., aminoglycosides).

Liver

CT findings may be normal in the early stages of cirrhosis, but with advanced architectural changes, there are often characteristic tomographic changes. The liver may be small with irregular edges and demonstrate inhomogeneous contrast enhancement. The right lobe and left medial lobe are often disproportionately smaller relative to the caudate and left lateral lobes. CT scans may demonstrate portosystemic collaterals or ascites, which suggest portal hypertension. Contrast-enhanced scans also can define portal venous and hepatic venous thrombosis. Chronic portal vein thrombosis often is accompanied by an extensive network of porta hepatitis collaterals termed *cavernous transformation of the portal vein.*

A CT scan is of primary importance in diagnosing and defining the cause of hepatic mass lesions. Hepatocellular carcinoma may be characterized by the appearance of a solitary mass, multicentric masses, or an infiltrative pattern on the CT scan. Unfortunately, distinguishing hepatocellular carcinoma from the regenerative changes of cirrhosis is often challenging, and the overall sensitivity of CT is less than 70%. Both hepatocellular carcinoma and hepatic metastases typically have hypodense appearances in contrast-enhanced scans, but if the scans are obtained early during the arterial phase of enhancement, hepatocellular carcinomas may demonstrate marked contrast enhancement. Hemangiomas produce a characteristic pattern of enhancement that begins peripherally and progresses centrally over time. In noncontrast scans, hemangiomas appear hypodense relative to the surrounding parenchyma. Hepatic adenomas and focal nodular hyperplasia are also often identified by their hypodense appearance in delayed-contrast images. A minority of masses caused by focal nodular hyperplasia demonstrate a central stellate scar. CT is an extremely sensitive technique for detecting hepatic cysts and abscesses. Because the tomographic features of many hepatic mass lesions are similar, CT-guided needle aspiration is often necessary to establish a histological diagnosis.

Biliary Tract

Although clearly less sensitive than ultrasound for detecting gallbladder stones, CT scanning is equivalent to ultrasound in detecting biliary dilation, and it provides superior imaging of the distal common bile duct. A common bile duct larger than 8 mm in diameter or a common hepatic duct larger than 6 mm in diameter suggests biliary obstruction. CT is more sensitive than ultrasound in detecting distal bile duct stones. However, the absence of stones or biliary dilation on a CT scan does not exclude the presence of choledocholithiasis. Cholangiography remains the procedure of choice for examining distal bile ducts. CT scanning is often used in conjunction with cholangiography to detect bile duct carcinomas. Although less sensitive than endoscopic retrograde cholangiopancreatography (ERCP), CT scanning may also demonstrate saccular dilation and diffuse stricturing of the biliary tree consistent with primary sclerosing cholangitis.

Pancreas

A CT scan is the preferred noninvasive method for pancreatic imaging. Intravenous contrast enhancement is necessary to distinguish the major splanchnic vessels in the peripancreatic bed. Adenocarcinoma usually appears as a hypodense mass; the overall sensitivity of CT scanning for detecting these neoplasms approaches 90%. In addition to identifying the primary tumor, a CT scan can provide critical staging information. Demonstration of vascular invasion of the large splanchnic vessels in the peripancreatic bed or of distant metastatic disease establishes the tumor as incurable. A CT scan is highly sensitive in documenting liver metastases, and dual-phase helical scanning shows improved sensitivity (>80%) in detecting vascular invasion. CT has limited accuracy in detecting small endocrine tumors of the pancreas. Whereas nonfunctioning tumors are often large and easily demonstrated in CT scans, gastrinomas and insulinomas are often less than 2 cm in diameter and escape detection. Cystic masses of the pancreas are readily identified, but CT-guided needle aspiration may be necessary to distinguish neoplastic cysts from pancreatic pseudocysts. The ability of CT to distinguish between microcystic and macrocystic neoplasms and intraductal papillary neoplasms with their divergent risks is limited.

Although usually reserved for patients with severe disease, contrast-enhanced CT scanning often provides information critical in managing acute pancreatitis. The extent of pancreatic necrosis, as represented by unenhanced parenchyma, has been closely correlated with the risk of complications (e.g., infected fluid collections and abscesses). CT is the most sensitive means for detecting pseudocysts and peripancreatic fluid collections. CT-guided needle aspiration for Gram stain and culture can be used if the clinical signs suggest the presence of an infection. CT-guided catheter drainage is one of many therapies for patients with refractory pseudocysts.

Colon

CT is useful in evaluating many colonic disorders, including ischemia, inflammatory bowel disease, diverticulitis, and colon cancer. The ability of helical CT to acquire a continuous, three-dimensional volumetric data set has led to the development of CT colonography or "virtual colonoscopy." These studies, like routine colonoscopy, require bowel preparation (usually oral sodium phosphate solution) but use no sedation; this allows patients to return to normal activity immediately. Although the sensitivity and specificity of virtual colonoscopy vary considerably among studies and evaluation of its clinical effectiveness is ongoing, the technique is likely to have a future role in colon cancer screening.

Miscellaneous Abdominal Structures

CT has emerged as the most important preoperative staging procedure for many gastrointestinal malignancies. A CT scan is often used in staging esophageal, gastric, small intestinal, and colorectal malignancies. Although it is generally impossible to differentiate gastrointestinal wall thickening caused by inflammatory disorders from thickening caused by a neoplasm in a CT scan, CT is a sensitive technique for detecting distant metastatic disease, invasion of adjacent structures, and lymph node enlargement. CT is also useful in the surveillance for tumor recurrence after curative resection.

CT is the most sensitive means for detecting intra-abdominal abscesses. In patients with Crohn's disease or diverticulitis with palpable abdominal masses and systemic signs of infection, CT scans may reveal a localized fluid collection in addition to the nonspecific bowel wall thickening observed in these disorders. Distinguishing an abscess from a fluid-filled loop of bowel demands adequate preparation with an oral contrast agent. When an intra-abdominal abscess is identified, the initial therapeutic approach often involves CT-guided catheter drainage of the abscess cavity.

Although surgical exploration is recommended for patients with an established obstruction of the small intestine, a CT scan is often helpful in confirming the diagnosis and directing the management if the findings of an abdominal radiograph are equivocal. In addition, the various causes of obstruction (e.g., adhesions, lumenal mass lesions, extrinsic mass lesions, and inflammatory disorders) can usually be distinguished in CT scans.

MAGNETIC RESONANCE IMAGING

MRI relies on the magnetic properties of hydrogen nuclei in various tissues. MRI scanners apply a magnetic field to the body, and radiofrequency pulses disturb the alignment of hydrogen nuclei with the magnetic field. The signal intensity for generating an image is based on the time required for the hydrogen nuclei to return to the original magnetic orientation (T1 weighted) and the decay of the nuclear orientation imposed by the radiofrequency pulse (T2 weighted). Images can be reconstructed in multiple planes, but anatomic references are easier to establish in the transverse plane. Because acquisition time is often of the order of minutes, image quality is very susceptible to motion artifact. Therefore, MRI has not proved useful for examining lumenal structures. Future advances in scanning techniques and software may decrease the image acquisition time and improve the spatial resolution of the bowel.

MRI primarily has played a role secondary to CT scanning for abdominal imaging. Focal lesions of the liver and pancreas are readily identified by MRI, but there is no evidence that MRI is superior to contrast-enhanced CT scanning. However, MRI is particularly useful in characterizing focal liver masses and may detect metastases in patients with cirrhosis.

The specific capability for imaging fluid-filled and vascular structures is unique to MRI. Gradient echo techniques used to define the biliary tree provide images with good resolution. As the quality of these images improves, MRI cholangiography may replace ERCP as a diagnostic method for some patients with disorders of the biliary system. Gradient echo imaging techniques are also being used to define blood flow in vascular structures. This is particularly useful as a noninvasive means for detecting portal vein or hepatic vein thrombosis or atherosclerotic disease of the splanchnic circulation.

Any ferromagnetic particle may be accelerated toward the scanner's magnet. Therefore, a careful history of prior surgical procedures and metal exposures should be obtained. MRI is contraindicated in patients with intraocular metallic fragments or ferromagnetic cerebral aneurysm clips. Most orthopedic and cardiovascular prostheses are safe. The presence of a cardiac pacemaker, however, is a relative contraindication to MRI because the powerful magnetic field can inhibit pacemaker function. Recent studies suggest that MRI is safe for carefully selected patients with pacemakers.

ANGIOGRAPHY

MRI and CT scans provide images of the major splanchnic vessels, but angiography remains the standard for imaging the gastrointestinal vascular system. Standard techniques involve fluoroscopically guided injection of a contrast agent into the selected vessel followed by sequential radiographs. Digital subtraction techniques have gained popularity because they require smaller amounts of the contrast agent and can be viewed on a video monitor; however, standard fluoroscopic techniques continue to provide superior image resolution. Technical considerations vary with each procedure. Arterial vessels are usually accessed by transfemoral or transaxillary approaches. The systemic venous circulation is usually entered from an internal jugular cannula, whereas portal venous access requires a transhepatic puncture. Most procedures can be performed in an outpatient service. Patient preparation requires clearing any residual lumenal contrast agent, and oral intake should be limited to clear liquids for 6 to 8 hours before the study. A small dose of a benzodiazepine is usually administered immediately before the study, and throughout the procedure, the patient is monitored for changes in heart rate, blood pressure, pulse oximetry values, and cardiac rhythm. The overall complication rates vary from 1.8% to 3.3%. The most common complications are puncture site bleeding and catheter-induced hemorrhage or embolization. Reactions to contrast agents occur in less than 1 in 1000 patients and anaphylaxis is even less common. The risk of renal failure is related to the amount of contrast material used; the overall risk is 1 in 10,000 patients. Carbon dioxide has been used as a contrast agent to visualize abdominal vasculature and aid in diagnosing gastrointestinal bleeding.

Angiography is the cornerstone of diagnosing occlusive and nonocclusive diseases of the splanchnic circulation. Selective injection of the superior mesenteric artery can identify any of the causes of acute mesenteric ischemia, including an arterial embolus, an arterial thrombus, a venous thrombus, and arteriolar vasospasm. Similarly, injection of the celiac, superior mesenteric, and inferior mesenteric arteries demonstrates significant narrowing of at least two of these vessels in patients with intestinal angina. Percutaneous translumenal angioplasty is a safe and effective alternative to surgery for treating intestinal ischemia caused by arteriosclerotic occlusive disease. Less common vascular disorders (e.g., mesenteric vasculitis and aneurysms) can also be identified by angiography. Venous phase studies are necessary to detect thrombosis of the portal vein or one of its major tributaries. Hepatic vein balloon occlusion venography is the procedure of choice for identifying the hepatic vein occlusion responsible for the Budd-Chiari syndrome, and translumenal balloon angioplasty can be used to restore hepatic vein patency.

TABLE 77-1
Indications and Contraindications to a Transjugular Intrahepatic Portosystemic Shunt

Indications
　Control of esophageal, gastric, small intestinal, or colonic variceal bleeding
　Control of bleeding from portal gastropathy
　Treatment of intractable ascites

Contraindications
　Fulminant hepatic failure
　Severe preprocedure hepatic encephalopathy despite medical therapy
　Active hepatic infection or bacteremia
　Decompensated heart failure
　Complete portal vein thrombosis

Because many tumors have abnormal vascular patterns, angiography can be used to identify primary or metastatic lesions. The introduction of contrast-enhanced CT and MRI techniques has diminished the role of angiography in the primary diagnosis of tumors, but it remains a valuable tool for detecting vascular invasion. Angiographic techniques also have a role in neuroendocrine tumor localization using selective intraarterial secretin injections followed by hepatic vein gastrin measurements for gastrinomas and intraarterial calcium infusion with hepatic vein insulin measurements for insulinomas. Angiography is also instrumental in the therapy of a wide variety of hepatic metastases through the use of hepatic artery infusion catheters and chemoembolization techniques.

Angiography is an important supplement to endoscopic intervention for variceal and nonvariceal gastrointestinal hemorrhage. A patient with bleeding gastroesophageal varices who has failed to respond to endoscopic therapy should be considered for a transjugular intrahepatic portosystemic shunt (TIPS) (Table 77-1). A TIPS is created by channeling a needle catheter from a hepatic vein tributary through the liver parenchyma until a branch of the portal vein is encountered. The established tract is dilated, and a stent is positioned across the tract to maintain patency. Ten percent to 20% of TIPS procedures are complicated by encephalopathy, but most cases can be controlled with medical therapy. When the portosystemic gradient is reduced to less than 12 mm Hg, a TIPS is extremely effective in reducing the risk of further bleeding. However, long-term patency rates have been disappointing, and a TIPS has been viewed primarily as a bridge to liver transplantation.

Nonvariceal upper and lower gastrointestinal hemorrhage occasionally requires angiography to identify or treat the source of blood loss. Although usually not helpful in identifying the source of upper gastrointestinal bleeding, selective arterial embolization is an effective means for controlling arterial bleeding caused by peptic ulcer disease if endoscopic therapy fails and the patient is a poor surgical candidate. Angiography plays a more important role in localizing and treating bleeding below the ligament of Treitz. Bleeding from diverticula, vascular ectasias, tumors, and aneurysms can be identified by angiographic techniques. Intraarterial vasopressin can be infused to control bleeding once a source is identified. Although sources of chronic lower gastrointestinal blood loss are best treated by endoscopic or surgical interventions, angiography may be helpful in identifying the source of blood loss.

Subject Index

Page numbers followed by f indicate a figure; t following a page number indicates tabular material.

A

Abdomen. *See* Acute abdomen
Abdominal aortic aneurysm
  causing acute abdomen, 57
Abdominal cavity
  anatomy, 470–471
  developmental anomalies, 471–473
  embryology, 470–471
Abdominal mass, 94–100
  differential diagnosis, 95–97
  etiology, 96t–97t
  histopathological evaluation, 99
  history, 97–98
  laboratory studies, 98
  physical examination, 98
  structural studies, 98–99
  treatment, 99–100
  workup, 97–99
Abdominal pain, 45–54
  chronology, 48–49
  complications, 53–54
  differential diagnosis, 45–46
  etiology, 46t–47t
  history, 47–48
  intensity, 48
  localization, 48
  quality, 48
  skin conditions associated with, 594–595
  treatment, 52–53
  workup, 47–48, 51f
Abdominal paracentesis, 128
Abdominal radiographs
  with abdominal pain, 52
  for ascites, 129
  chronic pancreatitis, 438
  for gas and bloating, 65
  gastric emptying disorders, 235
  IBD, 365
  in nausea and vomiting, 42
  small intestine dysmotility, 293
  small intestine ischemia, 608
Abdominal wall hernias
  with ascites, 132
Abetalipoproteinemia, 568
Abnormal chemistry, 113–123
  complications, 123
  differential diagnosis, 113–114
  hepatic function tests, 116–117

  history, 115–116
  physical examination, 116
  treatment, 122–123
Abscesses, 477–478
Acalculous cholecystitis
  gallstones, 464
Acanthosis nigricans, 593
Acetaminophen
  with conjugated hyperbilirubinemia, 109
  hepatotoxicity, 500–502
Achalasia, 196–199
  causing nausea and vomiting, 41
  clinical presentation, 197
  diagnosis, 197–198
  epidemiology, 196
  etiology, 196–197
  incidence, 196
  pathogenesis, 196–197
  primary, 6
  secondary, 6
  surgery, 199
Acid peptic disorders, 240–253
  epidemiology, 240
  etiology, 241
  incidence, 240
  pathogenesis, 241
Acid reflux testing
  GERD, 208
Acinarization, 625
Acquired hypogammaglobulinemia, 581
Acquired hypopharyngeal diverticula, 194
Acquired immunodeficiency syndrome (AIDS)
  acute abdominal pain, 554
  with conjugated hyperbilirubinemia, 109
  diarrhea, 549–553
  epidemiology, 547
  esophageal disorders, 547–549
  etiology, 547
  gastrointestinal complications of, 547–554
  gastrointestinal hemorrhage, 554
  hepatobiliary diseases, 553–554
Acquired polyposis syndrome, 398
Acquired Zenker diverticula, 194
Acromegaly, 571
Actinomyces israelii
  esophagus, 215
Activated charcoal
  for gas and bloating, 67

Acute abdomen, 54–61
  complications, 61
  differential diagnosis, 54–55
  etiology, 55t
  history, 57–58
  physical examination, 58–59
  with pregnancy, 143–144, 143t
  treatment, 60–61
  workup, 57–60, 59f
Acute appendicitis, 54
  ultrasound, 632
Acute cholecystitis
  causing acute abdomen, 56
  gallstones, 463–464
Acute colonic pseudoobstruction, 347–348
Acute diarrhea
  testing, 83
Acute fatty liver of pregnancy, 146–147
Acute gallstones
  cholecystitis, 463–464
Acute gastritis, 263–264
Acute graft-versus-host disease, 586–588
  causing nausea and vomiting, 40
Acute ileus, 68
Acute intermittent porphyria, 568, 569t
  causing abdominal pain, 47
Acute lower gastrointestinal bleeding, 22–23
  complications, 26
  differential diagnosis, 22
  history, 23
  medications, 24–25
  physical examination, 23
  resuscitation, 24
  surgery, 26
  treatment, 24–25
  workup, 23–24, 25f
Acute megacolon, 347–348
Acute pancreatitis, 427–434
  causing acute abdomen, 56
  clinical features, 430–431
  complications, 432–433
  course, 432–434
  diagnosis, 431–432
  differential diagnosis, 428t
  epidemiology, 427
  etiology, 427–430
  incidence, 427
  pathogenesis, 427–430
  prognosis, 432, 433t
  risk factors, 429–430
  treatment, 432–434
Acute sickle cell crisis, 574
Acute suppurative peritonitis, 484
Acute upper gastrointestinal bleeding,
      15–17
  differential diagnosis, 15–16
  treatment, 19–22
  workup, 19f
Acyclovir
  for intestinal infections in HIV-1 infected
      adults, 551t
Addison disease, 571

Adenocanthomas
  esophagus, 222
Adenocarcinoma. *See* Colon adenocarcinoma;
      Ductal adenocarcinoma; Gastric
      adenocarcinoma
Adenomatous polyps, 383–390
  chemoprevention, 388
  clinical features, 386–387
  course, 387–388
  diagnosis, 387–388
  epidemiology, 383–394
  etiology, 385–386
  incidence, 383–394
  malignant, 389–390, 389t
  natural history, 387–388
  pathogenesis, 385–386
  risk factors, 386
  screening, 388–389
  treatment, 387–388
Adenosquamous carcinoma
  esophagus, 222
Adult rumination syndrome
  causing weight loss, 34
Aeromonas
  foodborne disease, 305
  health care workers, 181
Aerophagia, 65
  causing gas and bloating, 64, 67
AFP. *See* Alpha-fetoprotein (AFP)
AIDS. *See* Acquired immunodeficiency syndrome
      (AIDS)
Air travel, 168–169
ALA. *See* Aminolevulinic acid (ALA)
5-ALA. *See* 5-aminolevulinic acid (5-ALA)
Alanine aminotransferase, 117–118
Albendazole
  for intestinal infections in HIV-1 infected
      adults, 551t
Albumin, 117
Alcohol abuse
  causing weight loss, 33
  with conjugated hyperbilirubinemia,
      108–109
  drug interactions, 524t
  esophageal tumors, 217
Alcohol dependence syndrome, 163t
Alcohol dependency, 162–163
Alcoholic cirrhosis
  treatment, 528
Alcoholic hepatitis
  treatment, 527–528
Alcoholic liver diseases, 522–528
  clinical features, 525
  diagnosis, 525–526
  etiology, 523–524
  pathogenesis, 523–524
  treatment, 527–528
Alcoholic steatosis
  treatment, 527
Alkaline phosphatase, 118, 120–121, 121f
  with abdominal pain, 51
Alkaline reflux esophagitis, 212

Alosetron
    producing colonic ischemia, 378
Alpha-1 antitrypsin deficiency, 119, 516
    diagnosis, 114t
Alpha-fetoprotein (AFP), 119–120
Altitude illness, 173
AMAG. *See* Autoimmune metaplastic atrophic
        gastritis (AMAG)
Ambien, 168
Ambulatory pH monitoring
    for chest pain, 12
    GERD, 208
Amebiasis, 555
Amiloride
    for ascites, 129
Amine precursor uptake and decarboxylation
        (APUD), 328, 448
Amino acid
    absorption disorders, 316
    transport disorders, 316–317
5-aminolevulinic acid (5-ALA)
    for Crohn's disease, 370
    for IBD, 367
    for ulcerative colitis, 370
Aminolevulinic acid (ALA)
    dehydratase deficiency, 569t
Aminotransferase, 117–118, 120–121
Amitriptyline
    for chest pain, 14
Ameba
    causing occult gastrointestinal bleeding, 28
Amebic liver abscess, 556
Amphetamine abuse, 166
Amphotericin
    for esophageal fungal infection, 214
    for intestinal infections in HIV-1 infected
            adults, 552t
Ampicillin
    for intestinal infections in HIV-1 infected
            adults, 552t
Amylase
    with acute abdomen, 59
Amyloidosis
    cutaneous manifestations, 592
    with small intestine dysmotility, 291
Amyotrophic lateral sclerosis, 577
ANA. *See* Antinuclear antibody (ANA)
Anabolic steroid, 167–168
Anal fissure, 410–411
Analgesia
    chronic pancreatitis, 439
Anal malignancies, 417
Anal myotomy
    for constipation, 94
Anal stenosis, 412
Anal warts, 356
Ancylostoma braziliense, 563
Ancylostoma caninum, 563
Ancylostoma ceylanicum, 562
Ancylostoma duodenale (hookworms), 562
Anderson-Fabry disease, 568
Angel dust, 166

Angiodysplasia, 599–601
    with acute lower gastrointestinal bleeding, 22
    causing upper gastrointestinal bleeding, 17
Angiography, 636–637
    for acute lower gastrointestinal bleeding,
            25–26
    for hepatocellular carcinoma, 541
    for lower gastrointestinal bleeding, 24
    for pancreatic endocrine neoplasms, 451
    for small intestine ischemia, 608–609
    for upper gastrointestinal bleeding, 18, 21
Angiosarcomas
    cutaneous manifestations, 605
Angiostrongylus costaricensis, 563–564
Angular stomatitis
    with IBD, 591
Anisakiasis, 563
Annular pancreas, 421–422
Anorectal abscess and fistula, 411
Anorectal disease, 409–418
Anorectal manometry
    for constipation, 92
Anorectal syphilis, 356
Anorectal varices, 410
Anorexia nervosa
    causing weight loss, 33–34
    with cocaine use, 579
    with pain, 49
Antacids
    for dyspepsia, 246–247
Antibiotics
    for IBD, 369
Antibody defects, 580–584
Antibody testing
    for celiac disease, 311
Antibody to HBsAg (anti-HB), 118
Antibody to hepatitis A (anti-HAV), 118
Anticoagulants
    causing occult gastrointestinal bleeding, 28
Antiemetic agents, 237–238
    for nausea and vomiting, 43
Antinuclear antibody (ANA), 119
Anti-smooth muscle antibody (ASMA), 119
Antrectomy
    for duodenal ulcers, 254
Aortic aneurysm
    abdominal
            causing acute abdomen, 57
Aortoenteric fistula
    causing upper gastrointestinal bleeding, 17
APC gene in familial adenomatous polyposis, 385,
            391, 392t, 393–394
Aphthous ulcers
    with acquired immunodeficiency syndrome
            (AIDS), 547
    with IBD, 591
Appendicitis
    acute, 54
        ultrasound, 632
    causing pain, 48
Aprepitant
    for nausea and vomiting, 44

APUD. *See* Amine precursor uptake and
  decarboxylation (APUD)
Arsenic poisoning, 573–574
Ascaris
  causing occult gastrointestinal bleeding, 28
  in returning traveler, 174
Ascaris lumbricoides, 561–562
Ascites, 124–133
  blood and urine studies, 127–128
  with cirrhosis, 534
  complications, 131–132
  differential diagnosis, 124–125
  etiology, 125t
  with gas and bloating, 65
  history, 126–127
  with myxedema, 126
  physical examination, 127–128
  treatment, 129–131, 130t
  ultrasound, 632
Ascitic fluid
  analysis, 128–129
Ascorbic acid. *See* Vitamin C
ASMA. *See* Anti-smooth muscle antibody
  (ASMA)
Aspartate aminotransferase, 117–118
Aspergillus
  esophagus, 213
Aspirin
  causing nausea and vomiting, 38
  with ulcer bleeding, 568
Astrovirus, 307
Asymptomatic illness
  travelers, 173
Ataxia-telangiectasia, 570, 583
Atovaquone/proguanil (Malarone), 172
Atrophic gastritis, 265–267
Atrophic pangastritis. *See* Atrophic gastritis
Atropine
  for IBD, 369
Autoantibody testing
  for autoimmune liver disease, 519
Autoimmune hepatitis
  classification of, 518t
  clinical features, 518–519
  diagnosis, 114t
  scoring, 521t
Autoimmune liver disease, 517–522
  course, 520–522
  diagnosis, 519–520
  epidemiology, 517
  etiology, 517–518
  incidence, 517
  pathogenesis, 517–518
  treatment, 520–522
Autoimmune metaplastic atrophic gastritis
  (AMAG), 265
Azathioprine
  for autoimmune liver disease, 520
  for IBD, 139, 368
  for ulcerative colitis, 370
Azithromycin
  for *Cryptosporidia,* 559

Azotemia
  with upper gastrointestinal bleeding, 18

B
Bacillus cereus
  causing nausea and vomiting, 40
  causing secretory diarrhea, 80
  foodborne diseases, 299t
  small intestine, 298
Bacterial alpha-galactosidase (Beano)
  for gas and bloating, 67
Bacterial overgrowth
  causing osmotic diarrhea, 79
Bacteroides
  with conjugated hyperbilirubinemia, 109
Balantidium coli, 560
Bannayan-Riley-Ruvalcaba syndrome, 397
Bannayan-Zonana syndrome. *See*
  Bannayan-Riley-Ruvalcaba syndrome
Barbiturates
  abuse, 164
Barium examination
  of pharynx and esophagus, 628–629
Barium radiographs
  with abdominal pain, 52
  for celiac disease, 312
  for chest pain, 12
  colon, 631
  for dysphagia, 8
  for gas and bloating, 65
  for lower gastrointestinal bleeding, 24
  short bowel syndrome, 323
  small intestine dysmotility, 293
  small intestine, 629–630
Barium swallow
  oropharyngeal dysphagia, 195
Barrett esophagus, 202
Barrett metaplasia, 220
Bartonella henselae, 553
Beano
  for gas and bloating, 67
Beef tapeworm, 564
Behavioral disorders
  causing weight loss, 33
Behavior modification, 3
Behçet disease, 190, 579
  cutaneous manifestations, 591
Belsey fundoplication
  for GERD, 211
Benign mucous membrane pemphigoid, 191
Benign recurrent intrahepatic cholestasis (BRIC),
  108
Benzene
  abuse, 167
Benzodiazepines, 3
  abuse, 164
  for chest pain, 14
Bernstein test
  GERD, 208
Bile ducts
  cancer, 459–460
  strictures, 469

Bile salt diarrhea, 80
Biliary cirrhosis. *See* Primary biliary cirrhosis
Biliary colic
 gallstones, 463
Biliary cysts, 455–457
 clinical course of, 456
 course of, 456–457
 diagnosis of, 456
 epidemiology of, 455
 etiology, 455
 incidence, 455
 pathogenesis of, 455–456
 Todani classification of, 455
 treatment of, 456–457
Biliary disease
 with ascites, 125
Biliary fistula, 469
Biliary scintigraphy
 with acute abdomen, 60
Biliary sludge
 acute pancreatitis, 429
Biliary tract, 454–461
 anatomy, 454–455
 CT, 634
 developmental anomalies of, 455
 embryology of, 454–455
 stones, 462–470
  complications, 469–470
 ultrasound, 632
Bilirubin, 116–117, 120–121
 with abdominal pain, 51
 in jaundice, 105–106
Binge drinking, 579
 causing acute upper gastrointestinal bleeding, 16
Biofeedback, 3
 for constipation, 94
Biotin
 deficiency, 156
Bismuth
 for diarrhea, 86
 for dyspepsia, 247
 for traveler's diarrhea, 172
Blastocystis hominis, 559
Bloating. *See* Gas and bloating
Blood-borne pathogens
 health care workers, 177–180
Blood tests
 for celiac disease, 311
Blue rubber bleb nevus syndrome, 570
 skin disease, 592
B-lymphocyte (antibody) defects, 580–584
Boerhaave syndrome, 45, 57, 192
Bone marrow transplantation
 with conjugated hyperbilirubinemia, 108
 gastrointestinal complications, 587t
Botulinum toxin
 for achalasia, 198
 for nausea and vomiting, 44
Bowel decompression
 for ileus, 74–75

Breath tests
 small intestinal bacterial overgrowth, 297
BRIC. *See* Benign recurrent intrahepatic cholestasis (BRIC)
Bronchopulmonary foregut malformation, 185
Brooke ileostomy, 100–102
 complications, 102
 outcome, 102
Bruton hypogammaglobulinemia, 580
Budd-Chiari syndrome, 121, 575, 579
 with ascites, 124
 radiation injury manifesting as, 614
Budesonide
 for IBD, 368
Bulimia nervosa, 578
 causing weight loss, 33–34
Bullous disease
 gastrointestinal tract, 594
Bullous pemphigoid, 191, 594
Buspirone, 3
 for chest pain, 14
Butyrophenones
 for nausea and vomiting, 43

C

CAGE questionnaire, 162
Calcitonin
 for diarrhea, 86
Calcium channel antagonists
 for achalasia, 198
Caliciviruses
 classic human, 307
Cameron erosions
 causing occult gastrointestinal hemorrhage, 27
Campylobacter
 acquired immunodeficiency syndrome (AIDS), 553
 colon, 351
 foodborne diseases, 299t
 hemolytic uremic syndrome, 574
 in returning traveler, 174
Campylobacter jejuni
 diarrhea, 138, 549
 health care workers, 181
 traveler's diarrhea, 172
Cancer cachexia, 575
Candida albicans, 577
 with acquired immunodeficiency syndrome (AIDS), 547
 causing odynophagia, 7
 causing upper gastrointestinal bleeding, 17
 esophagus, 213
Candida esophagitis, 202, 571–572
Cannabis, 166
Capillaria philippinensis, 561
Capillary leak syndrome, 575
Carbohydrate maldigestion, 63
Carcinoid syndrome, 594
 causing secretory diarrhea, 80
Carcinoma erysipeloides, 593
Carcinosarcoma
 esophagus, 222

Cardiac surgery
  complications of, 568
Cardiospasm. *See* Achalasia
Cardiovascular disease
  with ascites, 125
  gastrointestinal manifestations, 567–568
Carnett test, 50
Caroli disease, 108
Casal necklace, 596
Cat hookworms, 563
Caustic esophageal injury, 187–188
CCK. *See* Cholecystokinin (CCK)
Cefotaxime
  for SBP, 131
Ceftriaxone
  for intestinal infections in HIV-1 infected
    adults, 551t
Celiac axis, 224
Celiac disease, 308–313, 309t
  clinical features, 310–311
  complications of, 312–313
  course, 312–313
  diagnosis, 311–312
  epidemiology, 308
  etiology, 308–310
  incidence, 308
  pathogenesis, 308–310
  treatment of, 312–313
Celiac plexus block
  for abdominal pain, 53
Celiac sprue
  causing osmotic diarrhea, 79
Celiac staging and prognosis, 270
Cereal chemistry
  celiac disease, 309
Cerebrovascular accident
  causing oropharyngeal dysphagia, 194
Ceruloplasmin, 119
Cervical esophagus
  disorders of, 193–196
Cervicitis, 148
Cestodes (tapeworms), 564
Chagas disease, 6, 559–560
  with small intestine dysmotility, 291–292
Charcot triad, 57
Chemical gastritis
  chronic, 265
Chemical-induced colonic injury, 376–377,
    376t
Chemical peritonitis, 485
Chenodeoxycholic acid
  for gallstones, 465
Chest pain, 9–14
  cardiac disease causing, 10–11
  complications, 14
  differential diagnosis, 9–11
  esophageal disease, 11
  etiology, 10t
  history, 11–12
  musculoskeletal causes, 11
  neuropsychiatric causes, 11
  physical examination, 12

  treatment, 13–14
  workup, 11–13, 13f
Chest radiographs
  with abdominal pain, 52
  achalasia, 197
  for ascites, 129
  small intestine dysmotility, 293
Childhood visceral myopathies (CVMs)
  with small intestine dysmotility, 290–291
Child-Turcotte-Pugh classification, 537t
Chlamydia trachomatis
  cervicitis, 148
  proctitis, 355–356
Chloroquine, 171
Chlorozotocin
  for pancreatic endocrine neoplasms, 453
Cholecystectomy, 465
Cholecystitis
  acalculous
    gallstones, 464
  acute
    causing acute abdomen, 56
  causing pain, 48
  chronic
    gallstones, 464
  in pregnancy, 572
Cholecystokinin (CCK), 196, 449
Choledochal cyst, 108
Choledocholithiasis, 465–467
  clinical features, 466
  course, 467
  diagnosis, 466–467
  epidemiology, 465
  etiology, 465
  incidence, 465
  pathogenesis, 465
  treatment, 467
Cholera vaccine, 170
Cholestasis, 498
  with systemic infection, 495
  with total parenteral nutrition, 495
Cholestasis of pregnancy, 108
Cholestatic disorders
  differential diagnosis, 114
Cholestatic liver disease
  diagnosis, 120–121
Cholestatic syndromes, 490–496
Cholestyramine
  for diarrhea, 86
Chromium deficiency, 155
Chromosomal abnormalities, 568–569
Chromosomal instability
  colon adenocarcinoma, 400
Chromosome 21 trisomy, 568
Chronic chemical gastritis, 265
Chronic cholecystitis
  gallstones, 464
Chronic diarrhea
  directed evaluation, 84–85
  screening evaluation, 83
Chronic duodenitis, 270–271
Chronic gastritis, 264–270

Chronic glutamate receptors, 583
Chronic graft-versus-host disease, 588
Chronic idiopathic intestinal pseudoobstruction
   rheumatologic disorders, 233–234
Chronic intestinal pseudoobstruction, 68–70
   etiology, 69t
Chronic mucocutaneous candidiasis, 582
Chronic obstructive pulmonary disease
   unintentional weight loss, 32
Chronic pancreatitis, 435–440
   clinical presentation, 436–437
   complications, 440
   course, 439–440
   diagnosis, 437–438
   epidemiology, 435
   etiology, 435, 436t
   incidence, 435
   pathogenesis, 435
   treatment, 439–440
CHRPE. *See* Congenital hypertrophy of the
   retinal pigment epithelium (CHRPE)
Churg-Strauss syndrome, 579
Chylous ascites, 126
Ciguatera fish poisoning, 299t
Cimetidine, 247
Ciprofloxacillin
   for intestinal infections in HIV-1 infected
      adults, 551t, 552t
   for traveler's diarrhea, 172
Cirrhosis, 499. *See also* Primary biliary cirrhosis
   clinical features, 531–532
   with conjugated hyperbilirubinemia, 108
   course, 534–538
   diagnosis, 532–533
   endocrine manifestations, 531–532
   etiology, 529–531, 530t
   pathogenesis, 529–531
   pulmonary manifestations, 532
   renal manifestations, 532
   treatment, 528, 534–538
Cisplatin
   causing nausea and vomiting, 38
   for gastric adenocarcinoma, 275
Clarithromycin
   for intestinal infections in HIV-1 infected
      adults, 552t
Classic human caliciviruses, 307
Clonorchis sinensis, 566–567
Clostridium botulinum
   foodborne diseases, 299t, 300
Clostridium difficile, 577
   colitis, 354t
   colon, 352–354
   diarrhea, 138, 354t, 549
   health care workers, 180
   returning traveler, 174
Clostridium perfringens
   foodborne diseases, 299t, 300
   nausea and vomiting, 40
   secretory diarrhea, 80
Clotting factors, 117
Club drugs, 167

CMV. *See* Cytomegalovirus (CMV)
Cobalamin (vitamin B$_{12}$)
   absorption disorders, 318–319
   deficiency, 156
Cocaine
   abuse, 165–166
Coccygodynia, 418
Codeine
   for diarrhea, 86
Cognitive-behavioral treatment, 3
Colchicine
   for constipation, 93
Colitis. *See also* Ulcerative colitis
   diversion, 375
   ischemic, 610–611
      with acute lower gastrointestinal bleeding,
         22–23
   microscopic, 374t
   neutropenic
      causing acute abdomen, 57
Colitis cystica profunda, 382–383
Collagenous and lymphocytic colitis, 373–384
Colon
   adenoma to carcinoma sequence, 401
   anatomy, 331–333
   bacterial infections, 349–356
   CT, 634–635
   developmental abnormalities, 333–335
   embryology, 331–333
   imaging, 630–631
   laxative effects on, 377
   malignant tumors, 399–408
   malrotation, 334–335
   radiation injury, 614
Colon adenocarcinoma, 399–407
   adjuvant therapy, 403–404
   clinical features, 401–402
   course, 403–404
   diagnosis, 402–403
   diseases associated with increased risk of, 401
   environmental factors, 399–400
   etiology, 399–400
   genetic factors, 399–400
   pathogenesis, 399–400
   pathological classification, 404t
   prognosis, 403
   screening, 405–407
   treatment, 403–404
   unresectable, 405
Colonic diverticulitis
   causing acute abdomen, 56
Colonic duplication, 334
Colonic dysmotility, 348
Colonic injury
   chemical-induced, 376–377, 376t
Colonic ischemia
   medications producing, 378
Colonic lymphoma, 407–408
Colonic neoplasms
   with acute lower gastrointestinal bleeding,
      23
Colonic obstruction. *See* Obstruction

Colonic polyposis
    treatment, 395
Colonic pseudoobstruction
    acute, 347–348
    slow transit constipation, 345–346
Colonic ulcers, 379–382
Colonoscopy, 621–623, 630–631
    with abdominal pain, 52
    IBD, 363–364, 364t
    indications, 622t
Colorectal polyps
    classification, 385t
Combined B- and T-lymphocyte defects, 582
Common bile duct
    anatomy of, 454
Common variable hypogammaglobulinemia
        (acquired or late-onset), 581
Complement deficiency, 583–584
Complete blood count
    for abdominal pain, 51
    for acute abdomen, 59
    for nausea and vomiting, 41
Computed tomography (CT), 633–634
    abdominal pain, 52
    acute abdomen, 60
    acute pancreatitis, 432
    ascites, 129
    cholestasis, 120
    chronic pancreatitis, 438
    ductal adenocarcinoma, 443
    gallstones, 464
    hepatocellular carcinoma, 541
    IBD, 365
    jaundice, 111–112
Condyloma acuminata, 356
Congenital esophageal duplication, 183–184
Congenital esophageal stenosis, 183–184
Congenital hypertrophy of the retinal pigment
        epithelium (CHRPE), 394
Congenital megacolon. See Hirschsprung disease
Congenital thymic hypoplasia (DiGeorge
        syndrome), 582
Congestive heart disease
    causing nausea and vomiting, 40
    unintentional weight loss, 32
Conjugated hyperbilirubinemia, 107–109
    acquired forms, 108–109
    congenital forms, 107–108
    etiology, 106t
    familial forms, 108
Connective tissue diagnosis, 569–570
Constipation, 87–94, 578
    causing weight loss, 33
    differential diagnosis, 87–88
    drug treatment, 93–94
    elderly, 90
    etiology, 88t–89t
    functional studies, 91–92
    with gas and bloating, 67
    history, 90
    laboratory studies, 91
    with pain, 49

    physical examination, 91
    pregnancy, 142–143, 572
    structural studies, 91
    treatment, 93–95
    workup, 90–91, 92f
Continent ileostomy, 102–103
    complications, 103
    outcome, 103
Contrast radiographs, 628–631
    in nausea and vomiting, 42
    pharynx, 628–629
    upper gastrointestinal tract, 629
Copper, 119
    deficiency, 155
Cordotomy
    for abdominal pain, 53
Corticosteroids
    for IBD, 367–368
Corynebacterium diphtheriae
    esophagus, 215
Cowden disease, 392t, 397, 570
    cutaneous findings, 593
CREST syndrome, 603
Cricopharyngeal bars, 194
Crigler-Najjar syndrome, 112
Crohn's colitis. See Inflammatory bowel disease
Crohn's disease, 138, 270, 579. See also
        Inflammatory bowel disease (IBD)
    causing osmotic diarrhea, 79
    clinical features, 361t
    cutaneous manifestations, 591
    esophagus, 189–190
    gastritis, 268
    IBD, 360–362
    medical management, 370
    pregnancy, 145–146
Cryptococcus neoformans, 554
Cryptosporidium, 558–559
    acquired immunodeficiency syndrome
        (AIDS), 553
    diarrhea, 549
    in returning traveler, 174
CT. See Computed tomography (CT)
Culdocentesis
    with abdominal pain, 52
Cullen sign, 72, 595
Cutaneous larva migrans, 563
CVMs. See Childhood visceral myopathies
        (CVMs)
Cyclic vomiting syndrome, 40
    with delayed gastric emptying, 234
Cyclophosphamide
    causing nausea and vomiting, 38
Cyclospora, 559
    diarrhea, 549
Cyclosporine
    for IBD, 368–369
Cystic fibrosis, 423–426, 578
    clinical characteristics, 423–424, 424t
    course, 425–426
    diagnosis of, 424–425
    epidemiology, 423

etiology, 423
incidence, 423
pathogenesis, 423
treatment of, 425–426
Cytomegalovirus (CMV)
causing nausea and vomiting, 40
causing odynophagia, 7
with colitis, 550
esophagitis, 548
esophagus, 214
health care workers, 180
Cytoprotection, 247

D

Decarboxylation, 328, 448
Deep vein thrombosis
IBD, 362
DEET. *See N,N*-diethyl-m-toluamide (DEET)
Deferoxamine
for hemochromatosis, 122
Degos disease, 592
Dehydroemetine (Mebadin)
for liver abscess, 556
Delayed gastric emptying
GERD, 206
nongastrointestinal disorders, 234–235
Dementia, 576
Depression
causing weight loss, 33
Dermal papillae, 183
Dermatologic diseases
gastrointestinal manifestations, 570–571
Dermatomyositis, 194, 570
cutaneous manifestations, 591
Dermatosis-arthritis syndrome, 591
DES. *See* Diffuse esophageal spasm (DES)
Desipramine
for chest pain, 14
Diabetes, 571
diarrhea, 80
gastroparesis, 231–232
Diaphragmatic hernia, 472
Diarrhea, 76–86
acute
testing, 83
after vagotomy, 257–258
bile salt, 80
chronic
directed evaluation, 84–85
screening evaluation, 83
with cocaine use, 579
complications, 86
differential diagnosis, 76–79
etiology, 77t–78t
history, 81–82
mucosal injury, 81
etiology, 78t–79t
osmotic
differential diagnosis, 76–79
etiology, 77t
with pain, 49
physical examination, 82–83

secretory, 80–81
etiology, 77t–78t
traveler's, 172–173
treatment, 85–86
with VIPoma, 448–449
workup, 81–83
Diazoxide
for pancreatic endocrine neoplasms, 452
Diethyl-m-toluamide, 171
Diet therapy
constipation, 93
functional dyspepsia, 260–261
irritable bowel syndrome, 343
small intestine dysmotility, 294
Dieulafoy lesion, 598–599
causing upper gastrointestinal bleeding, 17
Dieulafoy-type colonic ulceration, 379–380, 380f
Diffuse esophageal spasm (DES)
causing chest pain, 11, 199–202
DiGeorge syndrome, 582
Digestive tract. *See* Gastrointestinal tract
Digitalis
producing colonic ischemia, 378
Digoxin
causing nausea and vomiting, 38
Dimenhydrinate
for nausea and vomiting, 43
Diphenoxylate
for diarrhea, 86
for IBD, 369
for traveler's diarrhea, 172
Diphtheria boosters, 171
Diphyllobothrium latum, 564
Disopyrobezoar, 228
Distal esophagus
spastic motor disorders of, 199–202, 200t
Distention
with ileus, 71
Diversion colitis, 375
Diverticula, 185–186, 331–339. *See also* specific
diverticula
Zenker, 6, 185–186
acquired, 194
causing nausea and vomiting, 41
elderly, 134
Diverticular hemorrhage, 339
Diverticulitis, 337–339
colonic
causing acute abdomen, 56
treatment, 338f
Diverticulosis
with acute lower gastrointestinal bleeding, 22
jejunal, 292
uncomplicated, 336–337
Dog hookworms, 563
Domperidone, 237, 237t
for nausea and vomiting, 44
Doppler ultrasound
for ascites, 129
Double contrast barium enema
colon adenocarcinoma, 402
Double duct sign, 444

Down syndrome (chromosome 21 trisomy), 568
Doxorubicin
    for gastric adenocarcinoma, 275
Doxycycline, 172
Drinking
    binge, 579
        causing acute upper gastrointestinal
            bleeding, 16
Drug abuse
    urinary screening guidelines, 165t
Drug-induced hepatic injury, 496–501, 497t
    clinical features, 498
    diagnosis, 498–501
    epidemiology, 496
    etiology, 497
    incidence, 496
    pathogenesis, 497
    treatment, 498–501
Drug-induced hepatitis
    diagnosis, 114t
Drug metabolism
    pregnancy, 140–141
Dubin-Johnson syndrome, 108, 117
Duchenne muscular dystrophy, 576
    with small intestine dysmotility, 291
Ductal adenocarcinoma, 441–447
    clinical features, 442–443
    course, 444–446
    diagnosis, 443–444
    epidemiology, 441
    etiology, 441–442
    incidence, 441
    palliative therapy, 445–446
    pathogenesis, 441–442
    risk factors, 441–442, 442t
    staging, 444–446, 444t
    surgery, 445
    treatment, 444–446
Dumping syndrome, 257
Duodenal neoplasms
    treatment, 395
Duodenal pseudomelanosis, 579
Duodenal ulcers
    diseases associated with, 243t
    pathophysiology, 244
    perforated, 54–55
    surgery of, 253–254
Duodenitis
    chronic, 270–271
    functional dyspepsia, 260
Dwarf tapeworm, 565
Dynamic psychotherapy, 3
Dysmenorrhea, 149
Dysmotility syndromes, 63–64
Dyspepsia
    initial management, 246–247
Dysphagia, 4–9, 202. *See also* Esophageal
                dysphagia; Oropharyngeal dysphagia
    with acquired immunodeficiency syndrome
            (AIDS), 547–548
    differential diagnosis, 4
    etiology, 5t

    from left atrial enlargement, 568
    physical examination, 7
    workup, 7–8, 8f
Dysphagia lusoria, 185

E
EAC. *See* Esophageal adenoma carcinoma (EAC)
Early gastric cancer, 273
Early satiety, 38
Eating disorders
    causing weight loss, 33
    with delayed gastric emptying, 234
Echinostoma, 567
Ectopic pregnancy, 148
    causing acute abdomen, 57
Edwardsiella tarda
    foodborne disease, 305
EGG. *See* Electrogastrography (EGG)
EHEC. *See* Enterohemorrhagic *Escherichia coli*
            (EHEC)
Ehlers-Danlos syndrome, 569, 592
    cutaneous manifestations, 605
EIEC. *See* Enteroinvasive *Escherichia coli* (EIEC)
Elderly, 133–140
    atrophic gastritis, 135–136
    constipation, 90, 137–138, 137t
    diarrhea, 138–139
    food intake disorders, 134–135
    hepatobiliary disease, 139–140
    malabsorptive disorders, 136–137
    physiological and pharmacological alterations
            in, 133–134
    swallowing disorders, 134–135
    ulcer disease, 135–136
    unintentional weight loss, 32
Electrogastrography (EGG)
    gastric emptying disorders, 236
    nausea and vomiting, 43
Electrolytes
    transport disorders, 317–318
Elevated liver enzymes. *See* Hemolysis, elevated
                liver enzymes, and low platelets
                (HELLP)
ELISA. *See* Enzyme-linked immunosorbent assay
                (ELISA)
EMAG. *See* Environmental metaplastic atrophic
                gastritis (EMAG)
Emesis, 14, 37–45. *See also* Nausea
    differential diagnosis, 37–40
    gravidarum
        with pregnancy, 141–142
    with ileus, 71
    medications, 38
    with pregnancy, 141–142
EMR. *See* Endoscopic mucosal resection (EMR)
End ileostomy, 100–102
Endocrinologic disorders
    causing constipation, 89
    gastrointestinal manifestations, 571–572
Endometriosis, 150, 375–376
Endoscopic mucosal resection (EMR)
    gastric adenocarcinoma, 275

Endoscopic retrograde cholangiopancreatography
    (ERCP), 623–626
  abdominal pain, 52
  acute abdomen, 60
  acute pancreatitis, 432
  alcoholic liver disease, 526
  cholestasis, 120
  complications, 625–626
  contraindications, 623–624
  ductal adenocarcinoma, 444
  indications, 623–624, 624t
  jaundice, 112
  patient monitoring, 624–625
  patient preparation, 624–625
  procedure, 625
Endoscopic ultrasonography (EUS), 626–628,
    627t
  with acute abdomen, 60
  with chronic pancreatitis, 438
  complications, 628
  ductal adenocarcinoma, 444
  pancreatic endocrine neoplasms, 451
Endoscopy, 615–628
  See also Upper endoscopy
  acute lower gastrointestinal bleeding,
    25–26
  adenomatous polyps, 387–388
  antibiotic prophylaxis, 616, 617t
  coagulation disorders, 616–618
  colon adenocarcinoma, 402
  conscious sedation, 615–616
  dysphagia, 8
  gas and bloating, 65
  IBD, 363–364
  lower gastrointestinal bleeding, 23–24
  occult gastrointestinal hemorrhage, 30
  odynophagia, 8
  oropharyngeal dysphagia, 195
  utility of, 615
Entamoeba diagnosis, 556
Entamoeba histolytica, 555–556, 556t
  diarrhea, 549
  in returning traveler, 174
  traveler's diarrhea, 172
Enteral nutrition, 158–159
  complications, 160
Enteric adenovirus, 307
Enteric bacteria
  health care workers, 180–181
Enteric fistulae, 479t
Enteric viruses
  health care workers, 180
Enterobius vermicularis (pinworm), 560
Enteroclysis, 629–630
Enterocytozoon bieneusi, 560
Enterohemorrhagic *Escherichia coli* (EHEC)
  colitis, 354–355
Enteroinvasive *Escherichia coli* (EIEC)
  colitis, 354–355
Enterokinase deficiency, 316
Enteropathogenic *Escherichia coli*
  foodborne diseases, 303

Enterotoxigenic *Escherichia coli* (ETEC)
  foodborne diseases, 302
Environmental factors
  functional dyspepsia, 260–261
Environmental metaplastic atrophic gastritis
    (EMAG), 266
Enzyme-linked immunosorbent assay
    (ELISA)
  for hepatitis, 118–119
Enzyme replacement
  chronic pancreatitis, 439, 439t
Eosinophilia, 121
Eosinophilic gastritis, 267
Eosinophilic gastroenteritis, 585–586
Epidermolysis bullosa, 570, 594
Epidermolysis bullosa dystrophia, 191–192
Epigastric hernias, 473
Episcleritis
  IBD, 362
Epithelial transport, disorders in small intestine,
    313–319
Epithelioid hemangioendotheliomas
  cutaneous manifestations, 605
ERCP. *See* Endoscopic retrograde
    cholangiopancreatography (ERCP)
Ergonovine test, 12
Ergot
  producing colonic ischemia, 378
Erosive duodenitis
  causing upper gastrointestinal bleeding,
    17
Erythema multiforme
  with IBD, 589
Erythema multiforme major. *See* Stevens-Johnson
    syndrome
Erythema nodosum
  with IBD, 589
Erythromycin, 237, 237t
  causing nausea and vomiting, 38
  for intestinal infections in HIV-1 infected
    adults, 552t
  for nausea and vomiting, 44
Erythropoiesis
  unconjugated hyperbilirubinemia, 106–107
Escherichia coli
  causing secretory diarrhea, 80
  colitis, 354–355
  with conjugated hyperbilirubinemia, 109
  diarrhea, 138
  foodborne diseases, 299t, 302
  gastritis, 267
  health care workers, 180
  in returning traveler, 174
  SBP, 131
  traveler's diarrhea, 172
Esomeprazole, 247
  for GERD, 210
Esophageal adenoma carcinoma (EAC), 218–
    220
Esophageal candidiasis
  with acquired immunodeficiency syndrome
    (AIDS), 548

Esophageal dysphagia, 6
  complications, 9
  etiology, 5t
  treatment, 9
Esophageal foreign bodies, 188–189
Esophageal hiatal hernias, 186–187
Esophageal infection, 203–216
Esophageal injury
  caustic, 187–188
  medication-induced, 188
  medications associated with, 135t
Esophageal intramural hematomas, 192
Esophageal manometry
  achalasia, 197, 198t
  for chest pain, 12
  GERD, 207–208
Esophageal motility disorders
  associated with systemic disease, 202–203
Esophageal odynophagia. *See* Odynophagia
Esophageal rings and webs, 184–185
Esophageal rupture
  causing acute abdomen, 57
Esophageal spasm diffuse, 199–202
Esophageal tuberculosis, 215
Esophageal tumors, 216–223
  staging, 218
Esophagitis
  causing pain, 48
  radiation, 611–612
  reflux, 203–216
    alkaline, 212
Esophagus
  anatomy, 182–183
  bacterial infections, 215–216
  Barrett, 202
  benign tumors, 223
  cervical
    disorders of, 193–196
  developmental anomalies, 183–185
  distal
    spastic motor disorders of, 199–202,
      200t
  embryology, 182–183
  epithelial tumors, 222
  fungal infections, 212–214
  motor disorders of, 6–7, 193–203
  mycobacterial infections, 215–216
  nonepithelial tumors, 222–223
  obstructive lesions, 6
  radiation injury, 611–612
  submucosal neoplasms, 223
  systemic disease manifestations, 189–190,
    190t
  treponemal infections, 215–216
  tumors
    screening and surveillance, 220–221
    TNM staging, 219f
    treatment, 221–222
  vascular compression, 185
  viral infections, 214–215
Essential fatty acid deficiency, 157
Essential minerals, 154–155

ETEC. *See* Enterotoxigenic *Escherichia coli*
    (ETEC)
Ethanol
  causing acute upper gastrointestinal bleeding,
    16
  chronic pancreatitis, 435
  pathogenesis, 523
Ethanol-induced pancreatitis, 429
EUS. *See* Endoscopic ultrasonography (EUS)
Exercise
  for constipation, 93
Extracorporeal shock wave lithotripsy
  for gallstones, 465
Extramammary Paget disease, 593
Extremities
  with nutritional deficiencies, 153t
Eyes
  with nutritional deficiencies, 153t

F
Familial adenomatous polyposis, 391–395,
    392t
  diagnosis, 394–395
  epidemiology, 391
  etiology, 391–393
  extraintestinal manifestations, 394
  incidence, 391
  pathogenesis, 391–393
  screening and surveillance, 394
  treatment, 395–396
Familial Mediterranean fever, 568
  causing abdominal pain, 47
Familial visceral myopathies (FVMs)
  with small intestine dysmotility, 290
Familial visceral neuropathies (FVNs)
  with small intestine dysmotility, 290
Famotidine, 247
Fasciola buski, 567
Fasciola hepatica, 566–567
Fasting hypoglycemia
  differential diagnosis, 450t
Fat. *See* Obesity
Fecal blood testing
  for occult gastrointestinal bleeding, 29
Fecal incontinence, 413–415, 414t
Females, 140–151
Fentanyl
  abuse, 164
Ferrous fumarate
  for occult gastrointestinal bleeding, 31
Ferrous gluconate
  for occult gastrointestinal bleeding, 31
Fever
  with pain, 49–50
Fiber
  for constipation, 93
Fibrolamellar hepatocellular carcinoma, 545
Fistulae, 478–480
5-aminosalicylate acid (5-ALA)
  for Crohn's disease, 370
  for IBD, 367
  for ulcerative colitis, 370

5-fluorouracil (5-FU)
  for gastric adenocarcinoma, 275
Flatulence, 62
Flexible sigmoidoscope, 621
Fluconazole
  for esophageal fungal infection, 213, 548
Fluid management
  for ileus, 74
Flukes, 565–566
  liver, 566–567
Flunitrazepam (Rohypnol), 167
Fluoride, 155
5-fluorouracil (5-FU)
  for gastric adenocarcinoma, 275
Focal nodular hyperplasia, 546
Folate
  deficiency, 156
Foodborne diseases
  epidemiology, 299t
Food hypersensitivity, 584–586
Foreign bodies
  esophageal, 188–189
  rectal, 416–417
Foveolae, 224
Fresh frozen plasma
  for upper gastrointestinal bleeding, 20
Fructose
  malabsorption
    with gas and bloating, 66
Fructose deficiency, 63
5-FU. *See* 5-fluorouracil (5-FU)
Fumagillin
  for intestinal infections in HIV-1 infected
    adults, 551t
Functional bowel disorders
  causing bloating and gas, 64
Functional dyspepsia, 232, 259–262
  causing nausea and vomiting, 38
  clinical features, 261
  course, 261–262
  diagnosis, 261
  disturbed gastric sensory function, 259–260
  disturbed motor gastric function, 259
  etiology, 259–260
  pathogenesis, 259–260
  psychological factors, 260
  Rome II criteria, 260t
  treatment, 261–262
Functional water diarrhea. *See* Irritable bowel
    syndrome (IBS)
Furazolidone
  for *Blastocystis hominis*, 559
Furosemide
  for ascites, 129
FVMs. *See* Familial visceral myopathies (FVMs)
FVNs. *See* Familial visceral neuropathies
    (FVNs)

G
Gallbladder
  anatomy of, 454
  cancer, 460–461

Gallstone pancreatitis
  treatment, 434
Gallstones, 462–465
  clinical course of, 463
  with conjugated hyperbilirubinemia, 109
  course, 464–465
  diagnosis, 464
  epidemiology of, 462
  etiology of, 462
  incidence, 462
  pathogenesis, 462
  pregnancy, 145
  risk factors, 463t
  treatment of, 464–465
Gamma-glutamyltransferase (GGT), 118
Gamma-hydroxybutyrate, 167
Ganciclovir
  for cytomegalovirus esophageal infections,
    548
  for intestinal infections in HIV-1 infected
    adults, 551t
Gardner syndrome, 394
  cutaneous findings, 593
Gas and bloating, 61–67
  complications, 67
  differential diagnosis, 63–64
  etiology, 62t
  functional studies, 65–67
  history, 64–65
  laboratory studies, 65
  physical examination, 65
  structural studies, 65
  treatment, 67
  workup, 64–65, 66f
Gas-bloat syndrome, 65, 67
Gastric acid
  functional dyspepsia, 260
  secretion
    Zollinger-Ellison syndrome, 252
Gastric adenocarcinoma, 258, 271–276
  clinical features, 274
  course, 275–276
  diagnosis, 274–275
  etiology, 271–274
  histopathology, 273–274
  pathogenesis, 271–274
  risk factors, 271–272
  screening, 275–276
  staging, 275
  treatment, 275–276
Gastric antral vascular ectasia, 601–603
Gastric arteriovenous ectasia
  causing upper gastrointestinal bleeding, 17
Gastric atresia, 225
Gastric bezoars, 227–229
  treatment, 228t
Gastric cancer
  classification of, 273f, 273t
  early, 273
Gastric carcinoids, 278
Gastric diverticula, 226–227
Gastric duplication, 226

Gastric emptying, 231–240
  delayed
    GERD, 206
    nongastrointestinal disorders, 234–235
  disorders
    diagnosis, 235–236
    medication effects on, 233t
    medication-induced delays in, 232
  rapid
    disorders with, 238–240
    rheumatologic disorders, 233
  scintigraphy
    for gas and bloating, 65
Gastric foreign bodies, 229
Gastric lymphoma, 276–277
  Ann Arbor staging system, 276, 277t
Gastric mucosal membrane, 225
Gastric mucous cell metaplasia (GMCM),
    270
Gastric outlet obstruction, 38
Gastric pits, 224
Gastric polyps, 277–278
Gastric rupture, 229–230
Gastric scintigraphic quantitation
  gastric emptying disorders, 235
Gastric teratoma, 226
Gastric ulcers. *See also* Peptic ulcer disease
  benign
    surgery, 254
  pathophysiology, 244
Gastric varices
  with esophageal varices, 16–17
  with portal hypertension, 16–17
Gastric volvulus, 230–231
Gastritis, 262–263
  acute, 263–264
  chronic, 264–270
  classification, 263t
  stress
    causing acute upper gastrointestinal
      bleeding, 16
Gastroduodenal manometry
  gastric emptying disorders, 236
Gastroesophageal reflux
  causing nausea and vomiting, 38
  pregnancy, 142, 572
  pulmonary disease, 578
Gastroesophageal reflux disease (GERD),
    203–212
  causing chest pain, 11
  clinical features, 206
  diagnosis, 206–207
  endoscopic therapy, 211
  epidemiology, 203–204
  etiology, 204
  incidence, 203–204
  in infants and children, 212
  lifestyle modification, 209, 209t
  medications, 210
  pathogenesis, 204–205
  surgery, 211
  tests, 207t

  tissue resistance, 205–206
  treatment, 208–209
Gastrointestinal bleeding. *See also* Occult
    gastrointestinal bleeding; Upper
    gastrointestinal bleeding
  gross, 14–26
    etiology, 15t
Gastrointestinal carcinoid tumors, 408
  distribution, 408t
Gastrointestinal disorders
  causing weight loss, 33
  patient interviewing, 2–3
  pharmacotherapy, 3
  psychological treatments, 3–4
  psychosocial factors, 1–3
  treatment, 3–4
Gastrointestinal malignancy
  cutaneous signs of, 593–594
Gastrointestinal mass, 95–97
Gastrointestinal motor abnormalities, 340
Gastrointestinal polyposis, 393
  cutaneous findings, 593
Gastrointestinal sensory abnormalities, 340–341
Gastrointestinal stromal cell tumors (GISTs), 277
Gastrointestinal tract
  endoscopic evaluation of, 615–618
Gastroparesis, 258
  causing nausea and vomiting, 38
  causing weight loss, 33
  diabetes, 231–232
  symptoms of, 235
  treatment, 236–238
Gastropathy
  causing gross gastrointestinal bleeding, 16
Gastroschisis, 471–472
*Gastrospirillum hominis. See Helicobacter
    heilmannii*
Gaucher disease, 568
Gaviscon
  for GERD, 210
Genetic abnormalities, 568–569
Genetics
  celiac disease, 309–310
  IBD, 357–358
Genetic testing
  cystic fibrosis, 425
GERD. *See* Gastroesophageal reflux disease
    (GERD)
GGT. *See* Gamma-glutamyltransferase (GGT)
Gianotti syndrome
  cutaneous signs associated with, 595
Giardia
  in returning traveler, 174
Giardia lamblia, 557, 558t
  diarrhea, 549
  traveler's diarrhea, 172
Gilbert syndrome, 112
Ginger
  for nausea and vomiting, 44
GISTs. *See* Gastrointestinal stromal cell tumors
    (GISTs)
Globus syndrome, 578

Glucagonoma, 449
Glucose
    malabsorption
        with gas and bloating, 66
Glucose-galactose malabsorption, 315
GMCM. *See* Gastric mucous cell metaplasia
        (GMCM)
Gold-induced enterocolitis, 574
Gold salts
    inducing colitides, 378
Gonorrheal proctitis, 355
Gorlin syndrome, 392t, 397
Graft-versus-host disease (GVHD), 190–191
Granisetron
    for nausea and vomiting, 44
Granulomatous cholangiopathy, 572
Granulomatous disease, 572
Granulomatous gastritis, 268
Granulomatous peritonitis, 484–485
Gravid women. *See* Pregnancy
Grey Turner sign, 72, 595
GRFoma, 449
Groin hernias, 474, 474t
Gross gastrointestinal bleeding, 14–26
    etiology, 15t
GVHD. *See* Graft-versus-host disease (GVHD)
Gynecological disease
    causing lower abdominal pain, 147–151,
        148t

H

Haemophilus
    gastritis, 267
Hair
    with nutritional deficiencies, 153t
Hallucinogens, 166–167
Hamartomatous polyposis syndrome, 396–397
Hawaii agents
    causing nausea and vomiting, 40
Health care workers
    gastrointestinal pathogens, 180–181
    immunizations, 175–176
    nosocomial infections, 174–181
Heart
    with nutritional deficiencies, 153t
Heartburn
    causing chest pain, 11
    with GERD, 206
Heart failure
    gastrointestinal manifestations, 567–568
Heavy metal toxicity, 573–574
Helicobacter heilmannii
    gastritis, 267
Helicobacter pylori
    acid peptic disorders, 241
    causing peptic ulcer, 16
    gastric adenocarcinoma, 271–272
    gastritis, 264–270
        clinical manifestations, 264–265
        diagnosis, 264–265
        etiology, 264
        pathogenesis, 264

GERD, 204
    granulomatous gastritis, 268
    with hyperemesis gravidarum, 142
    peptic ulcer disease
        treatment, 248–249, 248t
    testing, 245–246
HELLP. *See* Hemolysis, elevated liver enzymes,
        and low platelets (HELLP)
Helminths, 560–565
Hemangiomas, 546, 603–604
Hemangiopericytomas
    cutaneous manifestations, 605
Hematemesis, 14
Hematobilia, 469–470
    causing upper gastrointestinal bleeding, 17
Hematochezia, 14
Hematocrit
    for upper gastrointestinal bleeding, 18
Hematologic disorders
    gastrointestinal manifestations, 574–575
Hematomas
    esophageal intramural, 192
Hemoccult card test, 29
Hemochromatosis, 514–516
    diagnosis, 114t
    treatment, 122
Hemolysis
    unconjugated hyperbilirubinemia, 106–107
Hemolysis, elevated liver enzymes, and low
        platelets (HELLP), 572
    pregnancy, 147
Hemolytic uremic syndrome, 574
HemoQuant, 29
Hemorrhage
    with PUD, 255
Hemorrhoids, 409–410
Hemosuccus pancreaticus
    causing upper gastrointestinal bleeding, 17
Henoch-Schönlein purpura, 579
Hepatic adenoma, 545–546
Hepatic artery embolization
    for pancreas endocrine neoplasms, 453
Hepatic encephalopathy
    with cirrhosis, 536–538
Hepatic granulomas, 573t
Hepatic hydrothorax
    with ascites, 132
Hepatic injury. *See* Drug-induced hepatic injury
Hepatic porphyrias, 569t
Hepatic sarcoidosis, 572
Hepatic tumors, 499–500
Hepatitis, 498–499. *See also* Autoimmune
        hepatitis
    alcoholic
        treatment, 527–528
    drug-induced
        diagnosis, 114t
        treatment, 122
Hepatitis A, 502–504
    health care workers, 177
    prophylaxis, 179t
    vaccine, 170

Hepatitis B, 504–507
  health care workers, 177–178
  vaccine, 170
Hepatitis C, 507–510
  clinical features, 508–509
  course, 510
  diagnosis, 509
  epidemiology, 507–508
  etiology, 508
  health care workers, 178
  incidence, 507–508
  pathogenesis, 508
  treatment, 510
Hepatitis D, 510–511
Hepatitis E, 511
  travelers, 173
Hepatobiliary dysfunction serum markers, 117–118
Hepatobiliary system
  radiation injury, 614–615
Hepatoblastoma, 545
Hepatocellular carcinoma, 539–544
  chemotherapy, 544
  clinical features, 540
  course, 542–544
  diagnosis, 114t, 540–541
  epidemiology, 539
  etiology, 539–540
  hormone therapy, 544
  incidence, 539
  pathogenesis, 539–540
  surgery, 542–543
  treatment, 542–544, 543f
Hepatocellular diseases, 494
Hepatocellular injury, 120–121
  differential diagnosis, 114–115
Hepatorenal syndrome
  with ascites, 132–133
Hereditary angioedema, 568, 583–584
Hereditary complications, 569t
Hereditary hemochromatosis (HHC), 514
Hereditary hemorrhagic telangiectasia
        (Osler-Weber-Rendu syndrome), 571, 602
  causing upper gastrointestinal bleeding, 17
  skin disease, 592
Hereditary mixed polyposis syndrome, 392t
Hereditary nonpolyposis colorectal cancer
        (HNPCC), 150
  microsatellite instability, 400–401
Hereditary ovarian cancer, 150
Hereditary pancreatitis, 426
Hernias. See also specific hernias
  in adults, 473–476
Heroin
  abuse, 164
Herpes simplex virus (HSV)
  causing nausea and vomiting, 40
  causing odynophagia, 7
  with colitis, 550
  proctitis, 356

Herpes simplex virus type 1 (HSV-1)
  esophagus, 214
Heterotopic gastric mucosa, 185
Heterotopic pancreas, 422
HHC. See Hereditary hemochromatosis (HHC)
Hiatal hernias
  esophageal, 186–187
Hiccups, 576
Hidradenitis suppurativa, 418
Highly selective vagotomy
  for duodenal ulcers, 253–254
Hill gastropexy
  for GERD, 211
Hirschsprung disease, 92, 333–334, 347
  with constipation, 87
Histoplasma
  esophagus, 213
HIV. See Human immunodeficiency virus (HIV)
HIV-1. See Human immunodeficiency virus-1 (HIV-1)
HNPCC. See Hereditary nonpolyposis colorectal cancer (HNPCC)
Hookworms, 562–563
  causing occult gastrointestinal bleeding, 28
Hospital epidemiology, 174–175
Hospital infections. See Nosocomial infections
24-hour esophageal pH recording
  distal esophagus spastic motor disorders, 201
Howel-Evans syndrome, 594
HSV. See Herpes simplex virus (HSV)
HSV-1. See Herpes simplex virus type 1 (HSV-1)
Human immunodeficiency virus-1 (HIV-1)
  intestinal infections
    treatment, 551t–552t
Human immunodeficiency virus (HIV)
  esophagitis, 548
  health care workers, 177
  travelers, 173
Human papillomavirus, 356
Hydrea
  for gastric adenocarcinoma, 275
Hydrocortisone
  for pruritus ani, 415
Hydrogen breath test
  for gas and bloating, 66
Hydrogen receptor antagonists, 247
Hydroxyurea (Hydrea)
  for gastric adenocarcinoma, 275
Hymenolepis nana (dwarf tapeworm), 565
Hyperbilirubinemia, 105–106, 116–117. See
        Conjugated hyperbilirubinemia
Hypercoagulability states, 574
Hyperemesis gravidarum
  with pregnancy, 141–142
Hypergastrinemia
  differential diagnosis, 251t
Hyperimmune bovine colostrum
  for Cryptosporidium, 559
Hyperlipidemia, 569
Hyperparathyroidism, 572
Hyperplastic polyposis syndrome, 398
Hyperplastic polyps, 390

Hyperthyroidism, 572
    with small intestine dysmotility, 292
Hypertrichosis lanuginosa acquisita, 594
Hypertrophic gastropathies, 269–270
Hypertrophic pyloric stenosis, 227
Hypnotherapy, 3
Hypocalcemia, 154
Hypokalemia, 154
    with VIPoma, 448–449
Hypopharyngeal diverticula
    acquired, 194
Hypopharynx
    disorders of, 193–196
Hypophosphatemia, 154
Hypotension
    with pain, 50
Hypothyroidism
    with small intestine dysmotility, 292

I

Iatrogenic hernias, 476
IBD. *See* Inflammatory bowel disease (IBD)
IBS. *See* Irritable bowel syndrome (IBS)
Idiopathic gastroparesis, 232
Ig. *See* Immunoglobulin (Ig)
IgA. *See* Immunoglobulin A (IgA) deficiency
Ileal pouch, 100–105
    characteristics, 101t
Ileal pouch-anal canal anastomosis, 103–105
    complications, 104
    contraindications, 104t
    indications, 104t
    outcome, 104–105
Ileostomies, 100–105
    characteristics, 101t
Ileus, 68–75
    acute, 68
    complications, 75
    differential diagnosis, 68–71
    etiology, 69t
    history, 71
    laboratory studies, 72
    physical examination, 71–72
    plain radiograph studies, 72–73
    treatment, 74–75
    workup, 71–74, 73f
Illness experience, 2
Imaging procedures, 628–637
Imipramine
    for chest pain, 14
Immune factors
    celiac disease, 309
    IBD, 358–359
Immune serum globulin (ISG), 169
Immunodeficiency diseases
    gut, 580–584
Immunoglobulin (Ig)
    for *Cryptosporidium,* 559
Immunoglobulin A (IgA) deficiency, 580, 581t
Immunologic disorders
    gastrointestinal manifestations, 580–588
Immunologic tests, 119

Immunomodulators
    for IBD, 368–369
Immunosuppression
    for autoimmune liver disease, 520
Imperforate anus, 335
Indomethacin
    for diarrhea, 86
Infection control, 175–176
Infectious disease
    with ascites, 126
Infectious duodenitis, 270
Infectious gastritis, 267–268
Infiltrative diseases
    differential diagnosis, 115
Inflammatory bowel disease (IBD), 357–373
    adolescents, 373
    children, 373
    clinical features, 359–363
    colonic neoplasms, 372
    complications
        management, 371–372
    course, 366–373
    cutaneous manifestations of, 589–591, 590t
    diagnosis, 363–366
    diarrhea, 138
    epidemiology, 357
    etiology and pathogenesis, 357–358
    extraintestinal features, 362–363
    hepatobiliary complications, 362–363
    incidence, 357
    laboratory studies, 363
    medications, 367–368
    nutritional management, 366
    pathology, 365–366
    potential triggers, 358
    pregnancy, 145–146, 372–373
    surgery, 370–371
    treatment, 366–373
Inflammatory polyps, 390
Infliximab
    for Crohn's disease, 370
    for IBD, 369
Inhalants, 167
Insulinoma, 448
Intentional weight loss. *See* Eating disorders
Interferon
    for pancreatic endocrine neoplasms, 453
Internal hernias, 476
Intestinal flukes, 567
Intestinal hemangiomatosis, 603
Intestinal lymphangiectasia
    causing osmotic diarrhea, 79
Intestinal pseudoobstruction
    causing nausea and vomiting, 38
Intrahepatic cholestasis of pregnancy, 146,
        494–495
Intralumenal electrical impedance
    GERD, 208
Intussusception, 283–284
Iodine deficiency, 155
Iodoquinol
    for *Blastocystis hominis,* 559

Iron, 119
Iron deficiency, 154–155
  tests for occult gastrointestinal bleeding, 29
Iron deficiency anemia, 28
  with occult gastrointestinal bleeding, 30
Irritable bowel syndrome (IBS), 1, 340–345
  with abdominal pain, 53
  central nervous system dysfunction, 341
  clinical features, 341–342
  with constipation, 90
  course, 343–344
  diagnosis, 342–343
  epidemiology, 340
  etiology, 340–341
  food and flatus, 344t
  incidence, 340
  pathogenesis, 340–341
  psychological therapy, 344–345
  Rome II criteria, 341t
  treatment, 343–344
Ischemic colitis, 610–611
  with acute lower gastrointestinal bleeding,
    22–23
Ischemic hepatitis, 512
ISG. *See* Immune serum globulin (ISG)
Isomalt
  malabsorption, 63
Isoniazid
  prophylaxis, 176, 176t
Isopora belli, 559
  diarrhea, 549
  in returning traveler, 174
Isotretinoin
  inducing colitides, 378
Itraconazole
  for esophageal fungal infection, 548
  for intestinal infections in HIV-1 infected
    adults, 552t

J

Jamaican vomiting sickness, 40
Japanese encephalitis vaccine, 171
Jaundice, 105–113
  cutaneous signs associated with, 595
  differential diagnosis, 105–106
  evaluation, 111f
  history, 109–119
  imaging, 111–112
  laboratory studies, 110–111
  with pain, 49
  physical examination, 110
  treatment, 112–113
Jejunal diverticulosis, 292
Jet lag, 168–169
Juvenile polyposis, 392t, 396–397
Juvenile polyps, 390–391

K

Kaolin-pectin
  for diarrhea, 86
Kaposi sarcoma
  skin disease, 592

Ketamine
  abuse, 166
Ketoconazole
  for esophageal fungal infection, 213, 548
Klebsiella
  with conjugated hyperbilirubinemia, 109
  in returning traveler, 174
Klebsiella pneumoniae
  SBP, 131
Kock pouch, 102–103
  complications, 103
  outcome, 103
Kwashiorkor-marasmus syndrome, 577

L

Lactase deficiency, 63
  with gas and bloating, 67
  with osmotic diarrhea, 76–79
Lactobacillus acidophilus
  esophagus, 215
Lactose deficiency, 313–317
  ethnic distribution, 314t
Lansoprazole, 247
  for GERD, 210
LAP. *See* Leucine aminopeptidase (LAP)
Laparoscopic cholecystectomy, 465
Laparoscopy
  for duodenal ulcers, 254
Large gastric folds
  differential diagnosis, 269t
Large-volume paracentesis
  for ascites, 130
Late-onset hypogammaglobulinemia, 581
Laxatives
  causing secretory diarrhea, 80
Lead poisoning, 573
Left flank purpura (Grey-Turner sign), 72,
    595
Legionella
  with conjugated hyperbilirubinemia, 109
Legionella pneumophila, 174–175
Leiomyoma
  esophagus, 222–223
Leptospirosis, 172
LES. *See* Lower esophageal sphincter (LES)
Leucine aminopeptidase (LAP), 118
Leukemia, 575
Levator ani syndrome, 418
Linton-Nachlas tube
  with upper gastrointestinal bleeding, 21
Lipase
  with acute abdomen, 59
Listeria monocytogenes
  foodborne diseases, 301
Liver
  CT, 633–634
  ultrasound, 631–632
Liver abscess
  amebic, 556
Liver biopsy
  for alcoholic liver disease, 526
  for autoimmune liver disease, 519

cirrhosis, 533
with primary biliary cirrhosis, 492
Liver disease. *See also* Alcoholic liver disease;
　　Autoimmune liver disease
cholestatic
　diagnosis, 120–121
cutaneous signs associated with, 595–596
patient interviewing, 2–3
preeclampsia-associated
　pregnancy, 147
Liver enzymes. *See* Hemolysis, elevated liver
　　enzymes, and low platelets (HELLP)
Liver flukes, 566–567
Liver masses, 95
benign, 545–546
Liver-spleen scintigraphy
for ascites, 129
Liver transplant
for ascites, 130–131
Loperamide
for diarrhea, 86
for IBD, 369
for traveler's diarrhea, 172
Lorazepam
for nausea and vomiting, 44
Lower esophageal sphincter (LES), 204
substances modulating, 205t
Lower gastrointestinal bleeding. *See* Acute lower
　　gastrointestinal bleeding
Lower gastrointestinal endoscopy, 621–623
Low platelets. *See* Hemolysis, elevated liver
　　enzymes, and low platelets (HELLP)
LSD. *See* Lysergic acid diethylamide (LSD)
Lumbar hernias, 475
Lumenal acid clearance, 205
Lymphangiectasia, 284
Lymphocytic gastritis, 268–269
Lymphoma
esophagus, 222–223
Lysergic acid diethylamide (LSD), 166–167

M
Macrocystic adenomas
pancreas, 446
Magenblase syndrome, 62
Magnetic resonance angiography
small intestine ischemia, 608
Magnetic resonance cholangiopancreatography
　(MRCP)
with acute abdomen, 60
chronic pancreatitis, 438
with jaundice, 112
Magnetic resonance imaging (MRI), 635–636
hepatocellular carcinoma, 541
IBD, 365
jaundice, 111–112
Malabsorption
skin conditions from, 596
Malakoplakia, 383–384
Malaria
chemoprophylaxis, 171–172
Malarone, 172

Malignancy
with ascites, 125–126
Malignancy-related pseudoachalasia, 196
Malignant atrophic papulosis (Degos disease), 592
Malignant melanoma, 576
Mallory-Weiss syndrome
caused by nausea and vomiting, 45
Mallory-Weiss tears, 192
causing upper gastrointestinal bleeding, 17
Malnutrition
chronic pancreatitis, 435–436
skin conditions from, 596
Manganese, 155
Manometry
anorectal
　for constipation, 92
distal esophagus spastic motor disorders, 201
esophageal
　achalasia, 197, 198t
　for chest pain, 12
　GERD, 207–208
for gas and bloating, 65
gastroduodenal
　gastric emptying disorders, 236
in nausea and vomiting, 43
oropharyngeal dysphagia, 195
small intestine dysmotility, 293
Measles vaccine, 171
Mebadin
for liver abscess, 556
Mechanical colonic obstruction
with constipation, 87
Mechanical compression
for upper gastrointestinal bleeding, 21
Mechanical obstruction, 70
etiology, 69t
Meckel diverticulum, 280–281
with acute lower gastrointestinal bleeding, 23
Meclizine
for nausea and vomiting, 43
Medications
causing constipation, 89
causing delays in gastric emptying, 232
causing esophageal injury, 188
Mefloquine, 171–172
Megacolon
acute, 347–348
Meigs syndrome, 126
Melanoma
esophagus, 222
Melena, 14
Ménétrier disease
large gastric folds, 269
Ménière disease
causing nausea and vomiting, 40
Meningococcal vaccine, 171
6-mercaptopurine (6-MP)
for IBD, 139, 368
Merycism
causing weight loss, 34
Mesalamine
for IBD, 139

Mesenchymal tumors, 545
Mesenteric cysts, 482–483
Mesenteric diagnosis, 481t
Mesenteric fibromatosis, 482
Mesenteric granulomatous infection, 483
Mesenteric ischemia
    causing acute abdomen, 56–57
    clinical features, 607–608
    predisposing factors, 606t
Mesenteric panniculitis, 480–481
Mesenteric solid tumors, 482–483
Mesenteric vascular insufficiency, 605–611
Mesentery
    diseases of, 480–483
Metabolic disease
    causing constipation, 89
    gastrointestinal manifestations, 575
Methotrexate
    adverse effects, 570
Methyldopa
    inducing colitides, 378
Methylphenyltetrahydropyridine (MPTP)
    abuse, 164
Metoclopramide, 237, 237t
    for nausea and vomiting, 44
    for small intestine dysmotility, 294
    for upper gastrointestinal bleeding, 20
Metronidazole
    for *Blastocystis hominis,* 559
    for Crohn's disease, 370
    for *Giardia lamblia,* 557
    for IBD, 139
    for intestinal infections in HIV-1 infected
        adults, 551t, 552t
    for liver abscess, 556
Microcystic adenomas
    pancreas, 446
Microgastria, 226
Microlithiasis
    acute pancreatitis, 429
Microsatellite instability
    colon adenocarcinoma, 400–401
Microscopic colitis, 374t
Microvascular angina, 10
Microvillous inclusion disease, 318
Midcycle ovulatory pain, 148
Migraine, 576
Minerals
    deficiencies, 152–154
    transport disorders, 317–318
Mirtazapine, 3
Misoprostol, 248
    for constipation, 93
Mitomycin
    for gastric adenocarcinoma, 275
Molybdenum, 155
Monomicrobial bacterascites, 131
Motion sickness
    causing nausea and vomiting, 40
Mouth
    and nutritional deficiencies, 153t
6-MP. *See* 6-mercaptopurine (6-MP)

MPTP. *See* Methylphenyltetrahydropyridine
    (MPTP)
MRCP. *See* Magnetic resonance
    cholangiopancreatography (MRCP)
MRI. *See* Magnetic resonance imaging (MRI)
Mucoepidermoid carcinoma
    esophagus, 222
Mucosal injury diarrhea, 81
    etiology, 78t–79t
Multiple hamartoma syndrome
    cutaneous findings, 593
Multiple sclerosis, 576
Mumps vaccine, 171
Munchausen syndrome, 578
Mycobacterium avium
    diarrhea, 549
    gastritis, 267
Mycobacterium paratuberculosis
    IBD, 358
Mycobacterium tuberculosis
    causing occult gastrointestinal bleeding, 28
    granulomatous gastritis, 268
Myelofibrosis, 575
Myopathic disorders
    with constipation, 87–89
Myotonic dystrophy
    with small intestine dysmotility, 291

N
NAFLD. *See* Nonalcoholic fatty liver disease
    (NAFLD)
Nails
    with nutritional deficiencies, 153t
Nanophyetus salmincola, 567
Narcotics
    for abdominal pain, 53
NASH. *See* Nonalcoholic steatohepatitis
    (NASH)
Nausea, 37–45
    central nervous system causes, 38–40
    complications of, 44–45
    differential diagnosis, 37–40
    endocrinologic causes of, 40
    etiology, 39t
    functional studies, 43
    gastrointestinal disorders causing, 38
    history, 40–41
    infectious causes of, 40
    laboratory studies and diagnostic testing,
        41–42
    medications, 38
    metabolic causes of, 40
    with pain, 49
    peritoneal disorders causing, 38
    physical examination, 41
    with pregnancy, 141–142
    treatment, 43–44
    workup, 40–43, 42f
Necator americanus, 562
Neisseria gonorrhoeae
    cervicitis, 148
Nematodes, 560–565

Neonatal jaundice
  unconjugated hyperbilirubinemia, 107
Neoplasia
  gastrointestinal manifestations, 575
Nephrolithiasis
  causing pain, 48
Nephrotic syndrome
  with ascites, 124
Neurofibromatosis, 571
Neurofibromatosis 1 (NF1), 592
Neuroleptics, 3
Neuromuscular disorders
  gastrointestinal manifestations of, 576
Neuropathic disorders
  with constipation, 87–89
Neutropenic colitis
  causing acute abdomen, 57
Nevoid basal cell carcinoma syndrome. *See* Gorlin
    syndrome
NF1. *See* Neurofibromatosis 1 (NF1)
Niacin (vitamin B₃)
  efficiency, 156
Nicotine, 167
Niemann-Pick disease, 569
Nissen fundoplication
  for GERD, 211
Nitrates
  for achalasia, 198
Nitrous oxide
  abuse, 167
Nizatidine, 247
N,N-diethyl-m-toluamide (DEET), 171
Non-A, non-B hepatitis
  health care workers, 180
Nonadenomatous polyps, 390–391
Nonalcoholic fatty liver disease (NAFLD), 512
Nonalcoholic steatohepatitis (NASH), 512
Nonfamilial visceral myopathy
  with small intestine dysmotility, 291
Nonfamilial visceral neuropathy
  with small intestine dysmotility, 291
Nonsteroidal antiinflammatory drugs (NSAIDs)
  for abdominal pain, 52
  adenomatous polyps, 388
  causing acid peptic disorders, 242
  causing colitides, 378
  causing nausea and vomiting, 38
  causing occult gastrointestinal bleeding, 28
  causing peptic ulcer, 16
  causing peptic ulcer disease, 249
  with conjugated hyperbilirubinemia, 109
Nontyphoid salmonellosis, 303–304
Nonviral hepatitis, 512–516
Norfloxacin
  for traveler's diarrhea, 172
Nortriptyline
  for nausea and vomiting, 44
Norwalk agents
  causing nausea and vomiting, 40
  causing secretory diarrhea, 80
Norwalk-like caliciviruses
  foodborne diseases, 306–307

Norwalk virus
  foodborne diseases, 299t, 306
Nosocomial infections
  acquisition of, 174–175
NSAIDs. *See* Nonsteroidal antiinflammatory drugs
    (NSAIDs)
Nutritional deficiencies
  etiology, 152
  physical signs, 153t
Nutritional disorders
  gastrointestinal manifestations, 577
Nutritional support, 151–161
  differential diagnosis, 152–157
  history and physical, 157
  laboratory tests, 157
  treatment, 158–159
Nutritional therapy
  short bowel syndrome, 323–324
Nystatin
  for esophageal fungal infection, 214

O
Obesity, 577
  absorption disorders, 317
Obstruction
  with PUD, 255–256
Obstructive esophageal lesions, 6
Occult gastrointestinal bleeding
  complications, 32
  history, 28–29
  infectious causes, 28
  physical examination, 29
  treatment, 30–32
  tumors causing, 28
  vascular causes, 28
  workup, 28–29, 31f
Occult gastrointestinal hemorrhage, 26–32
  differential diagnosis, 26–27
  etiology, 27t
  inflammatory causes, 27
Octreotide, 240
  for diarrhea, 86
  for pancreatic endocrine neoplasms, 452,
    453t
  for small intestine dysmotility, 294
  for variceal hemorrhage, 535
Odynophagia, 4–9
  with acquired immunodeficiency syndrome
    (AIDS), 548
  physical examination, 7
  workup, 7–8
Omental cysts, 482–483
Omental diseases, 481t
Omental granulomatous infection, 483
Omental solid tumors, 482–483
Omental vascular accidents, 483
Omeprazole, 247
  for GERD, 210
  for upper gastrointestinal bleeding, 20
Omphalocele, 471–472
Ondansetron
  for nausea and vomiting, 44

Opiates
abuse, 164–165
Opioids
for abdominal pain, 52
Opisthorchis viverrini, 566–567
Oral contraceptives
with conjugated hyperbilirubinemia, 109
producing colonic ischemia, 378
Oral ferrous sulfate
for occult gastrointestinal bleeding, 31
Oral rehydration, 158
for traveler's diarrhea, 172
Organ transplantation
gastrointestinal complications, 586–588
gastrointestinal manifestations, 577
Oriental cholangiohepatitis, 470
Oropharyngeal dysphagia, 4–6
complications, 9
diagnosis, 195
etiology, 5t, 7
oral preparation defects, 4
oral transfer defects, 4
pharyngeal disorders, 4
treatment, 9, 195–196
Orthotopic liver transplantation
for cirrhosis, 538
Osler-Weber-Rendu syndrome, 571, 602
causing upper gastrointestinal bleeding, 17
skin disease, 592
Osmotic diarrhea
differential diagnosis, 76–79
etiology, 77t
Osteomalacia
with pulmonary disease, 578
Osteopenia
IBD, 362
Osteoporosis
IBD, 362
Ovarian cancer, 150, 576
Ovarian cysts
ruptured, 148
Ovarian torsion, 148–149
Overseas medical care, 169
Overseas water supplies, 169
Overweight. *See* Obesity

P

Packed erythrocytes
for upper gastrointestinal bleeding, 20
Pain. *See also* Abdominal pain; Chest pain
alleviating and aggravating factors, 49
associated symptoms, 49
midcycle ovulatory, 148
risk factors, 49–50
visceral, 45
Pancreas
agenesis or hypoplasia, 422
anatomy, 419–420
annular, 421–422
clinical features, 448–449
congenital cysts, 422–423
CT, 634

cystic neoplasms, 446–447
embryological development, 419–420
endocrine neoplasms of, 447–453
diagnosis, 450–451
treatment, 452–453
epidemiology, 447–448
epithelial neoplasms, 447
etiology, 448
hereditary diseases of, 423–427
incidence, 447–448
mucinous ductal ectasia, 447
nonfunctional tumors, 449–450
pathogenesis, 448
structural anomalies 420–423
ultrasound, 632
Pancreatic adenocarcinoma, 441–447
Pancreatic disease
with ascites, 125
cutaneous findings, 595
Pancreaticobiliary disease
with abdominal pain, 52
Pancreaticobiliary mass, 95
Pancreatic secretory trypsin inhibitor gene
mutation-associated pancreatitis, 426–427
Pancreatitis. *See also* Acute pancreatitis; Chronic pancreatitis
with conjugated hyperbilirubinemia, 109
Panic disorder
causing chest pain, 11
Pantoprazole, 247
for GERD, 210
Papular acrodermatitis of childhood, 595
Paralytic shellfish
foodborne diseases, 299t
Paraneoplastic syndrome, 576
Parasitic diseases, 555–567
Paregoric
for diarrhea, 86
Parenteral nutrition, 159–160
complications, 160–161
Parietal cells, 224
Parkinson disease, 576–577
Paromomycin
for *Cryptosporidium,* 559
for intestinal infections in HIV-1 infected adults, 551t
Paroxysmal nocturnal hemoglobinuria, 575
PCP. *See* Phencyclidine (PCP)
Pegylated interferon-alpha, 122
PEI. *See* Percutaneous alcohol injection (PEI)
Peliosis hepatis, 553
Pelvic hernias, 475
Pelvic inflammatory disease (PID), 147–148
Pemphigus, 571
Pemphigus vulgaris, 191, 594
Penicillamine
for Wilson disease, 514
Pentasa
for Crohn's disease, 370
Peptic duodenitis, 270
Peptic ulcer disease (PUD)

causing gross gastrointestinal bleeding, 16
clinical manifestations, 244–245
endoscopic studies, 245–246
Helicobacter pylori
    treatment, 248–249
pregnancy, 144–145
radiographic studies, 245
surgery of
    complications of, 256–257
    indications for, 254–256
    metabolic consequences, 258
    recurrence rates, 256t
    sequelae, 257t
Percutaneous alcohol injection (PEI)
    for hepatocellular carcinoma, 543
Percutaneous liver biopsy, 120
Percutaneous transhepatic cholangiography (PTC)
    for alcoholic liver disease, 526
    for cholestasis, 120
    with jaundice, 112
Perforated duodenal ulcer, 54–55
Perianal disease
    with acute lower gastrointestinal bleeding,
    23
Perineal skin lesions, 596–597, 597t
Peripheral parenteral nutrition (PPN), 159–160
Peritoneovenous shunts
    for ascites, 130
Peritoneum
    diseases, 483–486
Peritonitis, 483–484
    acute suppurative, 484
    with AIDS, 485–486
    with chronic peritoneal dialysis, 485
Periumbilical purpura (Cullen sign), 72, 595
Peutz-Jeghers polyps, 392t, 396
    cutaneous findings, 593
Phagocytic cell defects, 583
Pharmacobezoar, 228
Pharyngoesophageal diverticula, 185–186
Pharyngoesophagography, 628–629
Phencyclidine (PCP), 166
Phenolphthalein
    for constipation, 93
Phenothiazine
    for nausea and vomiting, 43
Phlebotomy
    for hereditary hemochromatosis, 516
PID. *See* Pelvic inflammatory disease (PID)
Pilonidal disease, 418
Pinworm, 560
Plague vaccine, 171
Plasmacytomas, 575
Plasmodium falciparum, 171
Platelets
    for upper gastrointestinal bleeding, 20
Plesiomonas shigelloides
    foodborne disease, 305
Plummer-Vinson syndrome, 574, 594
Pneumatic diagnosis
    for achalasia, 198–199
Pneumatosis cystoides intestinalis, 383

Pneumococcus
    SBP, 131
Poliomyelitis vaccine, 171
Polyarteritis nodosa
    cutaneous signs associated with, 595
Polycythemia vera, 575
Polyhydramnios
    superior mesenteric artery syndrome, 283
Polymyositis, 194, 570
Polypoid carcinoma
    esophagus, 222
Polyposis syndromes, 392t
Polyps. *See* specific polyps
Pork tapeworm, 564
Porphyria
    acute intermittent, 568, 569t
        causing abdominal pain, 47
    cutanea tarda, 569t
Portal hypertension, 500
    with acute lower gastrointestinal bleeding, 23
    with ascites, 124
    with cirrhosis, 530–531
    classification, 531t
    differential diagnosis, 531t
    hemorrhage secondary to, 16–17, 22
Portal venous pressure measurement
    cirrhosis, 533
Portocaval shunt
    for ascites, 130
Postcholecystectomy syndrome, 467–470
    clinical features, 468
    course, 468–469
    diagnosis, 468
    epidemiology, 467–468
    etiology, 468
    incidence, 467–468
    pathogenesis, 468
    treatment, 468–469
Postgastrectomy syndrome, 257–258
Postinfectious dyspepsia, 260
Postoperative cholestasis, 495–496
Postoperative gastroparesis, 232
Postsurgical dumping syndrome, 238–239
Postural hypotension
    with acute upper gastrointestinal bleeding,
    19–22
Potassium supplements
    for nausea and vomiting, 43
PPoma, 449–450
Prednisone
    for Crohn disease, 370
    for ulcerative colitis, 370
Preeclampsia-associated liver disease
    pregnancy, 147
Pregnancy
    acute fatty liver of, 146–147
    causing nausea and vomiting, 40
    cholestasis of, 108, 146
    ectopic, 148
        causing acute abdomen, 57
    gastrointestinal symptoms in, 141–144, 572
    physiology of, 140–141

Pregnancy testing
  with abdominal pain, 51
  with acute abdomen, 59
Pretravel preparations, 168
Primary achalasia, 6
Primary bile acid malabsorption, 319
Primary biliary cirrhosis, 490–494
  clinical features, 491
  course, 493–494
  diagnosis, 114t, 491–492
  differential diagnosis, 491t
  epidemiology, 490
  etiology, 490
  extrahepatic conditions associated with, 492t
  incidence, 490
  pathogenesis, 490
  treatment, 493
Primary hepatic neoplasms, 539–546
Primary mesothelioma, 486
Primary peristalsis, 6
Primary sclerosing cholangitis (PSC), 458t
  with conjugated hyperbilirubinemia, 109
Probenecid
  unconjugated hyperbilirubinemia, 107
Prochlorperazine, 237–238
Proctalgia fugax, 418
Proguanil, 172
Prokinetic agents, 237
Protein
  absorption disorders, 316
Protein-calorie malnutrition, 157
Protein-losing enteropathy, 288
  classification of, 287t
Proteus
  with conjugated hyperbilirubinemia, 109
Proton pump inhibitor, 247
  for upper gastrointestinal bleeding, 20
Protozoa, 555–560
Provocative tests
  GERD, 208
  Zollinger-Ellison syndrome, 251–252
Pruritus ani, 415, 416t
PSC. *See* Primary sclerosing cholangitis (PSC)
Pseudocysts
  acute pancreatitis, 433
Pseudohyponatremia, 154
Pseudomonas
  with conjugated hyperbilirubinemia, 109
Pseudomyxoma peritonei, 486
Pseudosarcoma
  esophagus, 222
Pseudoxanthoma elasticum, 569, 592
Psychogenic vomiting, 578
Psychological disorders
  gastrointestinal manifestations, 578
PTC. *See* Percutaneous transhepatic
    cholangiography (PTC)
PUD. *See* Peptic ulcer disease (PUD)
Puffer fish
  foodborne diseases, 299t
Pulmonary disease
  gastrointestinal manifestations, 578

Pulmonary emboli
  IBD, 362
Pyoderma gangrenosum
  IBD, 362
  with IBD, 590
Pyridoxine (vitamin B$_6$)
  deficiency, 156
  for nausea and vomiting, 44

R
Rabeprazole, 247
  for GERD, 210
Rabies vaccine, 170
Radiation esophagitis, 611–612
Radiation injury, 611–615
  etiology, 611–612
  pathogenesis, 611–612
Radiculopathy
  with pain, 50
Radiofrequency ablation (RFA)
  for hepatocellular carcinoma, 543–544
Radiographs. *See also* specific radiograph
  adenomatous polyps, 387
  colon adenocarcinoma, 402–403
  distal esophagus spastic motor disorders, 201
  familial adenomatous polyposis, 395
  gastric adenocarcinoma, 274
  GERD, 206–207
  IBD, 365
  for occult gastrointestinal hemorrhage, 30
Ranitidine, 247
Rapid gastric emptying
  disorders with, 238–240
Raves, 167
Raynaud phenomenon, 202
Recombinant immunoblot assay (RIBA)
  for hepatitis, 118–119
Rectal bleeding
  with pain, 49
Rectal foreign bodies and trauma, 416–417
Rectal prolapse, 412
Rectal radiation injury, 614
Rectoanal inhibitory reflex, 92
Reflux esophagitis, 203–212
  alkaline, 212
Refractory ulcers
  treatment, 249–250
Regurgitation, 38
Relaxation techniques, 3
Renal cell carcinoma, 576
Renal failure
  gastrointestinal manifestations, 578–579
Renal transplantation
  complications, 577–578
Retention polyps, 390–391
Retractile mesenteritis, 480–481
Retroperitoneal disease, 486–489
Retroperitoneal fibrosis, 488
Retroperitoneal fluid collection, 486–487
Retroperitoneal hemorrhage, 487
Retroperitoneal infection, 488–489
Retroperitoneal neoplasms, 489

Returning travelers, 173–174
RFA. *See* Radiofrequency ablation (RFA)
Rheumatoid arthritis, 570
Rheumatologic diseases
    cutaneous manifestations, 591–592
Rhizotomy
    for abdominal pain, 53
RIBA. *See* Recombinant immunoblot assay (RIBA)
Riboflavin (vitamin B_2)
    deficiency, 156
Rifabutin
    for intestinal infections in HIV-1 infected adults, 552t
Rifampin
    unconjugated hyperbilirubinemia, 107
Rifaximin
    for traveler's diarrhea, 172
Rohypnol, 167
Rotavirus
    causing foodborne diseases, 299t, 306
    causing nausea and vomiting, 40
    causing secretory diarrhea, 80
Rotor syndrome, 107–108, 117
Rubella vaccine, 171
Rumination, 38
Rumination syndrome, 578
Ruptured ovarian cysts, 148
Ruvalcaba-Myre-Smith syndrome. *See* Bannayan-Riley-Ruvalcaba syndrome

S

Salmonella
    acquired immunodeficiency syndrome (AIDS), 553
    causing nausea and vomiting, 40
    diarrhea, 549
    foodborne diseases, 299t
    health care workers, 180–181
    hemolytic uremic syndrome, 574
    in returning traveler, 174
Salmonella typhi
    foodborne disease, 304
Salmonellosis
    nontyphoid, 303–304
Sarcoidosis
    esophagus, 189
Satiety
    early, 38
SBP. *See* Spontaneous bacterial peritonitis (SBP)
Schistosoma intercalatum, 566
Schistosoma japonicum, 565–566
Schistosoma mansoni, 565–566
Schistosoma mekongi, 566
Schistosomiasis, 565–566
Schizophrenia, 578
Scintigraphy
    abdominal pain, 52
    achalasia, 198
    GERD, 207
    lower gastrointestinal bleeding, 24

nausea and vomiting, 43
oropharyngeal dysphagia, 195
upper gastrointestinal bleeding, 18
Scleroderma, 202, 233
    cutaneous manifestations, 591
    with small intestine dysmotility, 291
Sclerosing cholangitis, 457–459, 457t
Scopolamine
    for nausea and vomiting, 43
Scromboid, 299t
Seafood poisoning, 308
Sea travel, 168–169
Secondary achalasia, 6
Secondary immunodeficiencies, 584–586
Secretory component deficiency, 582
Secretory diarrhea, 80–81
    etiology, 77t–78t
Sedative-hypnotics
    abuse, 164
Selective immunoglobulin A deficiency, 580, 581t
Selenium deficiency, 155
Sengstaken-Blakemore tube
    with upper gastrointestinal bleeding, 21
Septata intestinalis, 560
    diarrhea, 549
Serositis
    with ascites, 126
Sertraline
    for chest pain, 14
Serum amylase
    with abdominal pain, 51
Serum ascites albumin gradient, 128
Serum bile acids, 117
Serum electrolytes
    with acute abdomen, 59
    in nausea and vomiting, 41
Serum gastrin
    Zollinger-Ellison syndrome, 251
Serum globulin, 117
Serum lipase
    with abdominal pain, 51
Severe combined immunodeficiency disease, 582
Sexually transmitted colorectal pathogens, 355–356
Shigella
    acquired immunodeficiency syndrome (AIDS), 553
    antibiotics for, 350t
    colon, 349–350
    foodborne diseases, 299t
    health care workers, 181
    hemolytic uremic syndrome, 574
    in returning traveler, 174
Shigella flexneri
    diarrhea, 549
Short bowel syndrome, 320–325
    clinical manifestations, 322
    diagnosis, 323
    epidemiology, 320
    etiology, 320, 321t

Short bowel syndrome (*contd.*)
  incidence, 320
  pathogenesis, 320
  treatment, 323–325
Shwachman-Diamond syndrome, 427
Sickle cell crisis
  acute, 574
Sigmoid colon
  cross-section, 337f
Sigmoidoscopy
  with abdominal pain, 52
Sigmoid volvulus, 75
Sildenafil
  for achalasia, 198
Simethicone
  for gas and bloating, 67
Sister Mary Joseph node, 593
6-mercaptopurine (6-MP)
  for IBD, 139, 368
Sjögren syndrome, 570
  with conjugated hyperbilirubinemia, 108
Skin
  with nutritional deficiencies, 153t
  lesions, 589–597
Skin disease
  gastrointestinal hemorrhage, 592–593
Small bowel enema (enteroclysis), 629–630
Small intestinal bacterial overgrowth, 63,
        294–297, 295t
  consequences, 296
  diagnosis, 296–297
  epidemiology, 294–295
  etiology, 295–296
  incidence, 294–295
  pathogenesis, 295–296
  treatment, 297
Small intestinal history
  for celiac disease, 311–312
Small intestinal ischemia, 605–610
  clinical features, 607–608
  course, 609–610
  diagnosis, 608–610
  epidemiology, 605
  etiology, 605–607
  incidence, 605
  pathogenesis, 605–607
  treatment, 609–610
Small intestinal obstruction. *See also* Obstruction
  causing acute abdomen, 55–56
Small intestine
  adenocarcinoma, 325–327
  anatomy of, 279–280
  atresia, 281–282
  bacterial infections, 293–308
  carbohydrate absorption disorders,
        313–316
  carcinoids, 327–329
  developmental abnormalities, 280–283
  drug-induced disease, 286–288
  duplications, 281
  dysmotility, 288–294
    diagnosis, 293–294

  etiology, 289–290, 289t
  pathogenesis, 289–290
  embryology of, 279–280
  epithelial transport, 313–319
  imaging, 629–630
  lymphomas, 330–331
  malrotation, 282–283
  medication-induced ulcers, 285–286
  mesenchymal tumors, 329–330
  radiation injury, 613–614
  stenosis, 281–282
  structural abnormalities, 283–284
  transplantation, 588
  tumors
    classification, 326t
    distribution, 327t
  ulcers, 285–286, 285t
    associated with systemic disease,
        286
  viral infections, 305–308
Smoking
  complications, 579
Snow Mountain agents
  causing nausea and vomiting, 40
Solitary rectal ulcer, 413
Solitary rectal ulcer syndrome, 381
Somatostatinoma, 449
Sorbitol
  deficiency, 63
  malabsorption
    with gas and bloating, 66
Sphincter of Oddi, 419, 429
Spigelian hernias, 475
Spinal cord injury, 577
Spindle cell carcinoma
  esophagus, 222
Spine radiographs
  IBD, 365
Spiral computed tomography
  hepatocellular carcinoma, 541
Spiramycin
  for *Cryptosporidium,* 559
Spironolactone
  for ascites, 129
Spontaneous bacterial peritonitis (SBP)
  with ascites, 131
Squamous cell cancer
  esophageal, 216–218
Squamous cell papillomas
  esophagus, 223
Staphylococcus
  causing nausea and vomiting, 40
Staphylococcus aureus
  causing secretory diarrhea, 80
  foodborne diseases, 299t
  small intestine, 298
  surgical wound infection, 175
Steatohepatitis, 499
Steatorrhea
  chronic pancreatitis, 439
Steatosis, 499
Stercoral ulcer, 380–381

Stevens-Johnson syndrome, 571
    with IBD, 589
Stomach
    adenocarcinoma, 271–276
    anatomy of, 223–225
    developmental abnormalities of, 225–226
    drugs with prokinetic effects on, 237t
    embryology, 223–225
    leiomyoma, 278
    leiomyosarcoma, 278
    metastatic tumors, 277
    radiation injury, 613
    tumors, 271–278
Streptococcus
    with conjugated hyperbilirubinemia, 109
Streptococcus viridans
    esophagus, 215
Streptozocin
    for pancreatic endocrine neoplasms, 453
Stress gastritis
    causing acute upper gastrointestinal bleeding,
      16
Strongyloides stercoralis, 562–563
Submucosal masses, 391
Substance abuse, 579. *See also* Alcohol abuse;
      Drug abuse
Sucralfate, 247
Sucrase isomaltase deficiency, 63, 315
Sulfadoxine-pyrimethamine
    for *Isospora belli,* 559
Sulfasalazine
    causing nausea and vomiting, 38
    for IBD, 139
Sulfobromophthalein, 117
Superior mesenteric artery, 224
Superior mesenteric artery syndrome, 283
    causing nausea and vomiting, 38
Swallowing
    testing of, 7–8
Sweat testing
    cystic fibrosis, 425
Sweet syndrome, 571
    with IBD, 590–591
Symptomatic illness
    travelers, 173–174
Syndrome X, 10
Syphilis
    anorectal, 356
Systemic diseases
    gastrointestinal manifestations, 567–579
Systemic lupus erythematosus, 202, 570
Systemic telangiectasia syndrome, 602–603

T
Tachycardia
    with pain, 50
Taenia saginata (beef tapeworm), 564
Taenia solium (pork tapeworm), 564
Tangier disease, 569
Tapeworms, 564–565
Tegaserod, 237t
    for constipation, 93

    for gas and bloating, 67
    for small intestine dysmotility, 294
Telangiectasia, 599
Tense ascites, 132
Tetanus boosters, 171
Therapeutic paracentesis
    for ascites, 129
Thiamine (vitamin B_1) deficiency, 156
Thrombocytopenia
    with upper gastrointestinal bleeding, 18
TIPS. *See* Transjugular intrahepatic portosystemic
      shunt (TIPS)
tLESR. *See* Transient LES relaxation (tLESR)
T-lymphocyte defects, 582
Tobacco, 167
    acid peptic disorders, 242
    complications, 579
    esophageal tumors, 217
Toluene
    abuse, 167
Total paracentesis
    for ascites, 130
Total parenteral hyperalimentation
    with conjugated hyperbilirubinemia,
      109
Total parenteral nutrition (TPN), 159–160
    complications, 161t
Toxic epidermal necrolysis
    with IBD, 589
Toxic megacolon, 68
Toxocara canis, 563
Toxocara cati, 563
Toxoplasma gondii, 554
TPN. *See* Total parenteral nutrition (TPN)
Tracheoesophageal atresia, 183
Tracheoesophageal fistula, 183
Tranquilizers, 3
Transcatheter arterial chemoembolization
    for hepatocellular carcinoma, 544
Transfusion
    for upper gastrointestinal bleeding, 20
Transient LES relaxation (tLESR), 204
Transjugular intrahepatic portosystemic shunt
      (TIPS)
    for ascites, 130
    contraindications, 637t
    indications, 637t
    for upper gastrointestinal bleeding, 21
Traumatic diaphragmatic hernias, 475–476
Traumatic esophageal injury, 192–193
Travel
    chemoprophylaxis, 171–172
    immunization, 169–171, 170–171
Travelers, 168–174
Traveler's diarrhea, 172–173
Trazodone
    for chest pain, 14
Trehalase deficiency, 315
Trematodes (flukes), 565–566
Treponema pallidum, 356
Triazolam, 168
Trichinella spiralis, 562

Trichloroethylene
abuse, 167
Trichobezoar, 228
Trichostrongylus, 561
Trichuris
in returning traveler, 174
Trichuris trichiura (whipworm), 560
Tricyclic antidepressants
for abdominal pain, 53
Trientine
for Wilson disease, 514
Trimethoprim-sulfamethoxazole
for *Cyclospora,* 559
for intestinal infections in HIV-1 infected
adults, 551t
for *Isospora belli,* 559
Trisomy 21, 568
Tropheryma whippelii, 79
Tropical sprue
causing osmotic diarrhea, 79
in the returning traveler, 174
Truncal vagotomy
for duodenal ulcers, 253
Trypanosoma cruzi, 6, 559–560
Tuberculosis, 572
esophageal, 215
nosocomial transmission, 176
Tumor markers
hepatocellular carcinoma, 541
Turcot syndrome, 394
Turner syndrome, 569
24-hour esophageal pH recording
distal esophagus spastic motor disorders, 201
Tylosis, 217, 571, 594
Typhlitis, 381–382
Typhoid fever vaccine, 170
Typhus, 173

U

UES. *See* Upper esophageal sphincter (UES)
Ulcerative colitis. *See also* Inflammatory bowel
disease (IBD)
classification of, 359t
IBD, 359–360
medical management, 369–370
pregnancy, 145–146
Ulcerative jejunoileitis, 286
Ulcers. *See* specific ulcers
Ultrasound, 631–632
with abdominal pain, 52
with acute abdomen, 60
acute pancreatitis, 432
ductal adenocarcinoma, 443
gallstones, 464
IBD, 365
Umbilical hernias, 473
Uncomplicated diverticulosis, 336–337
Unconjugated hyperbilirubinemia, 106–107
Upper endoscopy
with abdominal pain, 52
for ascites, 129
for chest pain, 12

distal esophagus spastic motor disorders,
201
in nausea and vomiting, 42
for upper gastrointestinal bleeding, 18,
20–21
Upper esophageal sphincter (UES)
disorders of, 193–196
Upper gastrointestinal bleeding
acute, 15–17
complications, 22
history, 17
laboratory studies, 18
mortality, 22
physical examination, 17–18
resuscitation, 19–20
workup, 17–22
Upper gastrointestinal endoscopy, 618–620
achalasia, 197
complications, 620
contraindications, 618
gastric adenocarcinoma, 274
gastric emptying disorders, 235
GERD, 207
indications, 618, 619t
patient monitoring, 618–619
patient preparation, 618–619
procedure, 619–629
Upper gastrointestinal tract
imaging, 629
Uremia, 578
Uridine diphosphate glucuronosyltransferase
unconjugated hyperbilirubinemia, 107
Urinalysis
with abdominal pain, 52
with acute abdomen, 59
Ursodeoxycholic acid. *See* Ursodiol
Ursodiol
for gallstones, 465
for PBC, 122
Urticaria, 571
cutaneous manifestations of, 589

V

Vanishing bile duct syndrome, 498
Variceal hemorrhage
with cirrhosis, 534–536
Varicella-zoster virus (VZV)
esophagus, 214
Varices
anorectal, 410
gastric, 16–17
Variegate porphyria, 594
Vascular ectasia
causing upper gastrointestinal bleeding,
17
Vascular lesions, 598–604, 599t
Vasculitides, 579
Vasoactive intestinal polypeptide (VIP)
causing secretory diarrhea, 80
Vasopressin
producing colonic ischemia, 378
for upper gastrointestinal bleeding, 20

Venlafaxine, 3
Verner-Morrison syndrome, 448–449
Verrucous carcinoma
    esophagus, 222
Vibrio cholerae
    causing secretory diarrhea, 80
    foodborne diseases, 299t, 301
    health care workers, 181
Vibrio parahaemolyticus
    foodborne diseases, 299t, 302
Video capsule endoscopy, 620–621
Videofluoroscopy
    oropharyngeal dysphagia, 195
VIP. *See* Vasoactive intestinal polypeptide
    (VIP)
VIPoma, 448–449
Viral encephalitis vaccine, 171
Viral gastroenteritis, 305
Viral hepatitis, 502–511
    diagnosis, 114t
    pregnancy, 146
Visceral larva migrans, 563
Visceral pain, 45
Vitamin A deficiency, 155
    skin conditions from, 596
Vitamin B$_1$
    deficiency, 156
Vitamin B$_2$
    deficiency, 156
Vitamin B$_3$
    deficiency, 156
Vitamin B$_6$
    deficiency, 156
    for nausea and vomiting, 44
Vitamin B$_{12}$
    absorption disorders, 318–319
    deficiency, 156
Vitamin C deficiency, 156
Vitamin D deficiency, 155
Vitamin E deficiency, 155–156
Vocal cord paralysis
    with dysphagia, 7
Volvulus, 283, 335–336
    gastric, 230–231
Vomiting (emesis), 14, 37–45. *See also* Nausea
    differential diagnosis, 37–40
    with ileus, 71
    medications, 38
    with pregnancy, 141–142
Von Hippel–Lindau disease, 569
VZV. *See* Varicella-zoster virus (VZV)

W

Watermelon stomach
    causing upper gastrointestinal bleeding, 17

Watery diarrhea, hypokalemia, and achlorhydria
    (WDHA), 448–449
    causing secretory diarrhea, 80
Weber-Christian disease, 480
Wegener granulomatosis, 579
Weight loss, 32–37, 578
    complications, 37
    differential diagnosis, 32–33
    etiology, 33t
    history, 34–35
    with pain, 49
    physical examination, 35
    treatment, 36–37
    workup, 34–35, 36f
Whipple disease
    causing osmotic diarrhea, 79
Whipworm, 560
Wilson disease, 119, 512–514
    diagnosis, 114t
    treatment, 122
Wiskott-Aldrich syndrome, 583

X

X-linked (Bruton) hypogammaglobulinemia, 580
Xylitol
    malabsorption, 63

Y

Yellow fever vaccination, 169
Yersinia
    foodborne disease, 299t, 304–305
Yersinia enterocolitica
    health care workers, 181
    traveler's diarrhea, 172

Z

Zenker diverticula, 6, 185–186
    acquired, 194
    causing nausea and vomiting, 41
    elderly, 134
Zinc
    deficiency, 155
    for Wilson disease, 514
Zoldipem (Ambien), 168
Zollinger-Ellison syndrome, 250–253
    clinical manifestations, 250–251
    course, 252–253
    diagnosis, 251–252
    epidemiology, 250
    etiology, 250
    incidence, 250
    large gastric folds, 269
    pathogenesis, 250
    treatment, 252–253
    tumor localization, 252